Sports and Exercise: Rehabilitation and Medicine

Sports and Exercise: Rehabilitation and Medicine

Edited by Brycen Laning

SYRAWOOD
PUBLISHING HOUSE
New York

Published by Syrawood Publishing House,
750 Third Avenue, 9th Floor,
New York, NY 10017, USA
www.syrawoodpublishinghouse.com

Sports and Exercise: Rehabilitation and Medicine
Edited by Brycen Laning

International Standard Book Number: 978-1-68286-550-7 (Hardback)

Cataloging-in-Publication Data

Sports and exercise : rehabilitation and medicine / edited by Brycen Laning.
p. cm.
Includes bibliographical references and index.
ISBN 978-1-68286-550-7
1. Sports. 2. Exercise. 3. Medical rehabilitation. 4. Sports medicine. I. Laning, Brycen.
GV707 .S66 2018
796--dc23

Printed in China.

TABLE OF CONTENTS

PREFACE

Sports science refers to the study of techniques and methodology that enables the care and well-being of athletes. This book on sports and exercise discusses topics related to interventional and rehabilitative therapies that are integral to athletic performance. There is a great emphasis paid to fitness and performance as well as routines that minimize the risk of injury. The objective of this book is to give a general view of the different areas of sports and medicine. It is a compilation of chapters that discuss the most vital concepts and emerging trends in this field. In this book, using case studies and examples, constant effort has been made to make the understanding of the difficult concepts of sports medicine and rehabilitation as easy and informative as possible, for the readers.

The researches compiled throughout the book are authentic and of high quality, combining several disciplines and from very diverse regions from around the world. Drawing on the contributions of many researchers from diverse countries, the book's objective is to provide the readers with the latest achievements in the area of research. This book will surely be a source of knowledge to all interested and researching the field.

In the end, I would like to express my deep sense of gratitude to all the authors for meeting the set deadlines in completing and submitting their research chapters. I would also like to thank the publisher for the support offered to us throughout the course of the book. Finally, I extend my sincere thanks to my family for being a constant source of inspiration and encouragement.

Editor

The Effectiveness of Pilates Exercise in People with Chronic Low Back Pain

Cherie Wells[1,2]*, Gregory S. Kolt[2], Paul Marshall[2], Bridget Hill[3], Andrea Bialocerkowski[4]

1 Faculty of Health, University of Canberra, Bruce, Australian Capital Territory, Australia, **2** School of Science and Health, University of Western Sydney, Campbelltown, New South Wales, Australia, **3** Epworth HealthCare, Richmond, Victoria, Australia, **4** Griffith Health Institute, Griffith University, Gold Coast, Queensland, Australia

Abstract

Objective: To evaluate the effectiveness of Pilates exercise in people with chronic low back pain (CLBP) through a systematic review of randomised controlled trials (RCTs).

Data Sources: A search for RCTs was undertaken using Medical Search Terms and synonyms for "Pilates" and "low back pain" within the maximal date range of 10 databases. Databases included the Cumulative Index to Nursing and Allied Health Literature; Cochrane Library; Medline; Physiotherapy Evidence Database; ProQuest: Health and Medical Complete, Nursing and Allied Health Source, Dissertation and Theses; Scopus; Sport Discus; Web of Science.

Study Selection: Two independent reviewers were involved in the selection of evidence. To be included, relevant RCTs needed to be published in the English language. From 152 studies, 14 RCTs were included.

Data Extraction: Two independent reviewers appraised the methodological quality of RCTs using the McMaster Critical Review Form for Quantitative Studies. The author(s), year of publication, and details regarding participants, Pilates exercise, comparison treatments, and outcome measures, and findings, were then extracted.

Data Synthesis: The methodological quality of RCTs ranged from "poor" to "excellent". A meta-analysis of RCTs was not undertaken due to the heterogeneity of RCTs. Pilates exercise provided statistically significant improvements in pain and functional ability compared to usual care and physical activity between 4 and 15 weeks, but not at 24 weeks. There were no consistent statistically significant differences in improvements in pain and functional ability with Pilates exercise, massage therapy, or other forms of exercise at any time period.

Conclusions: Pilates exercise offers greater improvements in pain and functional ability compared to usual care and physical activity in the short term. Pilates exercise offers equivalent improvements to massage therapy and other forms of exercise. Future research should explore optimal Pilates exercise designs, and whether some people with CLBP may benefit from Pilates exercise more than others.

Editor: François Hug, The University of Queensland, Australia

Funding: The authors have no support or funding to report.

Competing Interests: The authors have declared that no competing interests exist.

* Email: Cherie.Wells@canberra.edu.au

Introduction

Chronic low back pain (CLBP) is defined as pain for more than twelve weeks in the posterior lumbar region between the twelfth ribs and inferior gluteal folds [1]. CLBP is highly prevalent and associated with significant levels of disability [2–4]. As a consequence, CLBP places a large social and economic burden on society [2–4].

Pilates exercise is a commonly prescribed to people with CLBP [5–7]. Pilates exercise is named after its founder, Joseph Pilates, who developed a series of exercises in the 1920s to encourage physical and mental conditioning [8,9]. Core stability, strength and flexibility are emphasised in Pilates exercise, as is control of movement, posture, and breathing [9]. All of these aspects of Pilates exercise may benefit people with CLBP as exercises with similar features have been successful in reducing pain and improving functional ability [10–12].

When treating people with CLBP, it has been suggested in a Delphi survey that supervised Pilates exercise sessions should be undertaken 2–3 times per week for 3–6 months, and be supplemented by home exercises [13]. Individualised supervision has been advised in the first 2 weeks, but thereafter group sessions of up to 4 clients per therapist [13]. The use of specialised Pilates exercise equipment with spring resistance, such as a Reformer, has also been recommended for people with CLBP [13,14].

Despite the popularity of Pilates exercise in treating people with CLBP, its effectiveness in people with CLBP is yet to be established [15]. Six systematic reviews have investigated the effectiveness of Pilates exercise in people with CLBP, and a protocol for a Cochrane review has also been published [6,7,16–20]. Completed reviews, though, report different findings [6,7,16–

20]. Several reviews report a decrease in pain, but not all report improvements in functional ability [6,16–18]. Other reviews report no improvement in pain or functional ability or inconclusive findings [7,13,19]. The small number and mixed methodological quality of primary studies has made reporting of credible results difficult [15]. Several reviews have also conducted meta-analyses in the presence of significant clinical heterogeneity, resulting in misleading findings [15].

Recently, several randomised controlled trials (RCTs) have been published that are relevant to evaluating the effectiveness of Pilates exercise in people with CLBP [21–26]. The majority of these RCTs have not been included in prior reviews, so incorporating this new evidence in an updated systematic review is indicated. Given there is now a moderate volume of evidence available, it is also appropriate that this new systematic review includes only RCTs. This will ensure this review represents a high level of evidence and increases the credibility of results [15,27,28].

The aim of the following systematic review is to provide an update on the effectiveness of Pilates exercise in reducing pain and improving functional ability of people with CLBP based on the highest level and quality of research evidence available [28].

Materials and Methods

Study Design

A systematic review was undertaken to locate, evaluate and summarise findings from RCTs that have investigated the effectiveness of Pilates exercise in people with CLBP. A systematic review was chosen over a narrative review as it limits bias and error in the selection and appraisal of evidence [29,30]. In this systematic review, a comprehensive search of the literature was undertaken to answer a focused question, the methodological quality of primary studies was appraised, and findings were synthesised to address the study aim [29,30].

Search Strategy

A comprehensive literature search for evidence was undertaken on the 1st May, 2014 using 10 databases: Cumulative Index to Nursing and Allied Health Literature, Cochrane Library, Medline, Physiotherapy Evidence Database, ProQuest: Health and Medical Complete, Proquest: Nursing and Allied Health Source, Proquest: Dissertation and Theses, Scopus, Sport Discus, and Web of Science. To ensure relevant trials were not overlooked, the maximal date range available in each database was used. Medical Subject Headings terms of "Pilates", "Pilates method", and "Low Back Pain" and synonyms for low back pain were inputted in the title, abstract, and as able, the keyword fields to identify relevant evidence (Table 1).

Preliminary searching revealed that expanding the literature searches to include "exercise", "motor control", or "core stability" did not identify any additional Pilates specific exercise studies, nor did changing the Boolean operator to "or". Removing "low back pain" also did not identify any additional studies. Once RCTs were selected for inclusion, their reference lists were searched for additional, relevant studies that met inclusion criterion [16–19,24–29]. In addition, reference lists of previous systematic reviews of this topic were searched to ensure relevant studies were not missed [6,7,15–19].

Selection of Evidence

Selection of relevant studies was based on the study's title and the abstract, and as required, the full document. Two independent reviewers selected the evidence according to the selection criteria (CW, BH). Any disagreements were resolved through discussion with a third reviewer (AB). To be considered in this systematic review, studies needed to:

1. Be published in the English language, as access to interpreters was not available.
2. Be published in full so that the methodological quality of the study could be assessed alongside results. Abstracts were excluded as they contained insufficient data to enable analysis of methodological quality [31].
3. Be RCTs to limit the risk of bias in findings regarding efficacy [26]. If studies reported that they were RCTs but did not describe the randomisation procedure they were included in this review. If, however, studies reported that they were RCTs, but described a pseudo-random technique of allocating participants to groups, such as alternative allocation, they were excluded from this review [27,28].
4. Assess the effectiveness of Pilates exercise where the term "Pilates" was used to describe the type of prescribed exercise being investigated. Exercises described as "motor control" or "lumbar stabilisation" did not suffice for Pilates. This is because Pilates may include other features apart from motor control and lumbar stabilisation [9].
5. Include participants with CLBP, that is, localised pain in the lumbar region of more than 3 months in duration [1]. If studies only included participants with low back pain of less than 3 months duration, they were excluded. This is because people with CLBP respond differently to treatment compared to those with acute or subacute symptoms [32]. If studies included participants with acute or subacute low back pain and CLBP, the study was included as findings were still considered relevant.
6. Use outcome measures with appropriate psychometric qualities that evaluate pain and/or functional ability in people with CLBP [33]. For example, the Visual Analog Scale and Numerical Rating Scale for pain, and the Oswestry Disability Questionnaire and Roland Morris Disability Questionnaire for functional ability. RCTs with outcome measures for pain and/or functional ability that did not have sufficient validity, reliability, or responsiveness were excluded to avoid imprecise measurements of treatment effect [33].

Appraisal of Evidence

The methodological quality of included RCTs was evaluated by two independent reviewers using the McMaster Critical Review Form for Quantitative Studies (CW, BH) [34]. This critical appraisal tool was utilised because it is comprehensive in assessing methodological quality of quantitative evidence [35]. This critical appraisal tool also has good inter-rater reliability [36–38]. To confirm the reliability of scoring in this review, the percentage agreement and kappa score between the two reviewers was calculated [39]. Any disagreements between reviewers were resolved through discussion with a third reviewer (AB).

The McMaster Critical Review Form for Quantitative Studies directs reviewers to consider 16 items of methodological quality relating to the study's purpose, literature review, design, sample, outcomes, intervention, results and conclusions [34]. Guidelines for the appraisal of evidence in this review were created to assist reviewers in consistently evaluating methodological quality (Table 2). These were based on guidelines provided by the authors of the McMaster appraisal tool [34,38].

If RCTs met each criterion outlined in the appraisal guidelines, they received a score of "one" for that item, or, if they did not

Table 1. Search Strategy.

Database	Date Range	Key Words	Fields
Cochrane Library	1800–2014	(low back pain OR dorsalgia OR *spin* pain OR backache OR lumbago) AND (pilates OR pilates method)	Title, Abstract or Keyword
Cumulative Index to Nursing and Allied Health Literature	1970–2014	(low back pain OR dorsalgia OR *spin* pain OR backache OR lumbago) AND (pilates OR pilates method)	Title, Abstract, or Word in Subject Heading
Medline-	1928–2014	(low back pain OR dorsalgia OR *spin* pain OR backache OR lumbago) AND (pilates OR pilates method)	Title, Abstract or Keyword
Physiotherapy Evidence Database	1928–2014	low back pain AND pilates	Title and Abstract
Proquest (Dissertations and Theses, Medical and Health Complete, Nursing and Allied Health Source)	1928–2014	(low back pain OR dorsalgia OR *spin* pain OR backache OR lumbago) AND (pilates OR pilates method)	Title, Abstract, or Subject Heading
Scopus	1960–2014	(low back pain AND pilates) OR (dorsalgia AND pilates) OR (*spin* pain AND pilates) OR (backache AND pilates) OR (lumbago AND pilates)	Title, Abstract, or Keyword
Sport Discus	1975–2014	(low back pain OR dorsalgia OR *spin* pain OR backache OR lumbago) AND (pilates OR pilates method)	Title, Abstract, or Keyword
Web of Science	1977–2014	(low back pain OR dorsalgia OR *spin* pain OR backache OR lumbago) AND (pilates OR pilates method)	Topic or Title

meet the criteria, they received a score of "zero". Individual item scores were then summated to provide a total score of methodological quality out of 16, with higher scores reflecting greater methodological quality. Once quality scores were calculated, these were divided into five qualitative categories of poor (score = 0–8), fair (score = 9–10), good (score = 11–12), very good (score = 13–14) and excellent (score = 15–16) methodological quality, as defined in previous research [38].

Data Extraction and Syntheses

The number of included RCTs and their methodological quality were summarised using descriptive statistics. The author(s), year of publication, and details regarding participants, interventions, comparison treatments, outcome measures, were extracted from RCTs by the primary author (CW), and tabulated. To determine whether a meta-analysis of study findings could be performed, the clinical and statistical heterogeneity of RCTs was assessed [15,40–41].

Clinical heterogeneity of RCTs was assessed by comparing differences in the population, intervention, comparison treatments,

Table 2. Modified Guidelines for use of the McMasters Critical Appraisal Form for Quantitative Studies[34].

Item	Essential Criteria
1. Purpose	Do the authors clearly state that the aim of the study, which is to evaluate the effect of Pilates exercise in individuals diagnosed with chronic low back pain (CLBP)?
2. Literature review	Do the authors justify, by identifying gaps in the literature, the need to undertake further research into the effectiveness of Pilates exercise for individuals diagnosed with CLBP?
3. Study design	Have the authors used a randomised controlled trial to answer study aims, that is, to evaluate the effectiveness of Pilates exercise in people with CLBP?
4. Blinding	Have the authors used assessor blinding to minimise bias?
5. Sample description	Have the authors described the sample in terms of age, gender, and at least one measure of disability due to CLBP?
6. Sample size	Have the authors justified their sample size through a power calculation or post hoc analysis (and recruited sufficient numbers)?
7. Ethics and consent	Have the authors documented ethical approval for the research and gained informed consent by participants?
8. Validity of outcomes	Did the authors use outcome measures that are valid for use in people with CLBP to assess all outcome variables?
9. Reliability of outcomes	Did the authors use outcome measures that are reliable for use in people with CLBP to assess all outcome variables?
10. Intervention description	Did the authors provide sufficient information to enable reproduction of the intervention?
11. Statistical significance	Did the authors report the results for at least one outcome measure in line with study aim and in terms of statistical significance?
12. Statistical analysis	Did the authors use appropriate statistical analyses in evaluating results according to their aim?
13. Clinical importance	Did the authors reflect on the clinical importance of results for people diagnosed with CLBP?
14. Conclusions	Did the authors provide appropriate conclusions considering the study method and results?
15. Clinical implications	Did the authors discuss clinical implications of the results in terms of treatment of CLBP and in directing further research?
16. Study limitations	Did the authors identify limitations of the study methodology and results?

outcome measures, and timing of reassessment of individual studies [15]. Statistical heterogeneity was assessed by calculation of an i^2 statistic of studies with similar comparison treatment groups using the Cochrane Review Manager (version 5.2) software [41–43]. If i^2 was greater than 75%, studies were considered to have substantial heterogeneity [41]. If substantial clinical and statistical heterogeneity were present, pooling results in a meta-analysis was deemed inappropriate.

Key findings of RCTs were expressed in terms of between-group mean differences and 95% confidence intervals. If between-group mean differences and 95% confidence intervals were not provided by RCTs, these were calculated from post-treatment mean values and standard deviations using the Physiotherapy Evidence Database calculator [44]. For the randomised cross-over trial, the between-group mean difference and 95% confidence interval was calculated from the first comparison time period between the Pilates exercise and control group, as the carryover effect in relation to time of treatment and pain intensity was statistically significant [21].

Results for each outcome measures were considered to be statistically significant if the 95% confidence interval of the between group difference did not cross "zero" [45]. If a 95% confidence interval was unable to be calculated from results given, a p value less than 0.05 for the between group comparison was considered to indicate statistical significance [45]. Results were considered to be clinically significant in this review if the mean between-group difference was greater than the minimal clinically important difference reported in the literature [46,47].

Results

Search Results

A total of 267 "hits" were obtained with database searching, and an additional RCT was identified when reviewing reference lists of previous systematic reviews (Figure 1) [48]. The majority of studies identified by this search strategy were excluded due to being duplicates ($n = 115$) or not being an RCT ($n = 95$). Other studies were excluded as they were not published in the English language ($n = 16$), did not assess the effectiveness of Pilates exercise in people with CLBP compared to other treatment ($n = 17$), were published in an abstract format ($n = 8$).

There was 100% agreement between the 2 reviewers regarding the 14 RCTs included in this review (Figure 1) [21,23–26,48–56]. Four RCTs were described in academic theses [48,49,51,53] and 10 were published in academic journals [21,23–26,50,52,54–56]. It should be noted that 2 RCTs were reported across 2 papers but only 1 paper was included in this review to avoid duplication of findings [22,23,55,57]. For one RCT, the paper that was published in a peer-reviewed journal was selected over the thesis to extract results [55,57]. For the other RCT, the paper reporting on changes in pain and functional ability in the short and long term was included [23], rather than the paper reporting on outcomes only in the short term [22].

Methodological Quality

There was 95% agreement between the two reviewers regarding item scores of the McMaster Critical Review Form for Quantitative Studies. This represents "almost perfect" inter-rater reliability (kappa score $= 0.88$, $p = 0.00$) [39]. Discussion with the third reviewer was required to reach consensus regarding the adequacy of the description of Pilates exercise [27], presence of assessor bias [21], documentation of informed consent and ethical approval [51], use of valid and reliable outcome measures [51], and discussion of the statistical significance and clinical importance of results [48,49]. One of the RCTs was published by an author of this review (PM) [23]. To avoid bias, this author was not involved in the stages of review of this RCT [23].

The methodological quality of studies ranged from 4 to 16, representing "poor" to "excellent" methodological quality (Table 3). RCTs published in the past 2 years were generally of higher quality, as were those published in journals compared to academic theses. According to the McMaster Quantitative Review Form, strengths in the methodological quality of most RCTs related to the provision of a clear purpose (Item 1), description of participants (Item 5), and documentation of ethic approval and consent (Item 7) [34]. The majority of RCTs also provided results in terms of statistical significance (Item 11) and conducted appropriate statistical analyses (Item 12) [34].

Several RCTs, however, did not ensure assessor blinding (item 4), recruit an adequate sample size (Item 6), or document the validity and/or reliability of outcome measures (Item 8, 9) [34]. Other RCTs did not provide adequate detail of Pilates exercise programs for replication (Item 10), or discuss the clinical importance of results (Item 14) (Table 3) [34].

Description of Included Studies

A summary of the population, intervention, comparison, and outcome measures for each RCT is provided in Table 4 and 5. The number of participants per RCT ranged from 12 to 83, while the mean age of participants across RCTs ranged between 21 to 49 years of age. The ratio of female to male participants ranged from 5:1 through to 1:1, except in one study where only females were recruited [54].

In terms of the Pilates interventions, most RCTs described supervised exercise programs delivered in 30 to 60-minute sessions, 1–3 times per week, for 4–15 weeks (Table 4, 5). Home exercises were incorporated in 6 RCTs as part of the Pilates exercise intervention [25,26,48,52,54,55]. The supervision ratios of clients per therapist for supervised sessions ranged from 11:1 to 1:1, although not all RCTs provided this information. Use of specialised Pilates exercise equipment, such as a Reformer, was reported in 5 RCTs [21,23,26,49,55].

Pilates exercise was compared to usual care and physical activity in 9 RCTs, massage therapy in 1 RCT, and other forms of exercise in 4 RCTs (Table 4, 5). Usual care and physical activity could involve unknown other treatments [53,56], no treatment [25,50,52], education [24], medications [24,48,55], or consultations with health professionals, such as physiotherapists [48,55]. Other forms of exercise ranged from cycling [23], McKenzie exercise [54], traditional lumbar stabilisation exercise [51], and a mixed form of exercise including stretching, strengthening and stabilisation [26].

Variable outcome measures were used to investigate the effectiveness of Pilates exercise in reducing pain and improving functional ability in people with CLBP (Table 4, 5). These included the Visual Analog Scale and Numerical Rating Scale (11 and 101 point scales) for pain, and the Roland Morris Disability Questionnaire, Oswestry Disability Questions, Quebec Score, and the Miami Back Index for functional ability [33,47]. Treatment outcomes were measured at different time periods, ranging from 4 to 24 weeks.

Heterogeneity of Included Studies

Significant clinical heterogeneity was noted across RCTs in terms of the study population, intervention, and outcome assessment (Table 4, 5). Though all RCTs studied people with CLBP, some included people with acute and subacute symptoms, or other diagnoses [21,49,55]. Pilates exercise interventions also

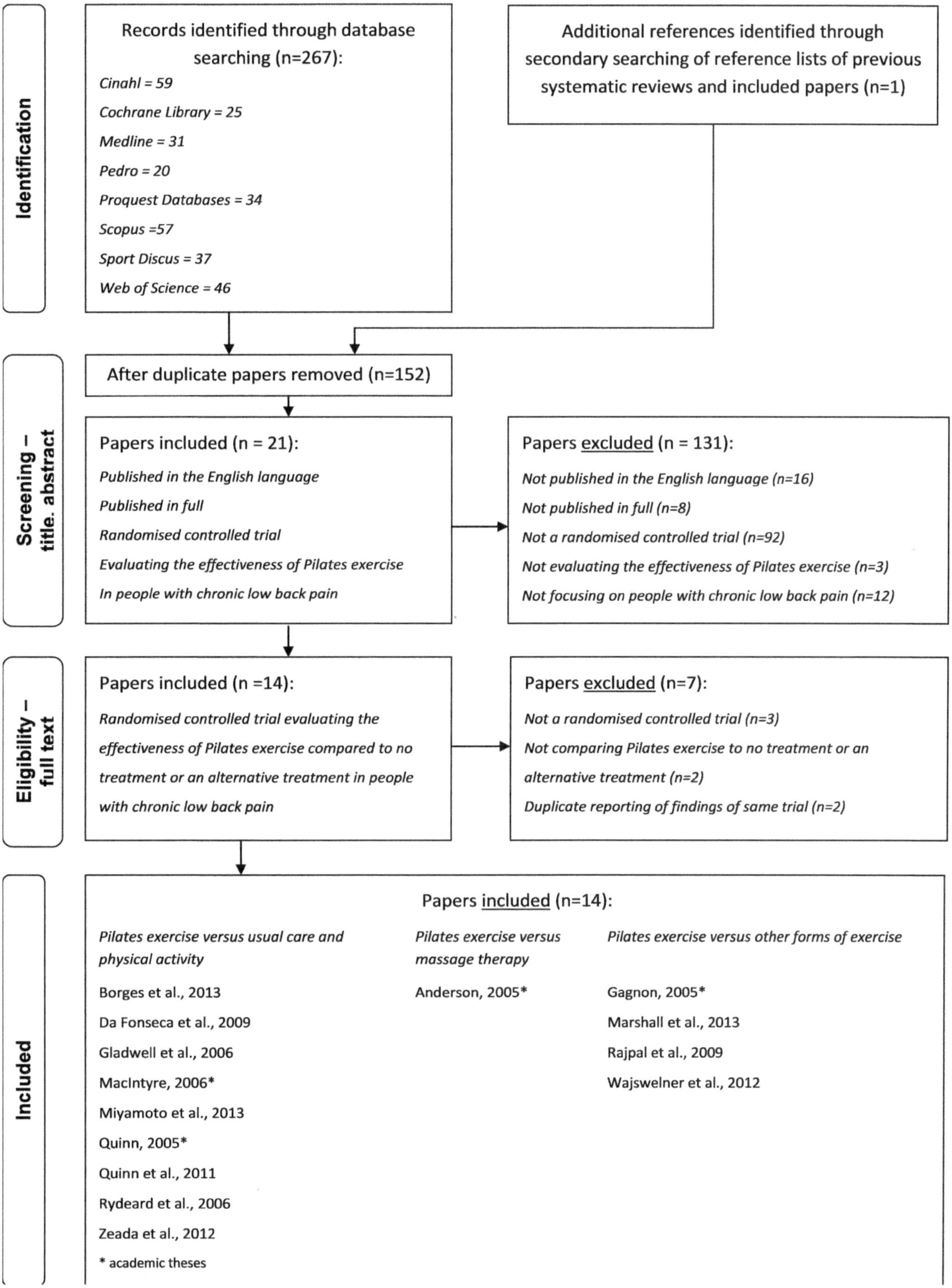

Figure 1. Results of Literature Search.

varied in terms of the duration of the intervention, level of supervision, incorporation of home exercises, education, and use of specialised equipment. Outcomes were also measured with different outcome measures at different time periods.

Comparison treatments also varied considerably across RCTs (Table 4, 5). When Pilates exercise was compared to usual care and physical activity, participants could access variable therapies depending on the RCT [24,48,55]. Usual physical activity also varied with some studies focusing on participants who were highly active [55,56], while the others did not. When Pilates exercise was compared to other forms of exercise, comparison exercise regimes were either similar to Pilates exercise [26,51], or quite distinct [23]. Also, in some studies, participants could access other interventions as well [26,51].

Significant statistical heterogeneity was also observed when comparing outcomes achieved with Pilates exercise versus usual care and physical activity for pain ($i^2 = 90\%$, $p<0.001$), and functional ability ($i^2 = 87\%$, $p<0.00001$) between 4 and 12 weeks. Similarly, significant statistical heterogeneity was noted when comparing pain relief achieved with Pilates exercise versus other forms of exercise ($i^2 = 83\%$, $p = 0.0006$) between 4 and 8 weeks. Pooling individual study findings in a meta-analysis, then, was deemed inappropriate for these variables in the short term, given the clinical and statistical heterogeneity of RCTs [40,41].

Moderate statistical heterogeneity was noted when comparing improvements in functional ability with Pilates exercise and other forms of exercise in the short term (4–8 weeks) ($i^2 = 44\%$, $p = 0.17$). At 24 weeks, mild statistical heterogeneity was evident when Pilates exercise was compared with other forms of exercise across the 2 RCTs for pain ($i^2 = 25\%$, $p = 0.25$) and functional ability ($i^2 = 9\%$, $p = 0.29$) [23,26]. Nevertheless, the clinical heterogeneity of RCTs comparing Pilates exercise to other forms of exercise suggested a meta-analysis would be of limited benefit [40,41].

Findings of Included Studies

Pilates exercise versus usual care and physical activity. Four high quality RCTs reported a statistically significant difference in pain relief with Pilates exercise in the short term (4–15 weeks) [21,24,25,55]. Two high quality RCTs, and one poor quality RCT, however, disagreed with these findings [48,50,52]. At 24 weeks, no statistically significance difference in pain relief with Pilates exercise and education versus education alone was reported (Table 6) [24].

The statistically significant improvements in pain reported in the short term were clinically significant in 3 out of 4 RCTs [21,24,25]. This is because mean difference scores exceeded the minimal clinically important difference for their respective outcome measures. For example, Borges et al. (2013) and Quinn, Barry, and Barry (2011) described a mean reduction (and 95% confidence interval) on the Visual Analog Scale of 4.1 (1.8 to 6.3) and 1.5 (0.9 to 2.1) points respectively [21,25]. The minimal clinically important difference for the Visual Analog Scale in people with CLBP has been reported in the literature as between 1.5 to 2 points [46,47].

Similarly, Miyamoto, Costa, Glavanin, and Cabral (2013) reported a mean reduction (and 95% confidence interval) of pain on the 11 point Numerical Rating Scale of 2.2 (1.1 to 3.2) points where the minimal clinically important difference was 2 points [47]. Meanwhile, Rydeard, Leger, and Smith (2006) did not report a clinically significant improvement in pain, that is a mean reduction (and 95% confidence interval) of 15.6 (13.4 to 17.8) points on the 101 point Numerical Rating Scale [55]. This is lower than the estimated minimal clinically important difference of 20 points [46].

With regards to functional ability, 3 high quality RCTs reported statistically significant improvements with Pilates exercise in the short term (4–12 weeks) [24,48,55]. In contrast, 2 high quality RCTs and 3 poor quality RCTs did not [25,50,52,53,56]. Meanwhile, at 24 weeks, no statistically significance difference in improvement in functional ability with Pilates exercise with education versus education alone was reported (Table 7) [24].

Statistically significant short-term improvements in functional ability with Pilates exercise were not clinically significant. For example, MacIntyre (2005) and Miyamoto et al. (2013) reported a mean improvement (and 95% confidence interval) of 2.6 (1.5 to 5.2) and 2.7 (1.0 to 4.4) on the Roland Morris Disability Questionnaire respectively. These changes were less than the minimal clinically important distance of 3.5 to 5 points [46,47]. Similarly, Rydeard et al. (2006) reported a mean change (and 95% confidence interval) of 1.2 (1.1 to 1.4) points on the Oswestry Disability Questionnaire which is below the minimal clinically important difference of 10 points [46,47].

Pilates exercise versus massage therapy. Only one RCT of fair quality compared the effectiveness of Pilates exercise to massage therapy [49]. This RCT did not report any statistically significant differences in pain or functional ability between groups at 6 weeks (Table 8, 9). As a consequence, there were no clinically significant differences noted between Pilates exercise and massage therapy.

Pilates exercise versus other forms of exercise. When Pilates exercise was compared to other forms of exercise, conflicting results in terms of pain relief were reported in the short term (4–8 weeks) [23,26,51,54]. One high quality and low quality RCT reported statistically significant improvements [23,54], while another high quality and low quality RCT did not [26,51]. At 24 weeks, though, there was agreement in 2 high quality RCTs that Pilates exercise resulted in equivalent improvements in pain as other forms of exercise (Table 8) [23,26].

The improvement in pain suggested in one high quality and low quality RCT in the short term was not clinically significant [23,54]. For example, Marshall, Kennedy, Brooks, and Lonsdale (2013) reported a mean decrease (and 95% confidence interval) of 1.1 (0.1 to 2.1) points on the Visual Analog Scale, and Rajpal, Arora, and Chauhan (2009) reported a mean decrease (and 95% confidence interval) of 1.4 (0.7 to 2.1) points on the Visual Analog Scale [23,54]. These scores were less than the minimal clinically important difference of 1.5–2 points on the Visual Analog Scale [46,47].

With regards to functional ability, one high quality RCT reported a statistically significant improvement with Pilates exercise over other forms of exercise in the short term [23]. In contrast, another high quality and low quality RCT did not report a statistically significant difference in improvement [26,51]. At 24 weeks, however, 2 high quality RCTs agreed that Pilates exercise offered similar improvements in functional ability as other forms of exercise (Table 9) [23,26].

The statistically significant improvement in functional ability reported by Marshall et al. (2013) in the short term was not clinically significant [23]. This is because the mean improvement (and 95% confidence interval) in functional ability was 6.5 (1.1 to 11.8) points on the Oswestry Disability Index which is less than the minimal clinically important difference of 10 points [23,46,47].

Discussion

This systematic review provides an update on the effectiveness of Pilates exercise in reducing pain and improving functional ability in people with CLBP based on current evidence. It provides

Table 3. Methodological Quality of Included Studies - McMaster Critical Review Form for Quantitative Studies [34].

Study	**Individual Item**																**Total (/16)**	**Qualitative Descriptor [38]**
	1	**2**	**3**	**4**	**5**	**6**	**7**	**8**	**9**	**10**	**11**	**12**	**13**	**14**	**15**	**16**		
Pilates exercise versus usual care and physical activity																		
1. Borges et al., 2013 [21]	1	1	1	1	1	1	1	0	0	1	1	1	0	1	1	1	**13**	Very good
2. da Fonseca et al., 2009 [50]	1	1	0	0	1	0	1	0	0	0	0	0	0	0	0	0	**4**	Poor
3. Gladwell et al., 2006 [52]	1	1	0	1	1	0	1	1	1	1	1	1	0	1	1	1	**13**	Very Good
4. MacIntyre, 2006 [48]	1	1	1	1	1	1	1	1	1	1	1	1	0	1	1	1	**15**	Excellent
5. Miyamoto et al., 2013 [24]	1	1	1	1	1	1	1	1	1	1	1	1	1	1	1	1	**16**	Excellent
6. Quinn, 2005 [53]	1	1	1	0	0	0	1	0	0	0	1	1	0	0	0	0	**6**	Poor
7. Quinn et al., 2011 [25]	1	1	1	1	1	0	1	0	1	1	1	1	1	1	1	0	**13**	Very good
8. Rydeard et al., 2006 [55]	1	1	1	1	1	0	1	1	1	0	1	1	1	1	1	1	**14**	Very good
9. Zeada et al., 2012 [56]	1	0	0	0	1	0	0	0	0	1	1	0	0	0	0	0	**4**	Poor
Pilates exercise versus massage or other forms of exercise																		
10. Anderson, 2005 [49]	1	1	1	1	1	0	0	0	0	1	0	1	0	1	1	1	**10**	Fair
11. Gagnon, 2005 [51]	1	1	1	0	1	0	1	0	0	0	1	1	0	1	1	1	**10**	Fair
12. Marshall et al., 2013 [23]	1	1	1	1	1	1	1	1	1	0	1	1	1	1	1	1	**15**	Excellent
13. Rajpal et al., 2009 [54]	0	0	0	0	0	0	1	0	0	1	1	1	0	0	0	1	**5**	Poor
14. Wajswelner et al., 2012 [26]	1	1	1	1	1	1	1	1	1	1	1	1	1	1	1	1	**16**	Excellent

Table 4. Description of Included Studies- Pilates exercise versus usual care and physical activity.

Study	Population	Intervention and Comparison	Outcome Measures [Timing]
1. Borges et al., 2013 [21]	22 participants with chronic low back pain (CLBP) and Human T-Lymphotrophic Virus	Pilates: 2 X 60 minute supervised sessions per week for 15 weeks; Equipment = Mat, Cadillac, Reformer; Supervision Ratio = ?11 clients: 1 therapist; Standardised protocol	Short Form – 36 - Pain
	Gender (Female: Male) = 2.7: 1.0	No Pilates: no change in daily activities for 15 weeks	Visual Analog Scale - Pain
	Age[&] (years) = 48.3 (10.0)		[0, 15 weeks]
	Baseline Pain Intensity[&] (/10)[a] = Pilates 7.2 (2.4); Comparison 6.9 (2.5)		
2. da Fonseca et al., 2009 [50]	17 people with CLBP	Pilates: 2 sessions per week for 15 sessions; Equipment = Mat	Visual Analog Scale – Pain
	Gender (Female: Male) = 2.4: 1.0	No Pilates: continue usual physical activity but no treatment apart from medications	[0, 7–8 weeks]
	Age[&] (years) = 33.1(11.6)		
	Baseline Pain Intensity[&] (/10)[a] = Pilates 5.9 (2.0); Comparison 6.1 (1.8)		
3. Gladwell et al., 2006 [52]	34 people with non-specific CLBP	Pilates: 60 minutes, 1 X per week for 6 weeks (as well as home exercises); Equipment: Mat	Oswestry Disability Questionnaire
	Gender (Female: Male) = 4:1	No Pilates: usual physical activity, no treatment apart from medication	Visual Analog Scale – Pain
	Age[&](years) = 40.6(9.7)		[0, 6 weeks]
	Baseline Pain Duration[&] (years) = 10.4 (10.1)		
4. MacIntyre, 2006 [48]	32 participants with CLBP	Pilates: 1 X 60 minute supervised mat session per week and 3 X 10 minute home exercises sessions per week for 12 weeks; General protocol	Roland Morris Disability Questionnaire
	Gender (Female: Male) Pilates = 3.0: 1.0; Comparison = 4.3: 1.0	No Pilates	Visual Analog Scale – Pain
	Age[&] (years) Pilates = 33.2 (7.7); Comparison = 46.7 (14.4)	(Both groups could undertake physiotherapy and exercise as required)	[0, 3, 12 weeks]
	Baseline Pain Intensity[&] (/10)[a] = Pilates 5.1 (2.0); Comparison 4.8 (1.7)		
	Baseline Disability[&] (/24)[t] = Pilates 7.0 (3.1); Comparison 7.4 (3.4)		
5. Miyamoto et al., 2013 [24]	86 participants with non-specific CLBP	Pilates: 2 X 60 minute supervised mat sessions per week for 6 weeks with education; Supervision ratio = 1:1; General protocol but graded to individual ability	Numeric Rating Scale (11 point) - Pain
	Gender (Female: Male) = Pilates 5.0: 1.0; Comparison 3.8: 1.0	No Pilates: Education booklet and physiotherapy advice 2X per week for 6 weeks (Both groups could take medication as required)	Roland Morris Disability Questionnaire
	Age[&] (years) = Pilates 40.7 (11.8); Comparison 38.3 (11.4)		[0, 6, 24 weeks]
	Baseline Pain Intensity[&] (/10)[+] = Pilates 6.6 (1.5); Comparison 6.5 (1.7)		
	Baseline Disability[&] (/24)[t] = Pilates 9.7 (4.5); Comparison 10.5 (5.4)		
6. Quinn, 2005 [53]	22 participants with CLBP	Pilates: 2 X 45–60 minute supervised mat sessions per week for 12 weeks; Standardised protocol	Oswestry Disability Questionnaire
	Age[&] (years) = Pilates 46.3 (6.7) years; Comparison 34.7 (7.3)	No Pilates: usual daily activities for 12 weeks, and no new exercise program	[0, 12 weeks]
	Baseline Disability[&] (/100)[s] = Pilates 25.9 (10.7); Comparison 22.0 (8.7)		
7. Quinn et al., 2011 [25]	29 participants with CLBP who had undergone physiotherapy treatment but had poor core stability and residual pain	Pilates: 1 X 60 minute supervised mat sessions and 5 X 15 minute home exercises per week for 8 weeks; Supervision ratio = 3–6:1; Standardised protocol but modified as required	Roland Morris Disability Questionnaire
	Age[&] (years) = Pilates 41.8 (13.8); Comparison 44.1 (12.5)	No Pilates: (or further treatment) for 8 weeks	Visual Analog Scale– Pain
	Baseline Pain Intensity[&] (/100)[^] = Pilates 40.4 (14.6); Comparison 39.9 (19.9)		[0, 8 weeks]

Table 4. Cont.

Study	Population	Intervention and Comparison	Outcome Measures [Timing]
	Baseline Disability[&] (/24) [t] = Pilates 6.9 (4.6); Comparison 7.7 (5.0)		
8. Rydeard et al., 2006 [55]	39 physically active participants with subacute, recurrent, or chronic low back pain	Pilates: 3 X 60 minute supervised sessions and 6 X 15 minute home exercises per week for 4 weeks; Equipment: Mat, Reformer; Standardised protocol	Numerical Rating Scale (101 point) - Pain
	Gender (Female: Male) = Pilates 2.0: 1.0; Comparison 1.6: 1.0	No Pilates: continued regular activity and consultation with medical and health care professionals	Roland Morris Disability Questionnaire - Hong Kong
	Age[&] (years) = Pilates 37.0 (9.0); Comparison 34.0 (8.0)		[0, 4 weeks]
	Baseline Pain Intensity[&] (/100)[b] = Pilates 23.0 (17.7); Comparison 30.4 (17.6)		
	Baseline Disability[&] (/24)[t] = Pilates 3.1(2.5); Comparison 4.2 (3.6)		
9. Zeada, 2012 [56]	20 athletes with chronic low back pain	Pilates: 4 sessions per week for 8 weeks; Equipment: Mat; Standardised protocol	Roland Morris Disability Questionnaire
	Age[&] (years) = Pilates 23.5 (2.4); Comparison 26.2(3.6)	No Pilates: 8 weeks	[0, 8 weeks]
	Baseline Disability[&] (/24)[t] = Pilates 7.4(1.2); Comparison 6.5 (0.9)		

[&]values represent Mean [Standard Deviation];
[a]as measured by Visual Analog Scale (11 point);
[t]as measured by Roland Morris Disability Questionnaire;
[+]as measured by Numerical Rating Scale (11 point);
[$]as measured by Oswestry Disability Index;
[^]as measured by Visual Analog Scale in mm;
[b]as measured by the Numerical Rating Scale (101 point).

a meta-synthesis of findings from 14 RCTs, including recently published RCTs that have not been included in other reviews [21,23–26,48–56]. A meta-analyses was not conducted due to the heterogeneity of RCTs [40,41].

Pilates exercise versus usual care and physical activity

Pilates exercise results in statistically significant improvements in pain and functional ability in the short term in people with CLBP. This conclusion is based on the balance of evidence, where more high quality RCTs have reported these findings [21,24,25,55]. In addition, short term improvements in pain may be clinically significant, but not improvements in functional ability [45–47].

Another conclusion of this review is that superior improvements with Pilates exercise compared to usual care and physical activity is unlikely at 24 weeks. This is based on research evidence of one high quality RCT that has investigated the longer term effect of Pilates exercise [24]. In this RCT, though, participants had ceased Pilates exercises at 6 weeks, and it is not known if a longer lasting effect may have been present if the intervention was continued for more than 6 weeks, as is recommended in the literature [13].

These systematic review findings are similar to those of another review in that a statistically significant reduction in pain with Pilates exercise was achieved when compared to no Pilates exercise [17]. This current review clarifies, though, that this improvement may only be in the short term, and that this change may be clinically significant. In relation to functional ability, these review findings contrast with other systematic reviews as a statistically significant improvement in functional ability in the short term was identified [6,7,17]. This difference may be due to inappropriate meta-analyses in some reviews and variable grouping of comparison treatments [13]. The size of functional improvements in RCTs in this review, however, do not appear to be clinically significant [46,47].

It should be acknowledged that not all RCTs in this review agreed regarding the effectiveness of Pilates exercise compared to usual care and physical activity [48,50,52,53]. Different results may be explained by the variable methodological quality of RCTs. For example, the majority of high quality RCTs reported statistically significant findings (4/6), while lower quality RCTs did not (2/2) [50,53].

Different results may also be due to small sample sizes or co-interventions within RCTs. Three of the 4 RCTs that did not find statistically significant findings were under-powered with small sample sizes, meaning that treatment changes may have been less easily detected [50,52,53]. The other RCT had a large sample size, but allowed the comparison group to access other interventions, such as physiotherapy and medications [48]. This may have led to the effectiveness of Pilates exercise being under estimated as the between group difference in outcome may have been reduced.

In addition, different RCT outcomes may have related to variable Pilates exercise regimes. For example, RCTs with statistically significant results prescribed supervised exercise sessions more than once a week, often with the use of specialised equipment [21,24,25,55]. It is therefore recommended that clinicians replicate Pilates exercise programs contained within RCTs with statistically significant results to maximise treatment outcomes.

Table 5. Description of Included Studies- Pilates exercise versus massage or other forms of exercise.

Study	Population	Intervention and Comparison	Outcome Measures [Timing]
1. Anderson, 2005 [49]	21 people with chronic or recurrent low back pain	Pilates: 2 X 50 minute supervised sessions per week for 6 weeks; Equipment = Reformer; Standardised protocol	Miami Back Index – Pain and Disability
	Gender (Female: Male) =0.9: 1.0	Massage: 2 X 30 minute sessions per week for 6 weeks	Oswestry Disability Questionnaire
	Age[&] (years) = Pilates 42.4 (12.0); Comparison 44.0 (13.7)		[0, 6 weeks]
	Baseline Pain Intensity[&] (/10)[#] = Pilates 6.4 (2.5); Comparison 7.3 (1.7)		
	Baseline Disability[&] (/100)[$] = Pilates 18.6 (5.9); Comparison 16.7 (4.2)		
2. Marshall et al., 2013 [23]	64 participants with CLBP	Pilates: 3 X 50–60 minute supervised sessions per week for 8 weeks; Equipment= Mat, Reformer; Supervision Ratio=10 clients: 1 therapist; Standardised protocol	Oswestry Disability Questionnaire
	Gender (Female: Male) =1.7: 1.0	Cycling: 3 X 50–60 minutes supervised indoor stationary cycle training for 8 weeks	Visual Analog Scale – Pain
	Age[&] (years) 36.2(6.2)		[0, 8, 24 weeks]
	Baseline Pain Intensity[&] (/10)[a] = Pilates 3.6 (2.1); Comparison 4.5 (2.5)		
	Baseline Disability[&](/100)[$] = Pilates 25.4 (11.2); Comparison 24.0 (11.9)		
3. Gagnon, 2005 [51]	12 participants with acute and chronic low back pain	Pilates: 1–2 X 30–45 minute supervised mat sessions per week for 6–7 weeks; Standardised protocol	Revised Oswestry Disability Index
	Gender (Female: Male) = Pilates 5.0: 1.0; Comparison 2.0: 1.0	Traditional lumbar stabilisation exercise: 1–2 X 30–45 minute supervised mat sessions per week for 6–7 weeks	Visual Analog Scale – Pain
	Age[&] (years) = Pilates 36.0 (11.4); Comparison 30.3 (12.4)	(Both groups could continue physiotherapy treatment and home exercises as indicated)	[0, 4, 6–7 weeks]
	Baseline Pain Intensity[&] (/10)[a] = Pilates 3.9 (2.5); Comparison 2.1 (1.7)		
	Baseline Disability[&] (/100)[$] = Pilates 17.2 (6.1); Exercise 15.8 (3.7)		
4. Rajpal et al., 2009 [59]	40 females 20–30 years old with postural CLBP	Pilates exercise: Daily home exercise (10 repetitions with 10 second hold) over 4 weeks – progressed from crook lying, 4 point kneeling and knee extension on fit ball	Visual Analog Scale – Pain
	Age (years): Mean =21.8	McKenzie exercise: Daily postural correction exercises (15–20 repetitions, 3 X per day) in sitting and standing	[0, 4 weeks]
5. Wajswelner et al., 2012 [26]	83 participants with CLBP or stiffness	Pilates: 2 X 60 minute supervised sessions per week, and daily home exercises for 6 weeks; Equipment: Mat, Reformer, Trapeze Table; Supervision Ratio: 4 clients: 1 therapist; Individualised, based on directional preferences	Numerical Rating Scale (11 point) - Pain
	Gender (Female: Male) = Pilates 1.3: 1.0; Comparison 1.2: 1.0	General exercise: 2 X 60 minute supervised sessions per week (including aerobic, stretching, strengthening, and stabilisation exercise) and daily home exercises for 6 weeks; Supervision Ratio: 4 clients: 1 therapist	Quebec Scale - Pain and Disability
	Age[&] (years) = Pilates 49.3 (14.1); Comparison 48.9(16.4)	(Both groups could utilise analgesic medication as required but no other form of treatment)	[0, 6, 12, 24 weeks]
	Baseline Pain Intensity[&] (/10)[+] = Pilates 4.9 (1.6); Comparison 4.6 (1.8)		
	Baseline Disability[&] (/100)[t] = Pilates 28.1 (11.4); Comparison 23.9 (14.0)		

[&]values represent Mean [Standard Deviation];
[#]as per Miami Back Index;
[$]as measured by Oswestry Disability Index;
[a]as measured by Visual Analog Scale (11 point);
[+]as measured by Numerical Rating Scale (11 point);
[t]as measured by Roland Morris Disability Questionnaire.

Pilates exercise versus massage therapy

Only one RCT compared Pilates exercise to massage therapy [49]. No statistically significant difference in improvements in pain or functional ability was noted at 6 weeks. More high quality RCTs, though, are required to confirm these findings due to the "fair" methodological quality of this RCT [34,38].

Table 6. Effectivenessof Pilates exercise versus usual care and physical activity in reducing pain in people with chronic low back pain.

Study	Methodological Quality [Score]	Population [Sample size]	Intervention and Comparison	Outcome Measure(s)	Assessment Timing	Mean Difference [95% confidence interval]
1. Borges et al., 2013 [21]	Very good [13/16]	Chronic low back pain [n = 64]	Pilates exercise versus no change in physical activity	Visual Analog Scale	15 weeks	−4.1 [−6.3 to −1.8][a]
2. da Fonseca et al., 2009 [50]	Poor [4/16]	Chronic low back pain [n = 17]	Pilates exercise versus no Pilates exercise	Visual Analog Scale	7–8 weeks	−1.9 [−5.0 to 1.2]
3. Gladwell et al., 2006 [52]	Very good [13/16]	Chronic low back pain [n = 34]	Pilates exercise versus usual care and physical activity	Visual Analog Scale – Present Pain	6 weeks	−0.2 [−0.8 to 0.4]
				Visual Analog Scale - Pain Diary	6 weeks	−0.3 [−0.9 to 0.3][+]
4. MacIntyre, 2006 [48]	Excellent [15/16]	Non-specific chronic low back pain [n = 86]	Pilates exercise versus no change in physical activity[$]	Visual Analog Scale	3 weeks	−0.4 [−1.7 to 0.9]
					12 weeks	−1.6 [−3.2 to 0.0]
5. Miyamoto et al., 2013 [24]	Excellent [16/16]	Chronic low back pain for more than 6 months [n = 22]	Pilates exercise and education versus education alone	Numerical Rating Scale (11 point)	6 weeks	−2.2 [−3.2 to −1.1][a]
					24 weeks	−0.9 [−1.9 to 0.1]
6. Quinn et al., 2011 [25]	Very good [14/16]	Chronic low back pain after physiotherapy [n = 29]	Pilates exercise versus no Pilates exercise	Visual Analog Scale	8 weeks	−1.5 [−2.1 to −0.9][a]
7. Rydeard et al., 2006 [55]	Very good [14/16]	Subacute, chronic, or recurrent low back pain, physically active [n = 39]	Pilates exercise versus no change in physical activity[$]	Numerical Rating Scale (101 point)	4 weeks	−15.6 [−17.8 to −13.4][a]

[a]statistically significant between group difference;
[+]reported as statistically significant in study, but not calculated in this review;
[$]with or without usual care.

Table 7. Effectiveness of Pilates exercise compared to usual care and physical activity in improving functional ability in people with chronic low back pain.

Study	Methodological Quality [Score]	Population [Sample size]	Intervention and Comparison	Outcome Measure(s)	Assessment Timing	Mean Difference [95% confidence interval]
1. Gladwell et al., 2006 [52]	Very good [13/16]	Chronic low back pain [n = 34]	Pilates exercise versus usual care and physical activity	Oswestry Disability Questionnaire	6 weeks	0.0 [−8.5 to 8.5]
2. MacIntyre, 2006 [48]	Excellent [15/16]	Non-specific chronic low back pain [n = 86]	Pilates exercise versus no change in physical activity[$]	Roland Morris Disability Questionnaire	3 weeks	−0.6 [−2.6 to 1.5]
					12 weeks	−2.6 [−5.2 to −0.1][a]
3. Miyamoto et al., 2013 [24]	Excellent [16/16]	Chronic low back pain for greater than 6 months [n = 22]	Pilates exercise and education versus education alone	Roland Morris Disability Questionnaire	6 weeks	−2.7 [−4.4 to −1.0][a]
					24 weeks	−1.4 [−3.1 to 0.0]
4. Quinn, 2005 [53]	Poor [6/16]	Chronic low back pain [n = 22]	Pilates exercise versus usual physical activity	Oswestry Disability Questionnaire	12 weeks	−7.1 [−17.6 to 3.4]
5. Quinn et al., 2011 [25]	Very good [14/16]	Chronic low back pain after physiotherapy [n = 29]	Pilates exercise versus no Pilates exercise	Oswestry Disability Questionnaire	8 weeks	1.3 [not given but p> 0.05]
6. Rydeard et al., 2006 [55]	Very good [14/16]	Subacute, chronic, or recurrent low back pain, physically active [n = 39]	Pilates exercise versus no change in physical activity[$]	Oswestry Disability Questionnaire	4 weeks	−1.2 [−1.4 to −1.0][a]
7. Zeada et al., 2012 [56]	Poor [4/16]	Athletes with chronic low back pain [n = 20]	Pilates exercise versus no Pilates exercise	Roland Morris Disability Questionnaire	8 weeks	1.7 [−0.4 to 3.8][+]

[$]with or without usual care;
[a]statistically significant between group difference;
[+]reported as statistically significant in the study.

Table 8. Effectiveness of Pilates exercise versus massage or other forms of exercise in reducing pain in people with chronic low back pain.

Study	Methodological Quality [Score]	Population [Sample size]	Intervention and Comparison	Outcome Measure(s)	Assessment Timing	Mean Difference [95% confidence interval]
1. Anderson, 2005 [49]	Fair [10/16]	Chronic or recurrent low back pain [n = 21]	Pilates exercise versus massage	Miami Back Index (Pain)	6 weeks	−10.8 [−25.9 to 4.3]
2. Marshall et al., 2013[23]	Excellent [15/16]	Chronic low back pain [n = 64]	Pilates exercise versus stationary cycling	Visual Analog Scale (Current pain)	8 weeks	−1.1 [−2.1 to −0.1][a]
					24 weeks	−1.4 [−2.6 to −0.2]
				Visual Analog Scale (Worst pain)	8 weeks	−0.4 [−1.4 to 0.6]
3. Gagnon, 2005 [51]	Fair [10/16]	Acute and chronic low back pain [n = 12]	Pilates exercise versus lumbar stabilisation	Visual Analog Scale	4 weeks	0.8 [−1.3 to 2.9]
					6–7 weeks	0.6 [−1.7 to 2.8]
4. Rajpal et al., 2009 [54]	Poor [5/16]	Females with chronic low back pain [n = 40]	Pilates exercise versus McKenzie exercise	Visual Analog Scale	4 weeks	−1.4 [−2.1 to −0.7][a, $]
5. Wajswelner et al., 2012 [26]	Excellent [16/16]	Chronic low back pain [n = 83]	Pilates exercise versus general exercise (mixed)	Numerical Rating Scale (11 point)	6 weeks	−0.5 [−1.3 to 0.3]
					12 weeks	−0.6 [−1.5 to 0.3]
					24 weeks	0.3 [−0.7 to 1.2]

[a]statistically significant between group difference;
[$]based on comparison of pre and post treatment scores.

Pilates exercise versus other forms of exercise

Based on current evidence, it is difficult to conclude on the short-term effectiveness of Pilates exercise in people with CLBP compared to other forms of exercise. Statistically significant improvements in pain and functional ability have been reported in one high quality RCT [23], but not in other high quality RCTs [26]. The clinical significance of reported statistically significant improvements is also unlikely [23,46,47]. There is consensus across high quality RCTs, though, that people with CLBP will experience equivalent improvements in pain and functional ability with Pilates exercise or alternative forms of exercise at 24 weeks [23,26].

Authors of this review therefore suggest that Pilates exercise is unlikely to provide superior improvements in pain and functional ability compared to other forms of exercise, at least in the long term. Findings of this review are similar to those of previous systematic reviews in that improvements in pain and functional ability with Pilates exercise compared to other forms of exercise have not been reported as statistically significant [6,7,17]. This

Table 9. Effectiveness of Pilates exercise versus massage or other forms of exercise in improving functional ability in people with chronic low back pain.

Study	Methodological Quality [Score]	Population [Sample size]	Intervention and Comparison	Outcome Measure(s)	Assessment Timing	Mean Difference [95% confidence interval]
1. Anderson, 2005 [49]	Fair [10/16]	Chronic or recurrent low back pain [n = 21]	Pilates exercise versus massage therapy	Miami Back Index (Disability)	6 weeks	−7.9 [−1.4 to 0.3]
				Oswestry Disability Questionnaire	6 weeks	−4.0 [−10.0 to 2.0]
2. Marshall et al., 2013 [23]	Excellent [15/16]	Acute and chronic low back pain [n = 12]	Pilates exercise versus stationary cycling	Oswestry Disability Index	8 weeks	−6.5 [−11.8 to −1.1][a]
					24 weeks	4.4 [−0.7 to 9.5]
3. Gagnon, 2005 [51]	Fair [10/16]	Chronic low back pain [n = 32]	Pilates exercise versus lumbar stabilisation	Oswestry Disability Index	4 weeks	−3.0 [−11.1 to 5.1]
					6–7 weeks	−2.2 [−10.9 to 6.5]
4. Wajswelner et al., 2012 [26]	Excellent [16/16]	Chronic low back pain [n = 83]	Pilates exercise versus general exercise	Quebec Score	6 weeks	1.8 [−3.1 to 6.7]
					12 weeks	−0.8 [−6.4 to 4.8]
					24 weeks	−1.1 [−5.8 to 3.6]

[a]statistically significant between group difference.

review is different, however, in that it acknowledges that there could be differences in the short term.

There are two reasons why authors of this review have not ruled out the possibility of Pilates exercise offering superior short-term benefit over other forms of exercise. First, one of the two RCTs that reported no difference in the short term was of "fair" methodological quality [34,38]. This meant that findings were likely to be more biased than that of higher quality RCTs [38]. Second, comparison exercise treatments were variable and it could be possible that Pilates exercise is more effective than some types of exercise, but not others. When Pilates exercise was compared to a distinctly different form of exercise, cycling, there was a statistically significant difference in outcome [23]. When compared to exercises involving lumbar stabilisation, however, no difference was noted [26,51]. Future research should investigate the relative effectiveness of Pilates exercise to different forms of exercise.

Limitations

Limitations of this systematic review relate to the inclusion of only RCTs published in the English language and consequent language bias. Of the 16 studies excluded based on their language, however, only 2 appeared to be potentially relevant RCTs when reviewing titles and abstracts translated into the English language [58,59]. Another limitation was the focus of this review on outcomes of pain and functional ability in people with CLBP. Other outcomes may have also been clinically important, such as quality of life [33,60]. In addition, the methodological quality of RCTs was summarised by a total score out of 16 using the McMaster Quantitative Review Form criteria [34]. This approach can lead to oversimplification of methodological quality as all items of the scale are weighted evenly [61].

The strength of the review findings was also influenced by the availability and diversity of primary evidence. The limited number of RCTs that had compared Pilates exercise to massage therapy and other forms of exercise lessened the certainty of results [15]. The small sample sizes and short term follow up of many RCTs also affected the precision of findings [62]. Moreover, the heterogeneity of study populations, interventions, comparison treatments, outcome measures, and timing of reassessment prevented conduction of meaningful meta-analyses of RCTs [40,41].

Conclusion

According to this systematic review, Pilates exercise results in statistically significant improvements in pain and functional ability in the short term compared to usual care and physical activity in people with CLBP [21,24,25,55]. Changes in pain are more likely to be clinically significant than improvements in functional ability. At 24 weeks, though, improvements with Pilates exercise and education may be equivalent to those achieved with education alone [24]. When Pilates exercise is compared to massage therapy or other forms of exercise, equivalent improvements in pain and functional ability have been reported in people with CLBP [23,26,49].

Implications

This systematic review provides an update on the effectiveness of Pilates exercise in people with CLBP that may be used to assist clinical decision-making. Future research should investigate optimal Pilates exercise regimes for people with CLBP, including appropriate frequencies and length of programs, supervision ratios, use of home exercises, and specialised equipment [13]. Future RCTs should also investigate the long term efficacy of Pilates exercise to other treatments, such as massage, and confirm if there is any difference in effectiveness between Pilates exercise and various forms of exercise, such as aerobic exercise versus lumbar stabilisation [15]. Research into whether some people with CLBP may benefit from Pilates exercise more than others may also assist in clinical decision-making on whether Pilates exercise is suitable for individual clients [63,64].

Author Contributions

Analyzed the data: CW BH. Wrote the paper: CW. Reviewed manuscript: CW BH AB GK PM.

References

1. Charlton JE (2005) Core Curriculum for Professional Education in Pain, 3rd ed. Seattle: International Association of the Study of Pain Press.
2. Dagenais S, Caro J, Haldeman S (2008) A systematic review of low back pain cost of illness studies in the United States and internationally. Spine J 8: 8–20.
3. Hoy D, March L, Brooks P, Woolf A, Blyth F, et al. (2010) Measuring the global burden of low back pain. Best Pract Res Clin Rheumatol 24: 155–165.
4. Woolf AD, Pflleger B (2003) Burden of major musculoskeletal conditions. Bull World Health Organ 81: 646–656.
5. Brennan S, French H (2008) A questionnaire survey of the knowledge and use of Pilates based exercise for chronic low back pain amongst Irish physiotherapists. Phys Ther Rev 13: 212–213.
6. Aladro-Gonzalvo AR, Araya-Vargas GA, Machado-Diaz M, Salazar-Rojas W (2013) Pilates-based exercise for persistent, non-specific low back pain and associated functional disability: A meta-analysis with meta-regression. J Bodyw Mov Ther 17: 125–136.
7. Pereira LM, Obara K, Dias JM, Menacho MO, Guariglia DA, et al. (2012) Comparing the Pilates method with no exercise or lumbar stabilization for pain and functionality in patients with chronic low back pain: Systematic review and meta-analysis. Clin Rehabil 26: 10–20.
8. Latey P (2001) The Pilates method: History and philosophy. J Bodyw Mov Ther 5:275–282.
9. Wells C, Kolt GS, Bialocerkowski A (2012) Defining Pilates exercise: A systematic review. Complement Ther Med 20: 253–262.
10. Hayden JA, van Tulder MW, Tomlinson G (2005) Systematic review: Strategies for using exercise therapy to improve outcomes in chronic low back pain. Ann Intern Med 142: 776–785.
11. Macedo LG, Maher CG, Latimer J, McAuley JH (2009) Motor control exercise for persistent, nonspecific low back pain: A systematic review. Phys Ther 89: 9–25.
12. Pillastrini P, Gardenghi I, Bonetti F, Capra F, Guccione A, et al. (2012) An updated overview of clinical guidelines for chronic low back pain management in primary care. Joint Bone Spine 79: 176–185.
13. Wells C, Kolt GS, Marshall P, Bialocerkowski A (2014) The definition and application of Pilates exercise to treat people with chronic low back pain: A Delphi survey of Australian physical therapists. Phys Ther 94, doi:10.2522/ptj.20130030
14. Da Luz MA, Costa LOP, Fuhro FF, Manzoni ACT, Oliveira NTB, et al. (2014) Effectiveness of mat Pilates or equipment-based Pialtes exercises in patiences with chronic nonspecific low back pain: A randomised controlled trial. Phys Ther 94: 623–631, doi 10.2522/ptj.20130277.
15. Wells C, Kolt GS, Marshall P, Hill B, Bialocerkowski A (2013) Effectiveness of Pilates exercise in treating people with chronic low back pain: A systematic review of systematic reviews. BMC Medical Research Methodology 13: 7. Available: http://www.biomedcentral.com/1471-2288/13/7. Accessed 4 February 2014.
16. La Touche R, Escalante K, Linares MT (2008) Treating non-specific chronic low back pain through the Pilates Method. J Bodyw Mov Ther 12: 364–370.
17. Lim ECW, Poh RLC, Low AY, Wong WP (2011) Effects of Pilates-based exercises on pain and disability in individuals with persistent non-specific low back pain: A systematic review with meta-analysis. J Orthop Sports Phys Ther 41:70–80.
18. Miyamoto GC, Costa LO, Cabral CM (2013) Efficacy of the Pilates method for pain and disability in patients with chronic nonspecific low back pain: A

systematic review with meta-analysis. Braz J Phys Ther 17:517–532, doi 10.1590/S1413-35552012005000127.
19. Posadzki P, Lizis P, Hagner-Derengowska M (2011) Pilates for low back pain: A systematic review. Complement Ther Clin Pract 17: 85–89.
20. Costa LOP, Hancock M, Maher C, Ostelo RWJG, Cabral CMN, et al. (2012) Pilates for low back pain (Protocol). Cochrane Database of Systematic Reviews 12:CD010265, doi: 10.1002/14651858.CD010265.
21. Borges J, Baptista AF, Santana N, Souza I, Kruschewsky RA, et al. (2014) Pilates exercises improve low back pain and quality of life in patients with HTLV-1 virus: A randomised crossover clinical trial. J Bodywork and Movt Ther 18: 68–74.
22. Brooks C, Kennedy S, Marshall PW (2012) Specific trunk and general exercise elicit similar changes in anticipatory postural adjustments in patients with chronic low back pain: A randomized controlled trial. Spine 37: E1543–E1550.
23. Marshall PW, Kennedy S, Brooks C, Lonsdale C (2013) Pilates exercise or stationary cycling for chronic nonspecific low back pain: Does it matter? A randomised controlled trial with 6 month follow-up. Spine 38: E952–959.
24. Miyamoto GC, Costa LOP, Glavanin T, Cabral CMN (2013) Efficacy of the addition of modified Pilates exercises to minimal intervention in patients with chronic low back pain: A randomised controlled trial. Phys Ther 93: 310–320. doi 10.2522/ptj.20120190.
25. Quinn K, Barry S, Barry L (2011) Do patients with chronic low back pain benefit from attending Pilates classes after completing conventional physiotherapy treatment? Physiotherapy Ireland 32:5–12.
26. Wajswelner H, Metcalf B, Bennell K (2012) Clinical pilates versus general exercise for chronic low back pain: Randomized trial. Med Sci Sports Exerc 44: 1197–1205.
27. Kunz R, Vist GE, Oxman AD (2007) Randomisation to protect against selection bias in healthcare trials. Cochrane Database Syst Rev 2: Article Number MR000012Article Number MR000012.
28. National Health and Medical Research Council (NHMRC) (2009) NHMRC additional levels of evidence and grades for recommendations for developers of guidelines. Canberra: National Health and Medical Research Council.
29. Collins J, Fauser B, Bart CJM (20050 Balancing the strengths of systematic and narrative reviews. Hum Reprod Update 11:103–104.
30. Cook D, Mulrow C, Haynes R (1997) Systematic reviews: Synthesis of best evidence for clinical decisions. Ann Intern Med 126: 376–380.
31. Hopewell S, Clarke M, Moher D, Wager E, Middleton P, et al. (2008) CONSORT for reporting randomised trials in journal and conference abstracts. Lancet 371:281–283.
32. Hayden JA, van Tulder MW, Malmivaara A, Koes BW (2005) Exercise therapy for treatment of non-specific low back pain. Cochrane Database Syst Rev 3: Article Number CD000335.
33. Chapman JR, Norvell DC, Hermsmeyer JT, Bransford RJ, DeVine J, et al. (2011) Evaluating common outcomes for measuring treatment success for chronic low back pain. Spine 36: S54–68.
34. Law M, MacDermid J (1998) Evidence-based rehabilitation (2nd Ed.). Thorofare, New Jersey: Slack.
35. Katrack P, Bialocerkowski AE, Massy-Westropp N, Kumar VSS, Grimmer KA (2004) A systematic review of the content of critical appraisal tools. BMC Med Res Methodol 4:22. Available: http://www.biomedcentral.com/1471-2288/4/22. Accessed 4 February 2014.
36. Lekkas P, Larson T, Kumar S, Grimmer K, Nyland L, et al. (2007) No model of clinical education for physiotherapy students is superior to another: A systematic review. Aust J Physiother 53: 19–28.
37. Schabrun SM, Hillier S (2009) Evidence for the retraining of sensation after stroke: A systematic review. Clin Rehabil 23: 27–39.
38. Daly A, Bialocerkowski A (2009) Does evidence support physiotherapy management of adult complex regional pain syndrome type one: A systematic review. Eur J Pain 13: 339–353.
39. Viera AJ, Carrett JM (2005) Understanding inter-observer agreement: The kappa statistic. Family Medicine 37: 360–363.
40. Fletcher J (2007) What is heterogeneity and is it important? BMJ 334:94–96.
41. Higgins JPT, Thompson SG, Deeks JJ, Altman DG (2003) Measuring inconsistency in meta-analyses. BMJ 327: 557–560. Available: http://www.bmj.com/content/327/7414/557. Accessed 7 May 2014.
42. Riley RD, Higgins JPT, Deeks J (2011) Interpretation of random effects meta-analyses. BMJ 342: d549. Available: http://www.bmj.com/content/342/bmj.d549. Accessed 7 May 2014.
43. The Cochrane Collaboration (2012) Review Manager (RevMan) [Computer program]. Version 5.2 Copenhagen: The Nordic Cochrane Centre.
44. Herbert R (2013) Confidence Interval Calculator. Available: http://www.pedro.org.au/english/downloads/confidence-interval-calculator/. Accessed 7 May 2014.
45. Van Tulder M, Malmivaara A, Hayden J, Koes B (2007) Statistical significance versus clinical importance: Trials on exercise therapy for chronic low back pain as example. Spine 32:1785–1790.
46. Ostelo RW, de Vet HC (2005) Clinically important outcomes in low back pain. Best Pract Res Clin Rheumatol 19: 593–607.
47. Ostelo RW, Deyo RA, Stratford P, Waddell G, Croft P, et al. (2008) Interpreting change scores for pain and functional status in low back pain: Towards international consensus regarding minimal importance change. Spine 33: 90–94.
48. MacIntyre L (2006) The effect of Pilates on patients' chronic low back pain: A pilot study [dissertation]. Johannesburg: University of the Witwatersrand.
49. Anderson B (2005). Randomised clinical trial comparing active versus passive approaches to the treatment of recurrent and chronic low back pain [dissertation]. Miami, Florida: University of Miami.
50. da Fonseca JL, Magini M, de Freitas TH (2009) Laboratory gait analysis in patients with low back pain before and after a Pilates intervention. J Sport Rehabil 18:269–282.
51. Gagnon LH (2005) Efficacy of Pilates exercises as therapeutic intervention in treating patients with low back pain [dissertation]. Knoxville: University of Tennessee.
52. Gladwell V, Head S, Haggar M, Beneke R (2006) Does a program of Pilates improve chronic nonspecific low back pain? J Sport Rehabil 15:338–350.
53. Quinn J (2005) Influence of Pilates-based mat exercise on chronic lower back pain [dissertation]. Boca Raton, FL: Florida Atlantic University.
54. Rajpal N, Arora M, Chauhan V (2008) The study on efficacy of Pilates and McKenzie exercise in postural low back pain – A rehabilitative protocol. Physiotherapy and Occupational Therapy Journal 1:33–56.
55. Rydeard R, Leger A, Smith D (2006) Pilates-based therapeutic exercise: Effect on subjects with nonspecific chronic low back pain and functional disability: A randomized controlled trial. J Orthop Sports Phys Ther 36: 472–484.
56. Zeada MA (2011) Ffects of Pilates on low back pain and urine catecholamine. Ovidius University Annals, Series Physiotherapy Education and Sport 12:41–47.
57. Rydeard RA (2001) Evaluation of a targeted exercise rehabilitation approach and its effectiveness in the treatment of pain, functional disability and muscle function in a population with longstanding unresolved low back pain [dissertation]. Kingston, Canada: Queens University.
58. Kawanishi CY, de Oliveira MR, Coelho VS, Parreira RB, de Oliveira RF, et al. (2011) Effect of Pilates exercise on trunk function and pain in patients with low back pain [Portuguese]. Revista Terapia Manual 9:410–417.
59. Montero-Camra J, Sierra-Silvestre E, Monteagudo-Saiz AM, Lepez-Fernandez J, Lopez-Lopez A, et al. (2013) Active eccentric stretch against passive analytical hamstring stretch in subacute or chronic non-specific low back pain: A pilot trial [Spanish]. Fisioterapia 35: 206–213, doi 19.1016/j.ft.2012.10.004.
60. Dworkin RH, Turk DC, Farrar JT, Haythornthwaite JA, Jensen MP, et al. (2005) Core outcome measures for chronic pain clinical trials: IMMPACT recommendations. Pain 113: 9–119.
61. Colle F, Rannou F, Revel M, Fermanian J, Poiraudeau S (2002) Impact of quality scales on levels of evidence inferred from a systematic review of exercise therapy and low back pain. Arch Phys Med Rehabil 83: 1745–1752.
62. Noordzij M, Tripepi Giovanni, Dekker FW, Zoccali C, et al. (2010) Sample size calculations: Basic principles and common pitfalls. Nephrol Dial Transplant 25: 1388–1393.
63. Stolze LR, Allison SC, Childs JD (2012) Derivation of a preliminary clinical prediction rule for identifying a subgroup of patients with low back pain likely to benefit from Pilates-based exercise. J Orthop Sports Phys Ther 42: 425–436.
64. Wells C, Kolt GS, Marshall P, Bialocerkowski A (2014) Indications, benefits, and risks of Pilates exercise for people with chronic low back pain: A Delphi survey of Pilates trained physical therapists. Phys Ther, doi 10.2522/ptj20130568.

2

Cardiorespiratory Optimal Point: A Submaximal Exercise Variable to Assess Panic Disorder Patients

Plínio Santos Ramos[1,2], Aline Sardinha[3], Antonio Egidio Nardi[3], Claudio Gil Soares de Araújo[1,4]*

1 Exercise Medicine Clinic – CLINIMEX, Rio de Janeiro, Rio de Janeiro, Brazil, **2** Maternity Hospital Therezinha de Jesus, Faculty of Medical and Health Sciences – SUPREMA, Juiz de Fora, Minas Gerais, Brazil, **3** Panic and Respiration Laboratory, Institute of Psychiatry, Federal University of Rio de Janeiro, National Institute for Translational Medicine (INCT-TM/CNPq), Rio de Janeiro, Rio de Janeiro, Brazil, **4** Heart Institute Edson Saad, Federal University of Rio de Janeiro, Rio de Janeiro, Rio de Janeiro, Brazil

Abstract

Panic disorder (PD) patients often report respiratory symptoms and tend to perform poorly during maximal cardiopulmonary exercise testing (CPX), at least partially, due to phobic anxiety. Thus, we hypothesized that a submaximal exercise variable, minimum VE/VO_2 - hereafter named cardiorespiratory optimal point (COP) -, may be useful in their clinical assessment. Data from 2,338 subjects were retrospectively analyzed and 52 (2.2%) patients diagnosed with PD (PDG) (70% women; aged 48±13 years). PD patients were compared with a healthy control group (CG) precisely matched to number of cases, age and gender profiles. PDG was further divided into two subgroups, based on having achieved a maximal or a submaximal CPX (unwilling to continue until exhaustion). We compared COP, VO_2 max, maximum heart rate (HR max) between PDG and CG, and also COP between maximal and submaximal PD subgroups. COP was similar between PDG and CG (21.9±0.5 vs. 23.4±0.6; p = 0.07), as well as, for PD subgroups of maximal and submaximal CPX (22.0±0.5 vs. 21.6±1.3; p = 0.746). Additionally, PD patients completing a maximal CPX obtained VO_2 max (mL.kg−1.min−1) (32.9±1.57 vs 29.6±1.48; p = 0.145) and HR max (bpm) similar to controls (173±2.0 vs 168±2.7; p = 0.178). No adverse complications occurred during CPX. Although clinically safe, it is sometimes difficult to obtain a true maximal CPX in PD patients. Normalcy of cardiorespiratory interaction at submaximal effort as assessed by COP may contribute to reassure both patients and physicians that there is no physiological substrate for exercise-related respiratory symptoms often reported by PD patients.

Editor: John Calvert, Emory University, United States of America

Funding: The experimental work was partially supported by Fundação de Amparo a Pesquisa do Rio de Janeiro - FAPERJ (Rio de Janeiro State Foundation for Scientifical Research) and Conselho Nacional de Desenvolvimento Científico e Tecnológico - CNPq (National Council for the Scientific and Technological Development and Instituto Nacional de Ciencia e Tecnologia - INCT-TM - Brazil. The funders had no role in study design, data collection and analysis, decision to publish, or preparation of the manuscript.

Competing Interests: The authors have declared that no competing interests exist.

* Email: cgaraujo@iis.com.br

Introduction

Patients reporting exercise-induced shortness of breath and/or palpitations are often anxious [1]. They could be a real diagnostic challenge since it is quite often difficult to distinguish between a real clinical abnormal respiratory or circulatory condition from one commonly seen during panic attacks (PA) [2,3]. Despite a very high lifetime prevalence of about 28% [4] for PA in adult subjects, It is worthwhile to note there are very limited amount of data about exercise and panic and, more specifically, about what role, if any, could cardiopulmonary exercise testing play in the clinical assessment of these patients.

Panic disorder (PD) is characterized by recurrent and unexpected anxiety or PA, without apparent cause, PA are characterized by the sudden appearance of four or more autonomic and respiratory symptoms, reaching peak in approximately 10 minutes and then disappearing [5]. Some evidence suggests that these patients may have subclinical respiratory and other abnormalities [3] related to body homeostasis during rest [2], as, for example, hyperventilation syndrome [6], with increased sensitivity to carbon dioxide (CO_2) [7,8]. This increased CO_2 sensitivity led to the most well accepted current hypothesis to explain the occurrence of PA, the theory of false suffocation alarm, that is related to abnormal control mechanisms of respiration in these patients [9].

It is well-established that expired gas data obtained during cardiopulmonary exercise testing (CPX) can be used in the diagnosis and prognosis of numerous pathologic conditions [10,11]. however, there are very limited data on CPX in PD patients [12]. In fact, preliminary evidence suggests that aerobic fitness may be reduced in this clinical condition [13,14,15]. Additionally, performance of maximal CPX could be particularly hampered by phobic anxiety, with autonomic manifestations naturally triggered by exercise, similar to those present in a PA [16]. Thus, due to the anticipatory anxiety related to a PA while performing a CPX, it is quite common that the patient will be unwilling to achieve the exhaustion that characterizes a maximal CPX [13,17].

In this study, we have used a recently proposed submaximal exercise variable, the cardiorespiratory optimal point (COP) [18], which represents the minimal ventilation (VE)/oxygen uptake (VO_2) value and reflects the best circulatory-respiratory interaction, to assess exercise ventilatory response in PD patients. So, in order to test the hypothesis that the exercise-related respiratory symptoms in PD patients are not due to a true abnormal cardiorespiratory interaction, we compared COP during CPX in PD patients and age and gender-matched healthy subjects. If our hypothesis is correct this will reassure both patients and physicians about the absence of a true physiological substrate for these frequent patients' complains.

Materials and Methods

Ethics statement

Both consent form and all study procedures and retrospective data analyses were previously approved by the Faculty of Medical and Health Sciences, SUPREMA institutional research ethics committee under number (protocol number 0166.0.000.399-11) in accordance with the Declaration of Helsinki of the World Medical Association Ethics Code. All subjects participated in the present study voluntarily, receiving no financial incentive. Participants were informed that they could withdraw at any time. Each subject (legal guardian if minor) read and signed a specific informed consent form.

All data are only available upon request to the senior author (legal guardian of the data). This option follows the local laws and ethical regulations that apply to confidentiality of clinical/medical data.

Sample

Among 2,338 subjects evaluated in our Exercise Medicine Clinic between January, 2006 and September, 2012, those who were previously diagnosed with PD by their doctors, according to the DSM-IV [5], and who met the following inclusion criteria: 1) absence of known cardiopulmonary diseases; 2) not under regular use of relevant medications; 3) body mass index <30 kg/m^2; 4) normal resting spirometry (FEV1/FVC>70%) [19]; 5) absence of clinical or electrocardiographic changes that characterize myocardial ischemia during CPX and 6) absence of locomotor limitations that can hinder the implementation of lower-limb cycling CPX. Among the 83 patients identified with PD (3.6% of total), 31 were excluded, nine for having performed treadmill CPX, 13 due to obesity, three due to a history and/or signs of coronary artery disease to CPX and six due to abnormal resting spirometry. To the remaining 52 patients, age was 48±13 years (mean± standard deviation), 36 (70%) were women, 36 (70%) had current clinical PD presentation and 16 (30%) had a history and a previous diagnosis of PD (without recurrence of PA in the last six months).

Control Group

A control group (CG) precisely matched with the same number of cases and the same age and sex profile as the PD patients was selected from a database of 624 healthy individuals evaluated during the same period that also attended all the inclusion criteria. Selection was performed from numbers assigned to each healthy subject belonging to the database by using the site www.randomizer.org.

Characterization of Subgroups

Two groups were so defined: healthy individuals (CG) and PD patients (PDG). For some further analyses, PDG was divided in two subgroups, MAX (maximal) and SUBMAX (submaximal) based on whether patients effectively concluded a truly maximal CPX.

Evaluation Protocol

Evaluation consisted of medical history, including specific questions about diagnosis, occurrence of PA events and treatment of PD and physical examination. Additionally, all medications in regular use were recorded. Anthropometric data was collected and resting spirometry and 12-lead electrocardiogram obtained. Subjects volunteered for the evaluation, typically performed under request of their attending physicians before to start an exercise program.

Resting Spirometry

At least three flow-volume curve maneuvers were performed using a pneumotachograph (SP-1 Spirometer, Schiller, Switzerland), periodically calibrated according to the standard recommendations [20]. Maximal voluntary ventilation was predicted by considering forced expiratory volume in one second (FEV1)×40 [21].

Maximal Cardiopulmonary Exercise Testing (CPX)

All subjects underwent a cycling maximal CPX (Cateye EC-1600, Cateye, Japan or Inbrasport CG-04, Inbrasport, Brazil), following an individualized ramp protocol aimed to obtain exhaustion between eight and 12 minutes [22]. The CPX's maximal nature was subjectively defined by the well-trained physician who supervised the procedure and supported by physiological indicators, such as the occurrence of anaerobic threshold (AT) [23], a U pattern of the ventilatory equivalent curves - and by – a score of 10 on the 0–10 Borg scale. The CPXs of patients who did not simultaneously achieve all of these criteria were considered submaximal [24,25]. Throughout CPX, electrocardiogram, heart rate, blood pressure and arterial oxygen saturation were also obtained.

Expired Gases Analyses

During CPX, expired gases were collected using a pneumotachograph Prevent (MedGraphics, USA) coupled to a mouthpiece, with concomitant nasal occlusion. A metabolic analyzer VO2000 (MedGraphics, United States) enabled the quantification of VE and partial fractions of oxygen and carbon dioxide, expressed every 10 s and later recalculated and expressed as mean values for each minute of CPX. These devices were regularly calibrated by a 2-L syringe and gases of known concentrations.

Cardiorespiratory Optimal Point (COP)

COP, a dimensionless variable, is defined as the minimal ventilation that is used for the consumption of one liter of oxygen, i.e, the identification of smallest value of the minute-by-minute ratio of VE and VO_2 during CPX and reflects the best possible cardiorespiratory interaction during exercise. The identification of COP is quite simple, objective, and independent from the evaluator's judgment. COP reference values for a wide age range among men and women are already available favoring its interpretation [18] and its measurement has been shown to be reliable in two separate CPX performed in the same subjects [26].

Statistical Analyses

Initially, normality (Kolmogorov-Smirnov) and homoscedasticity of the data distribution were tested. For descriptive purposes, central tendency and data variability were expressed as mean± standard deviation (minimal and maximal), and for statistical inference, as mean±standard error of the mean. Groups' comparisons were carried out by Student's t-test, except for between COP of the MAX and SUBMAX comparisons that due to the non-parametric distribution was carried out by Mann-Whitney test. Prism software version 6 (GraphPad, USA) was used for statistical analysis, considering a probability level of 5%.

Results

The most relevant demographic characteristics and the main results of resting spirometry and CPX, as a function of group/subgroup, are shown in Table 1.

When evaluating COP results, no differences between PD patients and control subjects (21.9±0.47 vs. 23.4±0.65; $p = 0.067$) nor between PDG SUBMAX and MAX CPX subgroups (22.0±0.50 vs. 21.6±1.31; $p = 0.736$) were found (Figure 1). In contrast, VO_2 max (mL.(kg.min)-1) of PDG was lower than in CG (27.2±1.35 vs. 32.9±1.57; $p<0.001$) and HR max (bpm) were higher for CG than for PDG (173±2.0 vs. 164±2.8; $p = 0.013$) (Table 1).

While comparing those who had performed a maximal CPX, i.e., CG and PDG MAX subgroup, there were no differences in VO_2 max (32.9±1.57 vs. 29.6±1.48 $mL.kg^{-1}.min^{-1}$; $p = 0.135$) or in HR max (173±2.0 vs. 168±2.7 bpm; $p = 0.168$).

Regarding COP results, except for one case (normality threshold value) all other 51 PD patients (98% of the total) had results that felt within the boundaries of two standard errors from the expected COP age-and-sex reference value [18]. (Figure 2).

It is noteworthy that none of PD patients had abnormal clinical, hemodynamic - blood pressure and heart rate - or respiratory responses to incremental exercise. Objectively, none of them achieved ventilatory limitation during CPX, as observed by VE maximal final values that were substantially below FEV1×40 [21]. (Table 1). Although minor ECG changes were eventually detected, such as isolated J point depression accompanied by rapid up slopping pattern of ST segment, it should be emphasized that there were no complaints of dyspnea or typical stress-induced precordial pain during or immediately following CPX by any of PD patients.

Discussion

Considering the initial sample of 2,338 adults, the prevalence of 3.6% of PD, tends to be slightly higher than reported by others [27]. This is consistent with the fact that our laboratory is a

Table 1. Characteristics and main results for spirometry and CPET in groups and subgroups.

Variables	Control	Panic Disorder		
Characteristics	**All(n = 52)**	**All (n = 52)**	**Maximal (n = 41)**	**Submaximal(n = 11)**
Sex (Female/Male)	31/21	31/21	20/21	11/0
Age (years)	47.7±13.2	48.5±13.4	47.5±13.6	52.5±12.0
	(19–75)	(17–78)	(17–74)	(34–78)
BMI (kg/m^2)	24.2±2.7	24.3±3.1	24.1±3.1	25.1-3.1
	(18.5–29.5)	(19.2–30.0)	(19.2–30.0)	(19.8–29.2)
HR at rest (bpm)	66.2±12.8	66.8±11.0	66.8±11.3	66.8±10.1
	(48–96)	(43–96)	(43–96)	(50–88)
Spirometry				
FEV1/FVC (%)	82.4±5.1	81.5±5.2	82.2±5.3	79.0±3.7
	(73.6–93.3)	(70.0–95.5)	(70.0–.5)	(70.1–83.2)
CPET				
Total Time (min)	10.6±2.3	9.5±2.4	10.3±1.8	6.7±1.8
	(6–15)	(3.4–14.0)	(7.0–14.0)	(3.4–9.5)
Maximum HR (bpm)	172.6±14.8	164.7±20.0	168.0±17.3	149.0±22.5
	(143–200)	(111–197)	(120–197)	(111–180)
Maximum predict VO_2 (%)	104.4±32.3	87.6±27.4	94.0±27.1	63.9±11.3
	(57.1–207.6)	(43.4–176.1)	(49.9–176.1)	(43.4–87.6)
Maximum VO_2 (mL.(kg.min)−1)	32.9±11.3	27.2±9.8	29.6±9.4	18.1±3.5
	(14.3–58.5)	(12.3–63.0)	(12.5–63.0)	(12.3–22.6)
VO2 AT (mL.(kg.min)−1)	23.0±8.6	19.2±6.6	20.5±6.7	14.5±2.9
	(9.1–45.5)	(5.4–48.0)	(5.4–48.0)	(7.5–18.0)
Maximum VE ($L.min^{-1}$)	81.9±31.7	61.1±27.3	68.1±25.7	35.0±14.4
	(34.9–160.2)	(21.1–139.0)	(23–139)	(21.1–61.4)
Maximal voluntary ventilation (VEF1×40) ($L.min^{-1}$)	117.6±30.2	109.1±27.1	115.6±25.0	84.7±20.1
	(62.4–184.4)	(48.4–168.8)	(60.0–168.8)	(48.8–114.4)
COP (VE/VO_2 min)	23.4±4.7	21.6±3.4	22.0±3.2	21.6±4.3
	(16.0–34.8)	(14.6–30.0)	(15.8–30.0)	(14.6–29.8)

BMI: Body mass index; HR: Heart Rate; FEV1: forced expiratory volume in 1 second; FVC: forced vital capacity; VO2: oxygen uptake; AT: Anaerobic Threshold; COP: cardiorespiratory optimal point.

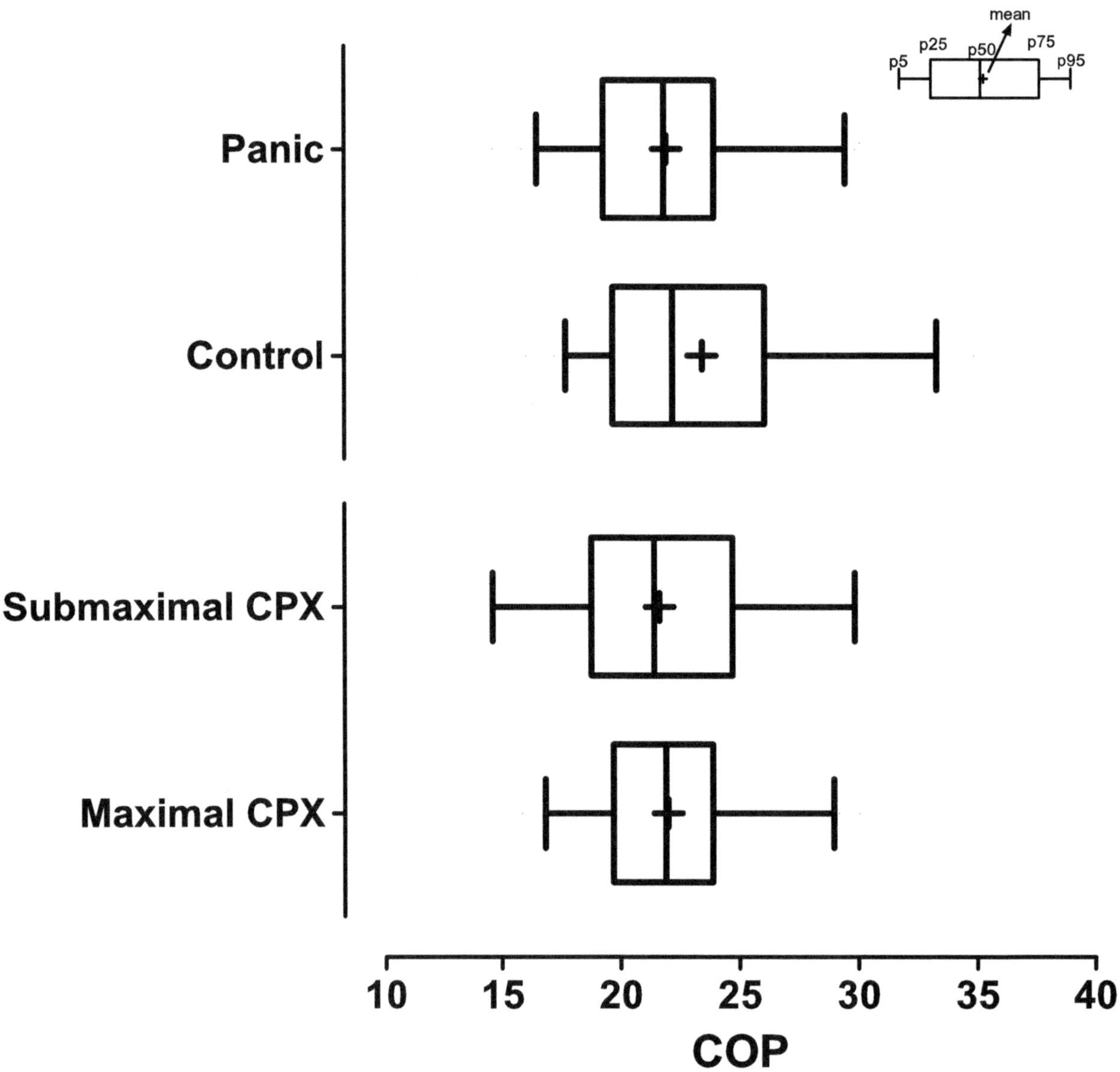

Figure 1. Comparison of COP for the control and PD groups and for the subgroups MAX and SUBMAX of patients with PD. * $p<0.05$.

reference center for referral of such patients. The present study has several relevant findings. First, it has a sample size considerably larger than other previous studies [13,14,28,29] in which the exercise response of PD patients was assessed. Additionally, the PD patients' results could be compared with those obtained in a set of healthy subjects with identical age and sex distribution, drawn randomly from a large database of the same laboratory.

Consistent with few existing studies of maximal exercise testing in PD patients [13,15,30], our data confirm that CPX is clinically safe in these patients and that the induction of PA seems to be very rare (no cases in the present study), occurring in less than 0.5% of cases, when all reported cases in the literature are combined [13,30]. Several studies have investigated respiratory symptoms in PD patients [2,31,32,33] and found that, during PA, respiratory complaints are common, such as dyspnea and tachypnea. Some specific respiratory tests aimed at inducing PA have been used, demonstrating that respiratory maneuvers, such as hyperventilation [34], carbon dioxide inhalation [35] and voluntary apnea [36], may increase anxiety in PD patients and thereby trigger a PA. In this regard, several studies have contributed to better understand the relationship between respiration and PA. In a recent review [31], it has been suggested that during hyperventilation, there are hypocapnia and vasoconstriction, with decreased cerebral blood flow, which may induces a PA. On the other hand, stimulation of chemoreceptors resulting from hypercapnia caused by CO_2 inhalation, may cause a hyperpnea that activates an abnormally sensitive fear network in the brainstem, and then also induce PA [31].

Exercise triggers physiological responses aimed to preserve homeostasis. In the respiratory system, there is increased VE mediated by a combination of hypercapnia, hypoxia, metabolic acidosis and afferent stimulation of joints and muscles [37,38], several of them may be directly involved in PA. Thus, it is possible that clinical characteristics of PD patients hinder the achievement of maximal CPX variables. In this sense, other studies subjecting PD patients to exercise testing showed lower HR max and aerobic

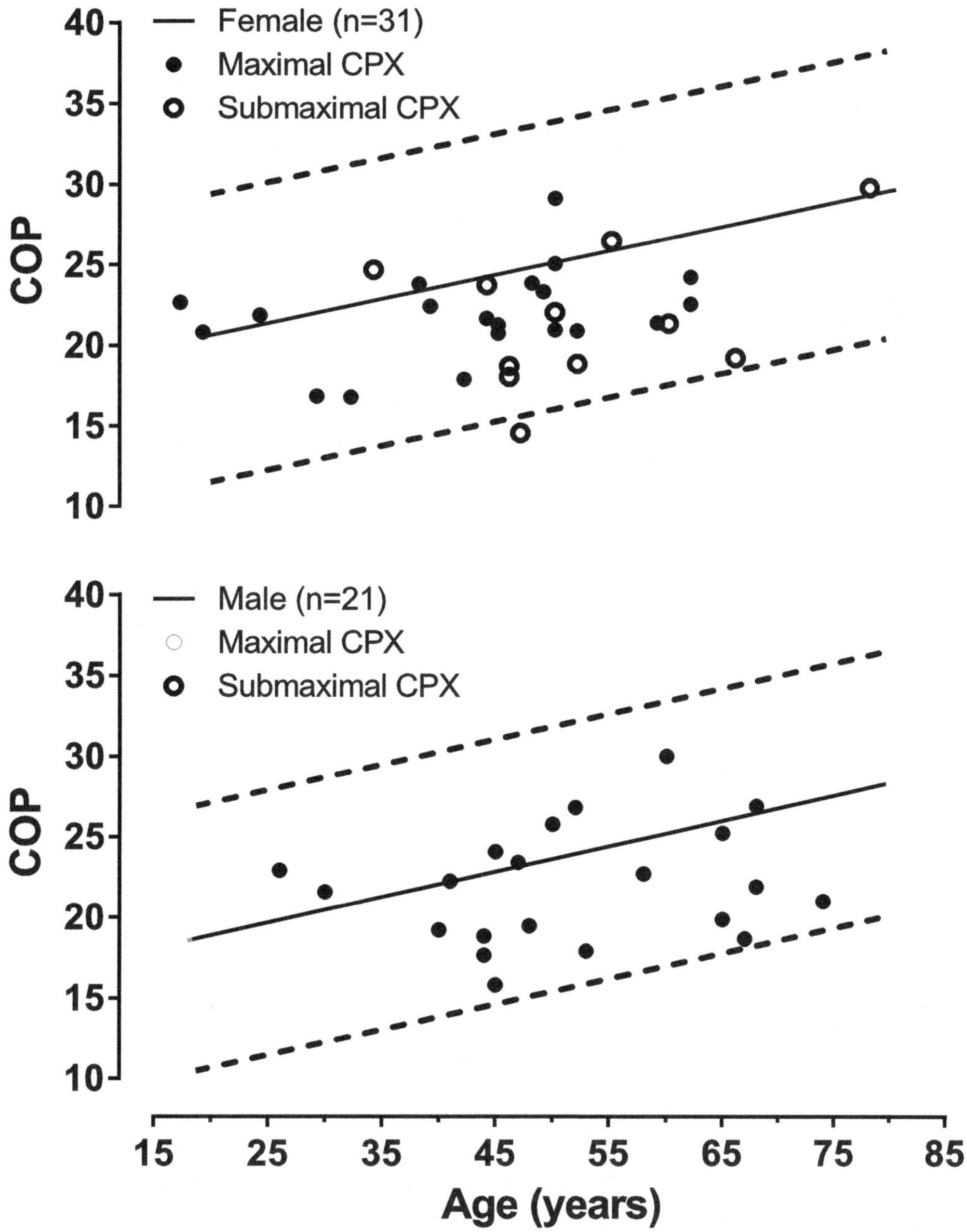

Figure 2. COP results for PD patients and maximal and submaximal CPET compared with the age and gender-predicted values.

fitness, and that this occurs, at least in part, by the difficulty in obtaining a truly maximal test [14].

PD patients commonly exhibit greater sensitivity to autonomic symptoms, which are potentially responsible for the phobic avoidance of situations that potentially trigger PA, such as intense exercise [29,39]. Since pre-exercise anxiety can lead to PAs, and some patients may require exercise discontinuation before reaching maximal effort, it could be difficult to determine the aerobic fitness of a PD patient. This issue can be further complicated during CPX when expired gases are collected. In fact, it has been previously reported [40] that breathing using a mouthpiece with occluded nose accompanied by the perception of increased HR can contribute to symptoms of discomfort, dyspnea, asphyxia and suffocation in PD patients. In the present study, approximately 20% of patients were unwilling to complete a truly maximal CPX, making submaximal cardiorespiratory data even more relevant. As previously stated, premature CPX interruption tends to do not affect COP determination, since COP occured at about 44% of VO_2 max and so, well before anaerobic threshold and maximal effort [18]. This is further corroborated by the fact that PDG and CG did not have different COP results, and there was no difference in COP when comparing between subgroups of PD patients (Figure 1).

When investigating COP behavior of PD patients (Figure 2) by using a regression equation [18], our results show that COP was about always (except in a single case), within the boundaries of estimate of error for healthy subjects. Therefore, it was observed that, from the point of view of cardiorespiratory integration, reflecting, at least partially, the quality of ventilation-perfusion ratio during exercise, PD patients exhibit no limitations and behave similarly to healthy subjects. Our data are in agreement with Caldirola et al. [13] who also observed that despite a high level of anxiety of PD patients at rest and a lower VO_2 followed by a higher HR during the exercise, treadmill ventilatory responses up to 65% of predicted HR max was similar between PD patients and healthy subjects.

In contrast, as already noted by other authors [13,14,28], VO_2 max tends to be lower in PD patients than in age and sex-matched healthy subjects. Nevertheless, when healthy subjects are compared with PD patients' subgroup who achieved maximal CPX, these differences disappeared. This lower aerobic fitness presented in many PD patients may be associated with the avoidance of potentially anxiogenic activities, leading to a reduction of exposure to exercise and outside activities that could somehow improve their aerobic fitness [13]. Nevertheless, it should be noted that regular exercise improves this condition, leading to levels similar to that of healthy subjects [14].

Another clinically relevant point is that in PDG SUBMAX, all patients were women. There are robust evidence of true sex differences in regards to the vulnerability and the psychopathology of panic. [41,42,43]. Few hypotheses have been advocated in recent decades to explain the etiology of these sex-related differences in the presentation of PD, including the progesterone receptor polymorphism [41], a lesser sensitivity of beta-adrenergic receptors [43] and distinct processes of fear conditioning [42]. In clinical terms, this greater female sensitivity to anxiety makes them to became highly responsive to the perception of autonomic symptoms as it occurs during a PA. This increased sensitivity also potentiates the panicogenic effects [16] and it has been previously associated with exercise avoidance in PD patients [13,39]. It is possible that this has contributed to explain why our female subjects prematurely stopped the CPX.

It should also be pointed that the present study has some limitations, such as the continued regular use of psychotropic drugs by PD patients. On the other hand, maintenance of the prescribed medication tends to increase the external validity of our results. Another potential limitation is the lack of a more detailed differentiation of the clinical condition of PD, as, for example, the classification of the PD patients in respiratory and non-respiratory subtypes, Nevertheless, a recent study [44] has found no significant differences in VO_2 max according to the subtype.

In conclusion, our study showed that cardiorespiratory interaction as assessed by COP – a submaximal variable obtained during CPX – was found to be within age- and sex-defined normal limits in PD patients, even of those unable to complete a truly maximal CPX. Additionally, it was confirmed that CPX is clinically safe, very unlikely to induce PA and is indicated for the assessment of cardiorespiratory symptoms of PD patients, even when a maximal CPX is not reached, being able to provide clinically relevant information and reassuring health professionals about the absence of a true physiological substrate for these often reported symptoms.

Author Contributions

Conceived and designed the experiments: PSR AS AEN CGSA. Performed the experiments: PSR AS AEN CGSA. Analyzed the data: PSR AS AEN CGSA. Contributed reagents/materials/analysis tools: PSR AS AEN CGSA. Contributed to the writing of the manuscript: PSR AS AEN CGSA.

References

1. von Leupoldt A, Taube K, Lehmann K, Fritzsche A, Magnussen H (2011) The impact of anxiety and depression on outcomes of pulmonary rehabilitation in patients with COPD. Chest 140: 730–736.
2. Sardinha A, Freire RC, Zin WA, Nardi AE (2009) Respiratory manifestations of panic disorder: causes, consequences and therapeutic implications. J Bras Pneumol 35: 698–708.
3. Perna G, Marconi C, Battaglia M, Bertani A, Panzacchi A, et al. (1994) Subclinical impairment of lung airways in patients with panic disorder. Biol Psychiatry 36: 601–605.
4. Kessler RC, Chiu WT, Jin R, Ruscio AM, Shear K, et al. (2006) The epidemiology of panic attacks, panic disorder, and agoraphobia in the National Comorbidity Survey Replication. Arch Gen Psychiatry 63: 415–424.
5. APA (2000) Diagnostic and Statistical Manual of Mental Disorders (DSM-IV). Washington, DC: APA.
6. Nardi AE, Lopes FL, Valenca AM, Nascimento I, Mezzasalma MA, et al. (2004) Psychopathological description of hyperventilation-induced panic attacks: a comparison with spontaneous panic attacks. Psychopathology 37: 29–35.
7. Freire RC, Lopes FL, Valenca AM, Nascimento I, Veras AB, et al. (2008) Panic disorder respiratory subtype: a comparison between responses to hyperventilation and CO2 challenge tests. Psychiatry Res 157: 307–310.
8. Nardi AE, Valenca AM, Lopes FL, Nascimento I, Veras AB, et al. (2006) Psychopathological profile of 35% CO2 challenge test-induced panic attacks: a comparison with spontaneous panic attacks. Compr Psychiatry 47: 209–214.
9. Klein DF (1993) False suffocation alarms, spontaneous panics, and related conditions. An integrative hypothesis. Arch Gen Psychiatry 50: 306–317.
10. Meneghelo RS, Araújo CGS, Stein R, Mastrocolla LE, Albuquerque PF, et al. (2010) Sociedade Brasileira de Cardiologia. III Diretrizes da Sociedade Brasileira de Cardiologia sobre Teste Ergométrico Arq Bras Cardiol 95: 1–26.
11. Myers J, Prakash M, Froelicher V, Do D, Partington S, et al. (2002) Exercise capacity and mortality among men referred for exercise testing. N Engl J Med 346: 793–801.
12. Zschucke E, Gaudlitz K, Strohle A (2013) Exercise and physical activity in mental disorders: clinical and experimental evidence. J Prev Med Public Health 46 Suppl 1: S12–21.
13. Caldirola D, Namia C, Micieli W, Carminati C, Bellodi L, et al. (2011) Cardiorespiratory response to physical exercise and psychological variables in panic disorder. Rev Bras Psiquiatr 33: 385–389.
14. Meyer T, Broocks A, Bandelow B, Hillmer-Vogel U, Ruther E (1998) Endurance training in panic patients: spiroergometric and clinical effects. Int J Sports Med 19: 496–502.
15. Taylor CB, King R, Ehlers A, Margraf J, Clark D, et al. (1987) Treadmill exercise test and ambulatory measures in panic attacks. Am J Cardiol 60: 48J–52J.
16. Telch MJ, Harrington PJ, Smits JA, Powers MB (2011) Unexpected arousal, anxiety sensitivity, and their interaction on CO(2)-induced panic: further evidence for the context-sensitivity vulnerability model. J Anxiety Disord 25: 645–653.
17. Sardinha AA, C G S; Nardi, A E (2011) Interval aerobic training as a tool in the cognitive behavioral treatment of panic disorder. J Bras Psiquiatr 60: 227–230.
18. Ramos PS, Ricardo DR, Araujo CG (2012) Cardiorespiratory optimal point: a submaximal variable of the cardiopulmonary exercise testing. Arq Bras Cardiol 99: 988–996.
19. Nathell L, Nathell M, Malmberg P, Larsson K (2007) COPD diagnosis related to different guidelines and spirometry techniques. Respir Res 8: 89.
20. Miller MR, Hankinson J, Brusasco V, Burgos F, Casaburi R, et al. (2005) Standardisation of spirometry. Eur Respir J 26: 319–338.
21. Campbell SC (1982) A comparison of the maximum voluntary ventilation with the forced expiratory volume in one second: an assessment of subject cooperation. J Occup Med 24: 531–533.
22. Araujo CG, Pinto VL (2005) Maximal heart rate in exercise tests on treadmill and in a cycloergometer of lower limbs. Arq Bras Cardiol 85: 45–50.
23. Araújo CGS (1983) Respostas cardiorespiratórias a um exercicio submáximo prolongado. Arq Bras Cardiol 41: 37–45.
24. Ramos PS, Araujo CG (2010) Normotensive individuals with exaggerated exercise blood pressure response have increased cardiac vagal tone. Arq Bras Cardiol 95: 85–90.
25. Ricardo DR, de Almeida MB, Franklin BA, Araujo CG (2005) Initial and final exercise heart rate transients: influence of gender, aerobic fitness, and clinical status. Chest 127: 318–327.
26. Ramos PS, Araújo CGS (2013) Analysis of the stability of a submaximal variable in the cardiopulmonary exercise testing: Cardiopulmonary optimal point. Rev Bras Ativ Fis Saúde 18: 585–593.
27. NIMH (1999) Facts About Panic Disorder.
28. Broocks A, Meyer TF, Bandelow B, George A, Bartmann U, et al. (1997) Exercise avoidance and impaired endurance capacity in patients with panic disorder. Neuropsychobiology 36: 182–187.
29. Sardinha A, Araujo CG, Soares-Filho GL, Nardi AE (2011) Anxiety, panic disorder and coronary artery disease: issues concerning physical exercise and cognitive behavioral therapy. Expert Rev Cardiovasc Ther 9: 165–175.

30. Martinsen EW, Raglin JS, Hoffart A, Friis S (1998) Tolerance to intensive exercise and high levels of lactate in panic disorder. J Anxiety Disord 12: 333–342.
31. Freire RC, Nardi AE (2012) Panic disorder and the respiratory system: clinical subtype and challenge tests. Rev Bras Psiquiatr 34 Suppl 1: S32–41.
32. Nardi AE, Freire RC, Zin WA (2009) Panic disorder and control of breathing. Respir Physiol Neurobiol 167: 133–143.
33. Nardi AE, Valenca AM, Nascimento I, Mezzasalma MA, Zin W (1999) Panic disorder and hyperventilation. Arq Neuropsiquiatr 57: 932–936.
34. Nardi AE, Valenca AM, Nascimento I, Zin WA (2001) Hyperventilation challenge test in panic disorder and depression with panic attacks. Psychiatry Res 105: 57–65.
35. Biber B, Alkin T (1999) Panic disorder subtypes: differential responses to CO2 challenge. Am J Psychiatry 156: 739–744.
36. Nardi AE, Nascimento I, Valenca AM, Lopes FL, Mezzasalma MA, et al. (2003) Panic disorder in a breath-holding challenge test: a simple tool for a better diagnosis. Arq Neuropsiquiatr 61: 718–722.
37. Bye PT, Farkas GA, Roussos C (1983) Respiratory factors limiting exercise. Annu Rev Physiol 45: 439–451.
38. Whipp BJ, Ward SA (1998) Determinants and control of breathing during muscular exercise. Br J Sports Med 32: 199–211.
39. Smits JA, Berry AC, Rosenfield D, Powers MB, Behar E, et al. (2008) Reducing anxiety sensitivity with exercise. Depress Anxiety 25: 689–699.
40. Antony MM, Ledley DR, Liss A, Swinson RP (2006) Responses to symptom induction exercises in panic disorder. Behav Res Ther 44: 85–98.
41. Ho HP, Westberg L, Annerbrink K, Olsson M, Melke J, et al. (2004) Association between a functional polymorphism in the progesterone receptor gene and panic disorder in women. Psychoneuroendocrinology 29: 1138–1141.
42. Kelly MM, Forsyth JP (2007) Sex differences in response to an observational fear conditioning procedure. Behav Ther 38: 340–349.
43. Kim YR, Min SK, Yu BH (2004) Differences in beta-adrenergic receptor sensitivity between women and men with panic disorder. Eur Neuropsychopharmacol 14: 515–520.
44. Muotri RW, Bernik MA (2014) Panic disorder and exercise avoidance. Rev Bras Psiquiatr 36: 68–75.

3

Impact of Walking on Glycemic Control and Other Cardiovascular Risk Factors in Type 2 Diabetes

Shanhu Qiu[1,2], Xue Cai[2], Uwe Schumann[1], Martina Velders[1], Zilin Sun[2]*, Jürgen Michael Steinacker[1]

1 Division of Sports and Rehabilitation Medicine, Department of Medicine II, Ulm University, Ulm, Germany, **2** Department of Endocrinology, Zhongda Hospital, Institute of Diabetes, Medical School, Southeast University, Nanjing, P. R. China

Abstract

Background: Walking is the most popular and most preferred exercise among type 2 diabetes patients, yet compelling evidence regarding its beneficial effects on cardiovascular risk factors is still lacking. The aim of this meta-analysis of randomized controlled trials (RCTs) was to evaluate the association between walking and glycemic control and other cardiovascular risk factors in type 2 diabetes patients.

Methods: Three databases were searched up to August 2014. English-language RCTs were eligible for inclusion if they had assessed the walking effects (duration ≥8 weeks) on glycemic control or other cardiovascular risk factors among type 2 diabetes patients. Data were pooled using a random-effects model. Subgroup analyses based on supervision status and meta-regression analyses of variables regarding characteristics of participants and walking were performed to investigate their association with glycemic control.

Results: Eighteen studies involving 20 RCTs (866 participants) were included. Walking significantly decreased glycosylated haemoglobin A1c (HbA1c) by 0.50% (95% confidence intervals [CI]: −0.78% to −0.21%). Supervised walking was associated with a pronounced decrease in HbA1c (WMD −0.58%, 95% CI: −0.93% to −0.23%), whereas non-supervised walking was not. Further subgroup analysis suggested non-supervised walking using motivational strategies is also effective in decreasing HbA1c (WMD −0.53%, 95% CI: −1.05% to −0.02%). Effects of covariates on HbA1c change were generally unclear. For other cardiovascular risk factors, walking significantly reduced body mass index (BMI) and lowered diastolic blood pressure (DBP), but non-significantly lowered systolic blood pressure (SBP), or changed high-density or low-density lipoprotein cholesterol levels.

Conclusions: This meta-analysis supports that walking decreases HbA1c among type 2 diabetes patients. Supervision or the use of motivational strategies should be suggested when prescribed walking to ensure optimal glycemic control. Walking also reduces BMI and lowers DBP, however, it remains insufficient regarding the association of walking with lowered SBP or improved lipoprotein profiles.

Trial Registration: PROSPERO CRD42014009515.

Editor: Lamberto Manzoli, University of Chieti, Italy

Funding: The authors have no funding or support to report.

Competing Interests: The authors have declared that no competing interests exist.

* Email: sunzilin1963@126.com

Background

Regular exercise is a key element in the management of type 2 diabetes [1–4]. Current guidelines and positions recommend that patients with type 2 diabetes should undertake moderate to vigorous aerobic exercise that includes running or bicycling to gain cardiovascular benefits [5,6]. However, most patients with type 2 diabetes are less likely to perform such high impact exercise because of their impaired tolerance of physical capacity [7,8] and somewhat hard feelings during the exercise.

Walking, as a typical low impact exercise, is the most popular and most preferred exercise among patients with type 2 diabetes [9,10]. It can be performed at a variety of speeds with different intensities [11], requires no specific skills or sophisticated preexercise evaluation [6], and has comparatively minimal adverse effects [12]. Although previous meta-analyses noted that walking could improve several known risk factors for cardiovascular disease such as blood pressure [13], body mass index (BMI) [14], and high-density lipoprotein cholesterol (HDL-C) [15], none of them had investigated the effects of walking on glycemic control, which is considered the mainstay of type 2 diabetes management.

Besides, it should keep in mind that those analyses were conducted mainly on sedentary but healthy adults, conclusions of which cannot be generalized to patients with type 2 diabetes, who are often more unwilling to exercise [16]. Moreover, there exists a large body of evidence that walking interventions can be very successfully implemented in patients with type 2 diabetes [17–34], but inconsistent results have been shown with regard to their beneficial effects on health outcomes, such as glycemic control [20,25,30,32], weight reduction [20,21], blood pressure [19,20] and lipoprotein profiles [19,22], questioning whether walking is the best medicine for diabetes [35].

Additionally, supervision is strongly recommended to optimize the exercise training effects on glycemic control [6,22]. Yet supervision is not always feasible in the primary-care exercise implementation due to the limited and unevenly distributed medical care resources [36]. Moreover, its necessity has been greatly challenged since several studies have pointed out that exercise such as walking in the free-living environment without supervision is also effective in improving glycemic control [18,20,23].

Therefore, the primary aim of this meta-analysis of randomized controlled trials (RCTs) was to examine the association of walking with glycemic control, and other cardiovascular risk factors including weight reduction, blood pressure, and lipoprotein profiles among patients with type 2 diabetes. The second aim was to evaluate whether supervised walking would lead to better improvement in glycemic control versus non-supervised walking among patients with type 2 diabetes.

Methods

Data sources and searches

The following databases were searched for primary articles: PubMed (from January 1, 1966 to August 8, 2014), the Cochrane Central Register of Controlled Trials (from January 1, 1966 to August 8, 2014) and Web of Science (from January 1, 1945 to August 8, 2014). The initial computer-based search strategies comprised common text words and Medical Subject Heading terms related to exercise, walking and type 2 diabetes, as well as entry terms associated with a highly sensitive search filter for RCTs. Searches were limited to human beings and the language was restricted to English. The reference lists of relevant systematic review/meta-analysis were hand-searched to find other potentially suitable studies. The complete search strategies are shown in Table S1. This meta-analysis is reported according to the Preferred Reporting Items for Systematic Reviews and Meta-Analyses (PRISMA) statement (Checklist S1), and adheres to a registered protocol (PROSPERO CRD42014009515; Table S2).

Study selection

Studies were eligible for inclusion if they fulfilled the following criteria: (i) enrolled participants diagnosed with type 2 diabetes; (ii) engaged in a structured walking programme; (iii) compared with a control group that received no walking training, but could maintain normal lifestyle or receive usual care; (iv) reported sufficient data to allow calculation of weighted mean difference (WMD) together with 95% confidence intervals (CIs) in the primary outcome – glycemic control as assessed by glycosylated haemoglobin A1c (HbA1c), or the secondary outcomes – weight reduction as indicated by BMI, blood pressure as measured by systolic blood pressure (SBP) or diastolic blood pressure (DBP), or lipoprotein profiles as determined by HDL-C or low-density lipoprotein cholesterol (LDL-C); (v) had a randomized, controlled design. Since the outcome of interest, HbA1c, reflects the average blood glucose concentration during the preceding 8–12 weeks, analyses were limited to studies in which the walking intervention lasted at least 8 weeks.

Studies were excluded if they (i) included participants diagnosed with pre-diabetes, gestational diabetes, or type 1 diabetes; (ii) had multiple exercise interventions that mixed/combined with other forms/modes of exercise, utilized interventions consisting only of recommending increased daily walking steps by motivational tools or lasting less than 8 weeks, or combined with dietary intervention; (iii) compared with the controls that received regular exercise training; (iv) reported only categorical data of outcomes; or (v) were non-randomized studies, posters or just abstracts. Studies that gave insufficient information regarding the forms of aerobic exercise interventions were also excluded if the related information could not be obtained from the corresponding authors.

Data extraction and quality assessment

Initial screen was based on titles or abstracts of retrieved publications; if they provided inadequate information with regard to inclusion or exclusion criteria, full-text articles were retrieved and evaluated. For each study, data regarding study sources (including author and publication year), characteristics of study population (including sample size, baseline mean age, BMI, sex [proportion of females] and duration of diabetes), characteristics of walking interventions (including frequency, intensity, time of each bout, length of intervention, and supervision status [that is, with or without]), outcomes (including at least one of the followings: HbA1c, BMI, DBP, SBP, HDL-C and LDL-C), adherence and dropout rates, were extracted.

The methodological quality of each eligible study was assessed using the Cochrane Collaboration's risk of bias tool [37], which includes random sequence generation, allocation concealment, blinding of participants and personnel, blinding of outcome assessment, incomplete outcome data and selective reporting. Risk of bias for each item was judged as low, unclear or high, based on the criteria in the Cochrane Handbook for Systematic Reviews [37].

Two authors (S.Q. and X.C.) independently performed the literature selection, data collection, and quality assessment. Discrepancies on the inclusion of studies or quality assessment were solved by consensus or discussion.

Data synthesis and analysis

For studies that reported standard error of mean, the standard deviation was obtained by multiplying by the square root of the corresponding sample size. For studies that compared 2 different walking interventions with a single control group, the "shared" group was split into 2 different groups with weighted smaller sample sizes in relation to different walking interventions. This was applied to give reasonably independent comparisons and to overcome a unit-of-analysis error [37]. For studies that gave outcomes at more than one time point during the intervention, data from the last time point were used for primary analyses.

Change scores from baseline or final values of each outcome variable were entered in the same meta-analysis, as suggested in the Cochrane Handbook for Systematic Reviews [37]. Data from intention-to-treat or per-protocol analyses were entered when available. The heterogeneity among studies was assessed using Cochran Q test, with a P value of $<.10$ being considered of statistical significance. The degree of inconsistency across studies due to heterogeneity was determined using I^2 statistic, where an I^2 value $\geq 50\%$ represented substantial heterogeneity. To account for between-study heterogeneity, the pooled-effect estimates expressed as WMD and the corresponding 95% CIs of each outcome were calculated using a random-effects model.

Subgroup analyses were performed to investigate the differences in outcome estimates across studies on the basis of supervision status. Univariate, weighted meta-regression analyses were conducted to determine whether the changes in outcome estimates were mediated by the characteristics of participants (baseline mean age [logarithmic transformation] BMI, sex and duration of diabetes) or walking interventions (length of intervention, frequency and volume [frequency × time of each bout]). The above analyses were conducted mainly on the primary outcome. Sensitivity analyses were used to assess the robustness of outcome estimates by removing each trial individually. Publication bias in the meta-analyses was detected and assessed by the Begg's test and Egger's test. Statistical analyses were performed using STATA Software (Version 12.0, College Station, Texas, USA).

Results

The flow diagram of literature search and study selection is shown in Figure 1. The initial search identified 2266 potentially suitable articles. One additional article was identified by analyzing the reference lists of relevant systematic review/meta-analysis papers searched. After careful screening and independent selection, 18 studies met all inclusion criteria. Among them, 2 studies had 2 different walking groups [20,34]; therefore, 20 trials were included in the final meta-analysis.

The detailed characteristics of these trials are summarized in Table 1. Of these 20 trials, a total of 866 participants were included, with sample sizes ranging from 16 to 149 in individual trials. All the participants were generally overweight or obese, with the baseline mean BMI ranging from 25.6 kg/m^2 to 32.7 kg/m^2. The walking structures varied among trials, with the length of interventions ranging from 8 weeks to 36 weeks. The time of each walking bout ranged from 20 minutes to 120 minutes, and the frequency differed from 3 times/week to 7 times/week, except 1 trial without indication [29]. The intensity of walking was moderate in general, except 3 trials without specification [18,19,27]. Eleven trials were conducted under supervision by qualified trainers, while among the remaining 9 trials that conducted without supervision, 5 of them had adopted strategies for promoting the training - that is, 1 had peer support [18] and the other 4 used step counters [20,23,32]. Three of the 20 trials were carried out in North America (U.S.) [18,21,30], 1 in South America (Brazil) [17], 11 in Asia (4 in South-Korea [24,26,32,33], 3 in India [23,27,31], 1 in Iran [28], 1 in Turkey [21] and 2 in Thailand [34]), 4 in Europe (3 in Denmark [19,20] and 1 in Italy [22]), and 1 in South Africa [25].

The risk of bias assessment for each trial is listed in Table S3. Among these 20 trials, 60% (12/20) reported adequate randomization sequence generation, 10% (2/20) provided proper allocation concealment, 75% (15/20) utilized proper methods in dealing with incomplete outcome data, and 100% (20/20) described losses to follow-up and exclusions. Because of the nature of walking intervention, none of the included trials had complete blinding of participants and personnel. Yet the outcome assessment for each trial is not likely to be influenced by lacking of blinding, given the outcome variables of interest were all measured in the standard approaches.

Only 9 of the 20 trials presented data on adherence to the walking intervention, with all the adherence rates more than 60%. Fifteen of the 20 trials reported dropout rates less than 10% (Table 1). No major adverse events related to walking, such as musculoskeletal injury or severe hypoglycemia, were reported; except 3 trials that reported mild hypoglycemia [19,22,31].

Primary outcome

Effect on glycemic control. Sixteen trials involving 724 participants were included in the meta-analysis. Compared with the non-walking control, the pooled estimate showed a significant decrease in HbA1c (WMD −0.50%, 95% CI: −0.78% to −0.21%; Figure 2), but with a substantial heterogeneity between trials ($P<.001$, $I^2=79.4\%$). Subgroup analyses showed supervised walking was associated with a significant decrease in HbA1c by 0.58% (9 trials, 391 participants; 95% CI: −0.93% to −0.23%), while the association between non-supervised walking and decreased HbA1c became statistically non-significant (7 trials, 333 participants; WMD −0.37%, 95% CI: −0.90% to 0.15%). Yet further subgroup analysis suggested that non-supervised walking with the use of motivational strategies was associated with a significant decrease in HbA1c (5 trials, 164 participants; WMD −0.53%, 95% CI: −1.05% to −0.02%), which made no difference from the supervised walking ($P=.88$). Univariate meta-regression analyses suggested that none of the covariates was the potential modifier of HbA1c change: baseline age (β coefficient, −0.90, $P=.62$), BMI (0.05, $P=.33$), sex (0.008, $P=.14$), duration of diabetes (−0.001, $P=.98$), walking frequency (0.16, $P=.16$), length of walking intervention (0.007, $P=.71$), or walking volume (0.001, $P=.23$). When individually removing each trial, pooled results were largely unchanged.

Secondary outcomes

Effect on weight reduction. Sixteen trials involving 649 participants compared walking with the controls. The overall, pooled data showed that walking was associated with a significant reduction in BMI by 0.91 kg/m^2 (95% CI: −1.22 to −0.59 kg/m^2; Table 2). Heterogeneity among trials was negligible ($P=.54$, $I^2<1\%$). When trials were individually removed, pooled results remained largely unchanged.

Effect on blood pressure. The overall, pooled estimates of trials reporting SBP (11 trials, 497 participants) showed a non-significant decrease in SBP among participants randomized to walking groups when compared with the controls (WMD −1.69 mmHg, 95% CI: −5.22 to 1.85 mmHg; P for heterogeneity = .001, $I^2=65.2\%$; Table 2). The pooled estimates of trials reporting DBP (12 trials, 509 participants) showed a bigger reduction in DBP among participants randomized to walking groups than those randomized to non-walking groups (WMD −1.97 mmHg, 95% CI: −3.94 to −0.00 mmHg; P for heterogeneity = .005; $I^2=59.3\%$; Table 2). Upon removal of trials individually from each meta-analysis, the overall WMD for DBP remained largely unchanged, while the WMD for SBP was changed to −3.20 mmHg (95% CI −5.35 to −1.05 mmHg) by removing the study by Gram *et al.* [19], a 16-week nordic walking intervention, which reported a larger increase in SBP (WMD 5.00 mmHg, 95% CI 2.67 to 7.33 mmHg) than any other trials.

Effect on lipoprotein profiles. Nine trials with 290 participants reported changes in HDL-C levels, and 8 trials with 270 participants reported changes in LDL-C levels. Walking training did not significantly increase the HDL-C levels (WMD 0.02 mmol/L, 95% CI: −0.06 to 0.10 mmol/L; P for heterogeneity = .03, $I^2=53.2\%$; Table 2) or change the LDL-C levels (WMD 0.04 mmol/L, 95% CI: −0.07 to 0.16 mmol/L; P for heterogeneity = .38, $I^2=7.0\%$; Table 2) among intervention participants. When trials were individually removed from each meta-analysis, pooled results regarding HDL-C or LDL-C were largely unchanged.

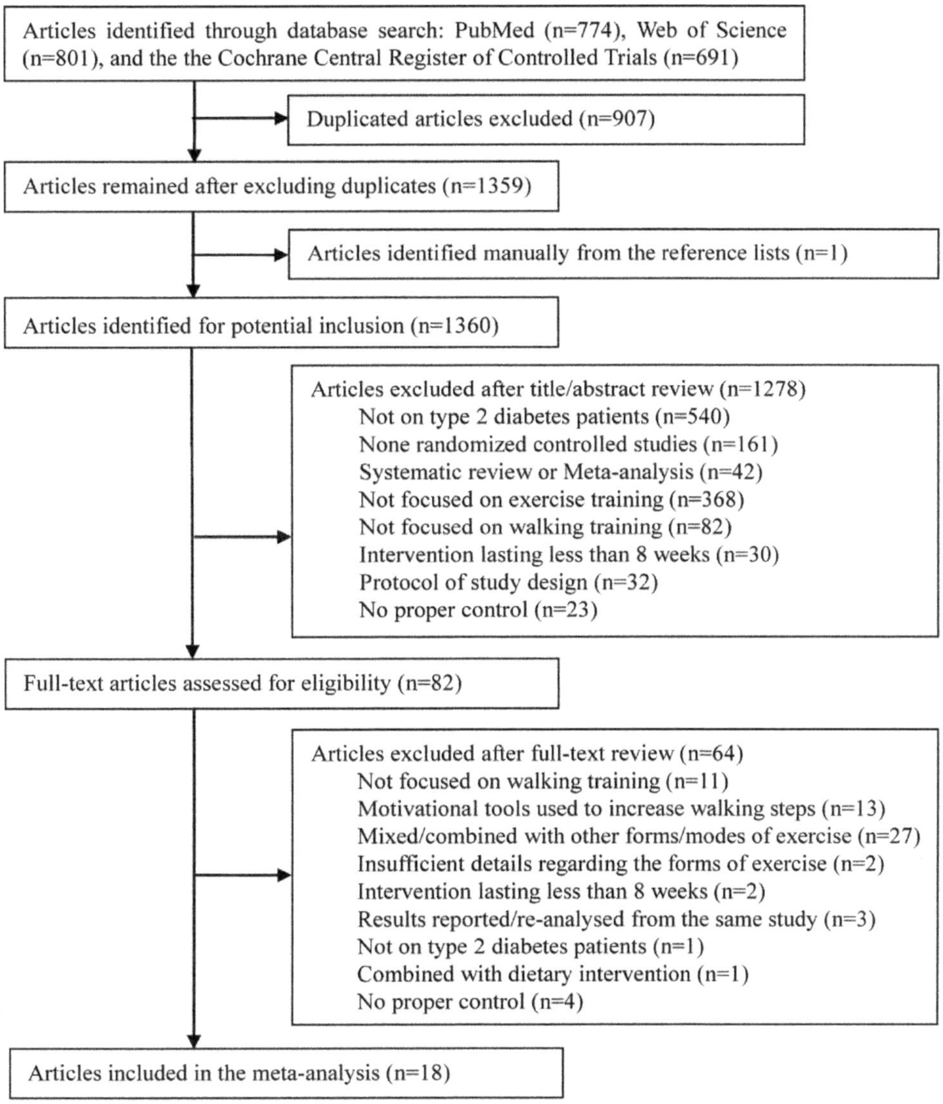

Figure 1. Flow diagram of search and selection processes.

Publication bias

There was no significant publication bias for all of the primary and secondary outcomes as evidenced by the Begg's test and Egger's test (all $P>.05$), except LDL-C (Egger's test, $P = .04$).

Discussion

The results of this meta-analysis suggest that in patients with type 2 diabetes, walking is associated with a significant decrease in HbA1c. The results further suggest that supervision is essential to walking training in decreasing HbA1c; while notably, the use of motivational strategies is also effective in decreasing HbA1c when performing non-supervised walking. The results also suggest that walking is associated with a reduced BMI and a lowered DBP. However, it shows inadequate evidence regarding the effects of walking in lowering SBP or altering lipoprotein levels in this meta-analysis.

Partly in line with our main results, a recent meta-analysis by Chudyk and Petrella [38] and another one by Snowling and Hopkins [39] demonstrated that aerobic exercise was associated with improved glycemic control in patients with type 2 diabetes. Yet it is worth noting that these meta-analyses included not only walking, but also other forms of aerobic exercise, such as bicycling or running. This could be prone to confounding when considering the possibility that physiological adaptations to exercise are specific to the stimulus applied [40], along with different physiological properties [41]. Since results from this meta-regression analysis did not find any modifier for HbA1c change, and given the common characteristics of the most trials, it is suggested to prescribe walking at a moderate intensity, 3–5 times/week, 120–150 minutes/week, for patients with type 2 diabetes to gain benefits on glycemic control.

Periodic supervision by qualified exercise trainers is recommended for patients with type 2 diabetes to ensure optimal glycemic control and to minimize injury risk when they undertake exercise training [6]. This recommendation has been further supported by a recently well-conducted meta-analysis [42], which noted that supervised exercise training was associated with a great decline in HbA1c level by 0.73% (95% CI: −1.06% to −0.40%). The observation from that meta-analysis is comparable to the

Table 1. Characteristics of included randomized controlled trials.

Source	Age, year[#]	No. of subjects	Intervention and control description[§]	Duration[$], weeks	Status of supervision	Adherence, %	Dropouts, %
Belli *et al.* 2011 [17]	53.4 (2.3)	9	Intervention: I: individual ventilatory threshold; F: 3 times/week; T: progressed from 20 minutes at week 1 to 60 minutes at week 5, and then maintained	12	With	92	25
	55.9 (2.2)	10	Control: continued normal lives without systematic exercise				16.7
Goldhaber-Fiebert *et al.* 2003 [18]	60 (10)	33	Intervention: I: not stated; F: 3 times/week; T: 60 minutes	12	Without	Not stated	17.5
	57 (9)	28	Control: continued normal lives without systematic exercise				20
Gram *et al.* 2010 [19]	62 (10)	22	Intervention: I: >40% of VO_{2max}; F: 3 times/week; T: at least 30 minutes	16	With	63.5	4.5
	61 (10)	22	Control: continued habitual lifestyle and advised to exercise				0
Karstoft *et al.* 2013a[*] [20]	60.8 (2.2)	12	Intervention: I: 55% of peak energy-expenditure rate; F: 5 times/week; T: 60 minutes (in total)	16	Without	89	8.3
	57.1 (3.0)	4	Control: continued habitual lifestyle				0
Karstoft *et al.* 2013b[*] [20]	57.5 (2.4)	12	Intervention: I: 70% of peak energy-expenditure rate; F: 5 times/week; T: 60 minutes (in total)	16	Without	89	8.3
	57.1 (3.0)	4	Control: continued habitual lifestyle				0
Kurban *et al.* 2011 [21]	53.77 (8.2)	30	Intervention: I: moderate; F: 3 times/week; T: 30 minutes	12	With	Not stated	0
	53.57 (6.6)	30	Control: continued habitual lifestyle				0
Negri *et al.* 2010 [22]	65.7 (4.9)	21	Intervention: I: increased gradually from low to moderate; F: 3 times/week; T: 45 minutes	16	With	60	20.5
	65.7 (5.2)	20	Control: continued habitual lifestyle and encouraged to exercise				4.8
Shenoy *et al.* 2010 [23]	53.15 (4.4)	20	Intervention: I: 50–70% of maximum heart rate; F: 5 times/week; T: 150 minutes/week (in total)	8	Without	Not stated	0
	51 (5.4)	20	Control: received no training				0
Sung *et al.* 2012 [24]	70.2 (4.7)	22	Intervention: I: 55–75% of maximum heart rate; F: 3 times/week; T: 30 minutes (1–4 weeks), 35 minutes (5–14 weeks) and 40 minutes (15–24 weeks)	24	With	Not stated	4.8 (in total)
	70.1 (3.6)	18	Control: received usual care				
van Rooijen *et al.* 2004 [25]	54	75	Intervention: I: moderate (12–14 PRE); F: ≥5 times/week; T: progressed from 10 to 45 minutes	12	Without	Not stated	6.3
	55	74	Control: received usual care without exercise				3.9
Ku *et al.* 2010 [26]	55.7 (7.0)	15	Intervention: I: moderate (3.6–5.2 METs); F: 5 times/week; T: 60 minutes	12	With	Not stated	0
	57.8 (8.1)	16	Control: continued habitual lifestyle				0
Arora *et al.* 2009 [27]	52.2 (9.3)	10	Intervention: I: not stated; F: 3 times/week; T: 30 minutes	8	Without	Not stated	0
	58.4 (1.8)	10	Control: continued habitual lifestyle				0

Table 1. Cont.

Source	Age, year#	No. of subjects	Intervention and control description§	Duration$, weeks	Status of supervision	Adherence, %	Dropouts, %
Moghadasi *et al.* 2013 [28]	43 (overall)	8	Intervention: I: 40–59% of VO_{2max}; F: 4 times/week; T: 30 minutes (for 2 miles)	12	With	Not stated	0
		8	Control: continued habitual lifestyle				0
Kaplan *et al.* 1985 [29]	54 (overall)	18	Intervention: I: 60–70% of maximal work capacity; F: not stated; T: progressed to 40–60 minutes	10	Without	Not stated	7.4 (in total)
		15	Control: received usual care				
Church *et al.* 2010 [30]	53.7 (9.1)	72	Intervention: I: about 65% of VO_{2max}; F: 3 times/week; T: 140 minutes/week (in total)	36	With	>70, for the most	4.2
	58.6 (8.2)	41	Control: continued normal lives without systematic exercise				9.7
Dixit *et al.* 2014 [31]	54.4 (1.2)	29	Intervention: I: 12–13 PRE; F: ≥3 times/week; T: ≥150 minutes/week (in total)	8	With	Not stated	27.5
	59.5 (1.2)	37	Control: received usual care				21.3
Koo *et al.* 2010 [32]	59 (4)	13	Intervention: I: moderate-to-vigorous; F: 7 times/week; T: 120 minutes	12	Without	≥80	0
	57 (8)	18	Control: received usual care				0
Kwon *et al.* 2010 [33]	55.5 (7.5)	13	Intervention: I: anaerobic threshold (moderate intensity); F: 5 times/week; T: 60 minutes	12	Without	Not stated	15.6 (in total)
	57.5 (8.6)	14	Control: continued normal lives				
Mitranun *et al.* 2014a** [34]	61.7 (2.7)	14	Intervention: I: 60–65% of VO2peak; F: 3 times/week; T: 30 minutes	12	With	≥80	6.7
	60.9 (2.4)	7	Control: continued sedentary lives				0
Mitranun *et al.* 2014b** [34]	61.2 (2.8)	14	Intervention: I: 50–80% of VO2peak; F: 3 times/week; T: 20–30 minutes	12	With	≥80	6.7
	60.9 (2.4)	8	Control: continued sedentary lives				0

I: intensity; F: frequency; T: time of each walking bout; PRE; perceived rate of exertion; VO_{2max}, maximal oxygen consumption; METs, metabolic equivalents.
#Age was represented as mean (SD), or mean if SD was not provided, or imputed with a mean.
§Characteristics of walking training described did not include warm-up or cool-down periods unless indicated.
$Duration meant length of walking intervention in this meta-analysis.
*The same study which included 2 different walking groups: "a" was a continuous walking training group; "b" was an energy expenditure–matched interval-walking training group.
**The same study which included 2 different walking groups: "a" was a continuous walking training group; "b" was a total oxygen consumption-matched interval-walking training group.

Source	Number of participants: Walking	Control	WMD (95% CI) [%]	Weight, %
Supervised walking				
Belli *et al.* 2011	9	10	-1.30 (-2.72, 0.12)	2.94
Gram *et al.* 2010	22	22	-1.00 (-1.15, -0.85)	10.57
Kurban *et al.* 2011	30	30	-0.29 (-0.82, 0.24)	7.94
Negri *et al.* 2010	21	20	-0.11 (-0.47, 0.25)	9.28
Sung *et al.* 2012	22	18	-0.95 (-1.71, -0.19)	6.11
Ku *et al.* 2010	15	16	-0.50 (-1.17, 0.17)	6.75
Church *et al.* 2010	72	41	-0.31 (-0.56, -0.06)	10.04
Mitranun *et al.* 2014a	14	7	-0.60 (-2.09, 0.89)	2.74
Mitranun *et al.* 2014b	14	8	-1.00 (-2.33, 0.33)	3.21
Subtotal estimates (*P* = .001)			-0.58 (-0.93, -0.23)	59.58
Non-supervised walking				
Goldhaber-Fiebert *et al.* 2003	33	28	-1.40 (-2.56, -0.24)	3.87
Karstoft *et al.* 2013a	12	4	-0.20 (-1.22, 0.82)	4.54
Karstoft *et al.* 2013b	12	4	0.00 (-1.02, 1.02)	4.54
Shenoy *et al.* 2010	20	20	-1.00 (-1.55, -0.45)	7.75
van Rooijen *et al.* 2004	75	74	0.73 (-0.01, 1.47)	6.28
Arora *et al.* 2009	10	10	-0.75 (-1.54, 0.04)	5.93
Koo *et al.* 2010	13	18	-0.13 (-0.71, 0.45)	7.51
Subtotal estimates (*P* = .17)			-0.37 (-0.90, 0.15)	40.42
Overall estimates (*P* = .001)			-0.50 (-0.78, -0.21)	100.00

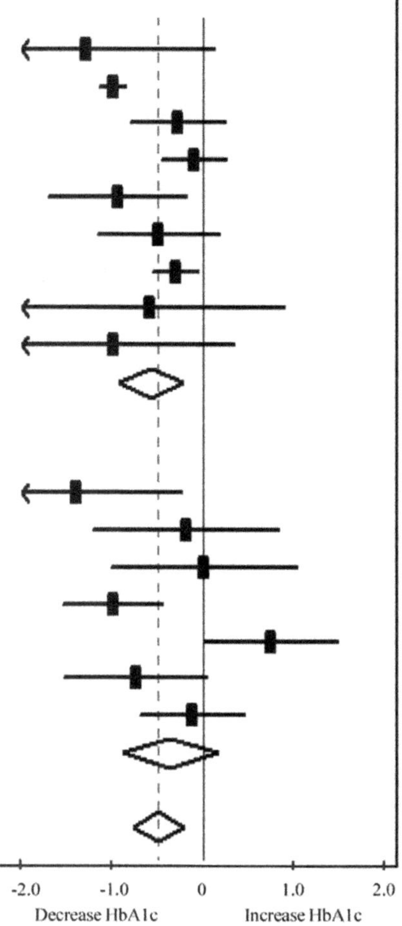

Figure 2. Forest plot of RCTs examining walking effects on HbA1c (%) in type 2 diabetes patients. RCTs, randomized controlled trials; HbA1c, glycosylated haemoglobin A1c; WMD, weighted mean difference; CI, confidence interval Summary estimates were analyzed with a random-effects model. HbA1c levels were converted from mmol/mol to % using the NGSP converter (available at http://www.ngsp.org/convert1.asp).

Table 2. Effects of walking training on secondary outcomes.

Outcome	No. of studies (No. of subjects)	Effect size[#]		Heterogeneity	
		WMD (95% CI)	***P* value**	**I^2 (%)**	***P* value**
Weight reduction					
BMI, kg/m^2	16 (649)	−0.91 (−1.22 to −0.59)	<.001	<1	=.54
Blood pressure, mmHg					
Systolic[§]	11 (497)	−1.69 (−5.22 to 1.85)	=.34	65.2	=.001
Diastolic	12 (509)	−1.97 (−3.94 to −0.0)	=.05	59.3	=.005
Lipoprotein, mmol/L					
HDL-C	9 (290)	0.02 (−0.06 to 0.10)	=.64	53.2	=.03
LDL-C	8 (270)	0.04 (−0.07 to 0.16)	=.49	7.0	=.38

WMD, weight mean difference; CI, confidence interval; BMI, body mass index; HDL-C, high-density lipoprotein cholesterol; LDL-C, low-density lipoprotein cholesterol. SI conversion factors: to convert HDL-C and LDL-C from mg/dl to mmol/L, multiply by 0.0259.

[#]Effect size was calculated using a random-effects model.

[§]The study of Karftoft *et al.* 2013a [20] was excluded because the baseline data of systolic blood pressure were not comparable between the intervention and control groups.

results from our subgroup analyses, where a decrease in HbA1c by 0.58% (95% CI: −0.93% to −0.23%) was found. However, it should be acknowledged that full supervision by a qualified exercise trainer may not always be feasible for a considerable amount of patients with type 2 diabetes, given the high prevalence of type 2 diabetes [43] and the limited medical resources [36]. Despite that non-supervised walking was associated with a non-significant decrease in HbA1c, evidence from our further subgroup analyses suggested that even without supervision, walking with the use of motivational strategies would be helpful in reducing HbA1c, in which the magnitude of HbA1c reduction was comparable to that of supervised walking ($P = .88$). The motivational strategies utilized in this meta-analysis included peer support and the use of step counters, both of which have been proved to be effective in increasing daily movement (unstructured activity) [44,45] and improving the training adherence or self-efficacy [44,46]. It is likely that these related factors have contributed to the observed decrease in HbA1c, at least partly.

In addition to glycemic control, the meta-analysis showed that walking was associated with a significant reduction in BMI when compared with the non-walking controls. This result is consistent with the finding from Kelley *et al.*, who reported a similar reduction in BMI from walking [15]. Since most patients with type 2 diabetes are overweight or obese, it therefore sounds reasonable to initially recommend walking to those patients to reduce body weight.

Snowling and Hopkins observed that aerobic exercise had minor effects in lowering SBP or DBP among patients with type 2 diabetes [39], although possibilities cannot be completely excluded that the overall effects would be masked by the different forms of aerobic exercise in that meta-analysis. In another meta-analysis, Kelley *et al.* noted that walking significantly reduced both SBP and DBP [13], yet this study enrolled sedentary adults other than patients with type 2 diabetes. Our meta-analysis showed that walking significantly lowered DBP but not SBP among patients with type 2 diabetes. In support of this, Murphy *et al.* showed that walking slightly reduced DBP but only had a tendency to lower SBP [14]. To some extent, this finding on DBP will help to prescribe walking to those type 2 diabetes patients who are especially vulnerable to elevated blood pressure [47]. This finding also provides evidence against the statement from the current guideline that reductions in DBP from aerobic exercise training are less common in patients with type 2 diabetes [6]. Our meta-analysis did not show a statistical support for the positive relationship between walking and increased HDL-C levels as well as decreased LDL-C levels among patients with type 2 diabetes. Partly in agreement with this, Kelley *et al.* found a non-significant increase in HDL-C associated with walking [15]. One possible explanation for this might be that all included trials had utilized walking training alone without weight reduction interventions, while the combination of both is more effective on lipids regulation [6,48].

This meta-analysis has several strengths. First, it is to date the most comprehensive analysis that systematically and quantitatively assesses the beneficial effects of a particular form of aerobic exercise – walking, on glycemic control and several other cardiovascular risk factors among patients with type 2 diabetes. Second, it enriches the knowledge for prescribing walking to patients with type 2 diabetes, aiming to optimise glycemic control, weight reduction or DBP. Third, it was registered a priori (PROSPERO CRD42014009515) that minimised the selection and recall bias, and utilised strict inclusion and exclusion criteria.

This meta-analysis also has several limitations. First, as with any meta-analysis, the internal validity depends on the methodological quality of the included trials. Although all trials were judged with low risk of detection bias and described losses to follow-up, insufficient reporting of the randomization sequence generation and improper dealing with incomplete outcome data addressed in some of the trials reviewed would increase the risk of selection bias and attribution bias. It is recommended that future RCTs should describe adequate information about randomization and report data with guidelines. Second, despite no significant publication bias was detected by the Begg's test and Egger's test for each outcome variable except LDL-C, the risk of publication bias still cannot be fully ruled out due to the language restriction to English, the selection of only published papers, as well as the potentially underpowered statistical tests. Third, substantial heterogeneity of HbA1c was identified among the included trials, and it cannot be explained by a single related variable in the meta-regression analyses. Fourth, while our subgroup analyses showed that supervised walking was superior to non-supervised walking in decreasing HbA1c, it should be noted that these comparisons were indirect and somewhat less reliable when compared with the head-to-head trials. Therefore, future research with a head-to-head design is needed on this topic. Finally, because of the short-term walking intervention (only up to 6 months) reported in all the included trials except one with a 9-month intervention [30], results of this meta-analysis largely represent the short-term effects of walking intervention among patients with type 2 diabetes. Future RCTs that extend length of walking intervention are required.

Conclusions

In conclusion, the meta-analysis shows that walking is associated with a decreased HbA1c among patients with type 2 diabetes. Supervision or the use of motivational strategies should be strongly recommended when prescribed walking to ensure optimal glycemic control. Walking is also effective in reducing BMI and lowering DBP, while evidence regarding its association with lowered SBP or improved lipoprotein profiles remains insufficient. Future RCTs with head-to-head designs comparing supervised walking versus non-supervised walking, and with extended length of walking interventions (>6 months), are required to strengthen the findings in this meta-analysis.

Supporting Information

Table S1 Search strategies.

Table S2 PROSPERO CRD42014009515.

Table S3 Bias assessment of each randomized controlled trial.

Checklist S1 PRISMA Checklist.

Author Contributions

Conceived and designed the experiments: SQ XC ZS JS. Performed the experiments: SQ ZS JS. Analyzed the data: SQ XC. Contributed reagents/materials/analysis tools: SQ XC US MV. Contributed to the writing of the manuscript: SQ XC US MV ZS JS.

References

1. Schellenberg ES, Dryden DM, Vandermeer B, Ha C, Korownyk C (2013) Lifestyle interventions for patients with and at risk for type 2 diabetes: a systematic review and meta-analysis. Ann Intern Med 159: 543–551.
2. Gregg EW, Gerzoff RB, Caspersen CJ, Williamson DF, Narayan KM (2003) Relationship of walking to mortality among US adults with diabetes. Arch Intern Med 163: 1440–1447.
3. Makura CB, Nirantharakumar K, Girling AJ, Saravanan P, Narendran P (2013) Effects of physical activity on the development and progression of microvascular complications in type 1 diabetes: retrospective analysis of the DCCT study. BMC Endocr Disord 13: 37.
4. Sigal RJ, Kenny GP, Boule NG, Wells GA, Prud'homme D, et al. (2007) Effects of aerobic training, resistance training, or both on glycemic control in type 2 diabetes: a randomized trial. Ann Intern Med 147: 357–369.
5. American Diabetes Association (2014) Standards of medical care in diabetes–2014. Diabetes Care 37 Suppl 1: S14–80.
6. Colberg SR, Sigal RJ, Fernhall B, Regensteiner JG, Blissmer BJ, et al. (2010) Exercise and type 2 diabetes: the American College of Sports Medicine and the American Diabetes Association: joint position statement. Diabetes Care 33: e147–167.
7. Gusso S, Hofman P, Lalande S, Cutfield W, Robinson E, et al. (2008) Impaired stroke volume and aerobic capacity in female adolescents with type 1 and type 2 diabetes mellitus. Diabetologia 51: 1317–1320.
8. Weinstock RS, Brooks G, Palmas W, Morin PC, Teresi JA, et al. (2011) Lessened decline in physical activity and impairment of older adults with diabetes with telemedicine and pedometer use: results from the IDEATel study. Age Ageing 40: 98–105.
9. Ford ES, Herman WH (1995) Leisure-time physical activity patterns in the U.S. diabetic population. Findings from the 1990 National Health Interview Survey-Health Promotion and Disease Prevention Supplement. Diabetes Care 18: 27–33.
10. Thomas N, Alder E, Leese GP (2004) Barriers to physical activity in patients with diabetes. Postgrad Med J 80: 287–291.
11. Murtagh EM, Boreham CA, Murphy MH (2002) Speed and exercise intensity of recreational walkers. Prev Med 35: 397–400.
12. Hootman JM, Macera CA, Ainsworth BE, Martin M, Addy CL, et al. (2001) Association among physical activity level, cardiorespiratory fitness, and risk of musculoskeletal injury. Am J Epidemiol 154: 251–258.
13. Kelley GA, Kelley KS, Tran ZV (2001) Walking and resting blood pressure in adults: a meta-analysis. Prev Med 33: 120–127.
14. Murphy MH, Nevill AM, Murtagh EM, Holder RL (2007) The effect of walking on fitness, fatness and resting blood pressure: a meta-analysis of randomised, controlled trials. Prev Med 44: 377–385.
15. Kelley GA, Kelley KS, Tran ZV (2005) Walking and Non-HDL-C in adults: a meta-analysis of randomized controlled trials. Prev Cardiol 8: 102–107.
16. Morrato EH, Hill JO, Wyatt HR, Ghushchyan V, Sullivan PW (2007) Physical activity in U.S. adults with diabetes and at risk for developing diabetes, 2003. Diabetes Care 30: 203–209.
17. Belli T, Ribeiro LFP, Ackermann MA, Baldissera V, Gobatto CA, et al. (2011) Effects of 12-week overground walking training at ventilatory threshold velocity in type 2 diabetic women. Diabetes Res Clin Pract 93: 337–343.
18. Goldhaber-Fiebert JD, Goldhaber-Fiebert SN, Tristan ML, Nathan DM (2003) Randomized controlled community-based nutrition and exercise intervention improves glycemia and cardiovascular risk factors in type 2 diabetic patients in rural Costa Rica. Diabetes Care 26: 24–29.
19. Gram B, Christensen R, Christiansen C, Gram J (2010) Effects of nordic walking and exercise in type 2 diabetes mellitus: a randomized controlled trial. Clin J Sport Med 20: 355–361.
20. Karstoft K, Winding K, Knudsen SH, Nielsen JS, Thomsen C, et al. (2013) The effects of free-living interval-walking training on glycemic control, body composition, and physical fitness in type 2 diabetic patients: a randomized, controlled trial. Diabetes Care 36: 228–236.
21. Kurban S, Mehmetoglu I, Yerlikaya HF, Gonen S, Erdem S (2011) Effect of chronic regular exercise on serum ischemia-modified albumin levels and oxidative stress in type 2 diabetes mellitus. Endocr Res 36: 116–123.
22. Negri C, Bacchi E, Morgante S, Soave D, Marques A, et al. (2010) Supervised walking groups to increase physical activity in type 2 diabetic patients. Diabetes Care 33: 2333–2335.
23. Shenoy S, Guglani R, Sandhu JS (2010) Effectiveness of an aerobic walking program using heart rate monitor and pedometer on the parameters of diabetes control in Asian Indians with type 2 diabetes. Prim Care Diabetes 4: 41–45.
24. Sung K, Bae S (2012) Effects of a regular walking exercise program on behavioral and biochemical aspects in elderly people with type II diabetes. Nurs Health Sci 14: 438–445.
25. van Rooijen AJ, Rheeder P, Eales CJ, Becker PJ (2004) Effect of exercise versus relaxation on haemoglobin A(1C) in Black females with type 2 diabetes mellitus. QJM 97: 343–351.
26. Ku YH, Han KA, Ahn H, Kwon H, Koo BK, et al. (2010) Resistance exercise did not alter intramuscular adipose tissue but reduced retinol-binding protein-4 concentration in individuals with type 2 diabetes mellitus. J Int Med Res 38: 782–791.
27. Arora E, Shenoy S, Sandhu JS (2009) Effects of resistance training on metabolic profile of adults with type 2 diabetes. Indian J Med Res 129: 515–519.
28. Moghadasi M, Mohebbi H, Rahmani-Nia F, Hassan-Nia S, Noroozi H (2013) Effects of short-term lifestyle activity modification on adiponectin mRNA expression and plasma concentrations. Eur J Sport Sci 13: 378–385.
29. Kaplan RM, Wilson DK, Hartwell SL, Merino KL, Wallace JP (1985) Prospective evaluation of HDL cholesterol changes after diet and physical conditioning programs for patients with type II diabetes mellitus. Diabetes Care 8: 343–348.
30. Church TS, Blair SN, Cocreham S, Johannsen N, Johnson W, et al. (2010) Effects of aerobic and resistance training on hemoglobin A1c levels in patients with type 2 diabetes: a randomized controlled trial. JAMA 304: 2253–2262.
31. Dixit S, Maiya AG, Shastry BA (2014) Effect of aerobic exercise on peripheral nerve functions of population with diabetic peripheral neuropathy in type 2 diabetes: a single blind, parallel group randomized controlled trial. J Diabetes Complications 28: 332–339.
32. Koo BK, Han KA, Ahn HJ, Jung JY, Kim HC, et al. (2010) The effects of total energy expenditure from all levels of physical activity vs. physical activity energy expenditure from moderate-to-vigorous activity on visceral fat and insulin sensitivity in obese Type 2 diabetic women. Diabet Med 27: 1088–1092.
33. Kwon HR, Min KW, Ahn HJ, Seok HG, Koo BK, et al. (2010) Effects of aerobic exercise on abdominal fat, thigh muscle mass and muscle strength in type 2 diabetic subject. Korean Diabetes J 34: 23–31.
34. Mitranun W, Deerochanawong C, Tanaka H, Suksom D (2014) Continuous vs interval training on glycemic control and macro- and microvascular reactivity in type 2 diabetic patients. Scand J Med Sci Sports 24: e69–76.
35. Hu FB, Manson JE (2003) Walking: the best medicine for diabetes? Arch Intern Med 163: 1397–1398.
36. Kravitz RL, Helms LJ, Azari R, Antonius D, Melnikow J (2000) Comparing the use of physician time and health care resources among patients speaking English, Spanish, and Russian. Med Care 38: 728–738.
37. Higgins JP, Green S (updated March 2011) Cochrane Handbook of systematic reviews, Version 5.1.0. Available: http://www.cochrane-handbook.org. Accessed 2014 August 20.
38. Chudyk A, Petrella RJ (2011) Effects of exercise on cardiovascular risk factors in type 2 diabetes: a meta-analysis. Diabetes Care 34: 1228–1237.
39. Snowling NJ, Hopkins WG (2006) Effects of different modes of exercise training on glucose control and risk factors for complications in type 2 diabetic patients: a meta-analysis. Diabetes Care 29: 2518–2527.
40. Goldberg AP (1989) Aerobic and resistive exercise modify risk factors for coronary heart disease. Med Sci Sports Exerc 21: 669–674.
41. Williams PT, Thompson PD (2013) Walking versus running for hypertension, cholesterol, and diabetes mellitus risk reduction. Arterioscler Thromb Vasc Biol 33: 1085–1091.
42. Umpierre D, Ribeiro PA, Schaan BD, Ribeiro JP (2013) Volume of supervised exercise training impacts glycaemic control in patients with type 2 diabetes: a systematic review with meta-regression analysis. Diabetologia 56: 242–251.
43. Xu Y, Wang L, He J, Bi Y, Li M, et al. (2013) Prevalence and control of diabetes in Chinese adults. JAMA 310: 948–959.
44. Dale JR, Williams SM, Bowyer V (2012) What is the effect of peer support on diabetes outcomes in adults? A systematic review. Diabet Med 29: 1361–1377.
45. Qiu S, Cai X, Chen X, Yang B, Sun Z (2014) Step counter use in type 2 diabetes: a meta-analysis of randomized controlled trials. BMC Med 12: 36.
46. Spence JC, Burgess J, Rodgers W, Murray T (2009) Effect of pretesting on intentions and behaviour: a pedometer and walking intervention. Psychol Health 24: 777–789.
47. The National High Blood Pressure Education Program Working Group (1994) National High Blood Pressure Education Program Working Group report on hypertension in diabetes. Hypertension 23: 145–158; discussion 159–160.
48. Look ARG, Pi-Sunyer X, Blackburn G, Brancati FL, Bray GA, et al. (2007) Reduction in weight and cardiovascular disease risk factors in individuals with type 2 diabetes: one-year results of the look AHEAD trial. Diabetes Care 30: 1374–1383.

4

Heart Rate Recovery in Asymptomatic Patients with Chagas Disease

Maria Clara Noman de Alencar[1], Manoel Otávio da Costa Rocha[1], Márcia Maria de Oliveira Lima[1], Henrique Silveira Costa[1], Giovane Rodrigo Sousa[1], Renata de Carvalho Bicalho Carneiro[1], Guilherme Canabrava Rodrigues Silva[2], Fernando Vieira Brandão[2], Lucas Jordan Kreuser[3], Antonio Luiz Pinho Ribeiro[1], Maria Carmo Pereira Nunes[1]*

1 Post-Graduate Program in Infectious Diseases and Tropical Medicine, School of Medicine, Universidade Federal de Minas Gerais, Belo Horizonte, MG, Brazil, **2** School of Medicine, Universidade Federal de Minas Gerais, Belo Horizonte, MG, Brazil, **3** University of Minnesota Medical School, Minneapolis, Minnesota, United States of America

Abstract

Background: Chagas disease patients with right bundle-branch block (RBBB) have diverse clinical presentation and prognosis, depending on left ventricular (LV) function. Autonomic disorder can be an early marker of heart involvement. The heart rate recovery (HRR) after exercise may identify autonomic dysfunction, with impact on therapeutic strategies. This study was designed to assess the HRR after symptom-limited exercise testing in asymptomatic Chagas disease patients with RBBB without ventricular dysfunction compared to patients with indeterminate form of Chagas disease and healthy controls.

Methods: One hundred and forty-nine subjects divided into 3 groups were included. A control group was comprised of healthy individuals; group 1 included patients in the indeterminate form of Chagas disease; and group 2 included patients with complete RBBB with or without left anterior hemiblock, and normal ventricular systolic function. A symptom-limited exercise test was performed and heart rate (HR) response to exercise was assessed. HRR was defined as the difference between HR at peak exercise and 1 min following test termination.

Results: There were no differences in heart-rate profile during exercise between healthy individuals and patients in indeterminate form, whereas patients with RBBB had more prevalence of chronotropic incompetence, lower exercise capacity and lower HRR compared with patients in indeterminate form and controls. A delayed decrease in the HR after exercise was found in 17 patients (15%), 9% in indeterminate form and 24% with RBBB, associated with older age, worse functional capacity, impaired chronotropic response, and ventricular arrhythmias during both exercise and recovery. By multivariable analysis, the independent predictors of a delayed decrease in the HRR were age (odds ratio [OR] 1.11; 95% confidence interval [CI] 1.03 to 1.21; $p = 0.010$) and presence of RBBB (OR 3.97; 95% CI 1.05 to 15.01; $p = 0.042$).

Conclusions: A small proportion (15%) of asymptomatic Chagas patients had attenuated HRR after exercise, being more prevalent in patients with RBBB compared with patients in indeterminate form and controls.

Editor: Larisa G. Tereshchenko, Johns Hopkins University SOM, United States of America

Funding: The authors have no support or funding to report.

Competing Interests: The authors have declared that no competing interests exist.

* Email: mcarmo@waymail.com.br

Introduction

Chagas disease remains a serious health problem in Latin America, being a leading cause of heart disease [1–3]. Although symptoms of chronic heart disease appear several years after initial infection, progressive myocardial damage occurs throughout early stages [4,5]. The development of electrocardiographic (ECG) abnormalities implies disease progression and usually precedes the appearance of symptoms [6–8]. In particular, patients with conduction system abnormalities expressed by right bundle-branch block (RBBB) are at risk for developing progressive myocarditis [6]. Nevertheless, there is a wide spectrum of Chagas disease patients with RBBB from asymptomatic with normal ventricular function to severe heart failure, and the prognosis depends mainly on left ventricular (LV) function [4,9,10]. Moreover, the subset of Chagas disease patients with RBBB and normal ventricular function encompasses a heterogeneous population with variable response to physical exercise in terms of functional performance and exercise-induced arrhythmias.

Autonomic disorder is an early alteration in the course of heart impairment in Chagas disease, which has also been implicated in the pathophysiology of the ventricular dysfunction [11–14]. A decline in heart rate (HR) after exercise is an index of autonomic activity that reflects parasympathetic reactivation [15,16]. An attenuated heart rate recovery (HRR) after exercise has been shown to be associated with impaired functional capacity and poor prognosis among people with and without cardiovascular disease [17–21].

We believe that HRR might be a useful tool for autonomic nervous system evaluation in the setting of Chagas disease. Therefore, the present study was designed to assess the HRR after maximal symptom-limited exercise test in asymptomatic Chagas disease patients with RBBB without ventricular dysfunction compared to patients in indeterminate form and healthy controls.

Methods

Study Population

Patients with the diagnosis of chronic Chagas disease, evaluated at our institution from October 2010 to April 2012, were initially considered for the study. Diagnosis of Chagas disease required at least two positive serologic tests for antibodies against *T. cruzi*. The study was approved by the Research Ethics Committee of the Federal University of Minas Gerais, Brazil, and an informed written consent was obtained from all subjects.

To be included in the study, patients should be asymptomatic, in sinus rhythm, and with normal left ventricular systolic function by echocardiography. Patients who were unable to perform an exercise test or had prior diagnosis of heart disease from other etiology were excluded. In addition, patients with other systemic diseases that can be associated with autonomic dysfunction, especially hypertension and diabetes, were not included.

Electrocardiography evaluation

ECG was analyzed by an experienced cardiologist who was blinded to the serological tests for Chagas disease following the recommendations for the standardization and interpretation of the electrocardiogram [22].

Diagnostic criteria for complete RBBB were QRS duration ≥120 ms, with prominent and notched R waves (rsr', rsR', or rSR' patterns) in right precordial leads (V_1 and V_2) and wide S waves that are longer in duration than the preceding R wave in left precordial leads (V_5 and V_6) with normal QRS axis (within $-30°$ and $90°$). Left anterior fascicular block (LAFB) was considered to be associated with RBBB when QRS axis was between $-45°$ and $-90°$ with qR pattern in lead aVL.

Patients meeting the inclusion criteria were further categorized into 2 groups according to ECG evaluation. Group 1 included patients in the indeterminate form of Chagas disease defined as those with positive serological tests with a normal chest radiograph and ECG [5,8] (Figure 1). In this group, patients with any minor ECG abnormalities including ST-T changes were not included.

Group 2 included patients with complete RBBB with or without LAFB, and normal left ventricular ejection fraction (Figures 2 and 3).

In addition, a control group comprised of healthy individuals referred for cardiovascular evaluation with normal exams was also included.

Exercise testing protocol

A symptom-limited exercise was performed on a treadmill (Digistress Pulsar, Micromed, Brazil) using a standard Bruce protocol [23]. A physician who was unaware of the echocardiogram results was present during all of the studies to encourage maximal exertion. A 12-lead ECG was continuously monitored and recorded in each minute, and cuff blood pressure was recorded manually at rest, during the last 30 seconds of each stage and during the 6-min recovery period. After achieving maximal workload, all patients spent 1 minute in a cool-down period at a speed of 2.4 km per hour and a grade of 2.5 percent [24]. After 1-min, all of them completed recovery phase in supine position.

Heart rate was measured at rest, peak exercise and at one minute recovery. Heart rate recovery (HRR) was defined as the difference between peak HR and HR registered at the end of active recovery. An abnormal HRR at minute 1 of recovery was defined as a change from the peak HR of 12 beats or less.

Chronotropic incompetence (CI) was defined accordingly the following criteria: (1) failure to achieve 85% of age-predicted maximal heart rate (220-age) [25] and/or (2) failure to attain 80% of HR reserve (HR reserve = age-predicted maximal heart rate – resting HR) [26]. The proportion of heart rate reserve achieved have been termed chronotropic index, considered abnormal <80% [26,27].

Echocardiographic Evaluation

A standard transthoracic two-dimensional (2D) echocardiogram was performed according to recommendations of the American Society of Echocardiography using a commercially available echocardiograph (GE Vivid 7, Horten, Norway). LV ejection fraction was calculated according to the modified Simpson's rule [28].

Diastolic function was assessed by pulsed-wave Doppler examination of mitral, and tissue Doppler imaging [28,29]. RV function was quantitatively assessed using the peak systolic tissue Doppler velocity acquired at the basal RV free wall [30].

Statistics analysis

Normally distributed variables are reported as mean ±_SD and compared with analysis of variance (ANOVA). Data that were not normally distributed are reported as median with interquartile range and compared with Mann Whitney test. Categorical variables are reported as number and percentage and compared with chi-square test.

A HRR ≤12 beats at 1 min post-exercise was defined as an abnormal response. Logistic regression analysis was performed to determine characteristics that were independently associated with abnormal HRR. Variables that were found to be significantly associated with abnormal HRR in univariable analysis or clinically relevant were included in the multivariable logistic regression analysis. To avoid colinearity among a subset of highly similar variables, only the clinically important variables were chosen to enter into the model. SPSS software (version 19.0) was used for statistical analysis.

Results

From 134 Chagas disease patients initially referred to the study, 23 patients (17%) were excluded: 15 patients in the indeterminate form and 8 with RBBB. Of the 15 patients excluded in the indeterminate form, 9 patients had hypertension, 4 patients had ST-T abnormalities, and 2 patients were found to have mild left ventricular enlargement on echocardiography examination. Of the 54 patients with RBBB, 5 had hypertension or diabetes, 2 had complete atrioventricular block, and one patient was unable to complete the exercise test. Therefore, a total of 111 Chagas disease patients and 38 controls who met all inclusion criteria were included.

The baseline characteristics of the patients and controls are shown in Table 1. All patients were asymptomatic, in NYHA functional class I, and 55 patients (50%) were male. Regarding medication, 9 patients (8%) were taking amiodarone (3 of whom were also taking beta-blockers). As expected, the mean QRS duration was 82.3±2.7 ms in patients in the indeterminate form compared to 136.3±15.8 ms in patients with RBBB.

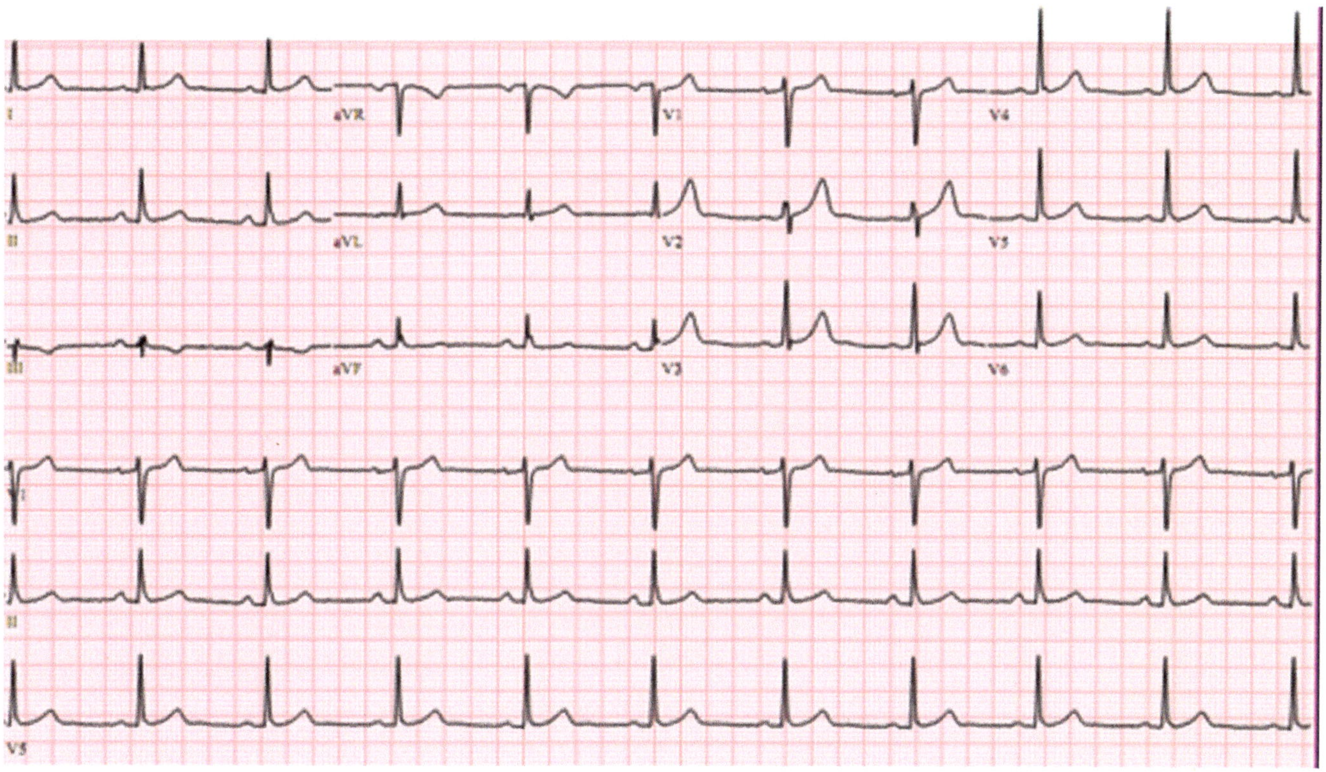

Figure 1. A normal ECG in a patient in the indeterminate form of Chagas disease.

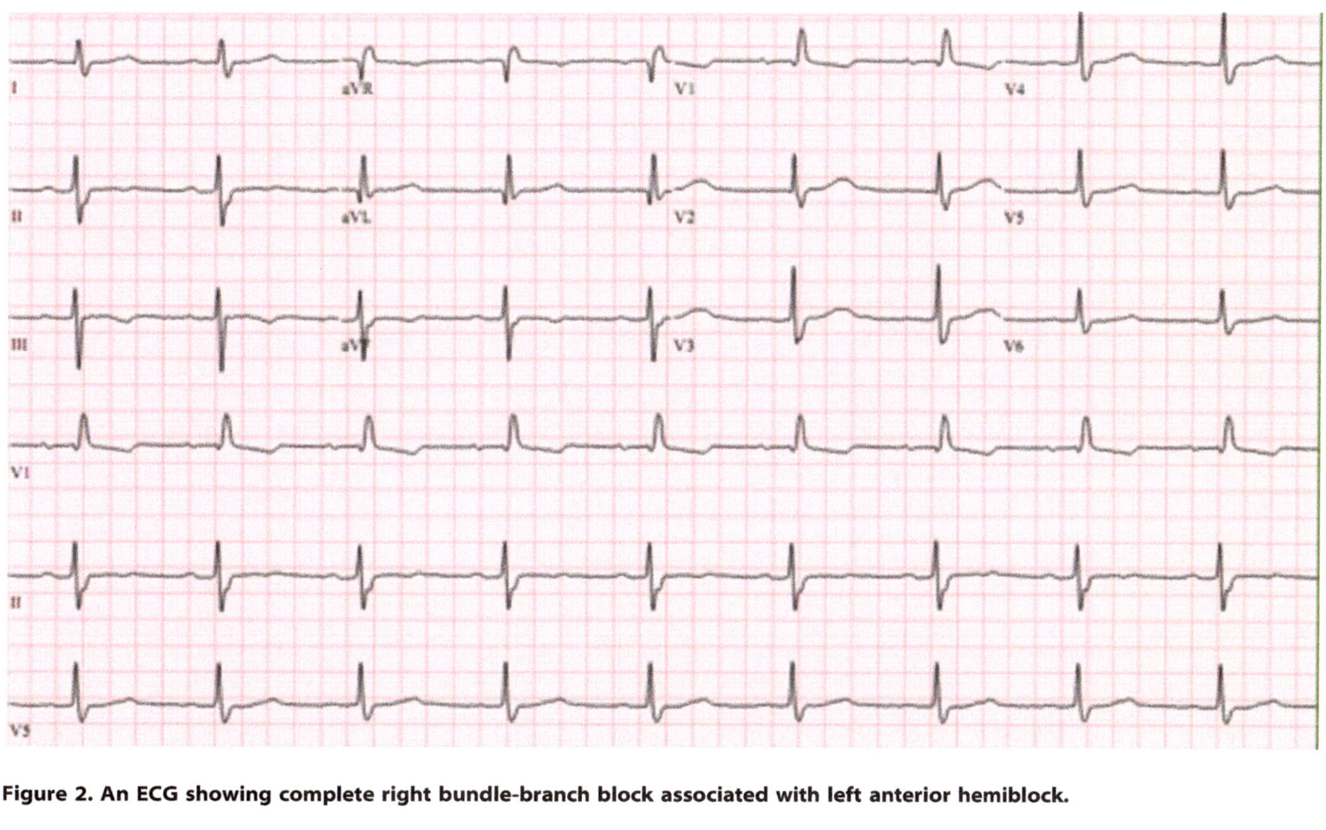

Figure 2. An ECG showing complete right bundle-branch block associated with left anterior hemiblock.

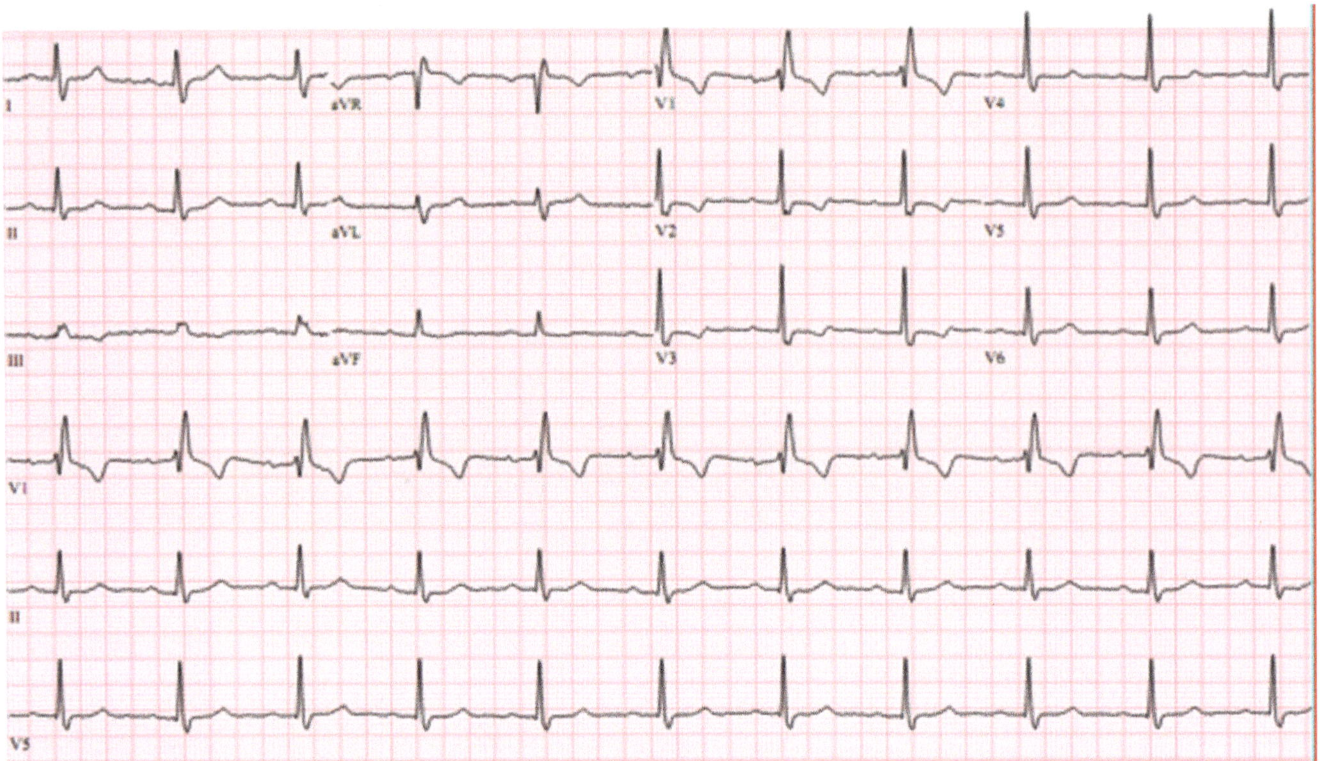

Figure 3. An ECG showing isolated right bundle-branch block.

Table 1. Characteristics of the Patients at rest.

Variable	Controls (n = 38)	Group 1 (n = 65)	Group 2 (n = 46)	p Value
Age (years)	44.1±9.2	46.9±7.9	50.9±9.9	0.001*
Male (n/%)	22 (58)	30 (46)	25 (54)	0.469
BSA (m^2)	1.79±0.2	1.75±0.1	1.75±0.2	0.476
SBP (mmHg)	125.8±14.7	120.6±13.2	122.4±8.3	0.127
DBP (mmHg)	86.3±8.5	84.5±7.1	80.8±6.2	0.002*
LVDd (mm)	47.2±5.6	48.2±4.6	46.6±3.2	0.171
LVSd (mm)	28.6±4.2	29.8±3.9	30.1±3.1	0.209
LVEF (%)	68 [66/73]	69 [64/72]	64 [61/67]	<0.001*
LA dimension (mm)	34 [30/36]	35 [31/37]	36 [34/38]	0.009*
E wave (cm/s)	79.6±20.0	73.7±17.6	78.6±14.6	0.192
A wave (cm/s)	53 [42/69]	55 [46/64]	75 [52/85]	<0.001*
DT (ms)	185 [171/214]	192 [171/208]	233 [215/273]	<0.001*
E/e' ratio	4.1±1.4	4.4±1.1	4.0±0.9	0.158
SPAP (mmHg)	20.7±3.5	20.3±4.2	24.8±7.4	0.398
RV systolic velocity† (cm/s)	11.3±1.4	11.6±1.5	11.9±1.7	0.202

Data are expressed as mean value ± SD or median [interquartile range] or), or absolute numbers (percentage).
*p<0.05 for comparison between controls and group 1 versus group 2.
†Maximal systolic velocity at the tricuspid annulus by tissue Doppler velocity
A= late transmitral flow velocity; BSA = body surface area; DBP = diastolic blood pressure; DT = deceleration time; E= early diastolic transmitral flow velocity; E/e' = ratio of the early diastolic transmitral flow velocity to early diastolic mitral annular velocity; LA = left atrium; LVDd = left ventricular end-diastolic diameter; LVEF = left ventricular ejection fraction; LVSd = left ventricular end-systolic diameter; SBP = systolic blood pressure, SPAP = systolic arterial pulmonary pressure.

Of the patients with RBBB, 26 patients had RBBB associated with left anterior fascicular block (56.5%), and 20 patients (43.5%) had isolated RBBB. Others conduction system abnormalities detected in these patients were first degree atrioventricular block in 7 patients (15.2%); Mobitz type I second degree atrioventricular block in 3 patients (6.5%). Minor ECG abnormalities including sinus bradycardia were detected in 19 patients (41.3%).

Control subjects and patients in the indeterminate form were younger than the patients with RBBB. Similarly, there were no difference in echocardiographic parameters between controls and patients in the indeterminate form (group 2) whereas patients in group 3 had lower LV ejection fraction, larger left atrial dimension, and impairment of diastolic dysfunction compared to other groups. Wall motion abnormalities were found in 11 patients: 6 patients in the indeterminate form (9%) and 5 with RBBB (11%), mainly in the apical, basal inferior and inferolateral walls.

Exercise testing

All patients completed the study protocol. No patient had angina during the exercise test or significant ischemic ST abnormalities in the electrocardiogram.

Exercise test responses according to the groups are shown in Table 2. There were no differences between controls and patients in group 1. On the other hand, patients in group 2 had more prevalence of chronotropic incompetence, lower exercise capacity and lower HRR (Figure 4) compared with controls and patients in group 1.

The median value for heart-rate recovery was 24 beats per minute, with a range from the 25th to the 75th percentile of 19 to 29 beats per minute. An abnormal value for heart-rate recovery was found in 17 patients (15%), 9% in indeterminate form and 24% with RBBB. No subjects in control group had HRR ≤12 beats/min (Figure 5).

Characteristics of the study participants according to HRR are summarized in Table 3.

There was a weak but significant correlation between the peak HR and HRR ($r = 0.2$; $p = 0.015$). However, no correlation was found when peak heart rate was expressed as a percentage of age-predicted maximal HR.

As compared with the patients with a normal value for HRR, those with an abnormal value (≤12 beats/min) were older, had more frequent abnormal rest ECG with RBBB, lower peak HR values in percentage of predicted, lower exercise capacity, and were more likely to have diastolic dysfunction and chronotropic incompetence as assessed by chronotropic index. Additionally, these patients had more frequent ventricular ectopy during both exercise and recovery. Likewise, use of amiodarone was more frequent in those with abnormal HRR. There were no differences in the LV ejection fraction or LV filling pressures between patients with normal and abnormal HRR (Table 3).

The variables included in the final multivariable model were age, use of amiodarone, resting HR, peak VO_2, left ventricular ejection fraction, E/e' ratio, and the presence of RBBB. The variables that remained independently associated with a delayed decrease in the HRR were age (OR 1.11; 95% CI 1.03 to 1.21; $p = 0.010$) and presence of RBBB (OR 3.97; 95% CI 1.05 to 15.01; $p = 0.042$).

Discussion

The present study addresses the value of recovery of the HR immediately after maximal symptom-limited exercise test as a marker of autonomic dysfunction in asymptomatic patients with Chagas disease. The principal findings of this study were (1) patients classified as in indeterminate form of the disease had heart-rate responses to exercise similar to healthy individuals; (2) abnormal HRR was detected in 17 patients (15%), 9% in indeterminate form and 24% with RBBB; and (3) a delayed

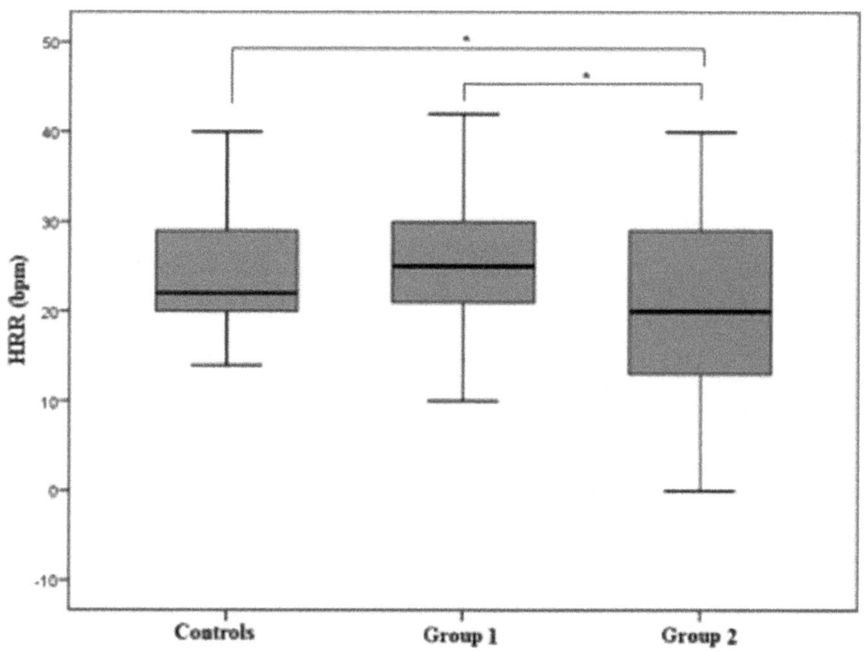

Figure 4. Heart rate response after exercise among the groups: healthy controls; group 1 = patients in the indeterminate form of Chagas disease; group 2 = patients with complete right bundle-branch block (RBBB) with or without left anterior hemiblock, and normal ventricular systolic function. Patients in group 2 had lower HRR compared to other groups. *p<0.05

Table 2. Exercise test responses according to the groups.

Variable	Controls (n = 38)	Group 1 (n = 65)	Group 2 (n = 46)	p Value
Resting HR (beats/min)	75.1±9.8	74.2±12.7	74.5±10.7	0.971
Peak HR (beats/min)	176 [166/187]	176 [165/184]	156 [136/168]	<0.001*
Peak HR (% predicted)	100 [97/103]	100 [94/107]	92 [81/99]	<0.001*
HRR (beats/min)	24.0±6.7	25.0±8.9	20.2±11.7	0.029*
HRR ≤12 bpm	0	6 (9)	11 (25)	0.001*†
Peak VO_2 ($ml.Kg^{-1}.min^{-1}$)	40.4±7.7	40.4±10.4	35.5±10.5	0.024*
METs	11.5±2.2	11.5±3.1	10.1±3.0	0.017*
Chronotropic index	0.99±0.1	0.98±0.2	0.82±0.2	<0.001*
Chronotropic index (<80%)	1 (3)	4 (6)	20 (43)	<0.001*
Peak exercise HR (<85% of the age-predicted HR	1 (3)	3 (5)	18 (39)	<0.001*

Data are expressed as mean value ± SD, number (percentage) of patients or median [interquartile range].
*p<0.05 for comparison between controls and group 1 versus group 2.
†p = 0.058 for comparison between controls and group 1.
HR = heart rate; HRR = heart rate recovery; MET = metabolic equivalents

decrease in the HR after exercise was associated with older age, worse functional capacity, impaired chronotropic response, and ventricular arrhythmias. These findings support the concept that abnormalities in autonomic balance may precede manifestations of cardiovascular disease in Chagas disease.

To the best of our knowledge, this is the first study to demonstrate abnormal HRR in asymptomatic Chagas disease patients. Previous study has shown that ECG during the early asymptomatic stage of infection is able to identify patients at high risk for developing progressive myocarditis. [6] In contrast, patients with normal ECG have a good prognosis with mortality rates similar to those of non-Chagas persons [6,31]. RBBB is a typical ECG abnormality of Chagas disease, unequivocally related to the cardiac involvement by the disease. However, in patients with RBBB the response to physical exercise is variable in terms of functional performance and exercise-induced arrhythmias. Therefore, even in RBBB Chagas disease patients with normal ventricular systolic function, physical effort can trigger arrhythmias, which might be associated with the changes in autonomic function during exercise. The HRR may provide further information regarding the risk for arrhythmias that occur in the setting of exercise or recovery. Our findings demonstrate that abnormal HRR was gradually more prevalent compared patients in the indeterminate form to patients with RBBB. This subset of chagasic patients who had abnormal HRR has a good prognosis in terms of symptoms and ventricular function, but they may be at risk for developing arrhythmias during exercise.

Autonomic Abnormalities in Chagas disease

The autonomic nervous system of patients with Chagas disease has been extensively studied [11,32,33]. Previous studies demonstrated destruction of the parasympathetic ganglions cells in the

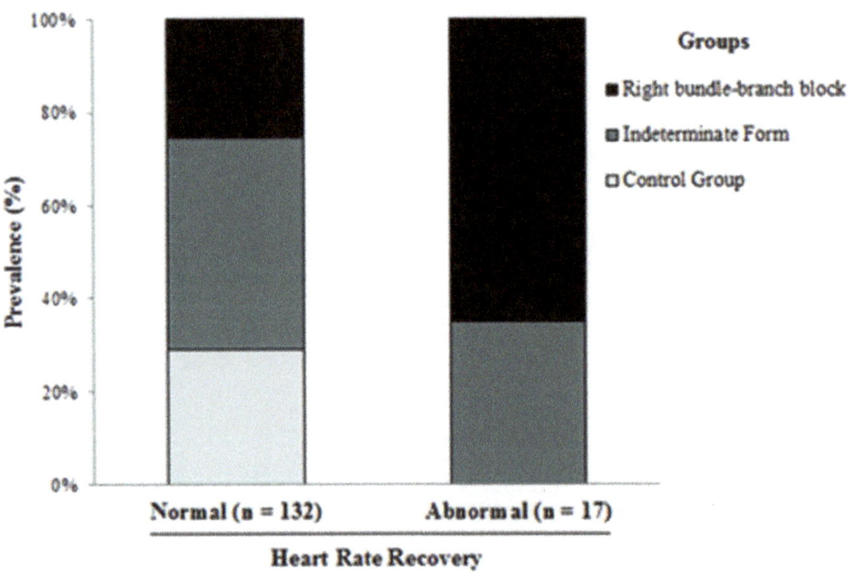

Figure 5. Proportion of abnormal HRR according to the groups. Abnormal HRR was gradually more prevalent across groups from controls, patients with the indeterminate form to patients with RBBB.

Table 3. Predictors of abnormal response of the HRR in the study population.

Variable	Normal (HRR>12bpm)	Abnormal (HRR≤12bpm)	OR (95%CI)	p Value
Age (years)	47.1±8.2	57.3±9.3	1.16 (1.08–1.25)	<0.001
Use of amiodarone	5 (5)	4 (24)	6.4 (1.59–25.48)	0.026
LVEF (%)	66.9±5.2	65.8±3.8	0.91 (0.82–1.02)	0.282
RBBB (n/%)	33 (35)	11 (65)	5.39 (1.85–5.72)	0.002
E (cm/s)	76.4±16.7	71.9±15.3	0.99 (0.99–1.00)	0.180
A (cm/s)	59.9±18.8	78.2±22.3	1.01 (1.00–1.01)	<0.001
DT (ms)	209.1±42.6	240.8±61.5	1.01 (1.00–1.02)	0.011
E/e' ratio	4.2±1.1	4.3±0.9	1.12 (0.69–1.83)	0.744
Resting HR (beats/min)	70.5±10.1	70.7±13.9	1.01 (0.97–1.06)	0.961
Peak HR (beats/min)	168.7±19.6	146.1±27.7	0.95 (0.93–0.98)	<0.001
Peak HR (% predicted)	97.9±10.6	89.5±15.7	0.93(0.89–0.98)	0.002
Peak VO_2 (ml.Kg^{-1}.min^{-1})	39.7±10.3	33.1±9.6	0.92 (0.86–0.98)	0.016
Frequent VPB during exercise*	17 (18)	7 (41)	3.97 (1.32–1.89)	0.014
Frequent VPB during recovery*	14 (15)	8 (47)	5.55 (1.80–7.11)	0.003
Peak exercise HR (<85% of the age-predicted HR)	15 (16)	5 (29)	2.97 (0.92–9.54)	0.200
Chronotropic index (<80%)	15 (16)	7 (41)	4.94 (1.65–4.83)	0.004

Data are expressed as mean value ± SD or number (percentage) of patients.
LVEF = left ventricular ejection fraction; RBBB = right bundle branch block; E= early diastolic transmitral flow velocity; A= late transmitral flow velocity; DT = deceleration time; ms = milliseconds; E/e' = ratio of the early diastolic transmitral flow velocity to early diastolic mitral annular velocity; HR = heart rate; VO_2 = oxygen uptake; VPB = ventricular premature beats.
*defined as more than 7 ventricular premature beats per minute [30].

heart due to the inflammatory process [32] and the presence of auto-antibodies with cholinergic antagonistic activity [13]. Patients presenting with chronotropic insufficiency in exercise test had both higher levels of anti-cholinergic autoantibodies [34] and reduced heart rate variability vagal indexes [35].

Abnormalities of autonomic HR control have been identified early in the course of the disease [11,12,33]. However, the implications of autonomic dysfunction in the pathogenesis of the chronic myocarditis, as well as its value in predicting adverse outcome remain a matter of debate. The destruction of the parasympathetic innervations may induce an increased sympathetic tone with a direct effect in the genesis of ventricular arrhythmias and sudden death [36]. In our study, chronotropic incompetence was found in asymptomatic patients with RBBB, whereas those patients in indeterminate form were similar to the controls. In agreement with previous investigation [35], our patients with the early manifestations of Chagas heart disease without ventricular dysfunction had impaired chronotropic response as defined by either a low percent of age-predicted HR achieved or a low percent HR reserve.

Azarbal et al [26] demonstrated that percent HR reserve was superior to the traditional percent of age-predicted HR in predicting cardiac death. Additionally, in that study percent HR reserve captured greater number of at-risk subjects that manifested a normal chronotropic response as assessed by the percent of age-predicted HR. In our study failure to reach 85% of the age-predicted maximum HR was similar between patients with normal and abnormal HRR. However, when the percent HR reserve was used as the criterion for CI, the prevalence of CI was greater in the patients with abnormal HRR compared to those with normal HRR. Therefore, the HR reserve approach has been used as the standard to assess the adequacy of HR response to exercise [37].

Heart rate response after exercise

In the present study we assessed the capacity of the HR to decelerate after exercise as an additional measurement of the autonomic nervous system function. The rapid decline in HR after exercise expresses sympathetic withdrawal and increased parasympathetic tone to the sino-atrial node. A low HRR value has been associated with increased all-cause mortality risk in a variety of asymptomatic and diseased populations [38], even after adjustment for severity of cardiovascular disease, LV function, and exercise capacity [39]. In the present study, the patients who had an abnormal value of HRR also presented with other markers of unfavorable prognosis, which includes worse exercise capacity, chronotropic incompetence, and ventricular arrhythmias. In particular, these patients had frequent ventricular ectopy either during exercise or recovery. In a large cohort of 29,244 patients from Cleveland Clinic, only the occurrence of frequent ventricular ectopy during recovery was independent predictor of death [40] which was superior in outcome prediction than ventricular ectopy occurring only during exercise. Similar to what occurs with ventricular ectopy, recovery of the HR immediately after exercise is a function of parasympathetic function, and might have a potential prognostic role in the setting of Chagas disease. It is important to note that this additional clinical information is derived at no additional cost or effort, and HRR is routinely measured during standard exercise testing.

Recently, Cahalin et al. [41] analyzing a cohort of heart failure patients demonstrated that HRR after the 6 min walk test (6MWT) is a powerful predictor of cardiac events that performs better than distance ambulated as the reference measure. Importantly, the predictive accuracy of HRR after the 6MWT is comparable with HRR after maximal exertion during cardiopulmonary exercise testing. In view of these findings, our study is particularity relevant since the HR response after exercise can be also evaluated at sub-maximal testing, especially for patients with Chagas disease who are unable to undergo a maximal symptom-limited evaluation. Additionally, even in those patients who had chronotropic incompetence, the HRR can be evaluated as an additional marker of autonomic dysfunction. Therefore, as the prognostic information of HRR is not only related to exercise performance or maximal HR achieved, this simple measure could be employed in clinical practice and is potentially applicable to the broad spectrum of Chagas disease patients.

The influence of the achieved maximal HR on HRR is not well understood. Myers et al. [42] found that both chronotropic incompetence and abnormal HRR are independent predictors for cardiovascular mortality and they may act as independent clinical predictors. Zaim et al. [43] found a direct correlation between the peak HR obtained during a symptom-limited exercise test and the subsequent HRR. In our study, although a weak correlation between maximal HR achieved and HRR was found, there was no correlation of percent-predicted maximal HR achieved and HRR. Further study and understanding of physiological mechanisms that control and possibly link the processes of maximal HR achieved and HRR are needed.

Study limitations

Heart rate variability, which represents the autonomic balance between the sympathetic and parasympathetic pathways acting on the intrinsic rhythm of the heart, was not assessed in this study. In addition, we did not exclude patients who were on medications that can alter the HR response to exercise. However, when we re-analyzed the data excluding 9 patients (8%) using amiodarone, the results did not change. Similarly, Cole et al [24] did not find associations between the use of beta-blockers or calcium-channel blockers and an abnormal value for HRR.

Clinical implications

Autonomic disorder is an early alteration in the course of heart impairment in Chagas disease, which has been implicated in the pathophysiology of the ventricular dysfunction. HRR proved to be a simple, reliable and noninvasive parameter to assess the autonomic balance during exercise, useful in detecting early changes in Chagas heart disease.

The results of the present study have great medical and social importance because Chagas disease patients often come from impoverished, poorly-educated backgrounds and work in physically demanding jobs including farming, construction, and housekeeping. Abnormal HRR during exercise may be helpful to clinical-decision making regarding patients management and labor counseling. As physical effort can trigger arrhythmias, assessment of HRR seems to offer important information by identifying patients who are at high risk of exercise-induced arrhythmias.

Conclusions

This study showed that a small proportion (15%) of asymptomatic Chagas patients had abnormal heart-rate responses to exercise, especially attenuated HRR after exercise, being more prevalent in patients with RBBB compared with patients in indeterminate form and controls. HRR assessment can identify autonomic dysfunction and could be helpful for clinical risk stratification in the setting of Chagas disease.

Author Contributions

Analyzed the data: MCPN ALPR. Contributed reagents/materials/analysis tools: MCNA RCBC. Wrote the paper: MCNA MOCR MCPN. Exercise test: HSC. Data collection: GCRS FVB LJK. Critical review of the manuscript: GRS MMOL.

References

1. World Health Organization (2010) First WHO report on neglected tropical diseases: working to overcome the global impact of neglected tropical diseases. World Health Organization ed.. Geneva. pp. 1–172.
2. Schmunis GA, Yadon ZE (2010) Chagas disease: a Latin American health problem becoming a world health problem. Acta Trop 115: 14–21.
3. Bern C, Kjos S, Yabsley MJ, Montgomery SP (2011) Trypanosoma cruzi and Chagas' Disease in the United States. Clin Microbiol Rev 24: 655–681.
4. Nunes MC, Carmo AA, Rocha MO, Ribeiro AL (2012) Mortality prediction in Chagas heart disease. Expert Rev Cardiovasc Ther 10: 1173–1184.
5. Nunes MC, Dones W, Morillo CA, Encina JJ, Ribeiro AL (2013) Chagas disease: an overview of clinical and epidemiological aspects. J Am Coll Cardiol 62: 767–776.
6. Maguire JH, Hoff R, Sherlock I, Guimaraes AC, Sleigh AC, et al. (1987) Cardiac morbidity and mortality due to Chagas' disease: prospective electrocardiographic study of a Brazilian community. Circulation 75: 1140–1145.
7. Ribeiro AL, Sabino EC, Marcolino MS, Salemi VM, Ianni BM, et al. (2013) Electrocardiographic abnormalities in Trypanosoma cruzi seropositive and seronegative former blood donors. PLoS Negl Trop Dis 7: e2078.
8. Ribeiro AL, Nunes MP, Teixeira MM, Rocha MO (2012) Diagnosis and management of Chagas disease and cardiomyopathy. Nat Rev Cardiol 9: 576–589.
9. Nunes MC, Reis RC, Colosimo EA, Ribeiro AL, Barbosa FB, et al. (2011) Risk estimation approach in Chagas disease is still needed. Int J Cardiol 147: 294–296.
10. Rassi A Jr, Rassi A, Rassi SG (2007) Predictors of mortality in chronic Chagas disease: a systematic review of observational studies. Circulation 115: 1101–1108.
11. Ribeiro AL, Moraes RS, Ribeiro JP, Ferlin EL, Torres RM, et al. (2001) Parasympathetic dysautonomia precedes left ventricular systolic dysfunction in Chagas disease. Am Heart J 141: 260–265.
12. Ribeiro AL, Lombardi F, Sousa MR, Rocha MO (2005) Vagal dysfunction in Chagas disease. Int J Cardiol 103: 225–226; author reply 227–229.
13. Ribeiro AL, Gimenez LE, Hernandez CC, de Carvalho AC, Teixeira MM, et al. (2007) Early occurrence of anti-muscarinic autoantibodies and abnormal vagal modulation in Chagas disease. Int J Cardiol 117: 59–63.
14. Molina RB, Matsubara BB, Hueb JC, Zanati SG, Meira DA, et al. (2006) Dysautonomia and ventricular dysfunction in the indeterminate form of Chagas disease. Int J Cardiol 113: 188–193.
15. Imai K, Sato H, Hori M, Kusuoka H, Ozaki H, et al. (1994) Vagally mediated heart rate recovery after exercise is accelerated in athletes but blunted in patients with chronic heart failure. J Am Coll Cardiol 24: 1529–1535.
16. Pierpont GL, Stolpman DR, Gornick CC (2000) Heart rate recovery post-exercise as an index of parasympathetic activity. J Auton Nerv Syst 80: 169–174.
17. Shetler K, Marcus R, Froelicher VF, Vora S, Kalisetti D, et al. (2001) Heart rate recovery: validation and methodologic issues. J Am Coll Cardiol 38: 1980–1987.
18. Jouven X, Empana JP, Schwartz PJ, Desnos M, Courbon D, et al. (2005) Heart-rate profile during exercise as a predictor of sudden death. N Engl J Med 352: 1951–1958.
19. Maddox TM, Ross C, Ho PM, Masoudi FA, Magid D, et al. (2008) The prognostic importance of abnormal heart rate recovery and chronotropic response among exercise treadmill test patients. Am Heart J 156: 736–744.
20. Tang YD, Dewland TA, Wencker D, Katz SD (2009) Post-exercise heart rate recovery independently predicts mortality risk in patients with chronic heart failure. J Card Fail 15: 850–855.
21. Ramos RP, Arakaki JS, Barbosa P, Treptow E, Valois FM, et al. (2012) Heart rate recovery in pulmonary arterial hypertension: relationship with exercise capacity and prognosis. Am Heart J 163: 580–588.
22. Surawicz B, Childers R, Deal BJ, Gettes LS, Bailey JJ, et al. (2009) AHA/ACCF/HRS recommendations for the standardization and interpretation of the electrocardiogram: part III: intraventricular conduction disturbances: a scientific statement from the American Heart Association Electrocardiography and Arrhythmias Committee, Council on Clinical Cardiology; the American College of Cardiology Foundation; and the Heart Rhythm Society: endorsed by the International Society for Computerized Electrocardiology. Circulation 119: e235–240.
23. Fletcher GF, Balady G, Froelicher VF, Hartley LH, Haskell WL, et al. (1995) Exercise standards. A statement for healthcare professionals from the American Heart Association. Writing Group. Circulation 91: 580–615.
24. Cole CR, Blackstone EH, Pashkow FJ, Snader CE, Lauer MS (1999) Heart-rate recovery immediately after exercise as a predictor of mortality. N Engl J Med 341: 1351–1357.

25. Lauer MS, Francis GS, Okin PM, Pashkow FJ, Snader CE, et al. (1999) Impaired chronotropic response to exercise stress testing as a predictor of mortality. JAMA 281: 524–529.
26. Azarbal B, Hayes SW, Lewin HC, Hachamovitch R, Cohen I, et al. (2004) The incremental prognostic value of percentage of heart rate reserve achieved over myocardial perfusion single-photon emission computed tomography in the prediction of cardiac death and all-cause mortality: superiority over 85% of maximal age-predicted heart rate. J Am Coll Cardiol 44: 423–430.
27. Kligfield P, Lauer MS (2006) Exercise electrocardiogram testing: beyond the ST segment. Circulation 114: 2070–2082.
28. Lang RM, Bierig M, Devereux RB, Flachskampf FA, Foster E, et al. (2005) Recommendations for chamber quantification: a report from the American Society of Echocardiography's Guidelines and Standards Committee and the Chamber Quantification Writing Group, developed in conjunction with the European Association of Echocardiography, a branch of the European Society of Cardiology. J Am Soc Echocardiogr 18: 1440–1463.
29. Nagueh SF, Appleton CP, Gillebert TC, Marino PN, Oh JK, et al. (2009) Recommendations for the evaluation of left ventricular diastolic function by echocardiography. J Am Soc Echocardiogr 22: 107–133.
30. Meluzin J, Spinarova L, Bakala J, Toman J, Krejci J, et al. (2001) Pulsed Doppler tissue imaging of the velocity of tricuspid annular systolic motion; a new, rapid, and non-invasive method of evaluating right ventricular systolic function. Eur Heart J 22: 340–348.
31. Ribeiro AL, Rocha MO (1998) [Indeterminate form of Chagas disease: considerations about diagnosis and prognosis]. Rev Soc Bras Med Trop 31: 301–314.
32. Junqueira Junior LF, Beraldo PS, Chapadeiro E, Jesus PC (1992) Cardiac autonomic dysfunction and neuroganglionitis in a rat model of chronic Chagas' disease. Cardiovasc Res 26: 324–329.
33. Villar JC, Leon H, Morillo CA (2004) Cardiovascular autonomic function testing in asymptomatic T. cruzi carriers: a sensitive method to identify subclinical Chagas' disease. Int J Cardiol 93: 189–195.
34. Talvani A, Rocha MO, Ribeiro AL, Borda E, Sterin-Borda L, et al. (2006) Levels of anti-M2 and anti-beta1 autoantibodies do not correlate with the degree of heart dysfunction in Chagas' heart disease. Microbes Infect 8: 2459–2464.
35. Rocha AL, Lombardi F, da Costa Rocha MO, Barros MV, Val Barros Vda C, et al. (2006) Chronotropic incompetence and abnormal autonomic modulation in ambulatory Chagas disease patients. Ann Noninvasive Electrocardiol 11: 3–11.
36. Junqueira Jr LF (2012) Insights into the clinical and functional significance of cardiac autonomic dysfunction in Chagas disease. Rev Soc Bras Med Trop 45: 243–252.
37. Lauer MS (2004) Chronotropic incompetence: ready for prime time. J Am Coll Cardiol 44: 431–432.
38. Lauer MS (2009) Autonomic function and prognosis. Cleve Clin J Med 76 Suppl 2: S18–22.
39. Vivekananthan DP, Blackstone EH, Pothier CE, Lauer MS (2003) Heart rate recovery after exercise is a predictor of mortality, independent of the angiographic severity of coronary disease. J Am Coll Cardiol 42: 831–838.
40. Frolkis JP, Pothier CE, Blackstone EH, Lauer MS (2003) Frequent ventricular ectopy after exercise as a predictor of death. N Engl J Med 348: 781–790.
41. Cahalin LP, Arena R, Labate V, Bandera F, Lavie CJ, et al. (2013) Heart rate recovery after the 6 min walk test rather than distance ambulated is a powerful prognostic indicator in heart failure with reduced and preserved ejection fraction: a comparison with cardiopulmonary exercise testing. Eur J Heart Fail 15: 519–527.
42. Myers J, Tan SY, Abella J, Aleti V, Froelicher VF (2007) Comparison of the chronotropic response to exercise and heart rate recovery in predicting cardiovascular mortality. Eur J Cardiovasc Prev Rehabil 14: 215–221.
43. Zaim S, Schesser J, Hirsch LS, Rockland R (2010) Influence of the maximum heart rate attained during exercise testing on subsequent heart rate recovery. Ann Noninvasive Electrocardiol 15: 43–48.

5

Impact of Physical Exercise on Substance Use Disorders

Dongshi Wang[1], Yanqiu Wang[1], Yingying Wang[1], Rena Li[1,2], Chenglin Zhou[1]*

1 Department of Sport Psychology, School of Kinesiology, Shanghai University of Sport, Shanghai, China, **2** Center for Hormone Advanced Science and Education, Roskamp Institute, Sarasota, Florida, United States of America

Abstract

Objective: The goal of this meta-analysis was to examine whether long-term physical exercise could be a potential effective treatment for substance use disorders (SUD).

Methods: The PubMed, Web of Science, Elsevier, CNKI and China Info were searched for randomized controlled trials (RCT) studies in regards to the effects of physical exercise on SUD between the years 1990 and 2013. Four main outcome measures including abstinence rate, withdrawal symptoms, anxiety, and depression were evaluated.

Results: Twenty-two studies were integrated in the meta-analysis. The results indicated that physical exercise can effectively increase the abstinence rate (OR = 1.69 (95% CI: 1.44, 1.99), $z = 6.33$, $p<0.001$), ease withdrawal symptoms (SMD = −1.24 (95% CI: −2.46, −0.02), $z = -2$, $p<0.05$), and reduce anxiety (SMD = −0.31 (95% CI: −0.45, −0.16), $z = -4.12$, $p<0.001$) and depression (SMD = −0.47 (95% CI: −0.80, −0.14), $z = -2.76$, $p<0.01$). The physical exercise can more ease the depression symptoms on alcohol and illicit drug abusers than nicotine abusers, and more improve the abstinence rate on illicit drug abusers than the others. Similar treatment effects were found in three categories: exercise intensity, types of exercise, and follow-up periods.

Conclusions: The moderate and high-intensity aerobic exercises, designed according to the Guidelines of American College of Sports Medicine, and the mind-body exercises can be an effective and persistent treatment for those with SUD.

Editor: Raghavan Raju, Georgia Regents University, United States of America

Funding: This work was supported by the ISP grant (No. 13490503600) from Scientific and Technological Commission of Shanghai, National Science Foundation of China (No. 31171004), and the Project of Scientific and Technological Innovation grant (No. yjscx201324) from Shanghai University of Sport. The funders had no role in study design, data collection and analysis, decision to publish, or preparation of the manuscript.

Competing Interests: The authors have declared that no competing interests exist.

* Email: chenglin_600@126.com

Introduction

Substance abuse, such as alcohol, nicotine, and illicit drugs, is one of the largest public health issues in the world. Figures from the World Health Organization (WHO) show that 2.5 million people die from alcohol abuse each year, and at least 15.3 million people have substance use disorders (SUD). Moreover, 120 countries have reported cases of HIV infection in drug addicts [1]. Substance abuse also increases the risk of spreading HIV and is an overall detriment to society, family, and individuals [2–4]. Currently, one of the most commonly used treatments for substance addiction is drug replacement therapy, using substances such as methadone or buprenorphine. Both methadone and buprenorphine are long-acting opioid agonists and used to treat opioid addiction, such as heroin, by reducing and/or eliminating the use of substances, relieving craving behavior, suppressing abstinence symptoms, and decreasing substance abuse-associated infective diseases transmission [5,6]. However, like all opioids, both methadone and buprenorphine have risk of addiction and often have potential of drug-drug interactions [7]. Opioid substitutes are also linked to diabetes, nicotine addiction, and premature death [8–10]. Therefore, there is a strong interest in finding alternative treatments for SUD.

In general, physical exercise is characterized as a planned, organized, and repeated body movement that aims to promote or maintain physical fitness [11–13]. The most common physical exercises include aerobics (brisk walking and running) and mind-body exercises (Tai Chi Quan, Qigong, and Yoga). Compared to methadone and buprenorphine drug-replacement therapies, physical exercise has been recognized as a potential add-on treatment for SUD. For example, studies showed that subjects with regular physical exercise showed lower rates of SUD compared to people with less exercise [14], and regular physical exercise in adolescence provided a preventive effect on alcohol and illicit drug use in adulthood [15]. Furthermore, exercise training caused a significant reduction in daily use and craving for cannabis in marijuana-dependent adults [16], and enhanced the healing effect on SUD [17–19]. The positive effects of physical exercise on SUD have also been confirmed in animal experiments. For example, wheel-running can ease withdrawal behavior in mice with morphine-addiction [20], while voluntary treadmill exercise [21,22] and mandatory treadmill exercise [23] can reduce cocaine, morphine, nicotine, and alcohol intake in various mouse models [22,24,25].

However, some contradictory findings were reported, such as exercise providing no significant effects on substance abusers. For example, one study reported that a 3- week regiment of aerobic exercise and strength training failed to increase the abstinence rate of alcohol abusers [26], and another study found that a 10-week physical exercise program caused no change in the abstinence rate of smokers or relief for emotional symptoms related to smoking [27]. As there is no clear answer for these controversial findings, more comprehensive analyses of physical exercise, such as the intensity and duration of exercise applied, are needed.

In the past two years, a number of articles reviewed whether physical exercise could be considered as a potential method for treating SUD [13,18,28–35]. These articles included preclinical and clinical literature of physical exercise-induced protective effects on the different transitional phases of SUD. These include the initiation of drug use, the progression from use to addiction, the drug withdrawal and relapse period [29] in alcohol, nicotine and illicit drug use disorders [32], and the improvement of mood and overall life quality of those with SUD [13]. A few articles also reviewed the relationship between various type of physical exercises as promising complementary therapies for SUD [33,34]. To further understand the relationship between physical exercise intervention and SUD, several statistical review articles have analyzed the effects of acute exercise on nicotine addiction. For example, Ussher *et al.* found that physical exercise can effectively intervene in symptoms related to smoking (RR: 0.97–4.96) using meta-analyses on thirteen [36] and fifteen [37] original research articles, while others reported similar results using analyses of individual participant data (IPD) or the systematic review method [38]. Together, these studies provide the support for using physical exercise as a treatment for SUD. However, there is a shortage of important evidence in previously published meta-analyses of physical exercise as treatments in SUD, such as the effect of mind-body exercise or chronic physical exercise on substance addiction with one or polydrugs, as well as a systematic evaluation of randomized controlled trials (RCT). A recent study reported that Yoga, a typical mind-body exercise, may improve mood status and quality of life for women undergoing detoxification for heroin dependence [39]. In addition, subjects who are addicted to more than one drug often develop more complicated symptoms related to the synergistic effect of drug-drug interaction on brain structures and functions [40]. It is known that acute exercise produces different effects on brain function, such as cognition, than long-term routing exercises, which can lead to improvement of object recognition memory and reduction of perceived stress [41]. Indeed, both acute and chronic aerobic exercises have been extensively used to treat SUD. The changes induced by acute exercise can be viewed as a transitory modulation of the arousal physiology [42], while effects of chronic physical exercise are generally explained by structural and durable changes in the organism, such as angiogenesis [43] and neurogenesis [44]. All of these may help to explain the contradictory findings on exercise intervention in SUD.

The aim of this meta-analysis is to verify the treatment effects of chronic physical exercise on various SUD by analyzing the current RCT studies. The abstinence rate, withdrawal symptoms, anxiety levels, and depression levels are included in this meta-analysis as outcomes of treatment. Furthermore, we also included the analyses of exercise intensities, exercise types, and lasting effects of physical exercise on SUD. Lastly, we performed sub-group analyses to provide details of potential optimal physical exercise therapies for specific drug addictions.

Methods

This meta-analysis followed the PRISMA guidelines [45] for conducting and reporting systematic reviews.

Search strategy

We conducted a search for relevant literature in the following electronic databases: PubMed, Web of Science, Elsevier, China National Knowledge Infrastructure (CNKI), and China Info. The key search words included exercise, physical activity, qigong, tai chi, yoga, heroin, morphine, opioid, opiate, cocaine, methadone, marijuana, cannabis, alcohol, drinker, cigarette, smoke, nicotine, drug abuse, drug dependence, and substance use. The search was limited to Chinese and English literature studying adults (≥18 years old) published from January 1990 to August 2013.

Study selection and quality assessment

During reviewing relevant papers, data extraction and analysis complied in accordance to the following standards: (1) The selected papers were studying physical exercise intervention's effect on drug abuse, excluding preventive studies. (2) All research use RCT. (3) Objects of the study were adults over 18 years old who were assessed as alcohol, nicotine, and illicit drug abusers through the DSM-III(R)/IV. (4) Excluding the studies on acute exercise, we selected results from chronic physical exercise experimental studies. (5) The primary outcome measures in the study included the rate of abstinence from drug addiction, withdrawal symptoms, the level of depression, and anxiety. (6) The baseline of the primary outcome measures in the study and descriptive statistical data after intervention must be obtainable.

The Delphi List Criteria was used to [46] assess the quality of each literature included in the meta-analysis. Our literature evaluation criteria included: randomness of grouping, concealment of treatment allocation, homogeneity of baseline data, clarity of various standards, viability of using the blind method for outcome measurement, assessment tools for the main outcome, and intent treatment analysis. In the current research, items 6 and 7 in the Delphi List are not integrated in the assessment. When measuring the effect of physical exercise on SUD, treatment providers need to guide and monitor patients to execute physical exercise intervention, making a blind method impossible.

Data extraction and statistical analysis

We used an Excel spreadsheet to extract the data from the integrated literature. The data included information of participants, intervention of experimental and control groups, types of drug addiction, and primary outcome measurements. We conducted a meta-analysis through the meta package in R software (R 3.0.1 version) [47]. We used the odd ratio (OR) to assess the abstinence rate under two different conditions. Due to different follow-up intervals, we defined follow-up periods of 1–3 months, 4–7 months, and ≥8 months as short, middle, and long term, respectively. We evaluated the treatment effect by measuring abstinence rates at the end of physical exercise and throughout different follow-up periods, and then conducted a sub-group analysis based on different follow-up phases. We also employed the standardized mean difference (SMD) to assess withdrawal symptoms, depression, and anxiety after physical exercise intervention. The confidence interval was set at 95%. A p value less than 0.05 is referred to the level of statistical significance. We used Q-test and I^2-test to assess heterogeneity. If the p value in Q-test was less than 0.05

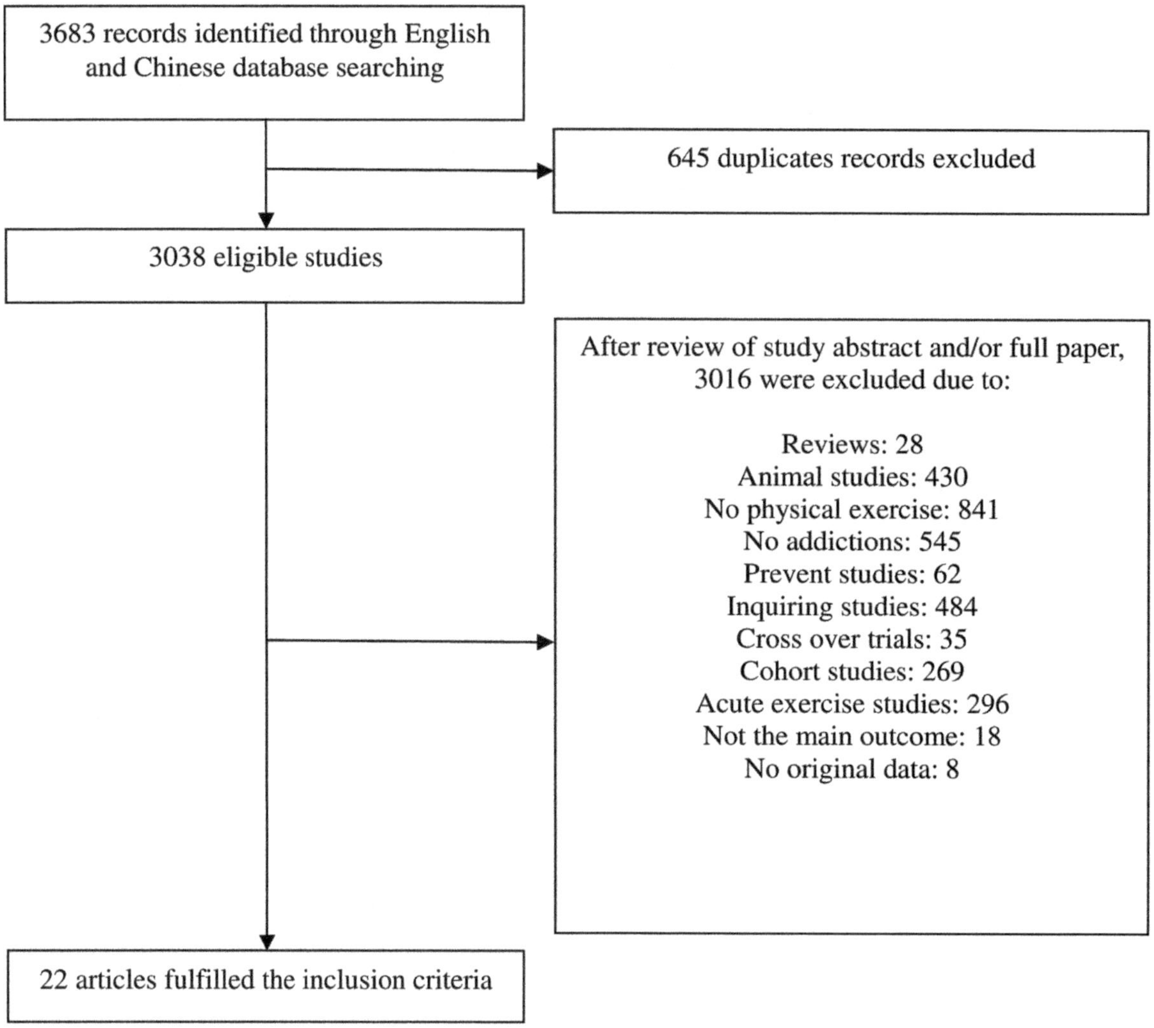

Figure 1. Flow chart of trials used in the study.

or if the I^2 index in I^2-test was more than 50%, the data was judged to achieve heterogeneity [48,49]. If there was heterogeneity, the random effects model was chosen in the meta-analysis; otherwise, the fixed effects model was used. Given the heterogeneity in the study, we rendered sensitivity analysis. We employed the funnel plot visual, Egger's test, and false safe number ($N_{fs0.05}$) to assess publication bias in the meta-analysis including more than ten papers [50]. In addition, we performed sub-group analysis according to certain characteristics of participants in the studies (physical exercise intensity, physical exercise type, addictive type, and follow-up period).

Authors WYQ and WYY completed the screening of the literature, data extraction, quality analysis, and statistical analysis process independently. Meetings were held regularly to minimize the risk of error in each link. In case of conflicts between two authors in any process, the final decision was made by another author.

Results

Included trials

Based on the selection criteria, we derived 22 out of 3683 studies for meta-analysis. The flow diagram of identification, screening and the inclusion of studies was shown (see Figure 1). One doctoral dissertation was selected [26], and the original data of one study was provided by contacting the author [51]. Five papers from 22 studies investigated the treatment effects of physical exercise on illicit drug abusers [39,51–54], eleven on nicotine abusers [27,55–64], three on alcohol abusers [26,65,66], and four on polydrug abusers of alcohol, nicotine, and illicit drugs [26,67–69]. Table 1 shows the specific characteristics of the included studies. Among all the studies, abstinence rate was regarded as the primary outcome measure with four reporting only the abstinence rate or abstinence population after physical exercise intervention [52,53,64,67]. Other papers reported abstinence conditions immediately after intervention and in different follow-up periods. Moreover, five papers reported withdrawal symptoms [51–54,57], seven papers described changes in anxiety levels before and after physical exercise intervention [26,51,53,57,63,66,69], and nine present variety in depression levels before and after physical exercise intervention [26,27,39,53,54,63,65,66,69].

Methodological Quality of Included Studies

Delphi List Criteria, which assesses the quality of RCT methodology [46], was used for quality assessment of all studies. Scores of quality ranged from 4 to 7 (see Table 2), which indicated

Table 1. Characteristics of included studies.

Article	Substance	Group	N	Age	Gender	Race	Physical Exercise					Outcome measure
							Type	Intensity	Duration	Frequency	Each time	
Burling (1992) [67]	Illicit drug, alcohol	Exp	34	38.8	2.9%F	50%Black; 41%Caucasian	Softball	NR	30 day	1/Wks	NR	Abstinent rate[a]
		Ctrl	61	NR	NR	NR	No Exercise	NR	30 day	NR	NR	
Marcus (1995) [55]	Nicotine	Exp	10	39	F	NR	Walking, rowing, cycle ergometry	70–85% HR max	12 week	3/Wks	30–45 min	Abstinent rate[a]
		Ctrl	10	36	F	NR	Education meeting	NR	12 week	1/Wks	30–45 min	
Donaghy (1997) [26]	Alcoholic,	Exp	80	41.3	25%F	NR	Aerobic exercise, strengthening	NR	3 week	3/Wks	30 min	Abstinent rate[a]; BDI; STAI(state)
		Ctrl	78	41.7	25%F	NR	Breathing	NR	3 week	3/Wks	30 min	
Martin (1997) [68]	Nicotine, alcohol, illicit drug	Exp	72	40.5	43%F	90.4%Caucasian	Walking	Moderate	8 week	3/Wks	15–45 min	Abstinent rate[a]
		Ctrl	70	41.5	46%F	95.7%Caucasian	Standard treatment	NR	8 week	NR	60–70 min	
Marcus (1999) [56]	Nicotine	Exp	134	40.7	F	NR	Walking, rowing, cycle ergometry	69–85% HR max	12 week	3/Wks	40 min	Abstinent rate[a]
		Ctrl	147	39.7	F	NR	Education meeting	NR	12 week	1/Wks	30 min	
Huang (2000a) [52]	Heroin	Exp	60	NR	30%F	Asia/Chinese	Jogging	40–70% $VO_{2\ max}$	10 day	3/Wks	40–60 min	Withdrawal symptoms[c]; Abstinent rate[a]
		Ctrl	60	NR	33%F	Asia/Chinese	Daily life	7–8 Borg[b]	10 day	NR	NR	
Huang (2000b) [53]	Heroin	Exp	60	27.0	30%F	Asia/Chinese	Brisk walking	50–60% $VO_{2\ max}$	6 month	3/Wks	40–60 min	Withdrawal symptoms[c]; Abstinent rate[a]; SAS; SDS
		Ctrl	50	28.2	27%F	Asia/Chinese	Daily life	9–10 Borg[c]	6 month	NR	NR	
Li (2002) [51]	Heroin	Exp	34	33.3	M	Asia/Chinese	Qi Gong	NR	10 day	4–5/D	25–30 min	Withdrawal symptoms[c]; HAS
		Ctrl	26	31.7	M	Asia/Chinese	NR	NR	10 day	NR	NR	
Ussher (2003) [57]	Nicotine	Exp	154	41.5	53%F	87.9%Caucasian	'Life-style' or more structured exercise	40% HR max	6 week	5/Wks	5–30 min	Withdrawal symptoms[d]; Abstinent rate[a] MPSS
		Ctrl	145	44.4	53%F	87.9%Caucasian	Health education	NR	6 week	1/Wks	5–30 min	
Marcus (2005) [58]	Nicotine	Exp	109	42.5	F	82.5%Caucasian; 6.9%Black	Aerobic training	50–69% HR max	8 week	4/Wks	30–45 min	Abstinent rate[a]

Table 1. Cont.

Article	Substance	Group	N	Age	Gender	Race	Physical Exercise					Outcome measure
							Type	Intensity	Duration	Frequency	Each time	
		Ctrl	108	43.0	F	82.5%Caucasian; 6.9%Black	Health education	NR	8 week	NR	30–45 min	
Vedamurthachar (2006) [65]	Alcohol	Exp	30	35.6	M	NR	Sudarshana Kriya Yoga	NR	2 week	NR	60 min	BDI
		Ctrl	30	37.7	M	NR	No intervention	NR	2 week	NR	NR	
Sareen (2007) [66]	Alcohol	Exp	26	50	14%F	NR	Iyengar Yoga	NR	12 week	2/Wks	60 min	POMS
		Ctrl	26	50	14%F	NR	Usual care	NR	12 week	NR	NR	
Prapavessis (2007) [59]	Nicotine	Exp	76	37.9	F	NR	Walking, rowing, cycle ergometry	60–75% HR max	12 week	3/Wks	45 min	Abstinent rate[a]
		Ctrl	66	38.2	NR	NR	Cognitive behavior therapy	NR	12 week	NR	NR	
Ussher (2007) [60]	Nicotine	Exp	154	41.5	53%F	87.9%Caucasian	'Life-style' or more structured exercise	40% HR max	6 week	5/Wks	5–30 min	Abstinent rate[a]
		Ctrl	145	44.4	53%F	87.9%Caucasian	Health education	NR	6 week	1/Wks	5–30 min	
Kinnunen (2008) [61]	Nicotine	Exp	92	38.3	F	81.5%Caucasian	Treadmill	60–80% HR max	19 week	1–2/Wks	30 min	Abstinent rate[a]
		Ctrl	34	39.9	F	75.8%Caucasian	Standard treatment	NR	19 week	NR	30 min	
Vickers (2009) [27]	Nicotine	Exp	30	41.8	F	Caucasian	Exercise	NR	10 week	5/Wks	30 min	Abstinent rate[a]; HRSD
		Ctrl	30	40.9	F	97%Caucasian	Health counseling	NR	10 week	1/Wks	30 min	
Williams (2010) [62]	Nicotine	Exp	29	41.5	F	83.3%Caucasian	Treadmill	70% HR max	8 week	3/Wks	50 min	Abstinent rate[a]
		Ctrl	30	43.3	F	86.7%Caucasian	Wellness videos	NR	8 week	3/Wks	30 min	
Bock (2012) [63]	Nicotine	Exp	32	43.8	F	88%Caucasian	Yoga	NR	8 week	2/Wks	60 min	Abstinent rate[a]; STAIT; CESD
		Ctrl	23	48.1	F	74%Caucasian	Wellness sessions	NR	8 week	NR	NR	
Whiteley (2012) [64]	Nicotine	Exp	166	44.1	F	NR	Aerobic & resistance training	77–85% HR max	12 week	1/Wks	40–60 min	Abstinent rate[a]
		Ctrl	164	42.9	F	NR	Wellness session	NR	12 week	NR	NR	
Li (2013) [54]	Heroin	Exp	17	30.3	F	Asia/Chinese	Tai Chi	NR	150 day	1–2/D	60 min	Withdrawal symptoms[c]; HRSD
		Ctrl	16	29.6	F	Asia/Chinese	Daily life	NR	150 day	NR	NR	
Smelson (2013) [69]	Cocaine, alcohol	Exp	51	30.6	4%F	60%Caucasian; 35%Black	Qi Gong	NR	14 day	2–3/Wks	15 min	SAIS(state); BDI
		Ctrl	50	40.4	4%F	60%Caucasian; 35%Black	Sham Qi Gong	NR	14 day	NR	15 min	

Table 1. Cont.

Article	Substance	Group	N	Age	Gender	Race	Physical Exercise					Outcome measure
							Type	Intensity	Duration	Frequency	Each time	
Zhuang (2013) [39]	Heroin	Exp	37	29.1	F	Asia/Chinese	Yoga	NR	6 month	5/Wks	50 min	POMS(depression)
		Ctrl	38	27.8	F	Asia/Chinese	Hospital routine care	NR	6 month	NR	NR	

Exp: Experimental; Ctrl: Control; F: Female subjects; NR: No Reported; HR: Heart Rate; $VO_{2\ max}$: maximal oxygen consumption; BDI: Beck Depression Inventory; SAIS: State-Trait Anxiety Inventory-State; TAIS: Trait Anxiety Inventory-State; SAS: Self-Rating Anxiety Scale; SDS: Self-rating depression scale; HAS: Hamilton Anxiety Scores; MPSS: Mood and Physical Symptoms Scale-anxiety; HRSD: Hamilton Rating Scale for Depression; CESD: Center for Epidemiologic Studies Depression Scale; POMS: Profile of Mood States.

[a] Continual abstinence;
[b] Borg index;
[c] Rating scale of heroin withdrawal symptoms;
[d] Tobacco withdrawal symptoms.

that the bias of the study was relatively low. Some authors did not clearly report the experimental information such as whether the assessment of outcome adopted the blind method, or if sufficient concealment was made in the allocation of participants.

Effect of physical exercise on abstinence rate

We conducted a meta-analysis of the abstinence rate for SUD at the end of the physical exercise treatment, the short-term (≤3 months), middle-term (4–7 months) and long-term (≥8 months) follow-up periods after the intervention. The Q test ($Q(31) = 36.64$, $p = 0.22$) and I^2 test ($I^2 = 15.4\%$) revealed no heterogeneity in any of the studies. The meta-analysis of the fixed effects model shows that physical exercise can significantly increase the abstinence rate in subjects with SUD (OR = 1.69 (95% CI: 1.44, 1.99), $z = 6.33$, $p < 0.001$) (see Figure 2). There was no evidence of publication bias upon using Egger's test ($z = 1.02$, $p = 0.31$) and a false safe number ($N_{fs0.05} = 351$). Table 3 shows the result of sub-group analysis indicating the effect of physical exercise intervention on the abstinence rate in various follow-up periods having no significant difference. The effect of physical exercise intensity and type of physical exercise on abstinence rate is not significantly different. However, there is strong evidence indicating the special effect of physical exercise on various addictive drugs. The treatment effect of physical exercise on drug abusers is better than its effect on alcohol and nicotine abusers (see Table 3).

Effect of physical exercise on withdrawal symptoms

We conducted a meta-analysis on withdrawal symptoms in drug abusers after physical exercise intervention. The Q test ($Q(4) = 151.4$, $p < 0.001$) and I^2 test ($I^2 = 97.4\%$) showed heterogeneity in the included studies. We chose the random effects model in meta-analysis and the result indicates that exercise can significantly ease withdrawal symptoms in subjects with SUD (SMD = −1.24 (95% CI: −2.46, −0.02), $z = -2.00$, $p < 0.05$) (see Figure 3). The sub-group analysis finds that different types of physical exercise affect withdrawal symptoms of SUD differently (see Table 3).

Effect of physical exercise on anxiety levels in subjects with SUD

We employed a meta-analysis on anxiety levels in subjects with SUD after physical exercise intervention. No evidence of heterogeneity was found based on the result of the Q test ($Q(6) = 4.17$, $p = 0.65$) and I^2 test ($I^2 = 0\%$). The meta-analysis of the fixed effects model showed that physical exercise can significantly attenuate anxiety symptoms in subjects with SUD (SMD = −0.31 (95% CI: −0.45, −0.16), $z = -4.11$, $p < 0.001$) (see Figure 4). The sub-group analysis finds that different types of physical exercise do not have significantly different effects on anxiety symptoms of addicts, and physical exercise does not differently influence the anxiety symptoms of all kinds of SUD (see Table 3).

Effect of physical exercise on depression levels in subjects with SUD

We conducted a meta-analysis on the depression level in SUD after physical exercise intervention. There was moderate heterogeneity exhibited in the studies demonstrated by the Q test ($Q(8) = 31.99$, $p < 0.001$) and I^2 test ($I^2 = 75\%$). The random effects model meta-analysis showed that physical exercise can significantly relieve depression symptoms in SUD (SMD = −0.47 (95% CI: −0.80, −0.14), $z = -2.76$, $p < 0.01$) (see Figure 5). The sub-group analysis indicated that the effect of physical exercise on the

Table 2. Assessment of Methodological Quality of Included Studies.

	Randomization[a]	Similar at baseline[b]	Criteria specified[c]	Assessor blinded[d]	Allocation concealment[e]	Variability outcome[f]	ITA[g]	Total score
Burling (1992) [67]	Unknown	YES	YES	Unknown	YES	YES	YES	5
Marcus (1995) [55]	YES	YES	YES	Unknown	Unknown	YES	YES	5
Donaghy (1997) [26]	YES	YES	YES	Unknown	Unknown	YES	YES	5
Martin (1997) [68]	YES	YES	YES	Unknown	YES	YES	NO	5
Marcus (1999) [56]	YES	YES	YES	YES	Unknown	YES	YES	6
Huang (2000a) [52]	YES	YES	YES	YES	Unknown	YES	NO	5
Huang (2000b) [53]	YES	YES	YES	YES	Unknown	YES	YES	6
Li (2002) [51]	YES	YES	YES	Unknown	Unknown	YES	YES	5
Ussher (2003) [57]	YES	YES	YES	Unknown	Unknown	YES	YES	5
Marcus (2005) [58]	YES	YES	YES	Unknown	Unknown	YES	YES	5
Char (2006) [65]	YES	YES	YES	YES	Unknown	YES	YES	6
Sareen (2007) [66]	YES	YES	YES	NO	Unknown	YES	YES	5
Prapavessis (2007) [59]	YES	YES	YES	YES	Unknown	YES	YES	6
Ussher (2007) [60]	YES	YES	YES	YES	YES	YES	YES	7
Kinnunen (2008) [61]	YES	YES	YES	Unknown	YES	YES	NO	5
Vickers (2009) [27]	YES	YES	YES	Unknown	YES	YES	NO	5
Williams (2010) [62]	YES	YES	YES	Unknown	Unknown	YES	NO	4
Bock (2012) [63]	YES	YES	YES	Unknown	Unknown	YES	YES	5
Whiteley (2012) [64]	YES	YES	YES	Unknown	YES	YES	YES	6

Table 2. Cont.

	Randomization[a]	Similar at baseline[b]	Criteria specified[c]	Assessor blinded[d]	Allocation concealment[e]	Variability outcome[f]	ITA[g]	Total score
Li (2013) [54]	YES	YES	YES	Unknown	YES	YES	NO	5
Smelson (2013) [69]	YES	YES	YES	Unknown	Unknown	YES	NO	4
Zhuang (2013) [39]	YES	YES	YES	Unknown	YES	YES	NO	5

[a] Was randomization performed?
[b] Were the groups similar at baseline regarding important prognostic indicators?
[c] Were the eligibility criteria specified?
[d] Was the outcome assessor blinded?
[e] Was allocation concealment adequate?
[f] Were point estimates and measures of variability presented for the primary outcome measures?
[g] Did the analysis include an intention to treat analysis?

depression symptoms of SUD is not significantly different. However, physical exercise does have a significant relief effect on depression symptoms in alcohol and illicit drug abusers (see Table 3).

Discussion

Summary of main results

Based on our knowledge, our statistical review of physical exercise in SUD is the first meta-analysis article on the treatment effects of chronic physical exercise on alcohol, nicotine, and illicit drugs in human studies. Our meta-analysis assesses the effects of various forms of physical exercises on SUD in the following four aspects: abstinence rate, withdrawal symptoms, anxiety, and depression level. Compared to the treatment effects on alcohol and nicotine abusers, chronic physical exercises can better increase the abstinence rate in illicit drugs abusers. Meanwhile, physical exercise (aerobic exercise and mind-body exercise) can effectively attenuate withdrawal symptoms and ease anxiety symptoms in alcohol, nicotine and illicit drug addictions, while physical exercise-induced improvement of depression symptoms was only observed in illicit drug abusers. Furthermore, there are no significant differences in exercise-induced treatment on SUD between exercise types (aerobics vs. mind-body exercise), nor among different levels of physical exercise intensities (low, moderate, and high intensity). Overall, physical exercise can effectively assist abusers with withdrawing from addictive drugs. The result of this meta-analysis is not only consistent with the previous meta-analysis results from a single acute physical exercise treatment for SUD [38,70], but it also complies with the result of several review articles [18,29,32].

Specificity of physical exercise on different addictive drugs. There are three types of addictive substances included in this analysis. They are alcohol, nicotine, and illicit drugs that induce strong dependence in human beings and could result in abuse. Since the different addictive mechanisms of these three substances may be involved, we performed sub-group analyses on each addictive substance independently. Indeed, we found that exercise affects the abstinence rate of illicit drugs more than that of alcohol and nicotine abuse. The possible cause for this result may be the difference in addictive mechanisms for each of the three addictive substances. For example, opioid drugs (morphine, heroin, etc.) take effect through β-endorphin neurotransmitters activating the μ and δ opium receptors [71]. Alcohol takes effect through promoting the reaction of the GABAA receptor [72] and increasing stimulation to the dopamine and opiate receptor [73,74]. Nicotine takes effect through acetylcholine neurotransmitters activating the α2β4nACh receptor [75–77].

Physical exercise intensity for effectively treating drug abuse. The sub-group analysis indicated no significant difference in the abstinence rate among low-, moderate-, and high-intensity long-term physical exercise. It is mean that all three exercise intensities induce similar levels of abstinence rate reduction in alcohol, nicotine and illicit drug abusers. Correspondingly, non-RCT studies presented that long-term treadmill exercise at moderate-intensity (55–69% HR max) can effectively ease the craving for cannabis [16] and increase abstinence rate of other drugs in SUD [17]. And non-RCT studies also show that high- and moderate-intensity long-term physical exercise can significantly treat alcohol abuse. A pilot study on the treatment effects of aerobics on alcohol abusers [78] reported that 35 minutes of moderate- (HR = 50–60% VO2max) to high-intensity (HR = 80–90% VO2max) physical exercise for six weeks, can significantly reduce depression symptoms in alcohol abusers.

Study	Experimental Events	Experimental Total	Control Events	Control Total	OR	95%-CI	W(fixed)
Burling,1992 short	21	34	34	82	2.28	[1.01; 5.17]	3.4%
Marcus,1995 end	3	10	1	10	3.86	[0.33; 45.57]	0.3%
Marcus,1995 long	3	10	1	10	3.86	[0.33; 45.57]	0.3%
Donaghy,1997 middle	10	20	8	21	1.62	[0.47; 5.63]	1.7%
Donaghy,1997 short	11	35	9	29	1.02	[0.35; 2.95]	3.0%
Martin,1997 end	43	72	22	70	3.24	[1.62; 6.45]	4.0%
Martin,1997 middle	21	72	15	70	1.51	[0.70; 3.24]	4.7%
Martin,1997 long	19	72	18	70	1.04	[0.49; 2.19]	5.9%
Marcus,1999 end	26	134	15	147	2.12	[1.07; 4.20]	5.1%
Marcus,1999 short	22	134	12	147	2.21	[1.05; 4.66]	4.2%
Marcus,1999 long	16	134	8	147	2.36	[0.97; 5.70]	3.0%
Huang,2000a long	15	38	4	51	7.66	[2.28; 25.71]	0.9%
Huang,2000b long	27	60	6	50	6.00	[2.22; 16.20]	1.6%
Ussher,2003 end	73	154	63	145	1.17	[0.74; 1.85]	15.0%
Marcus,2005 end	16	109	12	108	1.38	[0.62; 3.07]	4.5%
Marcus,2005 short	8	109	4	108	2.06	[0.60; 7.05]	1.6%
Marcus,2005 long	1	109	1	108	0.99	[0.06; 16.04]	0.4%
Prapavessis,2007 end	17	49	16	59	1.43	[0.63; 3.25]	4.2%
Prapavessis,2007 short	7	20	9	33	1.44	[0.43; 4.75]	1.9%
Prapavessis,2007 long	3	9	4	15	1.38	[0.23; 8.30]	0.9%
Ussher,2007 long	14	154	18	145	0.71	[0.34; 1.48]	7.4%
Kinnunen,2008 end	22	91	5	34	1.85	[0.64; 5.36]	2.4%
Kinnunen,2008 long	9	92	2	34	1.73	[0.36; 8.47]	1.2%
Vickers,2009 end	3	19	4	20	0.75	[0.14; 3.90]	1.4%
Williams,2010 end	10	29	5	30	2.63	[0.77; 8.99]	1.4%
Williams,2010 short	6	29	4	30	1.70	[0.42; 6.77]	1.4%
Bock,2012 end	15	32	4	23	4.19	[1.16; 15.11]	1.1%
Bock,2012 short	7	32	2	23	2.94	[0.55; 15.70]	0.8%
Bock,2012 middle	7	32	3	23	1.87	[0.43; 8.16]	1.2%
Whiteley,2012 end	23	166	23	164	0.99	[0.53; 1.84]	8.8%
Whiteley,2012 short	12	166	9	164	1.34	[0.55; 3.28]	3.7%
Whiteley,2012 middle	10	166	6	164	1.69	[0.60; 4.76]	2.5%
Fixed effect model		**2392**		**2334**	**1.69**	**[1.44; 1.99]**	**100%**

Heterogeneity: I-squared=15.4%, tau-squared=0.0426, p=0.2234

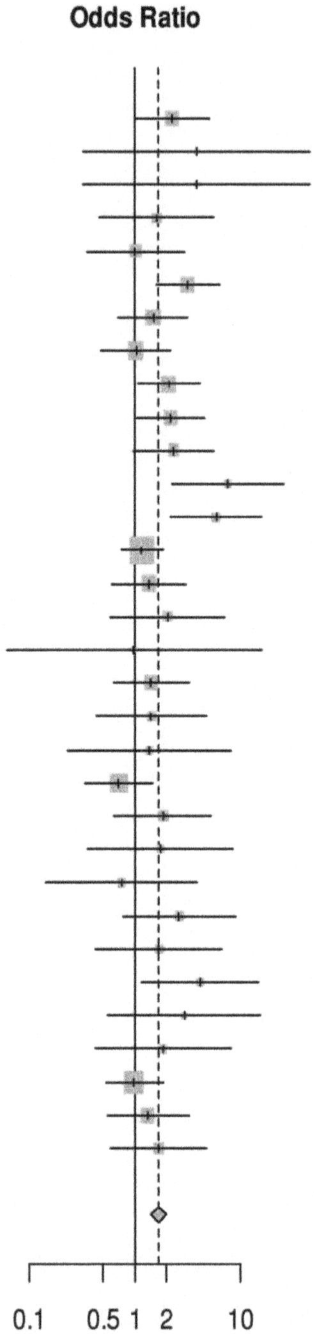

Figure 2. The forest plot about the effect of physical exercise on abstinence rate. The abstinence rate of past physical exercise treat, and differences follow-up periods were used odds ratio analysis.

Another cross-over design study showed that moderate-intensity fast walking can significantly enhance self-management techniques in alcohol abusers [79,80]. The results of the above-mentioned study further proved the findings of our meta-analysis. While the mechanisms underlying these results remain unclear, moderate- and high-intensity aerobic exercises have significant effects on SUD. Mind-body exercises are included as low-intensity physical exercise in this meta-analysis. Due to the different nature of mind-body exercises compared to classical running and walking, we have included the analyses of mind-body exercises in SUD independently in the sections below.

Persistency of treatment effects of physical exercise on SUD. To investigate the long lasting effects of exercise on SUD, we conducted a sub-group analysis to evaluate the treatment effects of physical exercise in different follow-up periods. As shown in Table 3, there is no significant difference in exercise-induced reduction of the abstinence rate among the different follow-up periods,suggesting that physical exercise leaves a long lasting treatment effect on SUD. The results of two meta-analyses [36,37]

Table 3. Sub-group analysis results.

	Sample size	N of studies	Meta-analytic effect size			Heterogeneity	
	(Exp/Ctrl)		SMD/OR(95%-CI)	Q(d.f.)	p	I^2	Q
Abstinence rate							
Intensity type							
low	96/69	3	2.96(1.29,6.83)	1.91(2)	0.3841	0%	0.66
moderate	1193/1244	19	1.62(1.32,1.98)			36.8%	28.49
high	1103/1021	10	1.71(1.28,2.29)			0%	5.47
Physical exercise type							
aerobic Ex	2296/2265	29	1.65(1.40,1.95)	1.82(1)	0.177	17.9%	34.10
mind-body Ex	96/69	3	2.96(1.29,6.83)			0%	0.66
Follow-up period							
end	865/810	11	1.60(1.26,2.02)	0.57(3)	0.9027	23.8%	13.12
short-term	559/616	8	1.79(1.25,2.56)			0%	2.65
middle-term	290/278	4	1.62(0.96,2.71)			0%	0.07
long-term	678/630	9	1.84(1.30,2.59)			60.9%	20.45
Addict type							
alcohol	271/260	5	1.65(1.14,2.39)	11.51(2)	0.0032**	33.1%	5.98
illicit drug	132/183	3	4.13(2.39,7.14)			43.9%	3.56
nicotine	1989/1891	24	1.51(1.24,1.83)			0%	16.40
Withdrawal symptoms							
Physical exercise type							
aerobic Ex	274/255	3	−1.67(−3.51, 0.17)	0.71 (1)	0.399	98.5%	2.59
mind-body Ex	51/42	2	−0.61(−2.25,1.03)			92.6%	1.30
Anxiety							
Addict type							
alcohol	61/55	2	−0.21(−0.58, 0.16)	1.03(2)	0.5975	37.9%	1.61
illicit drug	145/126	3	−0.40(−0.64, −0.16)			0%	1.41
nicotine	186/168	2	−0.26(−0.47, −0.05)			0%	0.13
Physical exercise type							
aerobic Ex	249/224	3	−0.29(−0.47, −0.11)	0.06(1)	0.8065	21.1%	2.54
mind-body Ex	143/125	4	−0.33(−0.57, −0.09)			0%	1.57
Depression							
Physical exercise type							
aerobic Ex	132/117	3	−0.43(−0.84, −0.03)	0.04(1)	0.838	59.4%	4.93
mind-body Ex	186/175	6	−0.50(−1.00, −0.01)			81.5%	27.03
Addict type							

Table 3. Cont.

	Sample size	N of studies	Meta-analytic effect size			Heterogeneity	
	(Exp/Ctrl)		SMD/OR(95%-CI)	*Q(d.f.)*	*p*	I^2	*Q*
alcohol	91/85	3	−0.77(−1.73,0.19)	8.21(2)	0.0165*	89.2%	18.52
illicit drug	165/154	4	−0.51(−0.73, −0.28)			0%	2.81
nicotine	62/53	2	0.10(−0.27, 0.46)			0%	0.01

Exp: Experimental; Ctrl: Control; Ex: Exercise; SMD: Standardized Mean Difference; OR: Odds Ratio; CI: Confidence Interval.
$*p<0.05$, $**p<0.01$

studies have also shown obvious treatment effects in 3 and 12 months follow-up periods. These results are likely due to the long lasting effect of physical exercise on changes in brain structure and function. For instance,studies showed that physical exercise can regulate the gene transcription of endogenous opium brain-derived neurotrophic factor (BDNF) by activating the cyclic AMP response element-binding (CREB) protein [81] and synaptic plasticity [82,83], which is critical for rehabilitation for patients with SUD via promoting repair of drug-induced neuronal damage [84] and improving corresponding brain functions [85]. This neuronal structural change induced by exercises might contribute a long lasting effect on SUD.

Different effects of various forms of physical exercises. In addition to aerobic exercises, mind-body exercises are also acceptable and easy to apply in treatment for drug abuse. The sub-group analysis showed that mind-body exercises and aerobic exercises induce similar beneficial effects on the abstinence rate, withdrawal symptoms, anxiety, and depression levels in subjects with SUD (see Table 3). The outcome from our analysis is consistent with previously published literatures, suggesting that mind-body exercises can also effectively facilitate the treatment of drug addiction [35].

In terms of exercise intensity, some studies have shown that the intensity of Tai Chi Quan is about 52–63% HR max [86], which is similar to low- or moderate-intensity aerobic exercises [87–89]. Meanwhile, Qigong [90] and Yoga [91,92] are also regarded as low- and moderate-intensity physical exercises. Therefore, both mind-body exercise and aerobic exercise show similar beneficial effects on drug addiction when administered at low- or moderate-intensities as shown in Table 3. In addition to exercise intensity, the particular characteristics of mind-body exercise, namely meditation and breathing exercises, may be the key reasons for producing significant exercise effectiveness [93,94].

Physical exercise inducing emotional improvement in SUD. The meta-analysis indicates that physical exercise can effectively ease anxiety and depression symptoms in subjects with SUD. The sub-group analysis shows that physical exercises reduce anxiety symptoms in nicotine, alcohol and illicit drug abusers, while significant exercise-induced improvement on depression symptoms was only found in alcohol and illicit drug abusers (see Table 3). Our findings are consistent with previously published review articles which also found that physical exercise can effectively ease anxiety symptoms in subjects with SUD [29,32,95].

However, we also included three studies that reported that physical exercise did not reduce depression symptoms in nicotine and alcohol abusers [27,63]. As the number of the RCT studies included in our meta-analysis is limited, it is insufficient to make a valid conclusion of whether exercise reduces depression symptoms in subjects with SUD. However, some review articles claim that physical exercise could attenuate depression symptoms in alcohol and nicotine abusers based on non-RCT studies [32,70]. Hence, subsequent studies are needed for further evidence of the effect of exercise on altering depression symptoms in SUD.

Limitations

There are some limitations that need to be considered in the current meta-analysis: (1) Addictive drugs involved in the studies often include participants with polydrug use disorders. Therefore, the specific treatment of exercise on a single drug abuse is difficult to analyze. Because there are insufficient RCT studies on exercise as an intervention for alcohol and drug abuse, the results in the present meta-analysis study may need further investigation. (2) Due to the limitation of available studies, only published RCT studies from 1990 to 2013 were included. There were no

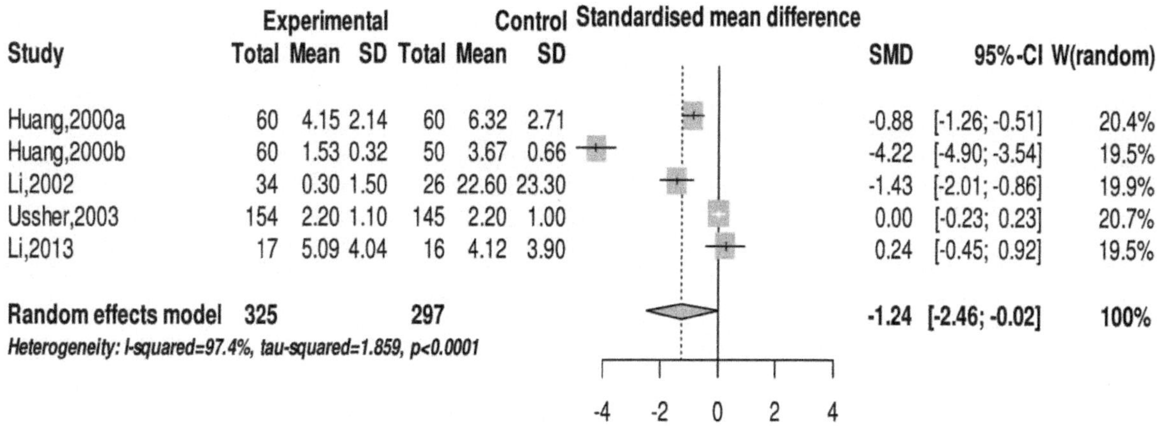

Figure 3. The forest plot about the effect of physical exercise on withdrawal symptoms.

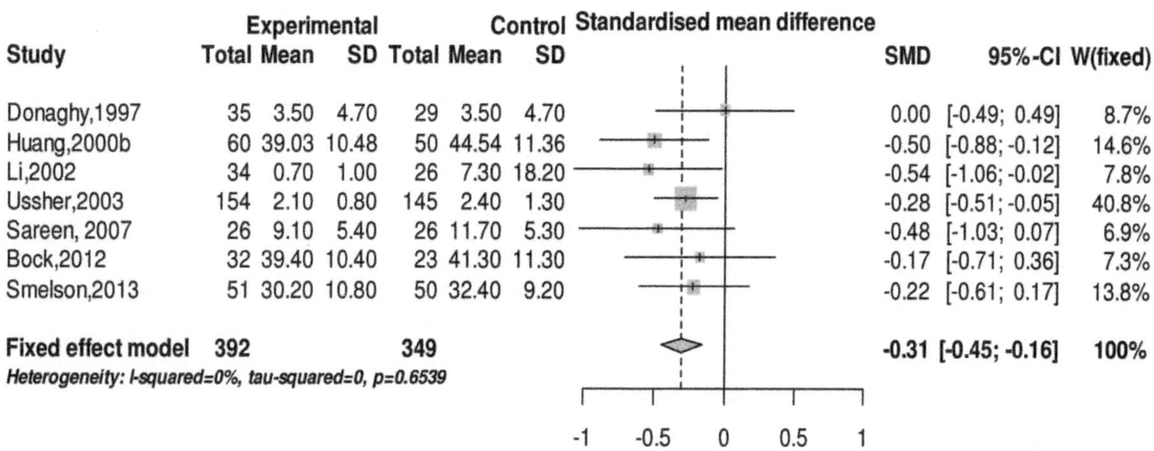

Figure 4. The forest plot about the effect of physical exercise on anxiety status.

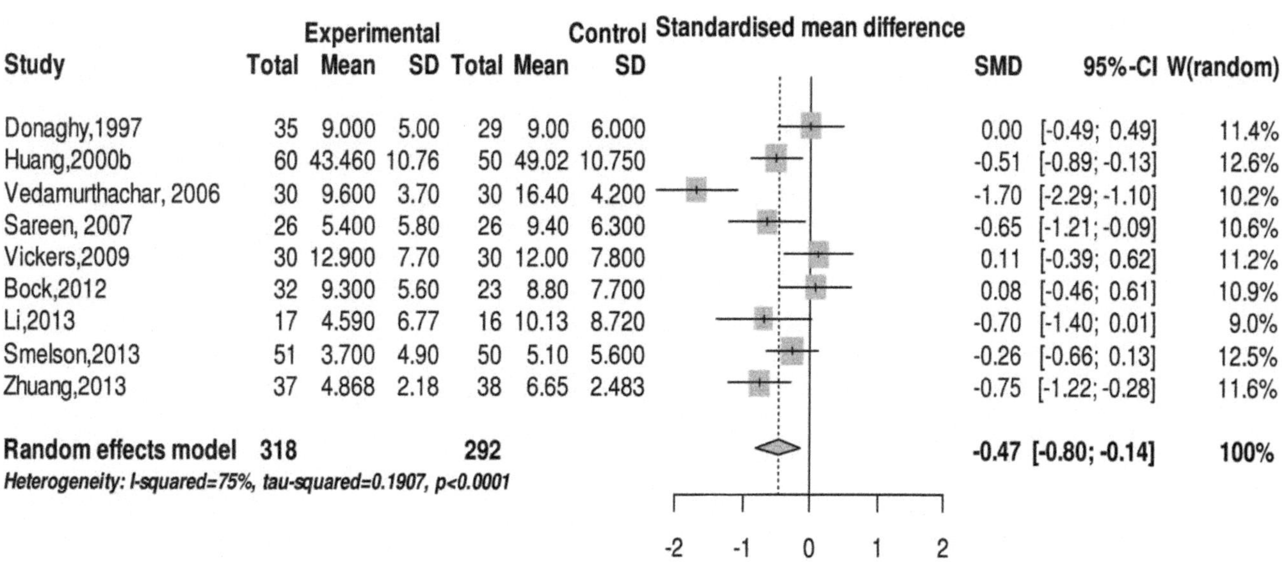

Figure 5. The forest plot about the effect of physical exercise on depression status.

unpublished papers and dissertations found. These limitations in the literature collection may cause publishing bias. (3) Some papers lack clear explanations on the study information. Such limitation affected the quality of study and the assessment of clinic-relevant data. (4) In the research, some studies comprised of mostly female participants, whereas male participants accounted for only a small part. We were unable to evaluate the differences in gender through a statistical method due to difficulty in obtaining individual data. Accordingly, compared with males, female participants have more difficulty in giving up drug addiction [95]. (5) The main outcome indices in meta-analysis include abstinence rate, withdrawal symptoms, anxiety, and depression levels; the assessment tools in the literature also varied. (6) The included studies have some risk of bias. Lacking of assessor blinding and allocation concealment was the most frequent shortcoming of these studies (See Table 2). Other limitations included the small sample size of two studies [54,55]. Although we adopted some methods (e.g., continuous variable adopts standardization mean difference method) for the assessment, certain biases listed above still exist.

Conclusions

The current meta-analysis provides strong evidence that physical exercise can be an effective adjunct treatment method for abstinence from alcohol, nicotine, and illicit drugs in abusers. Physical exercise not only increases the abstinence rate in subjects with SUD, but also eases withdrawal symptoms, anxiety, and depression symptoms. The treatment effects of physical exercise in these four aspects verify that physical exercise guidance by the American College of Sports Medicine (ACSM) [12] is an effective means for drug abstinence. Additionally, mind-body exercises (including Tai Chi Quan, Qigong, and Yoga) have similar treatment effects as to aerobic exercise. Although physical exercise has been proven effective in facilitating drug abstinence, its effects on alcohol, nicotine and illicit drug abusers are different. From the results of the meta-analysis, the effects of physical exercise on illicit drugs abusers are significantly greater compared to the others. Given the limitation of materials, these issues require further investigation.

Acknowledgments

The authors would like to thank all of the other authors for the research in which this meta-analysis was based upon; especially PhD Kevin Chen for original data resources support.

Author Contributions

Conceived and designed the experiments: DSW CLZ RL. Performed the experiments: DSW YQW YYW. Analyzed the data: DSW. Contributed reagents/materials/analysis tools: DSW YQW YYW. Wrote the paper: DSW RL YQW.

References

1. WHO (2013) Management of substance abuse. World Health Organization.
2. CNNCC (2013) Annual Report on Drug Control in China 2013. Beijing: Ministry of Public Security.
3. UNODC (2012) World Drug Report 2012. United Nations Publication.
4. Deng Q, Tang Q, Schottenfeld RS, Hao W, Chawarski MC (2012) Drug use in rural China: a preliminary investigation in Hunan Province. Addiction 107: 610–613.
5. Joseph H, Stancliff S, Langrod J (2000) Methadone Maintenance Treatment (MMT):A Review of Historical and Clinical Issues. The Mount Sinai Journal of Medicine 67: 347–364.
6. Mattick RP, Kimber J, Breen C, Davoli M (2014) Buprenorphine maintenance versus placebo or methadone maintenance for opioid dependence. Cochrane database of systematic reviews.
7. Fischer B, Rehm J, Rgen U, Kim G, Kirst M (2004) Eyes wide shut?-A conceptual and empirical critique of methadone maintenance treatment. European addiction research 11: 1–14.
8. Maruyama A, Macdonald S, Borycki E, Zhao J (2013) Hypertension, chronic obstructive pulmonary disease, diabetes and depression among older methadone maintenance patients in British Columbia. Drug and alcohol review 32: 412–418.
9. Fareed A, Casarella J, Amar R, Vayalapalli S, Drexler K (2009) Benefits of retention in methadone maintenance and chronic medical conditions as risk factors for premature death among older heroin addicts. Journal of Psychiatric Practice 15: 227–234.
10. Wapf V, Schaub M, Klaeusler B, Boesch L, Stohler R, et al. (2008) The barriers to smoking cessation in Swiss methadone and buprenorphine-maintained patients. Harm reduction journal 5: 1–7.
11. Corbin CB, Pangrazi RP, Franks BD (2000) Definitions: Health, Fitness, and Physical Activity. President's Council on Physical Fitness and Sports Research Digest.
12. Thompson WR, Gordon NF, Pescatello LS (2009) ACSM's guidelines for exercise testing and prescription: Hubsta Ltd.
13. Weinstock J, Wadeson HK, VanHeest JL (2012) Exercise as an adjunct treatment for opiate agonist treatment: review of the current research and implementation strategies. Substance Abuse 33: 350–360.
14. Ströhle A, Höfler M, Pfister H, Müller AG, Hoyer J, et al. (2007) Physical activity and prevalence and incidence of mental disorders in adolescents and young adults. Psychological medicine 37: 1657–1666.
15. Korhonen T, Kujala UM, Rose RJ, Kaprio J (2009) Physical activity in adolescence as a predictor of alcohol and illicit drug use in early adulthood: a longitudinal population-based twin study. Twin Research and Human Genetics 12: 261–268.
16. Buchowski MS, Meade NN, Charboneau E, Park S, Dietrich MS, et al. (2011) Aerobic exercise training reduces cannabis craving and use in non-treatment seeking cannabis-dependent adults. PLoS One 6: e17465.
17. Brown RA, Abrantes AM, Read JP, Marcus BH, Jakicic J, et al. (2010) A pilot study of aerobic exercise as an adjunctive treatment for drug dependence. Mental health and physical activity 3: 27–34.
18. Sarah EL, Joseph TC, Michael U, Bess HM (2013) Exercise-based smoking cessation interventions among women. Women's Health 9: 69–84.
19. Brown RA, Abrantes AM, Read JP, Marcus BH, Jakicic J, et al. (2009) Aerobic Exercise for Alcohol Recovery: Rationale, Program Description, and Preliminary Findings. Behavior modification 33: 220–249.
20. Miladi GH, Rashidy PA, Fathollahi Y (2012) Anxiety profile in morphine-dependent and withdrawn rats: effect of voluntary exercise. Physiology & behavior 105: 195–202.
21. Lynch WJ, Piehl KB, Acosta G, Peterson AB, Hemby SE (2010) Aerobic exercise attenuates reinstatement of cocaine-seeking behavior and associated neuroadaptations in the prefrontal cortex. Biol Psychiatry 68: 774–777.
22. Sanchez V, Moore C, Brunzell D, Lynch W (2013) Effect of wheel-running during abstinence on subsequent nicotine-seeking in rats. Psychopharmacology 227: 403–411.
23. Thanos PK, Stamos J, Robison LS, Heyman G, Tucci A, et al. (2013) Daily treadmill exercise attenuates cocaine cue-induced reinstatement and cocaine induced locomotor response but increases cocaine-primed reinstatement. Behav Brain Res 239: 8–14.
24. Engelmann AJ, Aparicio MB, Kim A, Sobieraj JC, Yuan CJ, et al. (2013) Chronic wheel running reduces maladaptive patterns of methamphetamine intake: regulation by attenuation of methamphetamine-induced neuronal nitric oxide synthase. Brain Structure and Function 219: 657–672.
25. Hashemi Nosrat Abadi T, Vaghef L, Babri S, Mahmood AM, Beirami M (2013) Effects of different exercise protocols on ethanol-induced spatial memory impairment in adult male rats. Alcohol 47: 309–316.
26. Donaghy ME (1997) The investigation of exercise as an adjunct to the treatment and rehabilitation of the problem drinker: University of Glasgow.
27. Vickers KS, Patten CA, Lewis BA, Clark MM, Ussher M, et al. (2009) Feasibility of an exercise counseling intervention for depressed women smokers. Nicotine & tobacco research 11: 985–995.
28. Hillman CH, Drobes DJ (2012) Physical Activity and Cognitive Control: Implications for Drug Abuse. Child Development Perspectives 6: 367–373.
29. Lynch WJ, Peterson AB, Sanchez V, Abel J, Smith MA (2013) Exercise as a novel treatment for drug addiction: A neurobiological and stage-dependent hypothesis. Neuroscience & Biobehavioral Reviews 37: 1622–1644.
30. Pareja GH, Sanchis GF, Mayero S (2013) Exercise as an adjuvant intervention in opiate dependence. Substance Abuse 34: 87–88.

31. Smith MA, Lynch WJ (2012) Exercise as a potential treatment for drug abuse: evidence from preclinical studies. Frontiers in Psychiatry 2: 1–8.
32. Zschucke E, Heinz A, Strohle A (2012) Exercise and physical activity in the therapy of substance use disorders. ScientificWorldJournal 2012: 1–19.
33. Khanna S, Greeson JM (2013) A narrative review of yoga and mindfulness as complementary therapies for addiction. Complementary therapies in medicine 21: 244–252.
34. Posadzki P, Choi J, Lee MS, Ernst E (2014) Yoga for addictions: a systematic review of randomised clinical trials. Focus on Alternative and Complementary Therapies 19: 1–8.
35. Carim TL, Mitchell SH, Oken BS (2013) Mind–body practices: An alternative, drug-free treatment for smoking cessation? A systematic review of the literature. Drug and alcohol dependence 132: 399–410.
36. Ussher M H TA, Faulkner G (2008) Exercise interventions for smoking cessation. Cochrane Database of Systematic Reviews.
37. Ussher MH, Taylor A, Faulkner G (2012) Exercise interventions for smoking cessation. Cochrane Database Syst Rev 1: 1–50.
38. Haasova M, Warren F, Ussher M, VanRensberg K, Faulkner GC, et al. (2013) The acute effects of physical activity on cigarette cravings Systematic review and meta-analysis with individual participant data (IPD). Addiction 108: 26–37.
39. Zhuang SM, An SH, Zhao Y (2013) Yoga Effects on Mood and Quality of Life in Chinese Women Undergoing Heroin Detoxification, a Randomized Controlled Trial Nursing Research 62: 260–268.
40. Pattison LP, McIntosh S, Sexton T, Childers SR, Hemby SE (2014) Changes in dopamine transporter binding in nucleus accumbens following chronic self-administration cocaine: Heroin combinations. Synapse.
41. Hopkins ME, Davis FC, Vantieghem MR, Whalen PJ, Bucci DJ (2012) Differential effects of acute and regular physical exercise on cognition and affect. Neuroscience 215: 59–68.
42. McMorris T, Graydon J (2000) The effect of incremental exercise on cognitive performance. International Journal of Sport Psychology 31: 66–81.
43. Swain RA, Harris AB, Wiener EC, Dutka MV, Morris HD, et al. (2003) Prolonged exercise induces angiogenesis and increases cerebral blood volume in primary motor cortex of the rat. Neuroscience 117: 1037–1046.
44. van Praag H (2008) Neurogenesis and exercise: past and future directions. Neuromolecular medicine 10: 128–140.
45. Moher D, Liberati A, Tetzlaff J, Altman DG (2009) Preferred reporting items for systematic reviews and meta-analyses: the PRISMA statement. Annals of internal medicine 151: 264–269.
46. Verhagen AP, de Vet HC, de Bie RA, Kessels AG, Boers M, et al. (1998) The Delphi list: a criteria list for quality assessment of randomized clinical trials for conducting systematic reviews developed by Delphi consensus. Journal of clinical epidemiology 51: 1235–1241.
47. Team RC (2013) R: A Language and Environment for Statistical Computing. Vienna, Austria: R Foundation for Statistical Computing.
48. Higgins JP, Thompson SG, Deeks JJ, Altman DG (2003) Measuring inconsistency in meta-analyses. BMJ: British Medical Journal 327: 557–560.
49. Higgins J, Thompson SG (2002) Quantifying heterogeneity in a meta-analysis. Statistics in medicine 21: 1539–1558.
50. Egger M, Smith GD, Schneider M, Minder C (1997) Bias in meta-analysis detected by a simple, graphical test. Bmj 315: 629–634.
51. Li M, Chen K, Mo Z (2002) Use of qigong therapy in the detoxification of heroin addicts. Alternative Therapies in Health and Medicine 8: 50–59.
52. Huang H, Yang F, Yang SS, Xiao DS, Nie AH, et al. (2000) Influence of aerobic training on recovery of herion sddicts. Chinese Journal of Physical Therapy 23: 267–270.
53. Huang H, Yang F (2000) Exercise therapy adjuvant treatment of herion dependence on clinical observation. Chinese Journal of Drug Abuse Prevention and Treatment 26: 30–31.
54. Li DX, Zhuang XY, Zhang YP, Guo H, Wang Z, et al. (2013) Effects of Tai Chi on the Protracted Abstinence Syndrome: A Time Trial Analysis. The American journal of Chinese medicine 41: 43–57.
55. Marcus BH, Albrecht AE, Niaura RS, Taylor ER, Simkin LR, et al. (1995) Exercise enhances the maintenance of smoking cessation in women. Addictive Behaviors 20: 87–92.
56. Marcus BH, Albrecht AE, King TK, Parisi AF, Pinto BM, et al. (1999) The efficacy of exercise as an aid for smoking cessation in women: a randomized controlled trial. Archives of Internal Medicine 159: 1229–1235.
57. Ussher M, West R, McEwen A, Taylor A, Steptoe A (2003) Efficacy of exercise counselling as an aid for smoking cessation: a randomized controlled trial. Addiction 98: 523–532.
58. Marcus BH, Lewis BA, Hogan J, King TK, Albrecht AE, et al. (2005) The efficacy of moderate-intensity exercise as an aid for smoking cessation in women: a randomized controlled trial. Nicotine Tob Res 7: 871–880.
59. Prapavessis H, Cameron L, Baldi JC, Robinson S, Borrie K, et al. (2007) The effects of exercise and nicotine replacement therapy on smoking rates in women. Addict Behav 32: 1416–1432.
60. Ussher M, West R, McEwen A, Taylor A, Steptoe A (2007) Randomized controlled trial of physical activity counseling as an aid to smoking cessation: 12 month follow-up. Addict Behav 32: 3060–3064.
61. Kinnunen T, Leeman RF, Korhonen T, Quiles ZN, Terwal DM, et al. (2008) Exercise as an adjunct to nicotine gum in treating tobacco dependence among women. Nicotine & Tobacco Research 10: 689–703.
62. Williams DM, Whiteley JA, Dunsiger S, Jennings EG, Albrecht AE, et al. (2010) Moderate intensity exercise as an adjunct to standard smoking cessation treatment for women: a pilot study. Psychology of Addictive Behaviors 24: 349–354.
63. Bock BC, Fava JL, Gaskins R, Morrow KM, Williams DM, et al. (2012) Yoga as a complementary treatment for smoking cessation in women. J Womens Health (Larchmt) 21: 240–248.
64. Whiteley JA, Williams DM, Dunsiger S, Jennings EG, Ciccolo JT, et al. (2012) YMCA commit to quit: randomized trial outcomes. Am J Prev Med 43: 256–262.
65. Vedamurthachar A, Janakiramaiah N, Hegde JM, Shetty TK, Subbakrishna D, et al. (2006) Antidepressant efficacy and hormonal effects of Sudarshana Kriya Yoga (SKY) in alcohol dependent individuals. Journal of affective disorders 94: 249–253.
66. Sareen S, Kumari V, Gajebasia KS, Gajebasia NK (2007) Yoga: a tool for improving the quality of life in chronic pancreatitis. World Journal of Gastroenterology 13: 391.
67. Burling TA, Seidner AL, Robbins-Sisco D, Krinsky A, Hanser SB (1992) Batter up! Relapse prevention for homeless veteran substance abusers via softball team participation. Journal of Substance Abuse 4: 407–413.
68. Martin JE, Calfas KJ, Patten CA, Polarek M, Hofstetter CR, et al. (1997) Prospective evaluation of three smoking interventions in 205 recovering alcoholics: One-year results of Project SCRAP-Tobacco. Journal of Consulting and Clinical Psychology 65: 190–194.
69. Smelson D, Chen KW, Ziedonis D, Andes K, Lennox A, et al. (2013) A Pilot Study of Qigong for Reducing Cocaine Craving Early in Recovery. The Journal of Alternative and Complementary Medicine 19: 97–101.
70. Roberts V, Maddison R, Simpson C, Bullen C, Prapavessis H (2012) The acute effects of exercise on cigarette cravings, withdrawal symptoms, affect, and smoking behaviour: systematic review update and meta-analysis. Psychopharmacology (Berl) 222: 1–15.
71. Sarkar DK, Sengupta A, Zhang C, Boyadjieva N, Murugan S (2012) Opiate antagonist prevents μ-and δ-opiate receptor dimerization to facilitate ability of agonist to control ethanol-altered natural killer cell functions and mammary tumor growth. Journal of Biological Chemistry 287: 16734–16747.
72. Silveri MM (2014) GABAergic contributions to alcohol responsivity during adolescence: Insights from preclinical and clinical studies. Pharmacology & Therapeutics 143: 197–216.
73. Gilman JM, Ramchandani VA, Davis MB, Bjork JM, Hommer DW (2008) Why we like to drink: a functional magnetic resonance imaging study of the rewarding and anxiolytic effects of alcohol. The Journal of Neuroscience 28: 4583–4591.
74. Berrettini W (2013) Opioid pharmacogenetics of alcohol addiction. Alcohol: Science, Policy and Public Health 3: 97–113.
75. Dajas-Bailador F, Wonnacott S (2004) Nicotinic acetylcholine receptors and the regulation of neuronal signalling. Trends in pharmacological sciences 25: 317–324.
76. Coe JW, Brooks PR, Vetelino MG, Wirtz MC, Arnold EP, et al. (2005) Varenicline: an α4β2 nicotinic receptor partial agonist for smoking cessation. Journal of medicinal chemistry 48: 3474–3477.
77. Sala M, Braida D, Pucci L, Manfredi I, Marks MJ, et al. (2013) CC4, a dimer of cytisine, is a selective partial agonist at α4β2/α6β2 nAChR with improved selectivity for tobacco smoking cessation. British journal of pharmacology 168: 835–849.
78. Roessler KK, Bilberg R, Jensen K, Kjaergaard A-S, Dervisevic A, et al. (2013) Exercise as Treatment for Alcohol Dependence. Sport Science Review 22: 205–216.
79. Taylor AH, Oh H, Cullen S (2013) Acute effect of exercise on alcohol urges and attentional bias towards alcohol related images in high alcohol consumers. Mental Health and Physical Activity 6: 220–226.
80. Karoly HC, Stevens CJ, Thayer RE, Magnan RE, Bryan AD, et al. (2013) Aerobic Exercise Moderates the Effect of Heavy Alcohol Consumption on White Matter Damage. Alcoholism: Clinical and Experimental Research 37: 1508–1515.
81. Koo JW, Mazei-Robison MS, Chaudhury D, Juarez B, LaPlant Q, et al. (2012) BDNF is a negative modulator of morphine action. science 338: 124–128.
82. Gomez PF, Hillman C (2013) The Influence of Exercise on Cognitive Abilities. Comprehensive Physiology 3: 403–428.
83. Coelho FG, Gobbi S, Andreatto CA, Corazza DI, Pedroso RV, et al. (2013) Physical exercise modulates peripheral levels of brain-derived neurotrophic factor (BDNF): a systematic review of experimental studies in the elderly. Arch Gerontol Geriatr 56: 10–15.
84. Thomas AG, Dennis A, Bandettini PA, Johansen-Berg H (2012) The effects of aerobic activity on brain structure. Frontiers in psychology 3: 1–9.
85. Lin TW, Kuo YM (2013) Exercise Benefits Brain Function: The Monoamine Connection. Brain Sciences 3: 39–53.
86. Lan C, Lai JS, Chen SY, Wong MK (1998) 12-month Tai Chi training in the elderly: its effect on health fitness. Medicine and Science in Sports and Exercise 30: 345–351.
87. Ahn S, Song R (2012) Effects of Tai Chi Exercise on glucose control, neuropathy scores, balance, and quality of life in patients with type 2 diabetes and neuropathy. The Journal of Alternative and Complementary Medicine 18: 1172–1178.

88. Wu Y, Wang Y, Burgess EO, Wu J (2013) The effects of Tai Chi exercise on cognitive function in older adults: A meta-analysis. Journal of Sport and Health Science 2: 193–203.
89. Pan L, Yan J, Guo Y, Yan J (2013) Effects of Tai Chi training on exercise capacity and quality of life in patients with chronic heart failure: a meta-analysis. European journal of heart failure 15: 316–323.
90. Kjos V, Etnier JL (2006) Pilot study comparing physical and psychological responses in medical qigong and walking. Journal of aging and physical activity 14: 241–253.
91. DiPietro L, Seeman TE, Stachenfeld NS, Katz LD, Nadel ER (1998) Moderate-intensity aerobic training improves glucose tolerance in aging independent of abdominal adiposity. Journal of the American Geriatrics Society 46: 875–879.
92. Ward S, McCluney N, Bosch P (2013) Heart Rate Response to Vinyasa Yoga in Healthy Adults. J Yoga Phys Ther 3: 1–15.
93. Khalsa SBS, Khalsa GS, Khalsa HK, Khalsa MK (2008) Evaluation of a residential Kundalini yoga lifestyle pilot program for addiction in India. Journal of ethnicity in substance abuse 7: 67–79.
94. Elibero A, Janse Van Rensburg K, Drobes DJ (2011) Acute effects of aerobic exercise and Hatha yoga on craving to smoke. Nicotine Tob Res 13: 1140–1148.
95. Kinnunen TH, Korhonen T, Craft LL, Perna FM (2010) Treating tobacco dependence in women with exercise: Review on effectiveness and mechanisms. International Journal of Sport and Exercise Psychology 8: 48–60.

6

Sex Differences in General Knowledge: Meta-Analysis and New Data on the Contribution of School-Related Moderators among High-School Students

Ulrich S. Tran*, Agnes A. Hofer, Martin Voracek

Department of Basic Psychological Research and Research Methods, School of Psychology, University of Vienna, Vienna, Austria

Abstract

Research from various countries consistently reported an advantage of boys over girls in general knowledge and was also suggestive of some overall trends regarding specific domains of general knowledge that were speculated to stem from biologically differentiated interests. However, results were heterogeneous and, as of yet, had not been evaluated meta-analytically. Moreover, previous research drew on overly homogeneous high-school or undergraduate samples whose representativeness appears problematic; mostly, likely moderators, such as school type, student age or parental education, were also not directly investigated or controlled for. We provide a meta-analytical aggregation of available results regarding sex differences in general knowledge and present new data, investigating the psychometric properties of the General Knowledge Test (GKT), on which previous research primarily relied, and explored sex differences in a large and heterogeneous Austrian high-school student sample ($N = 1088$). The aggregated sex effect in general knowledge was of medium size in previous research, but differences in specific domains were heterogeneous across countries and only modest at best. Large sex differences in our data could be explained to a large part by school-related moderators (school type, school, student age, parental education) and selection processes. Boys had a remaining advantage over girls that was only small in size and that was consistent with the magnitude of sex differences in general intelligence. Analysis of the GKT yielded no evidence of biologically differentiated interests, but of a specific interest in the humanities among girls. In conclusion, previous research likely overestimated sex differences in general knowledge.

Editor: Keith Laws, University of Hertfordshire, United Kingdom

Funding: The authors have no support or funding to report.

* Email: ulrich.tran@univie.ac.at

Introduction

Sex differences in cognitive abilities and intelligence are a much investigated topic, with a host of studies documenting an advantage of women in verbal tasks and perceptual speed, but an advantage of men in visuospatial and complex numerical abilities [1]. Moreover, evidence points towards an advantage of men over women in fluid intelligence (Gf) [2–4], but also in crystallized intelligence (Gc) and general knowledge [5,6].

Evidence from the standardization samples of information subtests of the Wechsler intelligence tests since 1958 consistently points towards an advantage of men in general knowledge [6,7]. Yet, research points out that general knowledge is an intellectual ability sui generis ('semantic long-term memory') that possibly needs to be regarded as another factor besides Gc and Gf, instead of being conceptualized as a verbal factor of Gc, and that may not be sufficiently explained by verbal ability, general intelligence, Gc or Gf alone [8–11].

Newer studies assessed general knowledge with a specific instrument, the General Knowledge Test (GKT) [9]. The original GKT consists of 216 items with an open response format that cover 19 different domains of knowledge. Its questions encompass "culturally valued knowledge, communicated by a range of non-specialist media" ([9], p. 859), like *Who discovered the double helix structure of DNA?* or *Which is the longest river in Asia?*, that are scored correct/incorrect, assigning half points to partly correct answers in some items. Irwing et al. [9] provided evidence that the 19 domains conform to a hierarchical second-order factor model, wherein six first-order factors (Current Affairs, Fashion, Family, Physical Health, Arts, and Science) load on the second-order factor general knowledge and account for the interrelations between the lower-order domains. Short forms, translations, and variants of the GKT were used in a number of further studies [10,12–18].

A number of studies with the GKT addressed sex differences explicitly and provided converging evidence on sizable sex differences in general knowledge, and sometimes also with regard to underlying domains. There seems to be a specific male advantage in domains that are concerned with competition for status and power (Current Affairs, Physical Health), and a female advantage in domains that are concerned with nurturance and family (Family). This pattern was interpreted by some authors as suggestive of biological, i.e., evolutionarily developed and genetically predisposed, differences in interest between men and women, besides being determined by socialization and societal norms [6,10,17,19]. Although there exists a systematic review on sex differences in general knowledge [19], there has been no attempt as of yet to aggregate the available evidence meta-analytically.

Previous studies on sex differences in general knowledge differed with regard to exact instrumentation, language and country, respondent age, socio-economic and educational background, and schooling. However, sex differences in intelligence and cognitive abilities may fluctuate from childhood to adolescence and adulthood [20,21]. Moreover, boys show an overall greater variability in cognitive ability than girls on the population level [22], which may in part explain better cognitive achievements of boys and men in university or high-school samples, wherein the distribution of cognitive ability is likely truncated at or above the overall mean, leaving an excess of above-average boys and men, but excluding the excess of below-average boys and men. Furthermore, contextual and sociocultural factors need to be taken into account that, via cultural norms and stereotyping, may promote gender inequality, hinder girls' access to specific areas of education, lead to differential patterns of course taking in school and academia, or directly lead to underperformance in standardized tests in terms of self-fulfilling prophecies [23–26].

Studies that directly assessed sex differences in general knowledge and its domains relied on overly homogeneous samples whose representativeness seems problematic [27]. For example, undergraduates in [6] and [10] attended one and the same university. Eighty-three percent of undergraduates in [28] stemmed from one of two universities that were also in close geographical proximity (approximately 10 km apart). Participants in [18] stemmed from five German high schools of Marburg and Gießen, cities with roughly equally sized populations, located in the same county, approximately 33 km apart. All participants were from twelfth grade and hence similar in age. Samples reported in [19] may have been more heterogeneous. However, the provided information is insufficient to state so with certainty.

Differences in schooling and selection processes within educational systems are known to moderate sex differences in school achievement [29,30]. Most bits of knowledge tested in the GKT have some affinity to contents typically taught in school. In agreement with this, general knowledge was found to predict school achievement [16] and to be higher in older students [15]. Moreover, parents' education may impact children's general knowledge, as it may also foster or limit school achievement [29,31]. Lynn and Irwing [10] found only small effects regarding fathers' education. However, tests may have been overly conservative, owing to their homogeneous sample. Even though apparently more students were recruited from groups of lower socio-economic status at their study site (the University of Ulster) compared with other UK universities, nearly two thirds (63%) of fathers had the same level of education (secondary school to age 16), and another 14% had a quite similar (secondary school to age 18) educational background. Thus, fathers' education apparently did not vary much in this sample, limiting its potential effects on general knowledge.

The present study set out to provide a systematic account and aggregation of previously published evidence on sex differences in general knowledge and its domains and to investigate general knowledge among high-school students with new data, exploring specifically likely contributions of school-related moderators, such as school type, student age, and parental education. Participants were drawn from different types of high schools, different grades, and different geographical areas in Austria's largest county, Lower Austria. Effects of different school curricula were thus for the first time directly tested. Catchment area was systematically varied to attain a higher variability of socio-economic status and educational background of participants and parents than previous research and to obtain thus a more representative sample.

Moreover, Lynn et al. [18] translated the GKT into German, but based their item selection on the test performance of a sample of adults. Being intended for adolescents and young adults (i.e., high-school students and undergraduates), application of this item selection appears questionable. Furthermore, some GKT items seem typical for an Anglo-American background and may not be readily applicable in German-speaking countries. We therefore based our analyses on a new German form of the GKT, specifically selecting items appropriate for German-speaking high-school students. Moreover, the structural properties of the German GKT were thoroughly reassessed, using, unlike [9] and [18], methods that are specifically suited to its ordered categorical (dichotomous) item response format. There is evidence that the use of factor scores may reduce spuriously large sex differences in sum scores of tests of various cognitive abilities [32]. Therefore, analyses were based on factor scores in the present study.

Meta-Analysis

Method

Study inclusion criteria and literature search. Published studies that reported sex differences in general knowledge as assessed with the GKT or instruments that could be readily likened to the GKT scheme, i.e., covered its lower-order domains or higher-order factors, were eligible for inclusion. Literature search drew on studies cited in [19] and on electronic databases (PubMed, PsycINFO, SCOPUS, Web of Science), using the search string (*general knowledge*) AND (*sex differences*). Six journal papers were identified for meta-analysis ([6,10,17–19,28]; see Figure 1 for study flow). Results of [19] and [28] were not obtained with the GKT, but could be readily likened to its domains. Results of [17] were omitted because the (composite) domains investigated there (General Culture: composed of National and World History, and Arts; Natural and Social Sciences: composed of Natural and Social Sciences, Medicine, World's Religions and customs; Current Affairs: composed of Politics, Business, Technology, Sports and Entertainment) did not clearly fit into the overall scheme here. Deviating from the presentation of sum score differences in extant studies, [10] reported estimates that were derived with structural equation modeling (SEM) and also controlled for Gf; these values were used in the present analysis. Similarly, [28] reported on results controlling for Gf and Gc in regression analysis besides sum score differences. However, these results were not presented in a way that lent to meta-analytical aggregation; thus, only sum score differences reported in [28] were included here.

The finally included five primary studies report data from four countries (Croatia, Germany, UK, and USA); three studies reported sex differences among undergraduates, two among high-school students and high-school graduates, and one among pupils. The Zarevski et al. [19] study presented data from four samples (three pupil samples, one high-school sample); pupil samples were combined for analysis. Study details and findings are displayed in Table 1.

Data synthesis. A fixed-effect model was used for meta-analytical effect size aggregation, with Cohen's d as effect size [33]. Because of the known low power of Cochran's Q test to detect between-study effect heterogeneity when the number of studies is small [34], effect heterogeneity was assessed descriptively with the

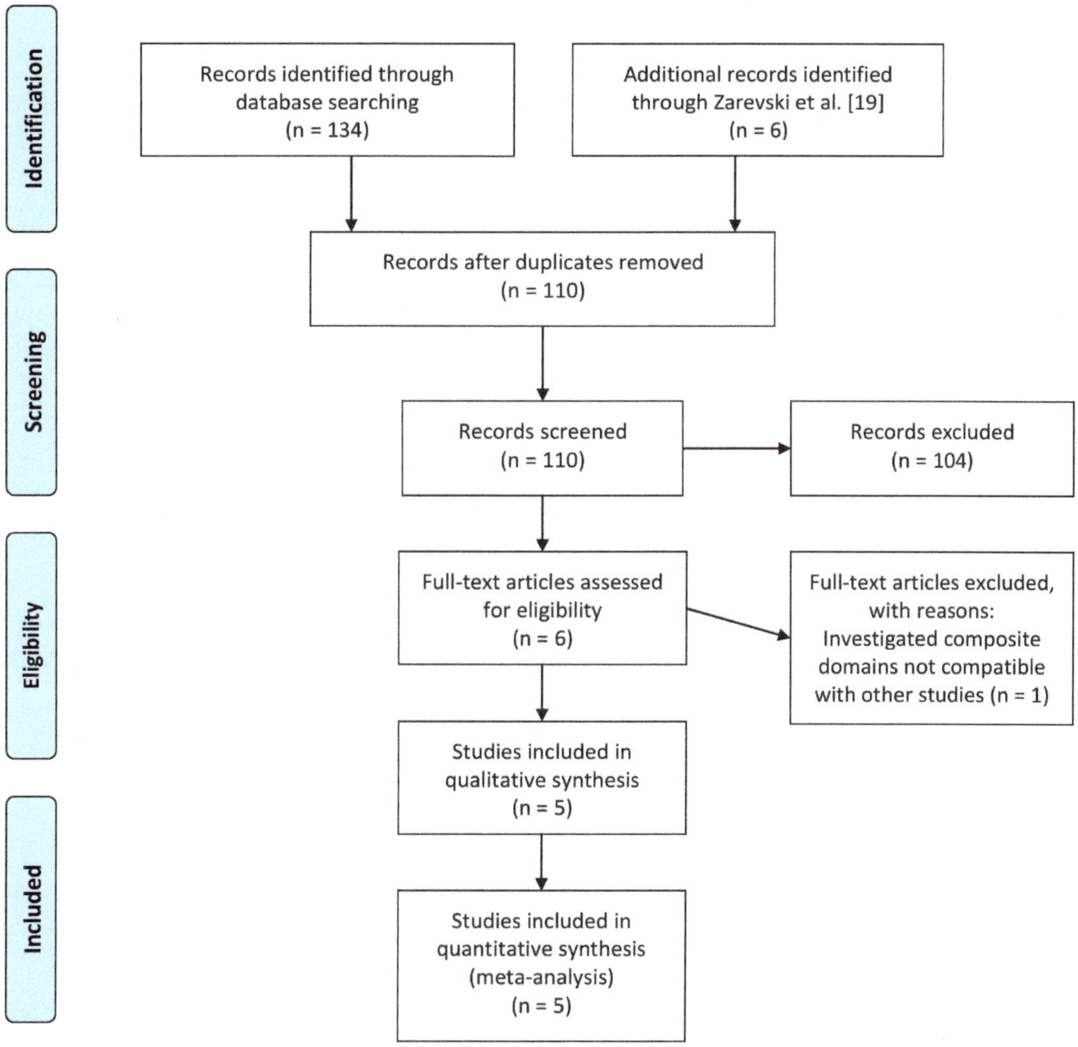

Figure 1. PRISMA flow diagram.

I^2 index. Heterogeneity was assumed small for $I^2 = 25\%$, moderate for $I^2 = 50\%$, and high for $I^2 = 75\%$ [34].

Results and discussion

Sex differences in general knowledge were consistently of at least nearly medium size (i.e., $|\ d\ | \geq 0.50$), but differences in domains varied across studies in size but also in direction (Table 1). Results for Fashion, Popular Music, Film, Biology, Literature, Art, and Classical Music were inconsistent. Otherwise, boys and men excelled girls and women in all remaining domains across all studies, with the exception of Medicine and Cookery, where girls and women consistently excelled boys and men. SEM-based effect sizes [10] were mostly smaller than effect sizes obtained from sum scores in otherwise similar studies [6]. Sex differences were also smaller in samples of younger respondents [19].

The aggregated effect in general knowledge was of medium size, but effects were mostly only small ($|\ d\ | < 0.20$) in the various domains (Table 1). Judging from the aggregated evidence, sex differences of at least medium size, favoring boys and men, were observable in Games, whereas small to medium effects were obtained in Sport, and in domains within Current Affairs and Science. Sex differences favoring girls and women were mostly negligible ($|\ d\ | \leq 0.11$); none were of even medium size. Effects that were at least small ($|\ d\ | \approx 0.20$) were obtained in Classical Music and in domains within Family. Domain-specific sex differences were thus mostly modest. Moreover, effect sizes in lower-order domains were considerable heterogeneous ($I^2 \geq 76\%$, except for Popular Music and Art, where $I^2 = 0\%$ and 19%, respectively), whereas with regard to general knowledge a homogeneous effect was observed ($I^2 = 0\%$).

In total, the available evidence suggests a robust medium-sized advantage of boys and men over girls and women in general knowledge, whereas differences in lower-order domains were markedly smaller and inconsistent, and appeared to increase with age. On the content level, differences in general knowledge appeared to be mostly driven by domains within Current Affairs, Physical Health, and Science. Even though considerable effect heterogeneity was observed within these domains, effects were overall largest there and already observable at a relatively low age. Girls and women had an advantage in domains within Family that was already also observable at a lower age; however, the aggregated effect size was only small and effects were heterogeneous. In conclusion, the available evidence corroborates a male

Table 1. Sex Differences in General Knowledge and its Domains in Previous Studies and Aggregated Effect Estimates.

Study	**Lynn et al. [6]**	**Ackerman et al. [28]**	**Lynn & Irwing [10]**	**Lynn et al. [18]**	**Zarevski et al. [19]**		
Sample	**Undergraduates, University of Ulster**	**Undergraduates**	**Undergraduates, University of Ulster**	**High-school students**	**Pupils, 3 samples combined***	**High-school graduates**	
Country	**Northern Ireland, UK**	**USA**	**Northern Ireland, UK**	**Germany**	**Croatia**	**Croatia**	**Aggregated mean effect**
Mean or median age	**20.4 years**	**19.0 years**	**20.5 years**	**18 years**	**15 years**	**18 years**	**[95% confidence interval]**
Total *N* (% female)	**635 (74%)**	**320 (53%)**	**1047 (57%)**	**302 (51%)**	**3156 (52%)**	**1174 (51%)**	
Current Affairs	0.82	–	–	–	–	–	–
Politics	0.69	0.28		0.33	0.21	0.30	0.28 [0.23, 0.34]***
Finance	0.69	0.33	(0.48)	0.85	0.21	-	0.35 [0.29, 0.40]***
History	0.72	0.50[a]	–	0.62	0.20	0.08	0.26 [0.21, 0.31]***
Discovery	0.69	–	–	0.56	0.25	–	0.33 [0.26, 0.39]***
Geography	0.41	0.66	–	0.67	0.16	0.30	0.27 [0.21, 0.32]***
Fashion	-0.01	–	–	–	–	–	–
Fashion	-0.05	–	(-0.09)	0.03	-0.13	0.19	-0.05 [-0.10, 0.00]
Popular Music	-0.15	–	–	0.04[e]	-0.02	-0.21	-0.07 [-0.13, -0.02]*
Film	0.13	–	–	0.06	-0.24	0.08	-0.11 [-0.17, -0.06]***
Family	-0.46	–	–	–	–	–	–
Medicine	-0.32	–	(-0.24)	-0.20	-0.23	–	-0.24 [-0.29, -0.18]***
Cookery	-0.48	–	–	-0.50	-0.15	–	-0.22 [-0.28, -0.15]***
Physical Health	0.75	–	–	–	–	–	–
Biology	0.42	0.25	–	0.49	-0.15	-0.49	-0.11 [-0.17, -0.06]***
Games	0.54	–	(0.41)	0.82	–	–	0.51 [0.42, 0.60]***
Sport	0.84	–	–	1.12	0.31	0.28	0.39 [0.34, 0.45]***
Arts	0.31	–	–	–	–	–	–
Literature	0.49	0.10[b]	(0.21)	-0.09	-0.07	-0.12	0.01 [-0.03, 0.06]
Art	0.07	0.09	–	-0.16	-0.05	-0.24	-0.08 [-0.13, -0.02]**
Classical Music	0.08	0.20	–	-0.03	-0.28	-0.21	-0.19 [-0.24, -0.14]***
Jazz and Blues	0.46	–	–	–	–	–	–
Science	0.58	–	–	–	–	–	–
General Science	0.63	0.55[c]	(0.45)	0.55[f]	0.19	–	0.32 [0.27, 0.38]***
History of Science	0.33	–	–	–	–	–	–
General knowledge	0.51	0.68[d]	0.48 (0.67)	0.60	–	–	0.53 [0.45, 0.62]***[g]

Note. Figures are standardized mean differences (Cohen's *d*) of sum scores. Positive values indicate that men/boys had higher scores than women/girls. Figures in parentheses were derived from structural equation modelling. * Weighted by inverse variance method. Mean of [a] 'U. S. History' and 'Western Civilization,' [b] 'U. S. Literature' and 'World Literature,' [c] 'Chemistry' and 'Physics.' [d] Composite of 19 domains of knowledge of which not all were commensurate to the domains of knowledge of the GKT. Composite scale of [e] 'Popular Music' and 'Jazz and Blues,' [f] 'General Science' and 'History of Science.' [g] Based on sum score estimates. * $p<.05$, ** $p<.01$, *** $p<.001$.

advantage in domains that are concerned with competition for status and power, and a female advantage in domains that are concerned with nurturance and family. However, there was also a considerable heterogeneity across different countries and studies with regard to these effects.

Psychometric Analysis of the GKT and Contribution of School-Related Moderators on Sex Differences in General Knowledge

Method

Ethical approval was obtained from the regional education authorities of Lower Austria (*Landesschulrat für Niederösterreich*), where the research was conducted. Ethic approval was then individually obtained from all participating schools as well, from the respective Head of School. Lastly, the parents of all participating students provided their written informed consent, as students were mostly underage and testing took place in a school context.

Construction of the German GKT. The GKT was translated, using forward and back-translation, into German and administered it to $N = 21$ (15 women) advanced and master thesis students of psychology at the University of Vienna. Instead of completing the test, raters rated item appropriateness on a 5-point scale (1 = *very appropriate* to 5 = *not appropriate*) with regard to whether each item represented "culturally valued knowledge but non-specialist information generally disseminated by the media" ([18], p. 1643) and whether each item was applicable to high school students (15–19 years) in Austria (neither too easy nor too difficult, suitable for German-speaking countries). Internal consistency (Cronbach's Alpha) of ratings was overall high (median $\alpha = .90$; minimum $\alpha = .73$ in Finance, maximum $\alpha = .96$ in Art). Using a cutoff of 2.5, items with worse ratings were eliminated, resulting in the elimination of 53 items (25%). 'Jazz and Blues' was merged with 'Popular Music', yielding 18 domains covered by a total of 163 items. The number of items per domain in the German GKT may be gleaned from Table 2. The full German GKT may be obtained from the authors.

Participants and procedure. Based on the register of education authorities, 21 high schools were identified in the southern region of Lower Austria and contacted for the purpose of this study. Twelve (57%) schools consented to participate. Permissions to carry out the study in these schools were obtained from state education authorities, head teachers and parents. Testing took place in class rooms, with a time restriction of 45 minutes (in [9] the 216-item GKT was administered in 60 minute sessions). Participants also answered questions on socio-demographics and their parents' education. Altogether, 62 classes of grades 10 to 12 completed the assessment.

In total, 1088 students (743 girls, 345 boys) participated, aged 15–21 years ($M = 16.6$, $SD = 0.9$). Of these, 54.8% attended a high school with a focus on natural sciences (*Realgymnasium* in German; 5 schools), 18.4% (general) high schools (*Gymnasium*; 3 schools), 17.6% vocational schools (3 schools), and 9.3% schools of commerce (1 school). Overall, 54.2% attended grade 10, 40.1% grade 11, and 5.7% grade 12. Sex was imbalanced within school types: relatively more boys (69.9%) than girls (47.8%) attended high schools with a focus on the natural sciences, and fewer boys (5.2%) than girls (23.3%) attended vocational schools ($\chi^2(3) = 66.45$, $p < .001$). Students in schools of commerce were slightly older than all other students ($M = 17.3$ years vs. 17.0 years; $F(3, 1079) = 5.79$, $p = .001$; post hoc Tukey tests: $ps \leq .026$).

With regard to living and catchment area, 29.0% of the students stemmed from communities with 5000+ residents, 53.0% from communities with 1000–5000 residents, and 16.3% from communities with less than 1000 residents; 1.7% provided no information. Of respondents' fathers and mothers, respectively, 46.0% and 47.9% had completed lower secondary school, 24.5% and 29.0% had completed upper secondary school, and 26.8% and 22.1% had a university diploma or a similar degree (2.7% and 1.1%, respectively, provided no information). Fathers' and mothers' educational background was fairly concordant (weighted kappa = .53, $p < .001$).

Analysis

Structure of the German GKT. Answers on the German GKT were scored 1 (*correct*) and 0 (*incorrect*). Partly correct answers (e.g., responding to *What are the chemical constituents of water?* solely 'hydrogen') were assigned half points. Unidimensionality of domains was investigated with confirmatory factor analysis, using Mplus 6.11 [35] and its weighted least square mean- and variance-adjusted (WLSMV) estimation option which is suited for ordered categorical variables and is based on the items' polychoric correlation matrix. Items were excluded where necessary to improve model fit.

In a second step, the higher-order factor model of [6] was fit onto the domain factor scores, using a robust maximum likelihood estimator (MLR) to guard against non-normality of data and to arrive at robust indices of model fit. As this model had no good fit on our data, and modification indices indicated a much more complicated loading pattern than originally assumed, a modified approach was chosen instead. In order to deal with the apparent cross-loadings of domains on first-order factors, exploratory structural equation modeling (ESEM [36]) was used, which estimates cross-loadings freely as in exploratory factor analysis, but also derives indices of model fit as in confirmatory factor analysis and structural equation modeling. ESEM was successfully utilized in previous research dealing with similar problems (e.g., [37]).

As of yet, it is technically not possible to fit a higher-order ESEM. Hence, analyses on the doubly-tiered hierarchical structure of the GKT were performed in two steps: first, with regard to domains and first-order factors, using domain factor scores; second, with regard to first-order factors and second-order general knowledge, using first-order factor scores. With regard to the former analysis, varying numbers of first-order factors were examined, selecting (1) the most parsimonious model (fewest factors) that had (2) a good model fit, (3) good interpretability, and (4) high factor determinacies (i.e., high correlations of factor score estimates with underlying factors).

Model fit was checked with CFI and TLI (comparative fit index, Tucker-Lewis index; acceptable fit: ≥.90, good fit: ≥.95), RMSEA (root mean square error of approximation; acceptable fit: <.08, good fit: <.06), and SRMR for MLR analyses (standardised root mean residual; acceptable fit: <.11, good fit: <.08) [38]. ESEM estimates a large number of parameters which may spuriously inflate the RMSEA [37] that penalizes for model complexity. This is similarly the case with the TLI. Hence, in ESEM analyses, model fit was primarily interpreted with regard to CFI values.

Sex differences and contribution of school-related moderators. Magnitude (Cohen's *d*) and significance of sex differences were assessed for domains, first-order factors, and second-order general knowledge with generalized linear models (GLM), using factor scores and investigating moderating effects of school type, school, parental education, and student age. Effect sizes were derived from GLM parameter estimates, presenting both naïve and unadjusted effect sizes (examining only sex in the GLM), and effect sizes adjusted for moderators (using the full

Table 2. Fit Statistics of Unidimensional Models in Domains.

Domain	Items	χ^2	*df*	CFI	TLI	RMSEA [90%-CI]
Politics	10	68.13	35	.975	.968	.029 [.019,.040]
Finance	11	53.88	44	.990	.987	.014 [.000,.026]
History	9	36.25	27	.990	.986	.018 [.000,.031]
Discovery	11	45.58	44	.992	.991	.006 [.000,.021]
Geography	11	67.27	44	.981	.976	.022 [.010,.032]
Fashion	9	43.21	27	.966	.954	.023 [.008,.036]
Popular Music	10	132.77	35	.922	.900	.051 [.042,.060]
Film	8	45.21	20	.883	.836	.034 [.021,.047]
without Item 6	7	23.16	14	.949	.924	.025 [.000,.042]
Medicine	9	41.42	27	.959	.945	.022 [.005,.035]
Cookery	8	37.39	20	.979	.970	.028 [.013,.042]
Biology	9	35.58	27	.987	.982	.017 [.000,.031]
Games	6	15.82	9	.959	.932	.026 [.000,.047]
Sport	7	16.29	14	.999	.998	.012 [.000,.033]
Literature	8	30.22	20	.919	.886	.022 [.000,.037]
without Item 5	7	20.46	14	.953	.930	.021 [.000,.039]
Art	6	28.02	9	.919	.865	.044 [.026,.063]
without Item 4	5	10.34	5	.971	.942	.031 [.000,.059]
Classical Music	9	33.29	27	.985	.990	.015 [.000,.029]
General Science	10	55.89	35	.978	.972	.023 [.011,.035]
History of Science	11	99.29	44	.927	.909	.034 [.025,.043]

Note. CFI = comparative fit index, TLI = Tucker-Lewis index, RMSEA = root mean square error of approximation.

GLM as outlined above). For first-order factors and second-order general knowledge, the dependent variable was modelled with a normal distribution in the GLM. For domain factor scores, Gamma distributions were used to account for observed skewness. The identity function was used as link function, the covariance matrix was estimated via a robust sandwich estimator. The GLM allowed to model heterogeneous variances (higher variance in boys) and the clustered nature of the data: students stemmed from different schools within the same school type. In the GLM, school was modelled as a nested factor within school type to account for the variability between schools and to safeguard against Type I errors due to cluster sampling.

A full (saturated) model was investigated with the GLM in order to avoid biased estimates of effect size [39]. However, instead of a main effect of age, the interaction of age by school type was tested in the GLM, to assess differences in years of schooling (age) between school types. Effects of fathers' and mothers' education were tested independently in separate GLMs. Post hoc comparisons were carried out utilizing sequential Bonferroni corrections.

Moreover, we also tested the association of parental education with school type (separate chi-square tests for mothers and fathers, and separately for boys and girls), to assess the overall contribution of parental education on their children's educational career. Significance was set to $p<.05$ (two-tailed).

Results and discussion

Unidimensionality of domains. Unidimensional factor models had an adequate fit in all domains, with the exception of Film, Art, and Literature (Table 2). In Literature, Item 3 (*Who wrote 'Doctor Zhivago'?*) had to be excluded beforehand, as no respondent knew the right answer. To improve model fit, Item 6 in Film (*Who played the leading male part in 'Titanic'?*), Item 4 in Art (*Who painted the 'Mona Lisa'?*), and Item 5 in Literature (*Who wrote 'Politeia'?*) had to be removed as well. Compared to the other items, knowledge on these items was probably overly influenced by popularity effects (Film), pervasiveness in the mass media (Art), or in not being a prototypical example of its subject (Literature). In all resulting scales unidimensional models had at least an acceptable fit, most had a good fit.

Structure and reliability of the GKT. The hierarchical model of [6] had no good fit on our data (Table 3). Modification indices indicated that a large number of domains should be allowed to cross-load on other factors besides their designated factor. ESEM analyses with six, five, four, and three factors (Table 3) suggested that a 4-factor model fitted the data best. In the 6-factor model, one factor had no, another only one, significant loading. In the 5-factor model, two factors had factor determinacies <.80, whereas in the 4-factor model only factor 4 had a factor determinacy that was only slightly below.80 (Table 4). Moreover, the overall fit of the 4-factor model could be considered good and was considerably better than that of a 3-factor model (Table 3). The seemingly low loadings in factor 4 need to be interpreted in context (Table 4): Loadings of Games, Literature, Arts, and Classical Music on factor 4 were lower by at most 37% (Literature) to as few as 15% (Arts) compared to the highest loadings of these domains on the other factors. Moreover, the negative loading of Sport on factor 4 was higher than its positive loading on factor 1 (.52). There was no indication for a need to model correlated residuals. Therefore, the 4-factor solution was kept as the final model as it appeared most parsimonious.

Factor 1 subsumed with highest loadings domains within Current Affairs and Art, but also Sport and History of Science

Table 3. Fit Statistics of the Higher-Order Factor Models.

Model	χ^2	*df*	CFI	TLI	RMSEA [90%-CI]	SRMR
Confirmatory hierarchical factor model of [6]	985.81	128	.862	.836	.078 [.074,.083]	.059
6-factor ESEM	98.64	60	.994	.984	.024 [.015,.033]	.010
5-factor ESEM	137.86	73	.990	.978	.029 [.021,.036]	.014
4-factor ESEM	**229.12**	**87**	**.977**	**.960**	**.039 [.033,.045]**	**.019**
3-factor ESEM	516.58	102	.934	.900	.061 [.056,.066]	.032

Note. CFI = comparative fit index, TLI = Tucker-Lewis index, RMSEA = root mean square error of approximation, SRMR = standardized root mean residual. The bold printed model was retained for further analysis.

(Table 4). Factor 2 subsumed with highest loadings domains within Fashion and Cookery, and factor 3 Medicine, Biology, Games, and General Science. Factors 1 to 3 incorporated a larger number of cross-loadings, some of them also negative, whereas factor 4 appeared special as it contained exceptionally large negative cross-loadings of Games and Sport. Medicine, Literature, Art, Classical Music, and History of Science all had positive cross-loadings on this factor. Moreover, factors 1 to 3 were positively inter-correlated (factor 1 with factor 2: $r = .65$, $p < .001$; factor 1 with factor 3: $r = .40$, $p < .001$; factor 2 with factor 3: $r = .19$, $p < .001$), but factor 4 had no associations of with any of the other factors (*rs* = .03,.11, and.05 with factors 1 to 3, $ps \geq .247$). In a further ESEM analysis with the four first-order factors, factors 1 to 3 had large and significant loadings (.97,.78,.47, $ps < .001$) on second-order general knowledge, but not factor 4 (loading = .04, $p = .321$). In this analysis, the variance of factor 1 had to be constrained to be positive to attain convergence. Fit of this 1-factor ESEM was good with regard to CFI, $\chi^2(2) = 51.17$, p<.001, CFI = .957, TLI = .871, RMSEA = .150, 90% confidence interval =

Table 4. Loadings in the 4-Factor ESEM.

	GEOMIN-rotated factors			
Domains	**1**	**2**	**3**	**4**
Current Affairs				
Politics	**<u>.85</u>**	.00	−.09	−.00
Finance	**<u>.60</u>**	**.12**	**.19**	**−.16**
History	**<u>.79</u>**	**−.19**	.01	.09
Discovery	**<u>.47</u>**	−.01	**.20**	−.08
Geography	**<u>.58</u>**	−.05	**.15**	−.07
Fashion				
Fashion	.02	**<u>.70</u>**	.01	.01
Popular Music	.04	**<u>.75</u>**	.02	**−.10**
Film	**.35**	**<u>.42</u>**	−.13	−.01
Family				
Medicine	.09	**.21**	**<u>.37</u>**	**.22**
Cookery	−.06	**<u>.43</u>**	**.35**	.11
Physical Health				
Biology	.00	.08	**<u>.69</u>**	−.02
Games	.03	−.01	**<u>.52</u>**	**−.38**
Sport	**<u>.52</u>**	.06	.01	**−.55**
Arts				
Literature	**<u>.30</u>**	**.18**	**.23**	**.19**
Art	**<u>.40</u>**	**.15**	.01	**.34**
Classical Music	**<u>.38</u>**	.07	.01	**.26**
Science				
General Science	.22	**−.15**	**<u>.64</u>**	−.00
History of Science	**<u>.48</u>**	−.02	**.18**	**.22**
Factor determinacies	.95	.89	.88	.78

Note. All bold printed loadings were significant at $p < .01$. Underlined loadings indicate where domains loaded highest positively.

[.116,.187]. Factor determinacy of second-order general knowledge was also high,.97.

With regard to interpretation, factors 1 to 3 appeared components of a common positive manifold of general knowledge. According to its high second-order factor loading, factor 1 was virtually identical to general knowledge itself. Factor 2 and 3 appeared to encompass more specific areas of knowledge, i.e., aspects of what could be termed 'recreational lifestyle' (factor 2) and the natural and the life sciences (factor 3). Factor 4 seemingly lay outside this manifold. Yet, it contained cross-loadings of domains that were themselves components of the manifold. However, positive and negative effects apparently cancelled each other out, resulting in no overall association of factor 4 with second-order general knowledge. With regard to its contents, factor 4 appeared to encompass increased knowledge of the arts, Medicine, and History of Science, reminiscent of a specialisation in the humanities, but accompanied by a specific lack of knowledge especially in Games and Sport.

Reliability indices of sum scores were excellent for the total GKT, but unacceptably low ($\alpha<.60$) in some domains (Table 5). However, given that domains were unidimensional, low reliabilities obviously stemmed from the dichotomous item format and the fact that there were only few items within some domains. Moreover, Cronbach's Alphas on the domain level in our study broadly matched previous figures [18].

Sex differences and contribution of moderators. In naïve estimation of sex differences, a large difference between boys and girls emerged in second-order general knowledge (Table 5). Even though effect size estimation was based on factors scores, we provide summary statistics on sum scores in Table 5 to enable direct comparisons with previous research. In first-order factors, the largest difference, favouring boys, was found in factor 1, closely followed by factor 2. However, differences were in favour of girls in factors 3 and 4; effect size was small in the former, but large in the latter. Differences in domain scores were mostly similar to differences in respective first-order factors. In sum scores, boys had a larger score variance in total general knowledge and most domains, with exceptions in Fashion, Family, Cookery, Physical Health, Biology, Literature, and Art, where girls had a larger score variance (Table 5). A similar pattern was observable in factor scores (not shown for brevity). Compared with [18] our results appeared to be on the large side on the domain level (+0.13*d* on average). Yet, a strong concordance was observable with regard to the relative magnitude of effect sizes across the different domains.

Adjusting for moderators, sex differences were greatly diminished in size. Overall, mothers' education had a stronger impact on general knowledge than fathers'; hence, we report here on results of GLMs incorporating only mothers' education ($N = 1071$ due to partially missing data). Table 6 displays effect tests with regard to investigated factors and interactions for first-order factors and second-order general knowledge. For brevity, only results on these higher-order factors, but not on domains, are detailed here. With regard to factor 1 and second-order general knowledge, we present details only for the latter, as findings were similar for both. Effects of sex robustly emerged in the analyses; however, they were systematically qualified by a number of interactions.

There was a main effect of school type on general knowledge, but not on first-order factors 2 to 4 (the effect on factor 3 was only small and negligible in size). In marginal means, general knowledge was highest in high schools, followed by high schools with a focus on the natural sciences, schools of commerce, and vocational schools ($d = -0.35$, -0.49, and -0.78, comparing the other school types, in the same order, to high schools; all pairwise comparisons were significant at an overall $p<.05$, except for the last two types of school, $p = .129$). Schools themselves impacted all first-order and the second-order factor significantly, indicating heterogeneity of individual schools that may stem from differences in catchment area, but also from differences between individual schools of the same type. Mothers' education exerted no significant main effect on any of the five dependent variables.

School type and individual schools qualified systematically, via first-order interactions, sex differences in all dependent variables. In marginal means, boys had higher factor scores in general knowledge than girls in all school types (largest difference in high schools, *d*s ranging from 0.52 to 1.11, *p*s $\leq.016$), but vocational schools ($d = 0.10$, $p = .681$), and higher scores in factor 2 in both types of high school (larger in high schools, $d = 0.99$, than in high schools with a focus on the natural sciences, $d = 0.72$, *p*s $<.001$), but not in vocational schools ($d = -0.15$, $p = .559$) or schools of commerce ($d = 0.35$, $p = .103$). In comparison, girls had higher scores than boys in factor 3 in all school types (largest difference in vocational schools, *d*s ranging from 0.34 to 0.64, *p*s $\leq.034$), but schools of commerce ($d = 0.07$, $p = .729$), and higher scores in factor 4 in all school types (largest difference in high schools, *d*s ranging from 0.61 to 1.40, *p*s $\leq.004$), but vocational schools ($d = 0.27$, $p = .227$). There was again systematic heterogeneity with regard to these effects on the level of individual schools.

Mothers' education impacted all dependent variables, except factor 4, via a first-order interaction with school type, altering the rank order of school types dependent on mothers' education, and with regard to general knowledge and factor 2 via a second-order interaction with sex and school. Factor scores were significantly higher in high schools than in all other school types, when mothers had completed upper secondary education, but, otherwise, differences were mostly significant only with regard to school of commerce (ranking last), when mothers had completed lower secondary education, and with regard to vocational schools (ranking last), when mothers had a university diploma.

Lastly, age affected general knowledge, and factors 2 and 3, dependent on school type. General knowledge increased systematically in high schools ($B = 0.18$, 95% confidence interval = [0.04, 0.33], $p = .015$) and vocational schools ($B = 0.25$ [0.17, 0.34], $p<.001$), but not in the other two school types (*p*s $\geq.077$). Factor 2 increased significantly only in vocational schools ($B = 0.21$ [0.06, 0.34], $p = .004$; other *p*s $\geq.296$). Factor 3 increased significantly in high schools with a focus on the natural sciences ($B = 0.09$ [0.01, 0.16], $p = .025$) and vocational schools ($B = 0.25$ [0.12, 0.37], $p<.001$; other *p*s $\geq.232$). Factor 4 remained unaffected by age.

School type was strongly dependent on mothers' and fathers' education. Associations were stronger for girls (mother: $\chi^2(6) = 37.80$, $p<.001$; father: $\chi^2(6) = 44.69$, $p<.001$) than for boys (mother: $\chi^2(6) = 17.59$, $p = .007$; father: $\chi^2(6) = 24.23$, $p<.001$). Fewer girls (13.8% vs. 25.8% with regard to mothers' education; 12.7% vs. 26.0% with regard to fathers' education) attended high schools, and more (13.6% vs. 4.7%, and 13.8% vs. 5.0%, respectively) schools of commerce, when parents had completed only lower secondary school, compared to higher educational levels. Vice versa, more girls (30.9% vs. 16.8%, and 26.9% vs. 16.9%, respectively) attended high schools, and fewer (2.6% vs. 11.0%, and 3.4% vs. 11.4%, respectively) schools of commerce, when parents had a university diploma, compared to lower educational levels. Similarly, fewer boys (0.0% vs. 12.3%, and 1.7% vs. 13.0%, respectively) attended schools of commerce, when parents had a university diploma; however, boys' attendance of high schools was unaffected by parental education.

Table 5. Scale Reliabilities, Sum Score Means and Standard Deviations, and Sex Differences in Factor Scores, Unadjusted and Adjusted for Moderators.

		Sum scores		Sex differences (Cohen *d*) in factor scores	
Domain	α	**Boys**	**Girls**	**Unadj.**	**Adj.**
Current Affairs					
Politics	.64	2.63 (1.78)	1.32 (1.30)	0.83***	0.15*
Finance	.60	3.61 (1.75)	1.99 (1.51)	1.05***	0.17*
History	.63	2.13 (1.87)	0.82 (1.11)	0.85***	−0.01
Discovery	.37	2.50 (1.19)	1.73 (0.92)	0.71***	0.11*
Geography	.66	2.52 (2.04)	1.34 (1.41)	0.69***	0.14*
Sport	.68	2.85 (2.01)	1.17 (1.10)	1.00***	0.19**
Fashion					
Fashion	.51	2.06 (1.36)	2.36 (1.59)	−0.36***	−0.11
Popular Music	.63	2.90 (1.86)	3.10 (1.74)	−0.10	−0.02
Film	.36	0.58 (0.89)	0.48 (0.72)	0.10	−0.01
Family					
Medicine	.41	3.14 (1.45)	3.27 (1.38)	−0.06	−0.01
Cookery	.58	3.06 (1.48)	3.30 (1.62)	−0.15*	−0.07
Physical Health					
Biology	.56	5.61 (1.66)	4.48 (1.82)	0.59***	0.15*
Games	.44	3.10 (1.33)	2.06 (1.28)	0.93***	0.05
Arts					
Literature	.34	1.12 (0.71)	0.94 (0.81)	0.26***	0.06
Art	.36	0.66 (0.77)	0.61 (0.85)	0.02	0.23***
Classical Music	.48	1.10 (0.93)	1.04 (0.91)	0.06	0.00
Science					
General Science	.60	5.44 (1.87)	3.72 (1.76)	0.96***	0.13*
History of Science	.45	2.12 (1.48)	1.52 (1.12)	0.42***	0.00
First-order factors					
Factor 1 (general knowledge)				1.03***	0.16*
Factor 2 (lifestyle)				0.94***	0.13
Factor 3 (sciences)				−0.27***	−0.05
Factor 4 (humanities)				−0.81***	−0.16*
Second-order general knowledge	.92	47.16 (15.02)	35.25 (13.41)	1.02***	0.16*

Note. α = Cronbach's Alpha; Unadj./Adj. = unadjusted/adjusted for moderators in GLM analyses. Positive effect sizes signify an advantage of boys over girls. * $p<.05$, ** $p<.01$, *** $p<.001$.

General Discussion

This study set out to investigate sex differences in general knowledge among high-school students in a more heterogeneous sample than previous research and by using a measure of general knowledge that was specifically tailored for German-speaking adolescents. Our study provides substantial evidence that the German GKT is a psychometrically sound and valid instrument. However, the higher-order structure proposed by [6] could not be fully replicated; second-order general knowledge was composed of four, not of six, first-order factors. Meta-analytical aggregation of previous studies suggested that sex differences were mostly heterogeneous and, across domains, of modest size at best. We obtained large sex differences in our data, but observed that general knowledge and its first-order factors were not independent of schooling and were moderated by parental education that also determined children's educational career. Sex differences in general knowledge could be explained to a large part in terms of selection processes, resulting in an overrepresentation of boys in school types where general knowledge was overall high, and an overrepresentation of girls in school types where general knowledge was overall low. Moreover, sex differences varied in size, dependent on school type, but also on individual schools. Broadly concordant with their specific curricula, increases in general knowledge and its first-order factors over time varied with school type. Controlling for these factors, sex differences were rendered small or even negligible, i.e., markedly less than 0.20*d* or insignificant.

Studies on school achievement [30,31] and cross-national data on sex differences in school achievement [29] highlight that differences in schooling, parental education, and parental involvement are major determinants of school success. Contextual and sociocultural factors may act as barriers with regard to educational success, especially for girls [23–26]. In the present

Table 6. Effect Tests in the GLMs.

	First-order factors				Second-order
	1	2	3	4	general knowledge
Sex	109.41(1)***	74.65(1)***	49.36(1)***	111.59(1)***	101.81(1)***
School type	18.83(3)***	6.26(3)	9.08(3)*	2.14(3)	17.90(3)***
School[a]	140.87(8)***	35.50(8)***	60.81(8)***	91.87(8)***	129.95(8)***
Mothers' education	2.41(2)	1.32(2)	6.77(2)*	3.09(2)	2.26(2)
Sex × school type	38.92(3)***	15.63(3)***	21.07(3)***	25.62(3)***	38.02(3)***
Sex × school[a]	88.69(8)***	27.50(8)***	46.84(8)***	54.87(8)***	97.48(8)***
Sex × mothers' education	2.16(2)	0.10(2)	7.22(2)*	1.10(2)	2.10(2)
School type × mothers' education	39.41(6)***	18.21(6)**	23.40(6)***	10.68(6)	37.63(6)***
School[a] × mothers' education	17.52(16)	23.30(16)	16.99(16)	26.79(16)*	17.37(16)
Sex × school type × mothers' education	7.24(5)	2.27(5)	10.39(5)	9.15(5)	7.09(5)
Sex × school[a] × mothers' education	28.40(12)**	24.99(12)*	15.51(12)	11.27(12)	27.60(12)**
School type × age	49.97(4)***	10.15(4)*	21.05(4)***	2.95(4)	44.83(4)***

Note. Entries are Wald χ^2 tests with degrees of freedom in parentheses. [a] Nested within school type. * $p<.05$, ** $p<.01$, *** $p<.001$.

study, parental education affected children's general knowledge on multiple levels, determining children's educational career and disadvantaging specifically girls. Moreover, parental education moderated children's general knowledge via interactions with school type and individual schools that likely mirrored effects of parental involvement on children's school success. Being mostly confined to samples that stemmed from one and the same, or from few but overly similar, institutions, previous research likely underestimated the variability of general knowledge that can be attributed to differences in schooling, but also catchment area, that was observed here.

Remaining sex differences, regarding an advantage of boys over girls in general knowledge, were in size comparable to sex differences in general intelligence, fluid intelligence, and crystallized intelligence, i.e., small. Previous research highlighted the important role of especially Gc for knowledge acquisition [40–43]. Hence, the advantage of boys observed here is in good agreement with prior evidence.

Unexpectedly, we obtained unique evidence of a first-order factor covering the humanities, where girls excelled boys by a small margin. We propose to interpret this result in view of specific interests that appear to be more pronounced among girls. A preference of women for the arts and the humanities is well-known from research in higher education [44]. More generally, interests were also found to affect knowledge acquisition besides Gc (e.g., [43,45]). However, the loading pattern in the humanities factor led to yet a further insight: positive knowledge in specific domains need not be accompanied by positive knowledge in other domains; i.e., governed by specific interests, various domains of general knowledge do not necessarily form a positive manifold (cf. [9]). In conclusion, the obtained results do not lend strong support to the interpretation that sex differences in general knowledge are driven by evolutionarily developed and genetically predisposed interests [6,10,17,19]. Moreover, in the absence of biological data, such an interpretation must remain speculative at best. Instead, sex differences were found to be associated with selection processes, schooling, and parental education; knowledge increases over time were broadly concordant with the curricula of the different school types. The very pattern of sex differences interpreted by some authors as indicative of biologically predisposed interests could thus be explained in large part by effects of social norms, socialization, and schooling. Controlling for these effects, remaining sex differences were only small and consistent with prior evidence on sex differences in general intelligence, Gf and Gc. Differences in Gc, i.e., concerning verbal ability, language development, reading comprehension, and verbal reasoning, may be the driving factors of remaining sex differences in general knowledge; with regard to the humanities factor, were girls excelled boys, specific interests that also show no obvious biological roots or functions appear to be the driving factor.

The larger score variance of boys in general knowledge and most domains observed in the current study is consistent with prior evidence regarding general intelligence [22]. Remaining sex differences in general knowledge may thus partially stem from this greater male variability, whose roots may lie in an X-chromosomal pathway of inheritance of genes affecting the development of mental abilities [46]. We suggest investigating the greater male variability in general knowledge in more detail in future studies, utilizing and examining tail ratios, i.e., ratios of the proportions of boys and girls above a predefined cutoff, which may be beneficially used to directly assess and quantify sex differences in the spread of variability (see [47]).

Limitations of the present study pertain to its cross-sectional design which precludes strong conclusions regarding causal relationships; i.e., apparent gains in general knowledge over time could have been, partly or fully, caused by cohort effects. Likewise, selection processes were inferred from outcome, but were not assessed with regard to the admission of student to individual schools. Associations between parents' education and children's general knowledge were also likely confounded by genetic effects, i.e., parents with higher educational levels and their children may have had a better general knowledge because of the same set of genes that had been passed on. These effects could not be controlled for in the present study. General intelligence, Gf, Gc, and personality traits and learning styles, reportedly affecting general knowledge [8,10–12,14,15,28,32], were not controlled in the present study, which may have influenced results. Finally, results of the present study are only valid with regard to the GKT and its variants. They may not generalize to other measures of general knowledge or domains of general knowledge that are not covered by the GKT.

In conclusion, the GKT was found a psychometrically sound and valid instrument that can therefore be recommended for use in further research. General knowledge was composed of four first-order factors, one of which referred to a specific interest in the humanities that was specifically pronounced among girls. Large naïve estimates of differences in general knowledge, favouring boys, could be explained to a large part by differences in schooling and selection processes that were moderated by parental education and specifically disadvantaged girls. Future research should focus of the effects of specific interests on the acquisition of general knowledge, controlling for general intelligence and Gc.

Acknowledgments

Thanks are extended to Richard Lynn and Jutta Margraf-Stiksrud for generously providing test materials for this research.

Author Contributions

Conceived and designed the experiments: MV. Performed the experiments: AAH. Analyzed the data: UST AAH. Wrote the paper: UST MV AAH.

References

1. Halpern DF (2000) Sex differences in cognitive abilities (3rd ed.). London: Lawrence Erlbaum. 440 p.
2. Irwing P, Lynn R (2005) Sex differences in means and variability on the Progressive Matrices in university students: A meta-analysis. Br J Psychol 96: 505–524.
3. Irwing P, Lynn R (2006) Is there a sex difference in IQ scores? Nature 442: E1.
4. Lynn R, Irwing P (2004) Sex differences on the Progressive Matrices: A meta-analysis. Intelligence 32: 481–498.
5. Hyde JS, Linn MC (1988) Gender differences in verbal ability: A meta-analysis. Psychol Bull 104: 53–69.
6. Lynn R, Irwing P, Cammock T (2001) Sex differences in general knowledge. Intelligence 30: 27–39.
7. Irwing P (2012) Sex differences in g: An analysis of the US standardization sample of the WAIS-III. Pers Indiv Diff 53: 126–131.
8. Ackerman PL, Rolfhus EL (1999) The locus of adult intelligence: Knowledge, abilities, and non-ability traits. Psychol Aging 14: 314–330.
9. Irwing P, Cammock T, Lynn R (2001) Some evidence for the existence of a general factor of semantic memory and its components. Pers Indiv Diff 30: 857–871.
10. Lynn R, Irwing P (2002) Sex differences in general knowledge, semantic memory and reasoning ability. Br J Psychol 93: 545–556.
11. Rolfhus EL, Ackerman PL (1999) Assessing individual differences in knowledge: Knowledge structures and traits. J Educ Psychol 91: 511–526.
12. Chamorro-Premuzic T, Furnham A, Ackerman PL (2006) Ability and personality correlates of general knowledge. Pers Indiv Diff 41: 419–429.
13. Furnham A (2009) The validity of a new, self-report measure of multiple intelligence. Curr Psychol 28: 225–239.
14. Furnham A, Chamorro-Premuzic T (2006) Personality, intelligence and general knowledge. Learning Indiv Diff 16: 79–90.
15. Furnham A, Christopher AN, Garwood J, Martin GN (2007) Approaches to learning and the acquisition of general knowledge. Pers Indiv Diff 43: 1563–1571.
16. Furnham A, Monsen J, Ahmetoglu G (2009) Typical intellectual engagement, Big Five personality traits, approaches to learning and cognitive ability predictors of academic performance. Br J Educ Psychol 79: 769–782.
17. Lynn R, Ivanec D, Zarevski P (2009) Sex differences in general knowledge domains. Coll Antropol 33: 515–520.
18. Lynn R, Wilberg S, Margraf-Stiksrud J (2004) Sex differences in general knowledge in German high school students. Pers Indiv Diff 37: 1643–1650.
19. Zarevski P, Ivanec D, Zarevski Z, Lynn R (2007) Gender differences in general knowledge: Four Croatian studies. Suvremena Psihologija 10: 213–221.
20. Keith TZ, Reynolds MR, Patel PG, Ridley KP (2008) Sex differences in latent cognitive abilities ages 6 to 59: Evidence from the Woodcock-Johnson III tests of cognitive abilities. Intelligence 36: 502–525.
21. Reynolds MR, Keith TZ, Ridley KP, Patel PG (2008) Sex differences in latent general and broad cognitive abilities for children and youth: Evidence from higher-order MG-MACS and MIMIC models. Intelligence 36: 236–260.
22. Deary IJ, Thorpe G, Wilson V, Starr JM, Whalley LJ (2003) Population sex differences in IQ at age 11: The Scottish mental survey 1932. Intelligence 31: 533–542.
23. Dykiert D, Gale CR, Deary IJ (2009) Are apparent sex differences in mean IQ scores created in part by sample restriction and increased male variance? Intelligence 37: 42–47.
24. Hyde JS (2005) The gender similarities hypothesis. Am Psychol 60: 581–592.
25. Hyde JS, Mertz JE (2009) Gender, culture, and mathematics performance. PNAS 106: 8801–8807.
26. Madhyastha TM, Hunt E, Deary IJ, Gale CR, Dykiert D (2009) Recruitment modeling applied to longitudinal studies of group differences in intelligence. Intelligence 37: 422–427.
27. Deary IJ (2012) Intelligence. Ann Rev Psychol 63: 453–482.
28. Ackerman PL, Bowen KR, Beier ME, Kanfer R (2001) Determinants of individual differences and gender differences in knowledge. J Educ Psychol 93: 797–825.
29. Organisation for Economic Co-operation and Development (OECD) (2009) Equally prepared for life? How 15-year-old boys and girls perform in school. Available: http://www.oecd-ilibrary.org/education/equally-prepared-for-life_9789264064072-en.
30. Wong KC, Lam YR, Ho LM (2002) The effects of schooling on gender differences. Br Educ Res J 28: 827–843.
31. Hill NE, Castellino DR, Lansford JE, Nowlin P, Dodge KA, et al. (2004) Parent academic involvement as related to school behaviour, achievement, and aspirations: Demographic variations across adolescence. Child Dev 75: 1491–1509.
32. Steinmayr R, Beauducel A, Spinath B (2010) Do sex differences in a faceted model of fluid and crystallized intelligence depend on the method applied? Intelligence 38: 101–110.
33. Borenstein M, Hedges LV, Higgins JPT, Rothstein HA (2009) Introduction to meta-analysis. Chichester: Wiley. 421 p.
34. Higgins J, Thompson SG (2002) Quantifying heterogeneity in a meta-analysis. Stat Med 21: 1539–1558.
35. Muthén LK, Muthén BO (2008) Mplus user's guide. Los Angeles, CA: Muthén & Muthén. 676 p.
36. Asparouhov T, Muthén B (2009) Exploratory structural equation modeling. Struct Equ Modeling 16: 397–438.
37. Marsh HW, Lüdtke O, Muthén B, Asparouhov T, Morin AJS, et al. (2010). A new look at the Big-Five factor structure through exploratory structural equation modeling. Psychol Assess 22: 471–491.
38. Hu L, Bentler PM (1999) Cutoff criteria for fit indexes in covariance structure analysis: Conventional criteria versus new alternatives. Struct Equ Modeling 6: 1–55.
39. Forstmeier W, Schielzeth H (2011) Cryptic multiple hypotheses testing in linear models: Overestimated effect sizes and the winner's curse. Behav Ecol Sociobiol 65: 47–55.
40. Ackerman PL, Beier ME (2006) Determinants of domain knowledge and independent study learning in an adult sample. J Educ Psychol 98: 366–381.
41. Beier ME, Ackerman PL (2005) Age, ability, and the role of prior knowledge on the acquisition of new domain knowledge: Promising results in a real-world learning environment. Psychol Aging 20: 341–355.
42. Hambrick DZ, Meinz EJ, Pink JE, Pettibone JC, Oswald FL (2010) Learning outside the laboratory: Ability and non-ability influences on acquiring political knowledge. Learning Indiv Diff 20: 40–45.
43. Hambrick DZ, Pink JE, Meinz EJ, Pettibone JC, Oswald FL (2008) The roles of ability, personality, and interests in acquiring current events knowledge: A longitudinal study. Intelligence 36: 261–278.
44. Rhoten D, Pfirman S (2007) Women in interdisciplinary science: Exploring preferences and consequences. Res Policy 36: 56–75.
45. Evans EM, Schweingruber H, Stevenson HW (2002) Gender differences in interest and knowledge acquisition: The United States, Taiwan, and Japan. Sex Roles 47: 153–167.
46. Johnson W, Carothers A, Deary IJ (2009) A role for the X chromosome in sex differences in variability in general intelligence? Perspect Psychol Sci 4: 598–611.
47. Voracek M, Mohr E, Hagmann M (2013) On the importance of tail ratios for psychological science. Psychol Rep 112: 872–886.

7

Effects of Exercise Modalities on Arterial Stiffness and Wave Reflection

Ammar W. Ashor[1,2]*, Jose Lara[1], Mario Siervo[1], Carlos Celis-Morales[1], John C. Mathers[1]

1 Human Nutrition Research Centre, Institute of Cellular Medicine, Newcastle University, Campus for Ageing and Vitality, Newcastle on Tyne, United Kingdom, **2** College of Medicine, University of Al-Mustansiriyah, Baghdad, Iraq

Abstract

Background and Objectives: Physical activity is associated with lower cardiovascular and all-cause mortality. However, the effects of different exercise modalities on arterial stiffness are currently unclear. Our objectives were to investigate the effects of exercise modalities (aerobic, resistance or combined) on pulse wave velocity (PWV) and augmentation index (AIx), and to determine whether the effects on these indices differed according to the participants' or exercise characteristics.

Methods: We searched the Medline, Embase and Cochrane Library databases from inception until April 2014 for randomized controlled trials lasting ≥4 weeks investigating the effects of exercise modalities on PWV and AIx in adults aged ≥18 years.

Results: Forty-two studies (1627 participants) were included in this analysis. Aerobic exercise improved both PWV (WMD: −0.63 m/s, 95% CI: −0.90, −0.35) and AIx (WMD:−2.63%, 95% CI: −5.25 to −0.02) significantly. Aerobic exercise training showed significantly greater reduction in brachial-ankle (WMD: −1.01 m/s, 95% CI: −1.57, −0.44) than in carotid-femoral (WMD: -0.39 m/s, 95% CI: −0.52, −0.27) PWV. Higher aerobic exercise intensity was associated with larger reductions in AIx (β: −1.55%, CI −3.09, 0.0001). In addition, aerobic exercise had a significantly larger effect in reducing PWV (WMD:−1.0 m/s, 95% CI: −1.43, −0.57) in participants with stiffer arteries (PWV ≥8 m/s). Resistance exercise had no effect on PWV and AIx. There was no significant effect of combined exercise on PWV and AIx.

Conclusions: We conclude that aerobic exercise improved arterial stiffness significantly and that the effect was enhanced with higher aerobic exercise intensity and in participants with greater arterial stiffness at baseline.

Trial Registration PROSPERO: Database registration: CRD42014009744,.

Editor: Yan Li, Shanghai Institute of Hypertension, China

Funding: AA is funded by the Ministry of Higher Education and Scientific Research of Iraq. JL and JCM acknowledge support from the LiveWell Programme a research project funded through a collaborative grant from the Lifelong Health and Wellbeing (LLHW) initiative, managed by the Medical Research Council (MRC) (grant number G0900686). The funders had no role in study design, data collection and analysis, decision to publish, or preparation of the manuscript.

Competing Interests: The authors have declared that no competing interests exist.

* Email: a.w.ashor@ncl.ac.uk

Introduction

Physical activity (PA) are associated with 35% reduction in cardiovascular disease (CVD) mortality and 33% reduction in all-cause mortality in comparison with sedentary lifestyle [1]. Moreover, there is an inverse dose-response relationship between PA and CVD mortality or risk of coronary artery diseases [2]. Changes in known CVD risk factors such as body weight, blood pressure and serum lipids explain a large proportion (59%) of the observed beneficial effect of exercise on major CVD outcomes [3]. The remaining 40% of risk reduction may be attributed to effects on vascular hemodynamics including endothelial function (EF), arterial remodelling and compliance [4].

Arterial stiffening is a hallmark of ageing and is closely associated with many pathological conditions including atherosclerosis, dyslipidaemia, diabetes and chronic kidney diseases [5]. Reduced arterial compliance (i.e. increased stiffness) leads to faster reflection of the systolic wave from the peripheral small arteries to the heart, causing augmentation of the central aortic pressure [6]. This augmentation in central pressure leads to increased ventricular afterload and reduced coronary perfusion pressure which, eventually, may cause myocardial hypertrophy, ischaemia and infarction [7]. Thus, arterial stiffness appears to contribute to the complex etiology of CVD and is regarded as a predictor of increased CVD risk and all-cause mortality [8].

Evidence from randomized controlled trials (RCT) demonstrated a beneficial effect of various exercise modalities (aerobic,

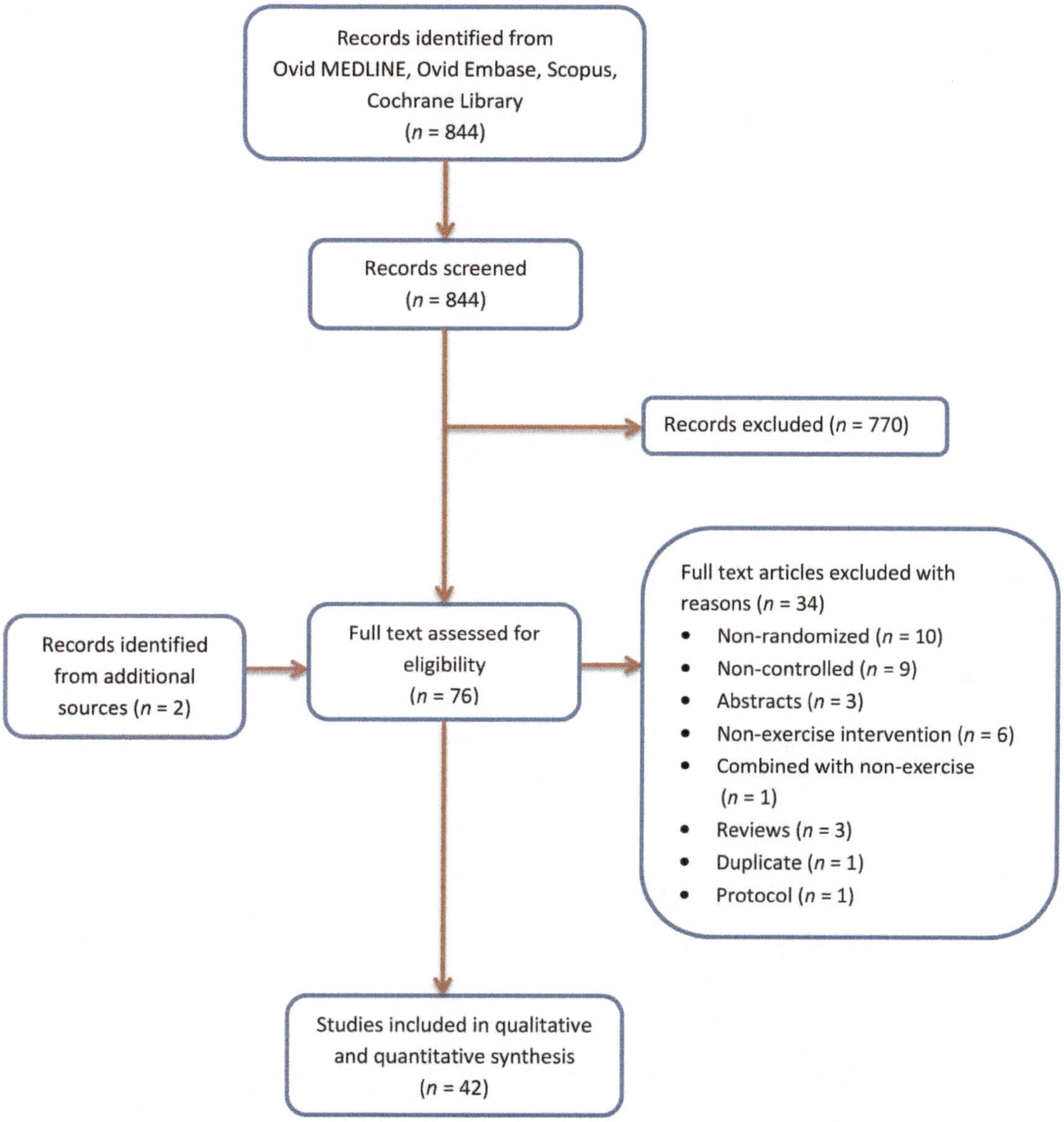

Figure 1. Flow diagram of the process used in selection of the randomized controlled trials included in this systematic review and meta-analysis.

resistance and combined) on endothelial function [9–11] but there is controversy about the effects of different exercise modalities on indices of arterial stiffness and wave reflection [12–14].

This systematic review aimed to investigate the effects of various exercise modalities on both PWV and AIx. The secondary aims were to determine whether the effects of exercise training on PWV and AIx were modified by participants (age, sex, health status, body mass index (BMI), heart rate, blood pressure, or baseline values of PWV) or exercise characteristics (intensity, frequency, duration of sessions or duration of intervention).

Methods

This systematic review was conducted according to the Cochrane guidelines and is reported according to PRISMA guidelines [15,16].

Data sources

The search for relevant studies was conducted via electronic searches of three databases (MEDLINE, Embase, and Cochrane library from inception until April 2014). Additionally, we searched for eligible studies in the reference lists of the relevant articles and reviews. The following keywords were used to search the above databases: exercise, training, physical activity, arterial stiffness, pulse wave velocity, augmentation index.

Study selection

The inclusion criteria for eligible studies were as follows: 1) RCT of exercise with comparative non-exercise, usual care or sedentary groups; 2) prescribed structured exercise intervention of ≥4 weeks duration; 3) adult humans aged ≥18 years; 4) studies that measured arterial stiffness by PWV or AIx before and after intervention. The selection of eligible studies was conducted by two reviewers independently (AA, JL). If consensus was reached,

Table 1. Characteristics of aerobic exercise studies included in the systematic review and meta-analysis.

Author	Health Status	Sample size	Age (years)	Male%	Basal BMI (kg/m^2)	Basal SBP (mmHg)	Basal DBP (mmHg)	Type of Exercise	Intensity	Session duration (minutes)	Frequency of sessions	Duration of Intervention (weeks)	Jadad's Score
Beck et al. 2013 [12]	Prehypertension	28	20.1±0.9	68	28.7±1.4	132±3	81±1	W/R	65–85%	45	3	8	3
Choi et al. 2012 [24]	Diabetes II	75	53.8±7.2	0		120 (118–130)	80 (79–80)	W	3.6–6 MET	60	5	12	5
Ciolac et al. 2010 AIT [25]	Risk of Hypertension	17	24.4±3.8	0	23.5±4.8	106±9.9	65±9.5	W/R	80–90%peakO2	40	3	16	3
Ciolac et al. 2010 CMT [25]	Risk of Hypertension	17	26.6±4.9	0	24.3±4.6	106±8.3	64.9±6.8	W/R	60–70%peakO2	40	3	16	3
Ferrier et al. 2001[26]	Systolic hypertension	10	64±7	50	29.5±1.3	154±7		C	65%Hrmax	40	3	8	3
Goldberg et al. 2012 [35]	Risk of Hypertension	30	20.5±0.5	100	23.3±0.5	115±1.4	69±1.6	C	65%Hrmax	30	3	4	2
Gumaraes et al. 2010 AIT [44]	Hypertension	22	45±9	77	29±5	125±9	81±5	R	65%Hrmax	40	3	16	5
Gumaraes et al. 2010 CMT [44]	Hypertension	21	50±8	62	28±4	124±9	81±9	R	65–80%Hrmax	40	3	16	5
Heydari et al. 2013 [36]	Healthy	34	24.4±4.7	100	28.4±0.6	120±2.4	64±1.8	C	80–90%Hrmax	20	3	12	2
Heydari et al. 2013 [37]	Healthy	38	26.5	100	28.4±2.4	119.6±9.9	63.7±7.3	C	80–90%Hrmax	20	3	12	5
Ho et al. 2012 [14]	Overweight/Obese	31	55 (44–62)	13	33 (25–46)	120 (96–159)	67 (55–86)	W	60%Hrr	30	5	12	4
Kearney et al. 2014 [45]	Overweight	65	45±6.2	77	29.2±4	122±12	85±7.4	W			5	26	4
Koh et al. 2010 ID [46]	CKD	23	52.3±10.9	61	27.6±7	148±22	82±10	C	12–13 Borg	30–45	3	26	2
Koh et al. 2010 HB [46]	CKD	23	52±14	65	27.9±4.9	143±32	78±16	W	12–13 Borg	30–45	3	26	2
Krustrup et al. 2010 FG [27]	Premenopausal	28	37±2	0	25±0.9	113±2	74±2	FB	80–84%Hrmax	60	2	16	3
Krustrup et al. 2010 RG [27]	Premenopausal	24	37±1	0	23.7±0.7	112±2	71±2	R	80–84%Hrmax	60	2	16	2
Krustrup et al. 2013 [38]	Hypertension	33	46	100	30±3.3	151	92	Soccer	85–90%Hrmax	60	2	26	2
Madden et al. 2009 [47]	Diabetes II	34	71.4	53	30±1.1	150±6	83±2	C	65–80%Hrmax	40	3	13	5
Madden et al. 2013 [48]	Diabetes II	52	68.5±0.9	58	30.9±1	148±4	82±3	C	60–75%Hrmax	40	3	26	4
Mustata et al. 2011 [49]	CKD	18	64 (55–73)	67	28 (25–32)	140 (130–150)	78 (70–80)	W/C	12–50 Borg	20–60	4	52	4
Nualnim et al. 2011 [50]	Hypertension	43	58±2	26	29±1	131±3	76±2	Swimming	60–75%Hrmax	20–45	3.5	12	4
Oudegeest-Sander et al. 2013 [51]	Healthy	22	68±3	50	27±2.6	131±9	76±6	C	70–85%Hrmax	30	3	52	4
Parnell et al. 2002 [52]	CHF	21	57±15	90	26±0.7	106±7	62±2	W/C	50–60%Hrmax	30–60	6	8	2
Sugawara et al. 2012 [31]	Post menopause	22	59±2	0	23.4±1	117±3	71±2	C	60–75%Hrmax	25–45	4.5	8	5
Toussaint et al. 2008 [62]	CKD	18	67 (60–83)	50	27±4	144±16	75±12	C		30	3	12	4
Westhoff et al. 2008 [53]	Hypertension	24	66.1±4	46	28.6±4.4	134±20	73±21.6	C	2±0.5 lactate	20	3	12	4
Yoshizawa et al. 2009 [33]	Healthy	24	47±2	0	24.6±1.1	120±3	74±3	C	60–70%peakO2	30	2	12	2

AIT, aerobic interval training; C, cycling; CHF, congestive heart failure; CKD, chronic kidney disease; CMT, continuous moderate-intensity training; HB, home-based; HRmax, maximum heart rate; Hrr, heart rate reserve; FB, football; FG, football group; ID, intradialytic; MET, metabolic equivalents; R, running; RG, running group; W, walking.

Table 2. Characteristics of resistance/combined exercises studies included in the systematic review and meta-analysis.

Author	Health Status	Sample size	Age (Years)	Male%	Body weight (kg)	Basal BMI (kg/m²)	Basal SBP (mmHg)	Basal DBP (mmHg)	Intensity	Session duration (minutes)	Frequency of Sessions	Duration of Intervention (weeks)	Jadad's Score
Resistance exercise													
Beck et al. 2013 [12]	Prehypertension	30	21.1±0.6	70	84.2±4.7	27.4±1.3	130.4±3	80±3	60% 1RM	45	3	8	3
Cortez-Cooper et al. 2008 [54]	Healthy	25	52±2	28	76±3	26.8±1.1	113±3	66±2	70% 1RM	30–45	3	13	2
Croymans et al. 2014 [34]	Overweight/Obese	36	21.5	100	97	31	132	81	100%1RM	60	3	12	3
Heffernan et al. 2013 [56]	Prehypertension	21	60±2	29		24±1	140±4	83±2	40–60%1RM		3	12	3
Ho et al. 2012 [14]	Overweight/Obese	32	52 (43–59)	12.5	89	33	126	71	70% 1RM	30	5	12	4
Miyachi et al. 2004 [40]	Healthy	28	22±1	100	66.5±2.4	22.2±0.7	116±3	69±1	80% 1RM	45	3	16	4
Okamoto et al. 2006 ERT [30]	Healthy	15	18.9±0.3	0	55.5±6.1	21.7±2.1	105	61	100%1RM	15	3	8	4
Okamoto et al. 2006 CRT [30]	Healthy	14	19±0.3	0	52.7±7.5	21.9±3.1	102	60	80% 1RM	15	3	8	4
Okamoto et al. 2008 [41]	Healthy	19	19.4	100					40% 1RM		2	8	3
Okamoto et al. 2009 UL [43]	Healthy	15	20±0.4	100	63±13	23±3.6	119±11	67±8	80% 1RM	75	2	10	3
Okamoto et al. 2009 LL [43]	Healthy	15	20±0.5	100	63±12	22±3.6	120±12	68±7	80% 1RM	75	2	10	3
Okamoto et al. 2009 ERT [42]	Healthy	15	19.6	100	62	21	118	66	80% 1RM	105	2	10	3
Okamoto et al. 2009 CRT [42]	Healthy	15	19	100	64	23	117	62	80% 1RM	105	2	10	3
Okamoto et al. 2011 [59]	Healthy	26	18.5	73	65.6±11.5	23.3±4.1	115±13	64±7	50% 1RM	50	2	10	3
Okamoto et al. 2013 ALRT [60]	Healthy	15	19	53	61	23	114	65	50–80%1RM	60	2	10	2
Okamoto et al. 2013 BLRT [60]	Healthy	15	19	47	58	22	115	65	50–80%1RM	60	2	10	2
Yoshizawa et al. 2009 [33]	Healthy	23	47±2	0	59±2	24.8±1	122±7	78±4	60% 1RM	30	2	12	2
Combined (aerobic and resistance) exercise													
Cortez-Cooper et al. 2008 [54]	Healthy	24	51±1	29	76±5	27±1.1	118±3	68±2	60–75%Hrr/ 70% 1RM	30–45	4	13	3
Dobrosielski et al. 2012 [55]	Diabetes II	114	57±6	68	97±2.1	33±0.6	127±1.6	72±1.1	60–90%Hrmax/ 50% 1RM	60	3	26	3
Figueroa et al. 2011[13]	Postmenopause	24	54±2	0	62	24			60%Hrmax/ 60% 1RM	40	3	12	3
Ho et al. 2012 [14]	Overweight/Obese	33	53 (43–64)	12	90	33	118	66	60%Hrr/75% 1RM	30	5	12	4
Kawasaki et al. 2011 [57]	Healthy	57	62±0.8	39	60±1.8	23.7±0.6	137±3.2	81±1.6	50%peakO2	100	2	26	3
Loimaala et al. 2009 [39]	Diabetes II	48	53.6±6.2	100	90±9.5	29±3.7	145±2.8		65–75%peakO2/ 60–80% 1RM	30	4	104	3
Miura et al. 2008 1DW [28]	Postmenopause	41	69±6.5	0	52±6.7	23±2.4	126±14	74±8	70%Hrmax	45	1	12	2
Miura et al. 2008 2DW [28]	Postmenopause	36	69.5±7	0	54±7	24±2.7	123±14	73±9	70%Hrmax	45	2	12	2
Ohta et al. 2012 [29]	Postmenopause	26	72±4	0		23±2.6	151±19	85±9.8	4 METs	20	5	12	3
Okamoto et al. 2007 BRT [58]	Healthy	17	18.5±0.2	65	58.4±3.2	22.1±0.7	113.6±3.4	62.5±2.2	60%Hrmax/ 80% 1RM		2	8	4

Table 2. Cont.

Author	Health Status	Sample size	Age (Years)	Male%	Body weight (kg)	Basal BMI (kg/m^2)	Basal SBP (mmHg)	Basal DBP (mmHg)	Intensity	Session duration (minutes)	Frequency of Sessions	Duration of Intervention (weeks)	Jadad's Score
OKamoto et al. 2007 ART [58]	Healthy	16	18.5±0.2	69	59±3	23±2	113.5±4	65±2	60%Hrmax/ 80% 1RM		2	8	4
Stewart et al. 2005 [61]	Prehypertension	104	63	49	83	29	140	77	60–90%Hrmax/ 50% 1RM	60	3	26	3
Wong et al. 2014 [32]	Postmenopause	30	57	0	88	34	133	77		50	3	8	4

1DW, 1 day per week, 2DW, 2 days per week; ALRT, low intensity after high intensity resistance training; ART, aerobic training after resistance training; BLRT, low intensity before high intensity resistance training; BRT, aerobic training before resistance training; CRT, concentric resistance training; ERT, eccentric resistance training; Hrmax, maximum heart rate; LL, lower limb; MET, metabolic equivalent; UL, upper limb; RM, repetition maximum;

articles were excluded or moved to the next stage (full-text screening) as appropriate. If consensus was not reached the article was moved to the next stage where the full-text of selected articles was appraised. Disagreements were resolved by discussion between the reviewers until consensus was reached.

Data extraction and quality assessment

The following information was extracted from eligible articles: 1) study design, quality, and sample size; 2) participants' characteristics (age, sex, health status, BMI, and baseline arterial stiffness and wave reflection indices, heart rate, systolic and diastolic blood pressure); 3) characteristics of exercise intervention (type, duration and frequency of sessions, and intensity and duration of intervention); 4) outcome measures and instruments; and 5) indices of study quality which was assessed by the modified Jadad's score (range 0–5) using three main items related to randomization, blinding and description of dropout or withdrawals [17]. Because it is difficult (if not impossible) to blind participants to an exercise intervention, we considered the blinding of the outcome assessment by the operator as a quality criterion.

Statistical analyses

The outcome of the meta-analysis is the net difference between the intervention and control group in PWV or AIx at the end of the study. PWV is defined as the speed of travel of the pressure pulse along the arterial segment, is calculated as the distance/transit time ratio and is expressed as meters per second [18]. The AIx is defined as the proportion of central pulse pressure due to the late systolic peak which, in turn, is attributed to the reflected pulse wave and is expressed as percentage [19]. Statistical analyses were performed using STATA 12 (StataCorp. 2011. College Station, TX, USA). The effect size was estimated as weighted mean differences (WMDs) with 95% confidence interval. Random effect models were used to take account of between-study heterogeneity for participant characteristics, study design and methods used to assess arterial stiffness and wave reflection. Data not provided in the main text or tables were extracted from the figures. For crossover trials, we used the mean and SD separately for the intervention and control conditions [20]. In trials with multiple treatment arms and a single control group, the sample size of the control group was divided by the number of treatment groups to avoid over-inflation of the sample size [15].

Subgroup analyses were undertaken to investigate the role of potential factors influencing the effect of exercise modalities on arterial stiffness and accounting for heterogeneity in the models. These factors included the age, gender and health status of participants, baseline values for BMI, blood pressure, PWV and AIx. However, in this investigation we restricted subgroup analysis to cases with $\geq$5 studies per subgroup [15]. Meta-regression analyses were conducted to examine the relationships between exercise characteristics (intensity, frequency and duration of sessions) and changes in PWV and AIx indices. Where studies reported a range of intensities across different time periods, exercise intensity was calculated as the mean intensity across all periods. Both relative (% maximum heart rate, %HRmax) and absolute (metabolic equivalents, METs) exercise intensities were calculated using the methods and formulae described by Howley [21]. Where studies used both aerobic and resistance exercise interventions, we estimated the exercise intensities for each type separately and then calculated the average of both exercise intensities.

Publication bias was evaluated by visual inspection of the funnel plot and by Egger's regression test [22]. Heterogeneity between

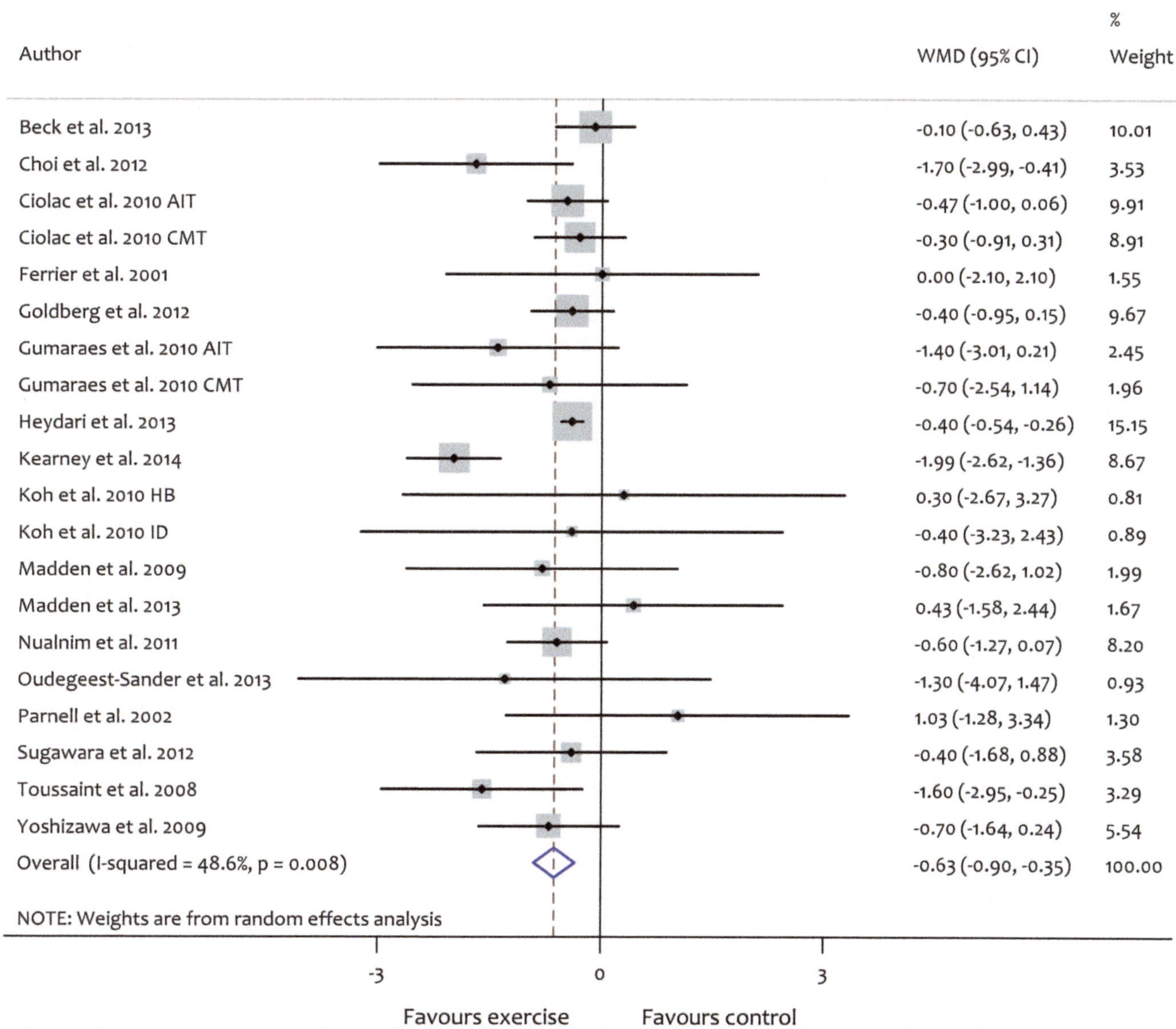

Figure 2. Forest plot showing the effect of aerobic exercise on pulse wave velocity (PWV). AIT, aerobic interval training; CMT, continuous moderate-intensity training; ID, intradialytic; HB, home-based.

studies was evaluated using Cochrane Q statistics; $P>0.1$ indicates significant heterogeneity. The I^2 test was also used to evaluate consistency between studies where a value <25% indicates low risk of heterogeneity, 25–75% indicates moderate risk of heterogeneity and >75% indicates high risk of heterogeneity [23].

Results

Search results

The process followed in the selection of eligible studies is summarized in Figure 1. After full text examination, 42 randomized controlled trials (RCT) were included in the final analysis.

Study characteristics

Characteristics of the studies included in the systematic review and meta-analysis are summarized in Tables 1 and 2. Further characteristics of the included studies are also provided in Tables S1 and S2. The total number of participants was 1627 (801 males, 826 females) with a median sample size of 24 participants per study (range 10–114). Participant age ranged from 19 to 72 years (median 47 years). Eleven studies included females only [13,24–33] while 9 studies included males only [34–43]. The median duration of the studies was 12 weeks (range: 4–52 weeks). The quality of the included studies ranged from 2–5 with a median quality score of 3. The study design comprised 40 parallel [12–14,24,25,27–61] and 2 crossover studies [26,62]. Some of the articles included results from separate, independent trials testing the effects of two or more exercise modalities on arterial stiffness so that the 42 articles yielded a total of 46 trials that measured PWV (20 aerobic, 14 resistance and 12 combined) and 23 trials that measured AIx (16 aerobic, 5 resistance and 2 combined) for the final analysis. Of the 23 trials that measured AIx, only 6 studies reported heart rate-adjusted AIx [12,31,32,34,46,53]. The methods for quantification of PWV differed between studies and included 28 trials carotid-femoral (cf-PWV), 17 trials brachial-ankle (ba-PWV) and 1 trial femoral-ankle (fa-PWV) measure-

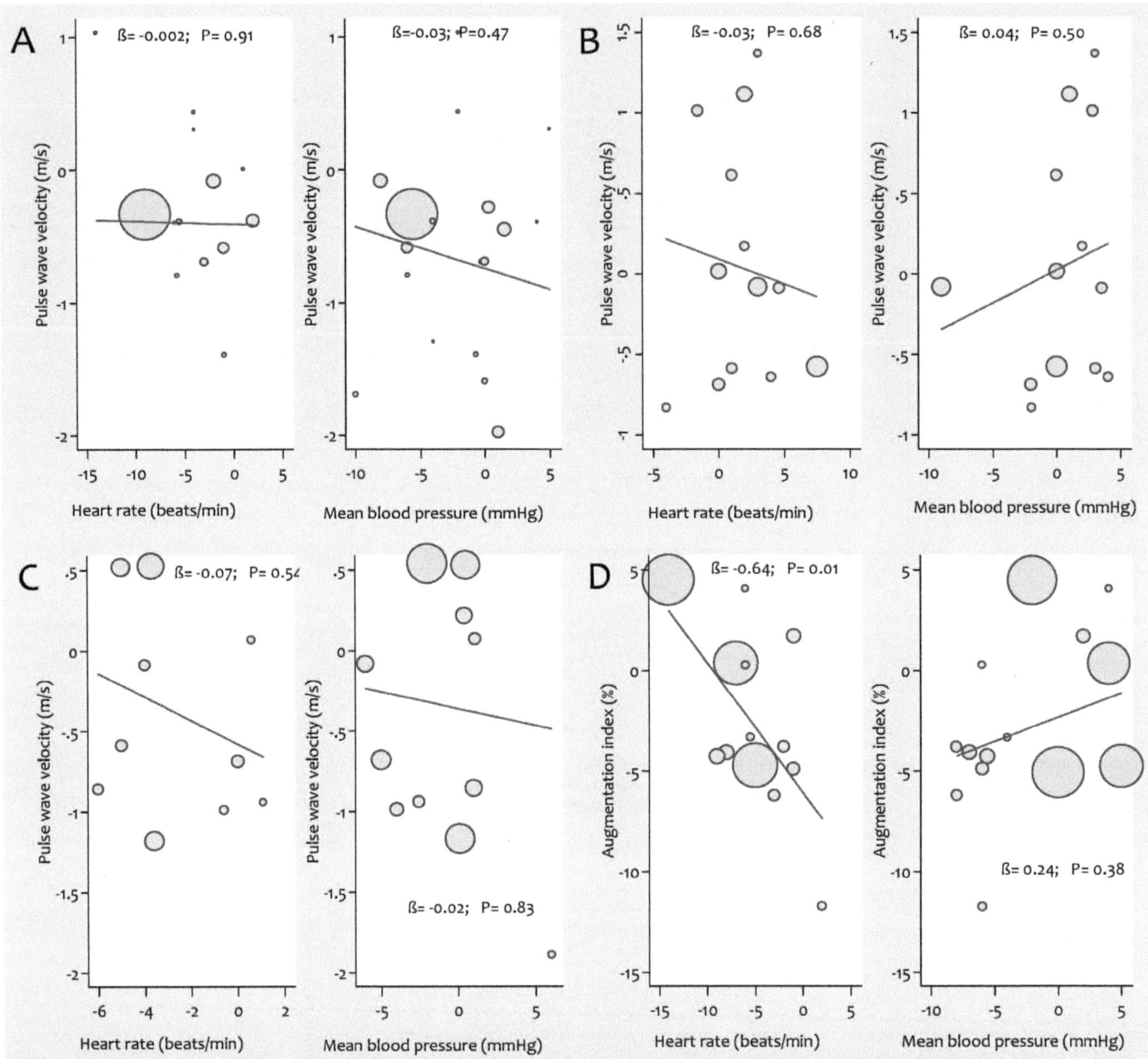

Figure 3. Associations between pulse wave velocity (PWV) and changes in heart rate and mean arterial blood pressure in response to (a) aerobic (b) resistance (c) combined aerobic and resistance exercise intervention. (d) Association between augmentations index (AIx) and changes in heart rate and mean arterial blood pressure in response to aerobic exercise intervention. Each study is depicted by a circle where the circle size represents the degree of weighting for the study based on participant numbers in the study.

ments. The relative intensity of exercise ranged from 55% to 100% with a median of 74% HRmax while the median of absolute intensity was 7.2 (range 4–12 METs). The duration of exercise sessions ranged from 20 to 100 minutes (median: 40 minutes) and the frequency from 1 to 6 sessions per week (median: 3 per week).

Aerobic exercise and PWV

Data synthesis from aerobic exercise trials revealed a significant reduction in PWV with exercise (WMD: −0.63 m/s, 95% CI: −0.90, −0.35, $P<0.01$). However, these studies were characterised by significant heterogeneity ($X^2 = 36.9$, $P<0.01$, $I^2 = 48.6\%$) (Figure 2). Aerobic exercise training showed significantly greater reduction in ba-PWV in comparison with cf-PWV (Table 3). Subgroup analysis showed significantly greater reduction in PWV after aerobic exercise intervention in participants with stiffer arteries (PWV >8 m/s) (Table 3). In addition, there was a tendency for larger reductions in arterial stiffness with aerobic exercise in studies lasting more than 10 weeks (Table 3). The outcomes of subgroup analyses according to participant health status are reported in Table 4. Meta-regression analyses did not show evidence of a relationship between exercise characteristics and PWV (Figure S1) and changes in PWV were not related to changes in heart rate or mean blood pressure after the interventions (Figure 3).

Table 3. Subgroup analyses of the effects exercise modalities on pulse wave velocity (PWV) using a random-effects model.

	Aerobic Exercise			Resistance Exercise			Combined (aerobic and resistance)		
	Trials (No.)[a]	WMD% (95% CI)	*P* value[b]	Trials (No.)[a]	WMD% (95% CI)	*P* value[b]	Trials (No.)[a]	WMD% (95% CI)	*P* value[b]
Outcome (m/s)			0.03			0.89			0.29
Carotid-femoral PWV	17 (422)	−0.39 (−0.52 to −0.27)		6 (144)	−0.12 (−0.67 to 0.43)		5 (320)	−0.07 (−0.66 to 0.51)	
Brachial-ankle PWV	10 (377)	−1.01 (−1.57 to −0.44)		12 (217)	−0.07 (−0.51 to 0.37)		8 (247)	−0.58 (−1.16 to 0.01)	
Age of participants (years)			0.96			0.36			0.99
≤ 50 years	9 (262)	−0.62 (−0.98 to −0.26)		13 (253)	0.001 (−0.39 to 0.39)		2 (33)	−0.35 (−2.01 to 1.31)	
> 50 years	11 (343)	−0.67 (−1.11 to −0.24)		1 (25)	−0.84 (−2.04 to 0.36)		10 (504)	−0.27 (−0.73 to 0.18)	
Gender			0.53			0.71			0.75
Female	5 (155)	−0.52 (−0.87 to −0.18)		3 (52)	0.09 (−0.81 to 1.01)		5 (157)	−0.47 (−1.14 to 0.19)	
Male	2 (68)	−0.40 (−0.53 to −0.26)		6 (115)	−0.14 (−0.74 to 0.45)		1 (48)	−0.70 (−1.77 to 0.37)	
Body mass index (kg/m^2)			0.47			0.15			0.35
≤ 24.9	5 (110)	−0.42 (−0.72 to −0.13)		10 (168)	0.20 (−0.25 to 0.66)		7 (217)	−0.57 (−1.26 to 0.11)	
≥ 25.0	14 (420)	−0.68 (−1.13 to −0.24)		3 (91)	−0.41 (−0.80 to −0.03)		5 (320)	−0.07 (−0.66 to 0.51)	
Baseline systolic pressure (mmHg)			0.27			0.16			0.67
≤ 120	8 (244)	−0.41 (−0.54 to −0.28)		10 (170)	0.20 (−0.27 to 0.67)		3 (57)	−0.50 (−1.67 to 0.67)	
> 120	12 (361)	−0.81 (−1.38 to −0.23)		3 (89)	−0.40 (−0.75 to −0.06)		8 (456)	−0.16 (−0.68 to 0.35)	
Baseline diastolic pressure (mmHg)			0.39			0.29			0.24
≤ 80	12 (350)	−0.43 (−0.55 to −0.30)		12 (223)	0.10 (−0.29 to 0.50)		8 (382)	−0.17 (−0.76 to 0.41)	
> 80	7 (245)	−0.80 (−1.71 to 0.10)		1 (36)	−0.60 (−1.09 to −0.10)		2 (83)	−1.21 (−2.54 to 0.11)	
Baseline PWV (m/s)			0.01						
≤ 8	6 (151)	−0.37 (−0.50 to −0.25)		4 (96)	0.07 (−0.60 to 0.76)		-	-	
> 8	14 (454)	−1.00 (−1.43 to −0.57)		10 (182)	−0.10 (−0.59 to 0.38)		12 (537)	−0.35 (−0.82 to 0.12)	
Intensity of exercise (METs)			0.51			0.63			0.59
≤ 7	10 (321)	−0.52 (−0.87 to −0.17)		6 (128)	−0.15 (−0.75 to 0.44)		7 (402)	−0.19 (−0.79 to 0.42)	
> 7	8 (201)	−0.39 (−0.52 to −0.26)		8 (150)	0.05 (−0.49 to 0.59)		4 (105)	−0.54 (−1.42 to 0.34)	
Duration of the study (weeks)			0.09			0.11			0.87
≤ 10	5 (111)	−0.21 (−0.57 to 0.13)		11 (194)	0.12 (−0.31 to 0.56)		3 (63)	−0.28 (−1.43 to 0.87)	
> 10	15 (494)	−0.80 (−1.16 to −0.44)		3 (84)	−0.62 (−1.03 to −0.22)		9 (474)	−0.33 (−0.85 to 0.18)	
Quality of studies (Jadad score)			0.37			0.86			0.91
< 3	5 (121)	−0.39 (−0.85 to 0.05)		4 (78)	−0.008 (−0.87 to 0.85)		2 (77)	−0.43 (−1.65 to 0.79)	
≥ 3	15 (484)	−0.70 (−1.04 to −0.36)		10 (200)	−0.08 (−0.50 to 0.34)		10 (460)	−0.35(−0.87 to 0.17)	

[a]Number of trials or subgroups (number of participants)
[b]*P* value for the meta-regression analyses between subgroups,
PWV pulse wave velocity, WMD weighted mean difference.

Table 4. Subgroup analyses of the effect exercise modalities (aerobic, resistance or combined) on indices of arterial stiffness (pulse wave velocity and augmentation index) according to the health status of the included participants.

	Trials (No.)[a]	WMD% (95% CI)	*P* value
Aerobic exercise (Pulse wave velocity)			
Healthy	3 (84)	−0.41 (−0.55 to −0.27)	< 0.01
Overweight/obese	1 (65)	−1.99 (−2.62 to −1.36)	< 0.01
Post-menopause	1 (22)	−0.40 (−1.68 to 0.88)	0.54
Pre-hypertension	4 (28)	−0.32 (−0.59 to −0.04)	0.03
Hypertension	4 (86)	−0.66 (−1.23 to −0.10)	0.02
Diabetes II	3 (161)	−0.89 (−2.09 to 0.32)	0.15
Congestive heart failure	1 (21)	1.03 (−1.28 to 3.34)	0.38
Chronic kidney disease	3 (64)	−1.14 (−2.26 to −0.01)	0.05
Aerobic exercise (Augmentation index)			
Healthy	2 (72)	−4.30 (−8.58 to −0.02)	0.05
Overweight/obese	1 (31)	1.57 (−4.75 to 7.89)	0.63
Pre-menopause	2 (52)	−2.55 (−7.55 to 2.44)	0.32
Post-menopause	1 (22)	−3.40 (−15.12 to 8.32)	0.57
Pre-hypertension	2 (28)	−7.16 (−14.79 to 0.46)	0.07
Hypertension	3 (100)	−4.60 (−9.44 to 0.24)	0.06
Congestive heart failure	1 (21)	4.07 (2.27 to 5.87)	< 0.01
Chronic kidney disease	4 (82)	−4.28 (−7.34 to −1.22)	< 0.01
Resistance exercise			
Healthy	12 (212)	0.03 (−0.43 to 0.47)	0.91
Overweight/obese	1 (36)	−0.60 (−1.09 to −0.11)	0.72
Pre-hypertension	1 (30)	−0.10 (−0.65 to 0.45)	0.02
Combined (resistance and aerobic) exercise			
Healthy	4 (114)	−0.59 (−1.55 to 0.37)	0.23
Post-menopause	5 (157)	−0.48 (−1.15 to 0.19)	0.16
Pre-hypertension	1 (104)	0.50 (−0.02 to 1.02)	0.06
Diabetes II	2 (162)	−0.32 (−1.19 to 0.55)	0.47

[a]Number of trials or subgroups (number of participants).

Visual inspection of the funnel plot for the aerobic exercise studies (Figure S2) together with Egger's regression test (β: −0.40, $P = 0.31$) suggest low likelihood of publication bias.

Resistance exercise and PWV

Overall, resistance exercise training was ineffective in improving PWV (WMD: −0.04 m/s, 95% CI: −0.42, 0.34, $P = 0.82$) but there was significant heterogeneity between studies ($X^2 = 39.9$, $P < 0.01$, $I^2 = 67.5$) (Figure 4). Subgroup analyses of resistance exercise studies showed no significant differences between groups based on participant or study characteristics (Table 3) and meta-regression analyses found no evidence for relationships between resistance exercise characteristics and arterial stiffness (Figure S3). Subgroup analyses according to participant health status are reported in Table 4. Changes in PWV were not related to changes in heart rate or blood pressure after the interventions (Figure 3).

Visual inspection of the funnel plot did not show evidence of publication bias for the resistance exercise studies included in the meta-analysis (Figure S2) and Egger's regression test outcomes (β: −0.54, $P = 0.50$) confirmed the likely absence of publication bias.

Combined (aerobic and resistance) exercise and PWV

Analysis of data from combined modalities exercise trials showed a non-significant reduction in PWV (WMD: −0.35 m/s, 95% CI: −0.82, 0.12, $P = 0.15$) with significant heterogeneity between studies ($X^2 = 24.3$, $P < 0.01$, $I^2 = 54.7$) (Figure 5). Subgroup analyses of combined (aerobic and resistance) exercise studies demonstrated no significant differences between groups based on participant characteristics (Table 3). The outcomes of subgroup analyses according to participant health status are summarized in Table 4. Meta-regression analyses showed no significant relationships between characteristics of the combined exercise interventions and PWV (Figure S4). Changes in PWV were not related to changes in heart rate or mean blood pressure after the interventions (Figure 3).

Neither funnel plot (Figure S2) nor Egger's regression test (β: 0.60, $P = 0.10$) suggested evidence of publication bias for the studies included in the combined exercise meta-analysis.

Effect of exercise modalities on AIx%

Aerobic exercise intervention lowered the AIx significantly (WMD: −2.63%, 95% CI: −5.25 to −0.02, $P = 0.05$) (Figure 6).

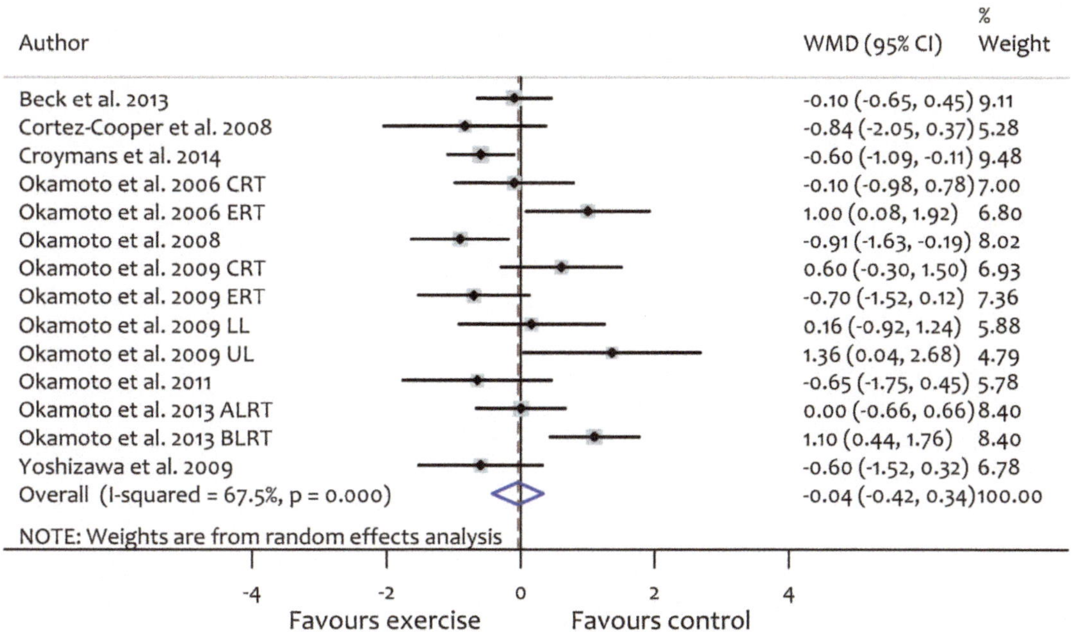

Figure 4. Forest plot showing the effect of resistance exercise on pulse wave velocity (PWV). ERT, eccentric resistance training; CRT, concentric resistance training; UL, upper limb; LL, lower limb; ALRT, low intensity after high intensity resistance training; BLRT, low intensity before high intensity resistance training.

There was significant heterogeneity between studies ($X^2 = 80.3$, $P<0.01$, $I^2 = 81.3$) but subgroup analyses did not reveal evidence of significant differences between groups based on participant or study characteristics (Table S3). Subgroup analyses according to participant health status are reported in Table 4. Meta-regression analyses showed that frequency of aerobic exercise sessions/week

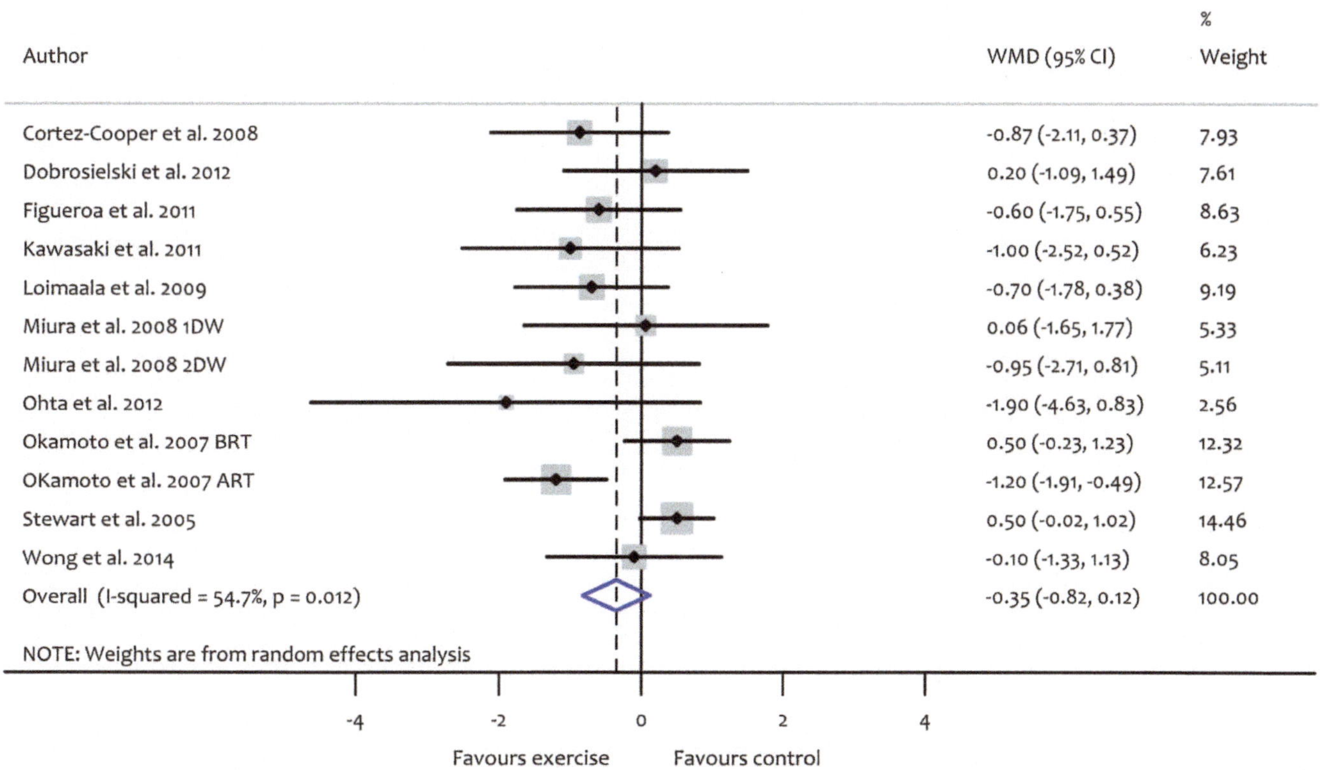

Figure 5. Forest plot showing the effect of combined (aerobic and resistance) exercise on pulse wave velocity (PWV). 1DW, 1 day per week, 2DW, 2 days per week; BRT, aerobic training before resistance training, ART, aerobic training after resistance training.

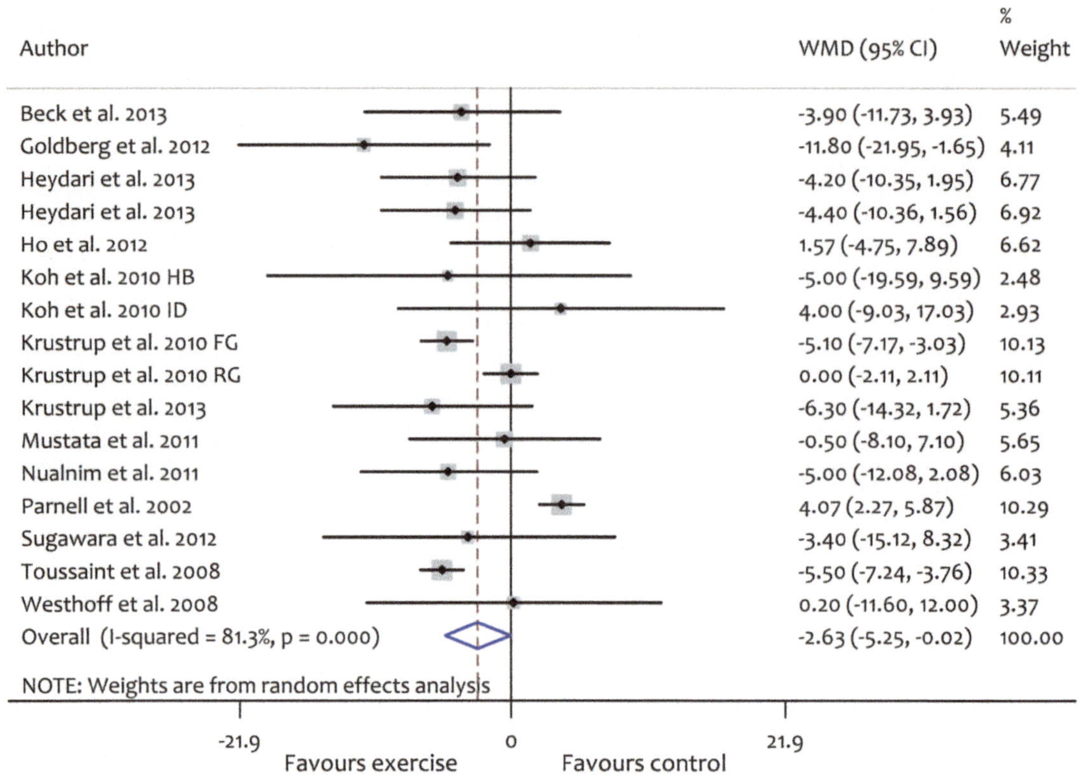

Figure 6. Forest plot showing the effect of aerobic exercise on augmentation index (AIx). intradialytic; HB, home-based; FG, football group, RG, running group.

was significantly associated with an increase in (worsened) AIx (β: 1.87, CI 0.34, 3.39, $P = 0.02$). Conversely, levels of absolute (β: −1.55, CI −3.09, 0.0001, $P = 0.05$) and relative (β: −0.19, CI: −0.40, 0.02, $P = 0.07$) exercise intensity were inversely associated with AIx (Figure 7). There was no evidence of publication bias in the included studies based on a funnel plot (Figure S2) and egger's regression test (β: −1.14, $P = 0.61$). Changes in AIx correlated significantly with changes in heart rate (β: −0.64, CI: −1.11, −0.17, $P = 0.011$) but not with changes in mean blood pressure (Figure 3).

Resistance exercise interventions did not reduce AIx significantly (WMD: −1.69%, 95% CI: −4.11 to 0.72, $P = 0.17$) (Figure 8). Furthermore, only two studies [14,32] investigated the effect of combined aerobic and resistance exercise on AIx and these showed non-significant improvement (WMD: −1.66%, 95% CI: −6.18 to 2.86, $P = 0.47$). Because of the small number of studies which addressed the effect of resistance (5 trials) or combined (2 trials) exercise on AIx, we were unable to perform subgroup or meta-regression analyses to investigate the potential modifying effects of participant or exercise characteristics on changes in AIx.

Discussion

In the current meta-analysis we observed a significant improvement in PWV and AIx in response to aerobic exercise intervention. This aerobic exercise effect tended to be greater in peripheral (ba-PWV) rather than in central (cf-PWV) indices. Additionally, larger effects observed in participants with more arterial stiffness at baseline and in trials with longer duration. Furthermore, intensity (relative and absolute) rather than volume of exercise (frequency and duration of sessions) was positively associated with improvement in AIx. However, resistance and combined (aerobic and resistance) exercise interventions produced no beneficial effects on PWV or AIx.

Oxidative stress and inflammation are the main insults causing stiffening of the vascular wall [63,64]. Fragmentation of elastin, deposition of collagen, and smooth muscle proliferation are the end result of continuous exposure to free radicals and inflammatory cytokines [65]. In addition, reduced nitric oxide (NO) and increased vasoconstrictor agents (angiotensin, endothelin, prostaglandins) exacerbate arterial stiffness [66]. Evidence from both animal and human studies shows the beneficial effect of physical activity (exercise) on vascular compliance and remodelling [67]. For example, the arteries of exercised animals had higher elastin and lower collagen than those from physically inactive animals [68]. Moreover, there is evidence that chronic exercise has anti-oxidative effects through up-regulation of superoxide dismutases (SOD1, SOD3) and down-regulation of NAD(P)H oxidase [69]. Furthermore, clinical investigations have documented the anti-inflammatory effect of regular physical activity by increasing the anti-inflammatory cytokines (interleukin 4, 10) and reducing pro-inflammatory cytokines (interleukin 6 and tumour necrosis factor alpha) [70]. Lastly, there is evidence that exercise enhances production of NO and reduces the concentrations of vasoconstrictor agents (endothelin I, angiotensin II) [71].

In our meta-analysis, aerobic exercise reduced PWV and AIx significantly. This finding is in contrast with findings from recently published meta-analyses which did not find a significant positive effect of aerobic exercise in pre-hypertensive, hypertensive and obese participants [72,73]. These 2 meta-analyses pooled the results from various measures of arterial stiffness and of wave

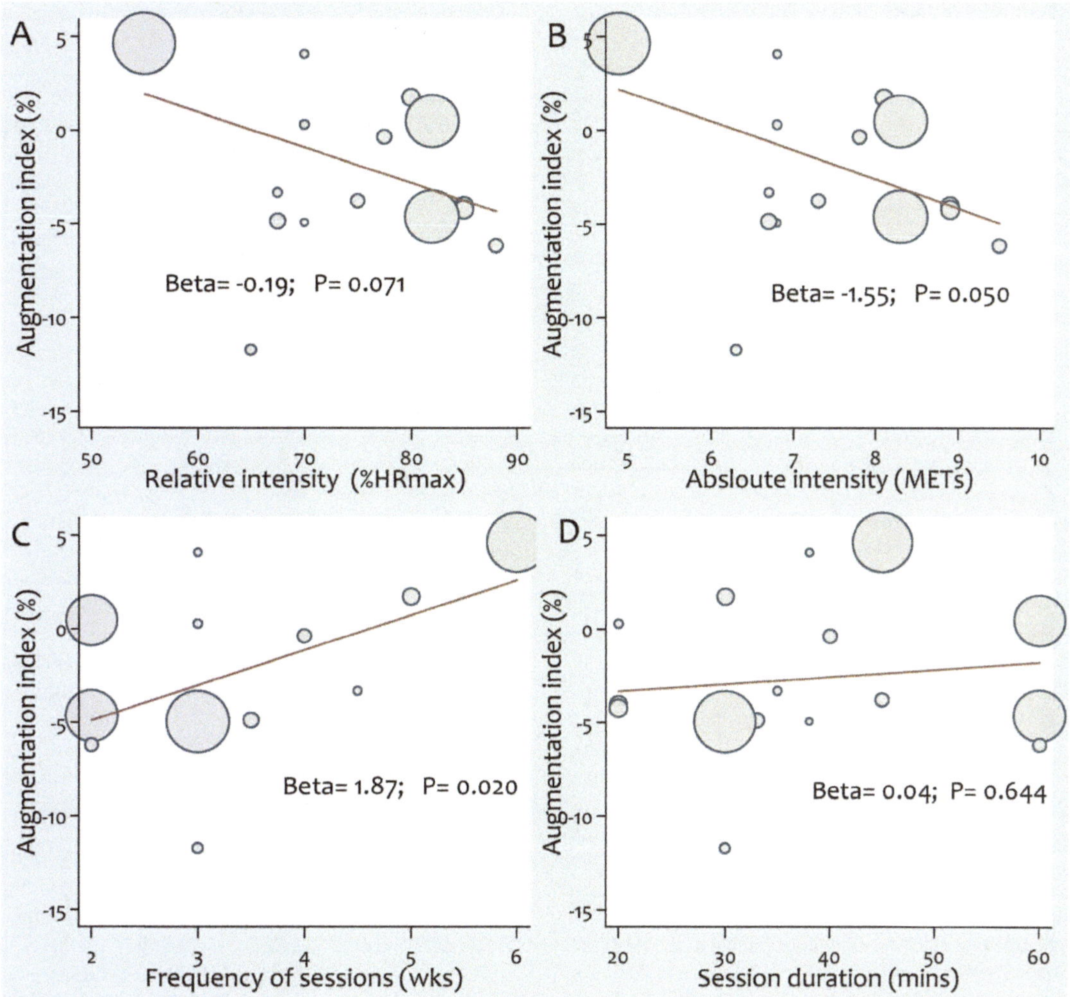

Figure 7. Associations between aerobic exercise intervention characteristics and augmentation index (AIx): (a) relative intensity; (b) absolute intensity; (c) session frequency; (d) session duration. Each study is depicted by a circle where the circle size represents the degree of weighting for the study based on participant numbers in the study.

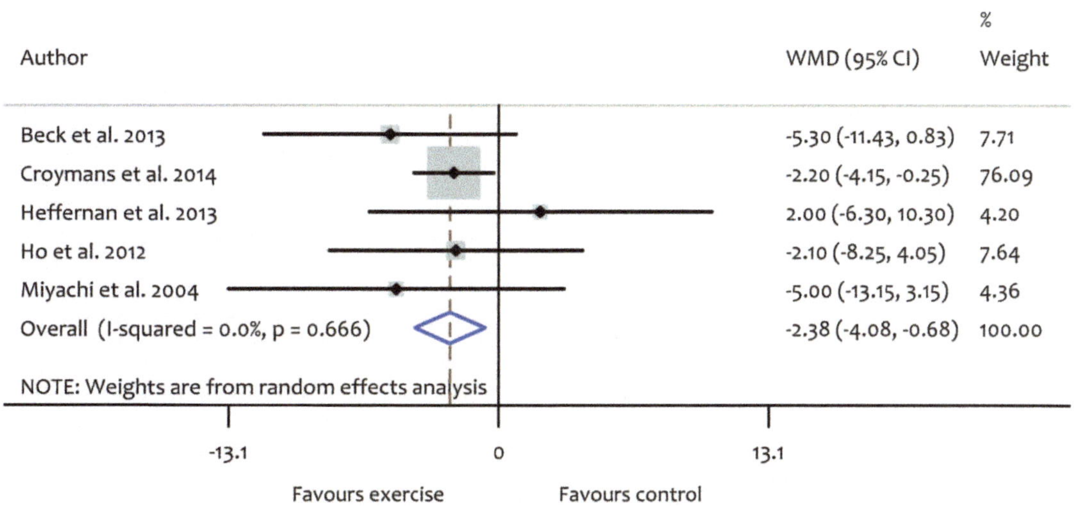

Figure 8. Forest plot showing the effect of resistance exercise intervention on augmentation index (AIx).

reflection as standardised mean differences. Furthermore, they included non-randomized controlled trials in their analysis. In the present meta-analysis we included only studies that reported the commonly used measures of arterial stiffness and wave reflection (PWV and AIx) [74,75] and we restricted our analysis to RCTs. Furthermore, we analysed the data as weighted mean difference so that the effect sizes obtained will be clinically applicable [76]. In contrast to the meta-analysis conducted by Montero et al. [72], we observed significant improvement in PWV with aerobic exercise intervention in pre- and hypertensive participants but we suggest that these results are interpreted cautiously because of the small number of studies included in the subgroup analyses (Table 4).

The magnitude of the effect of aerobic exercise training on PWV was greater in peripheral (ba-PWV) rather than in central (cf-PWV) indices of arterial stiffness. This difference might be explained by the apparently-greater shear stress-enhanced release of NO in the peripheral exercising limbs and the nitric oxide-producing small conduit arteries [4,77].

In the present study, we observed a tendency for a positive dose-response relationship between exercise intensity and improvement in AIx. Previous studies demonstrated that AIx is inversely associated with blood pressure and with peripheral vascular resistance [78]. Exercising with higher intensity might result in augmented release of NO as a consequence of greater shear stress on the vascular endothelium. This augmented release of the vasodilatory and protective molecule NO may leads to greater reduction in peripheral vascular resistance and, eventually, AIx [79]. These findings support the emerging evidence that high intensity physical activity may be more beneficial for cardiovascular health than low intensity exercise and PA guidelines published by the American College of Sports Medicine emphasise the benefit of high intensity exercise for maintaining and improving cardiovascular health [80,81]. Furthermore, we observed significant correlations between changes in AIx and changes in heart rate after aerobic exercise intervention. Previous studies have shown that AIx is influenced by changes in heart rate or blood pressure [78]. Unfortunately, in the present meta-analysis, only 6 studies reported the measurement of heart-rate adjusted AIx [12,31,32,34,46,53].

Overall, there was no effect, positive or negative, of resistance exercise interventions on PWV and AIx. This is contrary to the findings from a previous meta-analysis which showed that resistance exercise increased arterial stiffness significantly [82]. However, in that meta-analysis, subgroup comparison showed that the increased stiffness was observed only in young participants or with higher intensity resistance exercise. One possible reason for the difference between our findings and those of Miyachi (2013) is our inclusion of more studies which have been published recently [14,34,56,59,60]. We observed that some forms of resistance exercise were associated with improvement, or at least no deterioration, in arterial stiffness. These included lower intensity rather than high intensity training [59], lower-limb rather than upper-limb training [43], eccentric rather than concentric resistance training [42] and the combination of resistance with aerobic training [58].

Combined aerobic and resistance exercise showed no significant improvement in arterial stiffness. However, the proven beneficial effects of resistance exercise on cardio-metabolic parameters make it an indispensable adjunct to aerobic exercise for those patients with cardio-metabolic disorders [83,84]. Therefore, future studies should focus on combinations of aerobic exercise with modes of resistance exercise that have beneficial, or at least non-harmful, effects on vascular hemodynamic.

Previous studies showed that every 1 m/s increase in PWV is associated with 12–14% increase in the risk of cardiovascular events and 13–15% increase in the risk of CVD mortality [74,85]. In the present meta-analysis, we observed that aerobic exercise reduced PWV by 0.63 m/s which may translate into a reduction of 8% in cardiovascular events and 9% in cardiovascular mortality. Furthermore, subgroup analyses suggested that there may be bigger effects on PWV and, consequently, on cardiovascular events and mortality of aerobic exercise in higher risk participants (those with PWV ≥8 m/s at baseline) and with longer duration aerobic exercise interventions (>10 weeks).

Our systematic review and meta-analysis has several limitations. The small sample size of most of the included studies may limit the generalizability of our findings. However, the included studies were characterised as good quality on Jadad's Score (more than 2/3 of the studies had ≥3 out of 5 total score). Furthermore, the participants of the included studies were characterised by diverse health status, age, gender and country of origin which may aid in generalizing our results to the general population. Nevertheless, most of the studies which employed resistance exercise interventions recruited healthy participants (**Table 4**). Therefore, further studies are required to assess the effect of resistance exercise in participants with cardio-metabolic diseases. Finally, our meta-analysis was based on summary data from each of the original studies. We did not have access to individual-level data which would have allowed more extensive adjustment for potential confounding factors.

In summary, aerobic exercise improved indices of arterial stiffness and wave reflection significantly. Aerobic exercise training had a greater effect in peripheral (ba-PWV) rather than in central (cf-PWV) indices of arterial stiffness. The effect of aerobic exercise was enhanced with higher intensity exercise, in participants with higher vascular stiffness and with longer duration studies. Resistance exercise had no overall effect on PWV and AIx. The study showed that some forms of resistance exercise may be associated with beneficial effect on arterial stiffness. Therefore, further studies are required to investigate the effect of these forms of resistance exercise alone, or in combination with aerobic exercise, on indices of arterial stiffness and wave reflection.

Supporting Information

Figure S1 Associations between aerobic exercise intervention characteristics and pulse wave velocity: (a) relative intensity; (b) absolute intensity; (c) session frequency; (d) session duration. Each study is depicted by a circle where the circle size represents the degree of weighting for the study based on participant numbers in the study.

Figure S2 Funnel plot for publication bias of the effect of (a) aerobic (b) resistance (c) combined aerobic and resistance exercise intervention on pulse wave velocity (PWV). (d) Funnel plot for publication bias of the effect of aerobic exercise intervention on augmentation index (AIx).

Figure S3 Associations between resistance exercise intervention characteristics and pulse wave velocity (PWV): (a) relative intensity; (b) absolute intensity; (c) session frequency; (d) session duration. Each study is depicted by a circle where the circle size represents the degree of weighting for the study based on the number of study participants.

Figure S4 Associations between combined (aerobic and resistance) exercise intervention characteristics and arterial stiffness measured by pulse wave velocity (PWV): (a) relative intensity; (b) absolute intensity; (c) session frequency; (d) session duration. Each study is depicted by a circle where the circle size represents the degree of weighting for the study based on the number of study participants.

Table S1 Further characteristics of aerobic exercise intervention studies included in the meta-analysis.

Table S2 Further characteristics of resistance/combined exercise intervention studies included in the meta-analysis.

Table S3 Subgroup analyses of the effects aerobic exercise on augmentation index using a random-effects model.

Checklist S1 PRISMA Checklist 2009.

Acknowledgments

The authors thank Dr. Takanobu Okamoto for his help in providing us with additional data from some eligible studies. AA is funded by the Ministry of Higher Education and Scientific Research of Iraq. JL and JCM acknowledge support from the LiveWell Programme a research project funded through a collaborative grant from the Lifelong Health and Wellbeing (LLHW) initiative, managed by the Medical Research Council (MRC) (grant number G0900686). The material presented in this manuscript is original and it has not been submitted for publication elsewhere while under consideration by **PLOS ONE**.

Author Contributions

Conceived and designed the experiments: AA JL JM. Performed the experiments: AA CM JL. Analyzed the data: AA MS JM JL CM. Wrote the paper: AA MS JL CM JM.

References

1. Nocon M, Hiemann T, Muller-Riemenschneider F, Thalau F, Roll S, et al. (2008) Association of physical activity with all-cause and cardiovascular mortality: a systematic review and meta-analysis. Eur J Cardiovasc Prev Rehabil 15: 239–246.
2. Schuler G, Adams V, Goto Y (2013) Role of exercise in the prevention of cardiovascular disease: results, mechanisms, and new perspectives. Eur Heart J 34: 1790–1799.
3. Mora S, Cook N, Buring JE, Ridker PM, Lee IM (2007) Physical activity and reduced risk of cardiovascular events: potential mediating mechanisms. Circulation 116: 2110–2118.
4. Green DJ, Maiorana A, O'Driscoll G, Taylor R (2004) Effect of exercise training on endothelium-derived nitric oxide function in humans. J Physiol 561: 1–25.
5. Shirwany NA, Zou MH (2010) Arterial stiffness: a brief review. Acta Pharmacol Sin 31: 1267–1276.
6. Cavalcante JL, Lima JA, Redheuil A, Al-Mallah MH (2011) Aortic stiffness: current understanding and future directions. J Am Coll Cardiol 57: 1511–1522.
7. Sakuragi S, Abhayaratna WP (2010) Arterial stiffness: methods of measurement, physiologic determinants and prediction of cardiovascular outcomes. Int J Cardiol 138: 112–118.
8. Laurent S, Boutouyrie P (2007) Arterial stiffness: a new surrogate end point for cardiovascular disease? J Nephrol 20 Suppl 12: S45–50.
9. Munk PS, Staal EM, Butt N, Isaksen K, Larsen AI (2009) High-intensity interval training may reduce in-stent restenosis following percutaneous coronary intervention with stent implantation A randomized controlled trial evaluating the relationship to endothelial function and inflammation. Am Heart J 158: 734–741.
10. Olson TP, Dengel DR, Leon AS, Schmitz KH (2006) Moderate resistance training and vascular health in overweight women. Medicine and Science in Sports and Exercise 38: 1558–1564.
11. Vona M, Codeluppi GM, Iannino T, Ferrari E, Bogousslavsky J, et al. (2009) Effects of different types of exercise training followed by detraining on endothelium-dependent dilation in patients with recent myocardial infarction. Circulation 119: 1601–1608.
12. Beck DT, Martin JS, Casey DP, Braith RW (2013) Exercise training reduces peripheral arterial stiffness and myocardial oxygen demand in young prehypertensive subjects. American Journal of Hypertension 26: 1093–1102.
13. Figueroa A, Park SY, Seo DY, Sanchez-Gonzalez MA, Baek YH (2011) Combined resistance and endurance exercise training improves arterial stiffness, blood pressure, and muscle strength in postmenopausal women. Menopause 18: 980–984.
14. Ho SS, Radavelli-Bagatini S, Dhaliwal SS, Hills AP, Pal S (2012) Resistance, aerobic, and combination training on vascular function in overweight and obese adults. Journal of Clinical Hypertension 14: 848–854.
15. Higgins JPT, Green S, editors. Cochrane Handbook for Systematic Reviews of Interventions Version 5.1.0 [updated March 2011]. The Cochrane Collaboration, 2011. Available from www.cochrane-handbook.org.
16. Liberati A, Altman DG, Tetzlaff J, Mulrow C, Gotzsche PC, et al. (2009) The PRISMA statement for reporting systematic reviews and meta-analyses of studies that evaluate healthcare interventions: explanation and elaboration. BMJ 339: b2700.
17. Crowther M, Lim W, Crowther MA (2010) Systematic review and meta-analysis methodology. Blood 116: 3140–3146.
18. Zoungas S, Asmar RP (2007) Arterial stiffness and cardiovascular outcome. Clin Exp Pharmacol Physiol 34: 647–651.
19. Yasmin, Brown MJ (1999) Similarities and differences between augmentation index and pulse wave velocity in the assessment of arterial stiffness. QJM 92: 595–600.
20. Elbourne DR, Altman DG, Higgins JP, Curtin F, Worthington HV, et al. (2002) Meta-analyses involving cross-over trials: methodological issues. Int J Epidemiol 31: 140–149.
21. Howley ET (2001) Type of activity: resistance, aerobic and leisure versus occupational physical activity. Med Sci Sports Exerc 33: S364–369; discussion S419–320.
22. Egger M, Davey Smith G, Schneider M, Minder C (1997) Bias in meta-analysis detected by a simple, graphical test. Bmj 315: 629–634.
23. Higgins JP, Thompson SG, Deeks JJ, Altman DG (2003) Measuring inconsistency in meta-analyses. BMJ 327: 557–560.
24. Choi KM, Han KA, Ahn HJ, Hwang SY, Hong HC, et al. (2012) Effects of exercise on sRAGE levels and cardiometabolic risk factors in patients with type 2 diabetes: a randomized controlled trial. Journal of Clinical Endocrinology & Metabolism 97: 3751–3758.
25. Ciolac EG, Bocchi EA, Bortolotto LA, Carvalho VO, Greve JM, et al. (2010) Effects of high-intensity aerobic interval training vs. moderate exercise on hemodynamic, metabolic and neuro-humoral abnormalities of young normotensive women at high familial risk for hypertension. Hypertension Research - Clinical & Experimental 33: 836–843.
26. Ferrier KE, Waddell TK, Gatzka CD, Cameron JD, Dart AM, et al. (2001) Aerobic exercise training does not modify large-artery compliance in isolated systolic hypertension. Hypertension 38: 222–226.
27. Krustrup P, Hansen PR, Randers MB, Nybo L, Martone D, et al. (2010) Beneficial effects of recreational football on the cardiovascular risk profile in untrained premenopausal women. Scandinavian Journal of Medicine & Science in Sports 20 Suppl 1: 40–49.
28. Miura H, Nakagawa E, Takahashi Y (2008) Influence of group training frequency on arterial stiffness in elderly women. European Journal of Applied Physiology 104: 1039–1044.
29. Ohta M, Hirao N, Mori Y, Takigami C, Eguchi M, et al. (2012) Effects of bench step exercise on arterial stiffness in post-menopausal women: contribution of IGF-1 bioactivity and nitric oxide production. Growth Hormone & Igf Research 22: 36–41.
30. Okamoto T, Masuhara M, Ikuta K (2006) Effects of eccentric and concentric resistance training on arterial stiffness. Journal of Human Hypertension 20: 348–354.
31. Sugawara J, Akazawa N, Miyaki A, Choi Y, Tanabe Y, et al. (2012) Effect of endurance exercise training and curcumin intake on central arterial hemodynamics in postmenopausal women: pilot study. American Journal of Hypertension 25: 651–656.
32. Wong A, Figueroa A (2014) Eight weeks of stretching training reduces aortic wave reflection magnitude and blood pressure in obese postmenopausal women. Journal of Human Hypertension 28: 246–250.
33. Yoshizawa M, Maeda S, Miyaki A, Misono M, Saito Y, et al. (2009) Effect of 12 weeks of moderate-intensity resistance training on arterial stiffness: a randomised controlled trial in women aged 32–59 years. British Journal of Sports Medicine 43: 615–618.
34. Croymans DM, Krell SL, Oh CS, Katiraie M, Lam CY, et al. (2014) Effects of resistance training on central blood pressure in obese young men. J Hum Hypertens 28: 157–164.
35. Goldberg MJ, Boutcher SH, Boutcher YN (2012) The effect of 4 weeks of aerobic exercise on vascular and baroreflex function of young men with a family history of hypertension. Journal of Human Hypertension 26: 644–649.
36. Heydari M, Boutcher YN, Boutcher SH (2013) The effects of high-intensity intermittent exercise training on cardiovascular response to mental and physical challenge. International Journal of Psychophysiology 87: 141–146.

37. Heydari M, Boutcher YN, Boutcher SH (2013) High-intensity intermittent exercise and cardiovascular and autonomic function. Clinical Autonomic Research 23: 57–65.
38. Krustrup P, Randers MB, Andersen LJ, Jackman SR, Bangsbo J, et al. (2013) Soccer improves fitness and attenuates cardiovascular risk factors in hypertensive men. Medicine & Science in Sports & Exercise 45: 553–560.
39. Loimaala A, Groundstroem K, Rinne M, Nenonen A, Huhtala H, et al. (2009) Effect of long-term endurance and strength training on metabolic control and arterial elasticity in patients with type 2 diabetes mellitus. American Journal of Cardiology 103: 972–977.
40. Miyachi M, Kawano H, Sugawara J, Takahashi K, Hayashi K, et al. (2004) Unfavorable effects of resistance training on central arterial compliance: a randomized intervention study. Circulation 110: 2858–2863.
41. Okamoto T, Masuhara M, Ikuta K (2008) Effects of low-intensity resistance training with slow lifting and lowering on vascular function. J Hum Hypertens 22: 509–511.
42. Okamoto T, Masuhara M, Ikuta K (2009) Effects of muscle contraction timing during resistance training on vascular function. Journal of Human Hypertension 23: 470–478.
43. Okamoto T, Masuhara M, Ikuta K (2009) Upper but not lower limb resistance training increases arterial stiffness in humans. European Journal of Applied Physiology 107: 127–134.
44. Guimaraes GV, Ciolac EG, Carvalho VO, D'Avila VM, Bortolotto LA, et al. (2010) Effects of continuous vs. interval exercise training on blood pressure and arterial stiffness in treated hypertension. Hypertension Research - Clinical & Experimental 33: 627–632.
45. Kearney TM, Murphy MH, Davison GW, O'Kane MJ, Gallagher AM (2014) Accumulated brisk walking reduces arterial stiffness in overweight adults: evidence from a randomized control trial. Journal of the American Society of Hypertension 8: 117–126.
46. Koh KP, Fassett RG, Sharman JE, Coombes JS, Williams AD (2010) Effect of intradialytic versus home-based aerobic exercise training on physical function and vascular parameters in hemodialysis patients: a randomized pilot study. American Journal of Kidney Diseases 55: 88–99.
47. Madden KM, Lockhart C, Cuff D, Potter TF, Meneilly GS (2009) Short-term aerobic exercise reduces arterial stiffness in older adults with type 2 diabetes, hypertension, and hypercholesterolemia. Diabetes Care 32: 1531–1535.
48. Madden KM, Lockhart C, Cuff D, Potter TF, Meneilly GS (2013) Aerobic training-induced improvements in arterial stiffness are not sustained in older adults with multiple cardiovascular risk factors. Journal of Human Hypertension 27: 335–339.
49. Mustata S, Groeneveld S, Davidson W, Ford G, Kiland K, et al. (2011) Effects of exercise training on physical impairment, arterial stiffness and health-related quality of life in patients with chronic kidney disease: a pilot study. International Urology & Nephrology 43: 1133–1141.
50. Nualnim N, Parkhurst K, Dhindsa M, Tarumi T, Vavrek J, et al. (2012) Effects of swimming training on blood pressure and vascular function in adults >50 years of age. American journal of cardiology. . pp1005–1010.
51. Oudegeest-Sander MH, Olde Rikkert MG, Smits P, Thijssen DH, van Dijk AP, et al. (2013) The effect of an advanced glycation end-product crosslink breaker and exercise training on vascular function in older individuals: a randomized factorial design trial. Experimental Gerontology 48: 1509–1517.
52. Parnell MM, Holst DP, Kaye DM (2002) Exercise training increases arterial compliance in patients with congestive heart failure. Clinical Science 102: 1–7.
53. Westhoff TH, Schmidt S, Gross V, Joppke M, Zidek W, et al. (2008) The cardiovascular effects of upper-limb aerobic exercise in hypertensive patients. Journal of Hypertension 26: 1336–1342.
54. Cortez-Cooper MY, Anton MM, Devan AE, Neidre DB, Cook JN, et al. (2008) The effects of strength training on central arterial compliance in middle-aged and older adults. European Journal of Cardiovascular Prevention & Rehabilitation 15: 149–155.
55. Dobrosielski DA, Gibbs BB, Ouyang P, Bonekamp S, Clark JM, et al. (2012) Effect of exercise on blood pressure in type 2 diabetes: a randomized controlled trial. Journal of General Internal Medicine 27: 1453–1459.
56. Heffernan KS, Yoon ES, Sharman JE, Davies JE, Shih YT, et al. (2013) Resistance exercise training reduces arterial reservoir pressure in older adults with prehypertension and hypertension. Hypertension Research - Clinical & Experimental 36: 422–427.
57. Kawasaki T, Sullivan CV, Ozoe N, Higaki H, Kawasaki J (2011) A long-term, comprehensive exercise program that incorporates a variety of physical activities improved the blood pressure, lipid and glucose metabolism, arterial stiffness, and balance of middle-aged and elderly Japanese. Hypertension Research - Clinical & Experimental 34: 1059–1066.
58. Okamoto T, Masuhara M, Ikuta K (2007) Combined aerobic and resistance training and vascular function: effect of aerobic exercise before and after resistance training. Journal of Applied Physiology 103: 1655–1661.
59. Okamoto T, Masuhara M, Ikuta K (2011) Effect of low-intensity resistance training on arterial function. European Journal of Applied Physiology 111: 743–748.
60. Okamoto T, Masuhara M, Ikuta K (2013) Low-intensity resistance training after high-intensity resistance training can prevent the increase of central arterial stiffness. International Journal of Sports Medicine 34: 385–390.
61. Stewart KJ, Bacher AC, Turner KL, Fleg JL, Hees PS, et al. (2005) Effect of exercise on blood pressure in older persons: A randomized controlled trial. Archives of Internal Medicine 165: 756–762.
62. Toussaint ND, Polkinghorne KR, Kerr PG (2008) Impact of intradialytic exercise on arterial compliance and B-type natriuretic peptide levels in hemodialysis patients. Hemodialysis International 12: 254–263.
63. Park S, Lakatta EG (2012) Role of inflammation in the pathogenesis of arterial stiffness. Yonsei Med J 53: 258–261.
64. Patel RS, Al Mheid I, Morris AA, Ahmed Y, Kavtaradze N, et al. (2011) Oxidative stress is associated with impaired arterial elasticity. Atherosclerosis 218: 90–95.
65. Correia ML, Haynes WG (2007) Arterial compliance and endothelial function. Curr Diab Rep 7: 269–275.
66. Seals DR, Desouza CA, Donato AJ, Tanaka H (2008) Habitual exercise and arterial aging. J Appl Physiol (1985) 105: 1323–1332.
67. Gielen S, Schuler G, Adams V (2010) Cardiovascular effects of exercise training: molecular mechanisms. Circulation 122: 1221–1238.
68. Roque FR, Briones AM, Garcia-Redondo AB, Galan M, Martinez-Revelles S, et al. (2013) Aerobic exercise reduces oxidative stress and improves vascular changes of small mesenteric and coronary arteries in hypertension. Br J Pharmacol 168: 686–703.
69. Kojda G, Hambrecht R (2005) Molecular mechanisms of vascular adaptations to exercise. Physical activity as an effective antioxidant therapy? Cardiovasc Res 67: 187–197.
70. Teixeira-Lemos E, Nunes S, Teixeira F, Reis F (2011) Regular physical exercise training assists in preventing type 2 diabetes development: focus on its antioxidant and anti-inflammatory properties. Cardiovasc Diabetol 10: 12.
71. Higashi Y, Yoshizumi M (2004) Exercise and endothelial function: role of endothelium-derived nitric oxide and oxidative stress in healthy subjects and hypertensive patients. Pharmacol Ther 102: 87–96.
72. Montero D, Roche E, Martinez-Rodriguez A (2014) The impact of aerobic exercise training on arterial stiffness in pre- and hypertensive subjects: A systematic review and meta-analysis. Int J Cardiol 173: 361–368.
73. Montero D, Roberts CK, Vinet A (2014) Effect of aerobic exercise training on arterial stiffness in obese populations : a systematic review and meta-analysis. Sports Med 44: 833–843.
74. Vlachopoulos C, Aznaouridis K, Stefanadis C (2010) Prediction of cardiovascular events and all-cause mortality with arterial stiffness: a systematic review and meta-analysis. J Am Coll Cardiol 55: 1318–1327.
75. Vlachopoulos C, Aznaouridis K, O'Rourke MF, Safar ME, Baou K, et al. (2010) Prediction of cardiovascular events and all-cause mortality with central haemodynamics: a systematic review and meta-analysis. Eur Heart J 31: 1865–1871.
76. Cummings P (2011) Arguments for and against standardized mean differences (effect sizes). Arch Pediatr Adolesc Med 165: 592–596.
77. Rakobowchuk M, Stuckey MI, Millar PJ, Gurr L, Macdonald MJ (2009) Effect of acute sprint interval exercise on central and peripheral artery distensibility in young healthy males. Eur J Appl Physiol 105: 787–795.
78. DeLoach SS, Townsend RR (2008) Vascular stiffness: its measurement and significance for epidemiologic and outcome studies. Clin J Am Soc Nephrol 3: 184–192.
79. Padilla J, Harris RA, Rink LD, Wallace JP (2008) Characterization of the brachial artery shear stress following walking exercise. Vasc Med 13: 105–111.
80. Haskell WL, Lee IM, Pate RR, Powell KE, Blair SN, et al. (2007) Physical activity and public health: updated recommendation for adults from the American College of Sports Medicine and the American Heart Association. Med Sci Sports Exerc 39: 1423–1434.
81. Whyte LJ, Gill JM, Cathcart AJ (2010) Effect of 2 weeks of sprint interval training on health-related outcomes in sedentary overweight/obese men. Metabolism 59: 1421–1428.
82. Miyachi M (2013) Effects of resistance training on arterial stiffness: a meta-analysis. Br J Sports Med 47: 393–396.
83. Marzolini S, Oh PI, Brooks D (2012) Effect of combined aerobic and resistance training versus aerobic training alone in individuals with coronary artery disease: a meta-analysis. Eur J Prev Cardiol 19: 81–94.
84. Snowling NJ, Hopkins WG (2006) Effects of different modes of exercise training on glucose control and risk factors for complications in type 2 diabetic patients: a meta-analysis. Diabetes Care 29: 2518–2527.
85. Vlachopoulos C, Aznaouridis K, Terentes-Printzios D, Ioakeimidis N, Stefanadis C (2012) Prediction of cardiovascular events and all-cause mortality with brachial-ankle elasticity index: a systematic review and meta-analysis. Hypertension 60: 556–562.

8

Does the Method of Weight Loss Effect Long-Term Changes in Weight, Body Composition or Chronic Disease Risk Factors in Overweight or Obese Adults?

Richard A. Washburn[1], Amanda N. Szabo[1], Kate Lambourne[1], Erik A. Willis[1], Lauren T. Ptomey[1], Jeffery J. Honas[1], Stephen D. Herrmann[2], Joseph E. Donnelly[1]*

1 Cardiovascular Research Institute, Department of Internal Medicine, The University of Kansas Medical Center, Kansas City, Kansas, United States of America, **2** Sanford Research, Department of Children's Health Research Center, Sioux Falls, South Dakota, United States of America

Abstract

Background: Differences in biological changes from weight loss by energy restriction and/or exercise may be associated with differences in long-term weight loss/regain.

Objective: To assess the effect of weight loss method on long-term changes in weight, body composition and chronic disease risk factors.

Data Sources: PubMed and Embase were searched (January 1990-October 2013) for studies with data on the effect of energy restriction, exercise (aerobic and resistance) on long-term weight loss. Twenty articles were included in this review.

Study Eligibility Criteria: Primary source, peer reviewed randomized trials published in English with an active weight loss period of >6 months, or active weight loss with a follow-up period of any duration, conducted in overweight or obese adults were included.

Study Appraisal and Synthesis Methods: Considerable heterogeneity across trials existed for important study parameters, therefore a meta-analysis was considered inappropriate. Results were synthesized and grouped by comparisons (e.g. diet vs. aerobic exercise, diet vs. diet + aerobic exercise etc.) and study design (long-term or weight loss/follow-up).

Results: Forty percent of trials reported significantly greater long-term weight loss with diet compared with aerobic exercise, while results for differences in weight regain were inconclusive. Diet+aerobic exercise resulted in significantly greater weight loss than diet alone in 50% of trials. However, weight regain (~55% of loss) was similar in diet and diet+ aerobic exercise groups. Fat-free mass tended to be preserved when interventions included exercise.

Editor: Darcy Johannsen, Pennington Biomed Research Center, United States of America

Funding: This review was funded by the International Life Sciences Institute. The funders had no role in study design, data collection and analysis, decision to publish, or preparation of the manuscript.

Competing Interests: JD and RW are investigators of individual trials included in this review. The authors declare that they have no other competing interests.

* Email: jdonnelly@ku.edu

Introduction

An energy restricted diet, aerobic exercise, and diet combined with aerobic exercise, have shown success in producing clinically significant (≥5%) [1] reductions in body weight [2–7]. However, the combined prevalence of overweight and obesity among US adults continues at approximately 69% [8], due in part to the inability of individuals who lose weight to maintain weight loss long term [9–14].

Nearly 25 years ago Pavlou et al [15] observed that aerobic exercise combined with an energy restricted diet during weight loss was essential for weight loss maintenance. It has been hypothesized that the type and magnitude of biological changes predisposing to weight regain may differ between weight loss induced by diet compared with aerobic exercise [16] which may explain the observation of Pavlou. Several excellent reviews have described the compensatory changes in biological systems involved in energy utilization/storage and appetite regulation induced by an energy restricted diet [17–21]. These changes act in concert to predispose individuals to regain lost weight. For example, weight loss by diet results in decreased resting and non-resting energy expenditure [22–24], fat oxidation [25], thyroid hormones [26–28] and increased cortisol [29,30]; changes which all are associated with increased energy storage. Energy restriction also results in increased gastric inhibitory peptide and ghrelin [31], decreased leptin [32], peptide YY [33,34], amylin, and insulin [35] and alterations in the sympathetic nervous system [36–38] that all promote increased energy intake. Changes in several of these hormones [32] as well as resting energy expenditure [39] may not be transient, but may persist for up to one year post diet induced weight loss. Given the complexity of the control of energy balance, which involves psychological, physiological and environmental factors, weight loss induced changes in any one of physiological parameters is unlikely to be individually predictive of weight regain [19].

In contrast to weight loss by an energy restricted diet alone, weight loss via aerobic exercise or a combination of diet and aerobic exercise results in beneficial changes on both sides of the energy balance equation which may be associated with better maintenance of lost weight. For example, weight loss by an energy restricted diet is associated with decreased resting metabolic rate (RMR) [40,41] which may [24,42,43] or may not [22,44,45] be greater than expected based on the loss of fat and fat-free mass. In contrast, weight loss achieved by aerobic exercise is composed predominantly of fat mass, while fat-free mass is preserved [6,7,46], and RMR is generally unchanged [47] or slightly increased [48]. In addition, reductions in RMR/kg weight loss may be greater for weight loss induced by energy restriction compared with weight loss by exercise [49] and potential metabolic adaptation in RMR may be eliminated when exercise is combined with energy restriction [43,50]. Weight loss by energy restriction has also been shown to result in significant decreases in both total daily energy expenditure and physical activity energy expenditure [51,52] which are eliminated when energy restriction is combined with aerobic exercise [11,43].

Aerobic exercise may also improve the coupling between energy intake and energy expenditure [16,53–57] which may be important in maintaining energy balance in a weight reduced state. In contrast, physical inactivity disrupts the homeostatic mechanisms associated with appetite control which could contribute to positive energy balance and weight gain [53,58–61]. While the mechanisms for this exercise effect are unclear, alterations in appetite regulatory hormones [62] [63] and reduced neuronal response in brain regions known to be associated with food intake regulation in a direction expected to lead to reduced EI [64] have been hypothesized.

Several earlier reviews/meta-analyses have provided evidence to support the hypothesis of better long-term weight loss for interventions using energy restriction plus exercise compared with energy restriction alone [65–67] while others have not [68–70]. The discrepancy in results among reviews is likely a function of differences in inclusion criteria in terms of study designs (observational vs. randomized trials), length of weight loss/follow-up periods, and participant characteristics including age, sex and baseline BMI. The objective of this systematic review was to update and expand upon previous reviews by identifying and evaluating randomized trials that have compared the effect of energy restriction, exercise (aerobic and resistance) and there various combinations, on long-term weight loss, changes in body composition and chronic disease risk factors.

Methods

This systematic review was performed and reported in accordance with the Preferred Reporting Items for Systematic Reviews and Meta-Analysis (PRISMA) guidelines [71,72].

Objectives

The objective of this systematic review was to address the question:

Does the method of weight loss, i.e., energy restriction, exercise (aerobic or resistance), and there various combinations effect long-term changes in weight, body composition or chronic disease risk factors in overweight or obese adults?

Eligibility criteria

Only primary source articles published in English in peer-reviewed journals utilizing a randomized design were included. Specific eligibility included: *Participants*: Overweight and obese (BMI≥25 kg/m^2) adults (age 18–65 yrs). Studies of participants with elevated chronic disease risk factors and/or type 2 diabetes (DM2) were included. *Types of studies*: Our original intent was to evaluate trials that included at least a 6 month active weight loss intervention followed by at least 12 months of active or passive weight maintenance. We were able to identify only 3 randomized trials that satisfied these criteria. Therefore, we expanded our criteria to include trials with an active weight loss and weight maintenance phase of any duration, as well as trials with an active weight loss intervention longer than 6 months. *Comparisons*: Weight loss by energy restriction alone, exercise alone (aerobic or resistance), and there various combinations with the comparisons in the same randomized trial. *Outcomes*: Body weight was required for inclusion. Other outcomes included, if available, were body composition (fat mass, fat-free mass, waist circumference) and chronic disease risk factors including total, HDL and LDL cholesterol, triglycerides, insulin, glucose, HbA_{1c}, and blood pressure.

Information Sources

Studies were identified by searching electronic data bases, related article reference lists, and consulting with experts in the field. The search was applied to PubMed (1990 – present) and adapted for EMBASE (1990—present). The last search was conducted on October 31st 2013. The search was developed as a collaborative effort of the research team in consultation with a Kansas University reference librarian and conducted by a co-author (AS). No attempts were made to contact study investigators or sponsors to acquire any information missing from the published article.

Search Strategy

Studies were identified by searching electronic data bases, related article reference lists, and consulting with experts in the field. The search was applied to PubMed (1990 – present) and adapted for EMBASE (1990—present). The last search was conducted on October 31st, 2013. The search was developed as a collaborative effort of the research team in consultation with a Kansas University reference librarian and conducted by a co-author (AS). No attempts were made to contact study investigators or sponsors to acquire any information missing from the published article.

Search Strategy

We used the following search terms for Pub Med to identify potential articles with abstracts for review: Physical Activity[Title/Abstract] OR Exercise[Title/Abstract] OR diet[Title/Abstract] OR calorie restriction[Title/Abstract] OR low calorie diet[Title/Abstract]) AND (weight loss[Title/Abstract] OR weight maintenance[Title/Abstract] OR weight regain[Title/Abstract]) NOT spinal[All Fields] NOT paraplegia[Title/Abstract] NOT stroke[-

Title/Abstract] NOT athletes[Title/Abstract] NOT Alzheimer's[Title/Abstract] NOT fibromyalgia[Title/Abstract] NOT wheelchair[Title/Abstract] NOT "surgical procedures, operative"[All Fields] NOT "general surgery"[MeSH Terms] NOT cancer[Title/Abstract] NOT dialysis[Title/Abstract] NOT pregnant[Title/Abstract] NOT injury[Title/Abstract] NOT HIV[Title/Abstract] NOT Parkinson[Title/Abstract] NOT depression[Title/Abstract] NOT Cancer[Title/Abstract] NOT pregnant[Title/Abstract] AND (("1990/01/01"[PDAT]: "3000/12/31"[PDAT]) AND "humans"[MeSH Terms] AND English[lang] AND ("adult"[MeSH Terms:noexp] OR "middle aged"[MeSH Terms])) AND (Clinical Trial[ptyp] OR Randomized Controlled Trial[ptyp]).

The search was then modified slightly for EMBASE: 'physical activity'/exp OR 'physical activity' OR 'exercise'/exp OR 'exercise' OR 'diet'/exp OR diet OR 'calorie restriction'/exp OR 'calorie restriction' OR 'low calorie' AND ('weight loss'/exp OR 'weight loss' OR 'weight maintenance' OR 'weight regain') NOT (spinal OR paraplegia OR depression OR stroke OR athletes OR fibromyalgia OR wheelchair OR pregnantOR lactation OR alzheimer OR parkinson OR 'cancer'/exp OR 'surgery'/exp OR 'general surgery') AND [adult]/lim AND [humans]/lim AND [embase]/lim AND [1990–2014]/py AND ([controlled clinical trial]/lim OR [randomized controlled trial]/lim) AND [english]/lim AND [2000–2014]/py. Word truncation and the use of wildcards allowed for variations in spelling and word endings.

Study Selection

Retrieved abstracts were independently assessed for inclusion in the review by 2 investigators and coded as "yes", "no" or "maybe." All investigators who participated in eligibility assessments were trained regarding study inclusion/exclusion criteria and completed practice eligibility assessments on 50 test abstracts prior to actual coding. Eligibility assessments on the practice abstracts were reviewed by the primary author (JED) and any coding problems were resolved. Disagreements regarding eligibility for inclusion were resolved via development of consensus among all co-authors. Full text articles for abstracts coded as "yes" or "maybe" were retrieved and reviewed independently by 2 co-authors prior to inclusion in the review. An excel spread sheet was developed and used to track eligibility status.

Data collection

Extracted data was entered into the University of Kansas secure, REDCap (Research Electronic Data Capture, Version 4.14.5) data base [73]. A REDCap data extraction form was developed, pilot tested on a sample of 10 studies and revised accordingly. Relevant data were extracted from each manuscript by one author and verified by a second author. Disagreements were resolved by discussion. Data extracted from each article included basic study information including design (long-term or weight loss with follow-up), sample size, groups compared, diet intervention, exercise intervention, compliance with the diet and exercise interventions, participant characteristics (age, sex, BMI, minority and health status), and results.

Risk of bias in individual studies

Risk of bias for randomized trials was independently evaluated by two authors using the Cochrane risk of bias tool [74]. Risk of bias was assessed in the following domains: selection bias, performance bias, detection bias, attrition bias, reporting bias, and other bias. A third reviewer resolved any discrepancies in bias coding. Studies were not excluded on the basis of risk of bias.

Synthesis of results

There was considerable heterogeneity across studies for several important parameters including: 1) participant characteristics (age, sex, BMI, health status), 2) diet (low calorie, very low calorie) and exercise prescriptions (mode, frequency, intensity, duration), 3) comparison groups (diet, aerobic exercise, resistance exercise and all possible combinations), 4) duration of the weight loss and/or follow periods, and type of intervention during the follow-up period. Given this heterogeneity, a meta-analysis was considered inappropriate. Results based on the extracted data were instead synthesized and presented grouped by comparisons (e.g. diet vs. aerobic exercise, diet vs. diet plus aerobic exercise etc.) and study design (long-term or weight loss with follow-up).

Results

The initial database search plus hand searching identified 2,857 unique records of which 2,760 were excluded based on review of title and abstract. Full-text articles for the remaining 97 citations were reviewed. Seventy seven articles did not satisfy our inclusion criteria and were excluded, thus 20 articles were included in the review (Figure 1). Six trials (30%) reported on long-term weight loss while 14 trials (70%) reported on weight loss with follow-up assessments. Study and participant characteristics are presented in Tables 1 and 2.

Diet vs. Aerobic Exercise

Seven trials, which represent 35% of the trials selected for this review, provided a comparison of long-term weight loss [5,75–78], or weight loss with assessments after a period of follow-up [77,79,80] achieved by diet alone or aerobic exercise alone.

Study Characteristics-Diet vs. Aerobic Exercise

Sample size. The median (range) sample size for diet groups with long-term comparison was 42 (18-118) and aerobic exercise groups was 24 (21-117) [5,75-78]. The median (range) sample size for trials with a follow-up period was 37(15-42) for diet groups, and 24 (17-37) for aerobic exercise groups [77,79,80].

Trial duration. All trials with long-term comparisons included a period of active weight loss of 12 months [5,75–78]. The length of the active weight loss and follow-up periods in the 3 trials with this design was variable. For example, Volpe et al [79] included a 6 month active intervention with a 6 month follow-up. Skender et al [77] included a 12 month active intervention with 12 month follow-up, while Wing et al [80] completed follow-up assessments 18 months after completing a 6 month active intervention.

Completion rate. Four trials with long-term comparisons provided completion rate by intervention group [5,75–77] The median (range) completion for diet groups was 89.5% (69%–95%) and aerobic exercise groups was 85% (70%–91%). Pritchard et al [78] reported an overall completion rate of 88%. Two of the three trials that included assessments after a follow-up period reported completion rates [77,80]. Skender et al [77] reported completion rates for the active intervention of 69% and 70% for the diet and aerobic exercise groups, respectively. The completion rate at follow-up was reduced to 36% and 58% for the diet and aerobic exercise groups, respectively. Wing et al [80] reported completion rates for the active intervention of 95% in the diet group and 89% in the aerobic exercise group and 95% for the diet group and 84% for the aerobic exercise group at follow-up.

Diet. All trials employed an energy restricted meal plan diet with behavioral counseling during the active intervention [5,75–80].

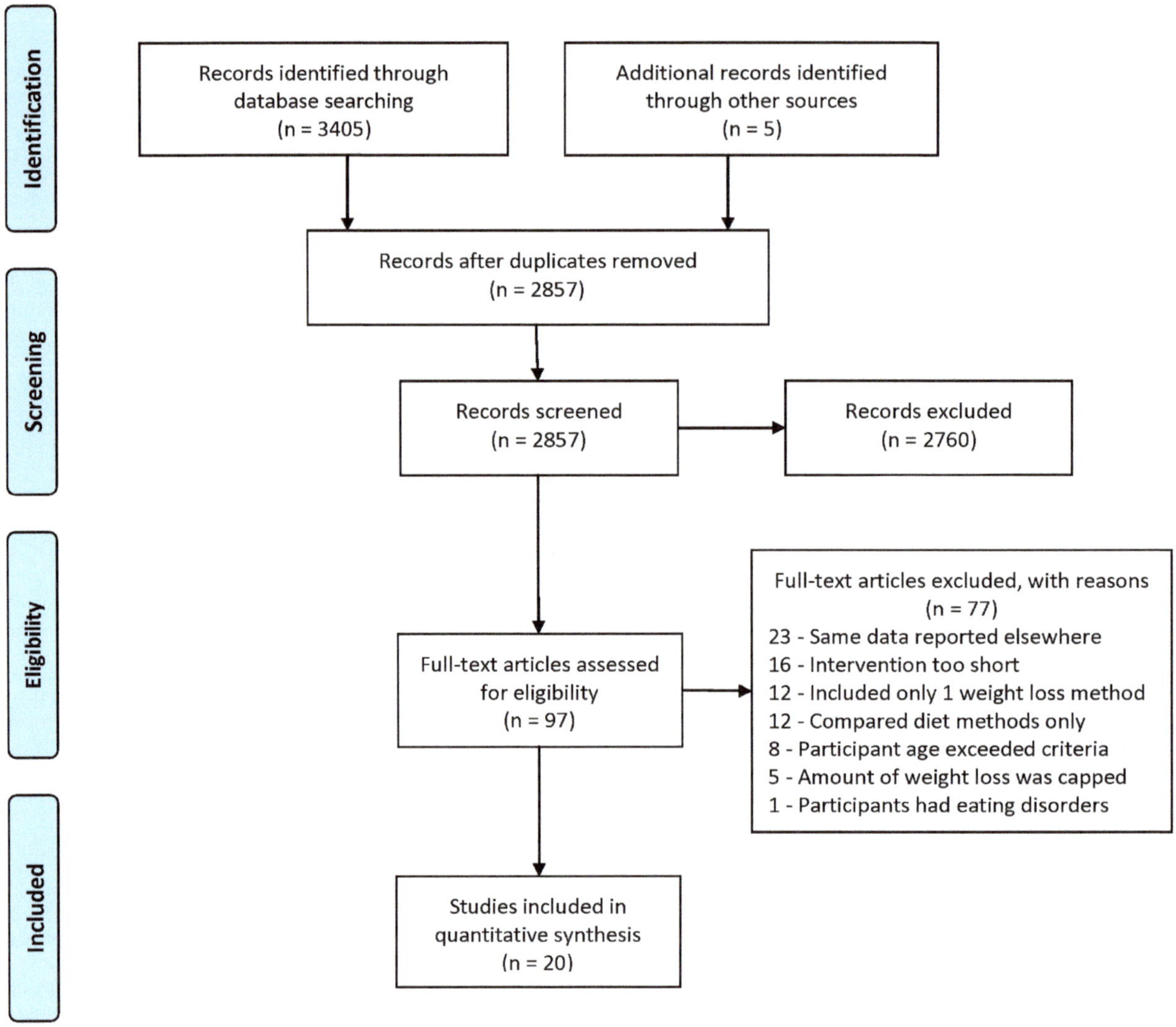

Figure 1. Flow diagram for identification, screening, assessing eligibility, and inclusion in systematic review.

Compliance with diet protocol. Four trials including long-term comparisons provided information on compliance with the prescribed diet [5,75,76,78]. Anderssen et al [75] and Pritchard et al [78] both reported decreased energy intake in the diet but not the aerobic exercise groups. Energy intake was assessed by food-frequency questionnaire [75] or a combination of food records and recalls [78]. Racette et al [5] reported a 12% decrease in energy expenditure assessed by doubly labeled water over the 12 month intervention. Foster-Schubert et al [76] found no significant changes in energy intake assessed by food-frequency questionnaire in any intervention group. Volpe et al [79] found no change in energy intake assessed by food records in either the diet or aerobic exercise groups while Wing et al [80] reported significantly lower energy intake assessed by food-frequency questionnaire in the diet compared with the aerobic exercise group during the active intervention.

Aerobic exercise mode/supervision. A variety of exercise modes were employed including brisk walking/jogging [5,75,77,78,80], treadmill or cycle ergometer [5,76,78] and Nordic Track exercise machine [79]. Exercise was supervised in two trials, [75,79], unsupervised in three trials [5,77,78] and partially supervised in two trials [76,80].

Aerobic exercise frequency. Exercise was prescribed at 3 days per week in 2 trials [75,78], 5 days/wk in three trials [76,79,80] and 3–5 days/wk in one trial [77]. Racette et al [5] individualized the number of weekly exercise sessions to achieve a target level of weekly exercise energy expenditure.

Aerobic exercise intensity. Exercise intensity was prescribed at between 60–85% of peak or maximum heart rate in three trials [75,76,78], and at a self-assessed "vigorous but never strenuous" level on one trial [77]. Exercise intensity was not specified in three trials [5,79,80].

Aerobic exercise duration. Five trials prescribed exercise duration by time; two trials prescribed 30 min/session [78,79], two trials prescribed 45 min/session [76,77], and one trial 60 min/session [75]. Racette et al [5] prescribed an exercise duration designed to achieve a 20% energy deficit designed to be comparable with the level of energy deficit prescribed for the diet group. Wing et al [80] prescribed walking at 3 miles/wk.

Compliance with exercise protocol. Five trials (5 of 7) provided data on compliance with the exercise intervention using a variety of metrics [5,75,76,78,80]. Anderssen et al [75] reported the aerobic exercise group attended 57% of scheduled exercise sessions. Participants in the Foster-Schubert [76] trial averaged

Table 1. Study Characteristics

Study	Intervention groups	Sample size/sex/health status/minority %	Age (yrs.)	BMI (kg/m^2)	Length weight loss	Length follow-up	Outcomes
Long-term trials							
Anderssen et al.(75)	D, AE, D+AE, C	D = 52	NR by group.	D = 29.5 (0.5) [a]	12 mos.	NA	WT, WC, BP, TC, HDL-C, LDL-C, TG
		AE = 49	Mean age ~40 yrs.	AE = 28.6 (0.5)			
		D+AE = 65		D+AE = 28.6 (0.4)			
		C = 43		C = 28.3 (0.5)			
		9.6% women					
		High BMI, DBP, TC, TG, low HDL-C					
		Minority-NR					
Dengel et al.(81)	D, D+AE, C	D = 85	D = 61.0 (1.7-SE)	D = 30.1 (0.5-SE)	10 mos.	NA	WT, BC (under water weight)
		D+AE = 37	D+AE = 57.1(1.4-SE)	D+AE = 30.1(0.6-SE)			
		C = 16	C = 63.6 (1.9-SE)	C = 29.5 (0.8-SE)			
		100% men					
		Healthy					
		Minority-0%					
Foster-Schubert et al. (76)	D, AE, D+AE, C	D = 118	D = 58.1 (6.0)	D = 31.1(3.9)	12 mos.	NA	WT, WC, BC (DXA)
		AE = 117	AE = 58.1 (5.0)	AE = 30.7(3.7)			
		D+AE = 117	D+AE = 58.0 (4.5)	D+AE = 31.0 (4.3)			
		C = 87	C = 57.4 (4.4)	C = 28.6 (2.8)			
		100% women					
		Healthy					
		Minority-15%					
Pritchard et al. (78)	D, AE, C	D = 18	D = 42.3(4.5)	D = 29.0(2.8)	12 mos.	NA	WT, BC (DXA)
		AE = 21	AE = 44.9(6.5)	AE = 29.2(2.8)			
		C = 19	C = 42.3(4.5)	C = 28.6(2.8)			
		100% men					
		Healthy					
		Minority-NR					
Racette et al. (5)	D, AE, C	D = 21	D = 55.6(0.8-SE)	D = 27.2 (0.6-SE)	12 mos.	NA	WT, BC (DXA/MRI)
		AE = 24	AE = 58.8(0.6-SE)	AE = 27.2(0.4-SE)			
		C = 13	C = 56.0(0.9-SE)	C = 27.9(0.4-SE)			
		62% women					

Table 1. Cont.

Study	Intervention groups	Sample size/sex/health status/minority %	Age (yrs.)	BMI (kg/m^2)	Length weight loss	Length follow-up	Outcomes
		Healthy					
		Minority-10.2%					
Wood et al. (82)	D, D+AE, C	D = 67	NR by group	NR by group	12 mos.	NA	WT, TC, HDL-C, LDL-C, TG, BP, BC (underwater weight)
		D+AE = 90	Men = 40.3 (6.3)	Men = 30.7 (2.2)			
		C = 87	Women = 39.1 (6.4)	Women = 27.9 (2.2)			
		49% women					
		Healthy					
		Minority-NR					
Follow-up trials							
Andreou et al. (83)	D, D+AE	D = 95	D = 33.0(10.1)	D = 31.4(5.9)	18 wks.	18 wks.	WT, WC, BC, (BIA)
		D+AE = 111	D+AE = 35 (11.2)	D+AE = 29.1(4.8)			
		100% women					
		Healthy					
		Minority-All from Cyprus					
Hunter et al. (84)	D, D+AE, D+RE	D = 30	D = 34.8 (5.6)	D = 29.3(1.1)[3]	154 days	12 mos.	WT, BC (DXA and MRI)
		D+AE[1] = 18	D+AE[1] = 34.1(7.2)	D+AE[1] = 23.5(1.0)			
		D+AE[2] = 14	D+AE[2] = 34.1 (5.3)	D+AE[2] = 24.1(1.2)			
		D+RE[1] = 21	D+RE[1] = 34.7 (8.4)	D+RE[1] = 23.9 (1.0)			
		D+RE[2] = 14	D+RE[2] = 36.2 (6.6)	D+RE[2] = 24.0 (1.2)			
		100% women					
		Healthy					
		Minority-54%					
Melanson et al. 2004 (91)	AE, D+AE	AE = 47	NR by group	AE = 30.6(0.5-SE)	12 wks.	12 wks.	WT, WC. BC(air displacement) TC, HDL-C,LDL-C, TG
		D+AE = 42	Mean age = 42.6(6.0)	D+AE+31.8(0.7-SE)			
		88% women					
		Healthy					
		Minority-NR					
Melanson et al 2006 (92)	AE, D+AE(cereal),	AE = 43	AE = 42.6(1.4-SE)	AE = 31.0(2.4-SE)	12 wks.	12 wks.	WT

Table 1. Cont.

Study	Intervention groups	Sample size/sex/health status/minority %	Age (yrs.)	BMI (kg/m^2)	Length weight loss	Length follow-up	Outcomes
	D+AE(no cereal)	D+AE(cereal) = 45	D+AE(cereal) = 42.5 (0.9-SE)	D+AE(cereal) = 31.1(2.5-SE)			
		D+AE(no cereal) = 46	D+AE(no cereal) = 41.7(1.2-SE)	D+AE(no cereal) = 30.5(2.4-SE)			
		79% women					
		Healthy					
		Minority-25.9%					
Molenar et al. (85)	D, D+AE, C	D = 67	D = 43 (9)	D = 31.3(2.0)	6 mos.	6 mos.	WT, WC
		D+AE = 67	D+AE = 43(10)	D+AE = 30.8(1.9)			
		C = 70	C = 41(11)	C = 30.2(1.9)			
		40% women					
		Healthy					
		Minority-NR					
Neumark-Sztainer et al. (86)	D, D+AE	D = 21	NR by group	NR by group	3 mos.	5 mos.	WT, WC, BC(skinfolds)
		D+AE = 21	Age range = 25-50	Mean BMI = 30.3 (SD-NR)			
		100% women					
		Healthy					
		70% Asian/North African					
Skender et al. (77)	D, AE, D+AE	D = 42	NR by group	NR	12 mos.	12 mos.	WT
		AE = 43	Age range (25-45)				
		D+AE = 42					
		47% women					
		Healthy					
		Minority-NR					
Snel et al. (87)	D, D+AE	D = 13	D = 59.0 (2.0-SE)	D = 37.9(1.4-SE)	4 mos.	14 mos.	WT, WC, BC (BIA), TC, HDL-C, LDL-C, TG, HbA$_{1C}$, INSULIN, GLUCOSE,
		D+AE = 14	D+AE = 56 (2.0-SE)	D+AE = 36.4(1.1-SE)			
		47% women					

Table 1. Cont.

Study	Intervention groups	Sample size/sex/health status/minority %	Age (yrs.)	BMI (kg/m²)	Length weight loss	Length follow-up	Outcomes
		Insulin dependent type 2 diabetics. Off medicine during weight loss.					
		Minority-0%					
Svendsen et al. (93)	D, D+AE+RE, C	D = 51	NR by group	NR by group	12 wks.	6 mos.	WT,BC (DXA) TC, HDL-C, LDL-C, TG
		D+AE+RT = 49	Sample mean = 53.8 (2.5)	Sample mean = 29.7(3.1)			
		C = 21					
		100% women					
		Healthy					
		Minority-NR					
Van Aggel-Leijssen et al. (88)	D,D+AE	D = 17	D = 38.6(6.5)	D = 32.0 (2.1)	12 wks.	40 wks.	WT, BC (underwater weight)
		D+AE = 20	D+AE = 39.3(7.7)	D+AE = 32.6 (2.5)			
		100% men					
		Healthy					
		Minority-NR					
Volpe et al.(79)	D, AE, D+AE	Women	Women	Women	6 mos.	6 mos.	WT, WC, BC (underwater weight), BP, TC, HDL-C, LDL-C, TG
		D = 15	D = 44.0(6.5)	D = 30.8(2.8)			
		AE = 17	AE = 42.4(7.3)	AE = 30.5(3.0)			
		D+AE = 14	D+AE = 45.1(4.8)	D+AE = 30.4(2.5)			
		Men	Men	Men			
		D = 13	D = 43.9(6.5	D = 31.1(3.3)			
		AE = 17	AE = 44.6(8.1)	AE = 30.5(3.6)			
		D+AE = 14	D+AE = 44.9(9.8)	D+AE = 30.5(3.2)			
		Healthy					
		Minority-NR					
Wadden et al. (89)	D, D+AE, D+RE, D+AE+RE	D = 29	D = 41.0 (8.8)	D = 36.4 (5.5)	48 wks.	52 wks.	WT, BC (underwater weight)
		D+AE = 31	D+AE = 40.8 (7.9)	D+AE = 37.3(5.1)			

Table 1. Cont.

Study	Intervention groups	Sample size/sex/health status/minority %	Age (yrs.)	BMI (kg/m²)	Length weight loss	Length follow-up	Outcomes
		D+RE = 31	D+RE = 40.0 (9.1)	D+RE = 36.5 (6)			
		D+AE+RE = 29	D+AE+RE = 42.8 (8.0)	D+AE+RE = 35.3(4.4)			
		100% women					
		Healthy					
		Minority-30%					
Wang et al. (90)	D, D+AE(low intensity), D+AE(high intensity)	D = 15	NR by group	BMI NR	20 wks.	52 wks.	WT
		D+AE(low intensity) = 13	Sample mean = 58.6 (2.5)	%fat by group			
		D+AE(high intensity) = 13		D = 43(4)			
				D+AE(low intensity) = 42.3(3.8)			
		100% women		D+AE(high intensity) = 43.1(3.4)			
		Healthy					
		Minority-34%					
Wing et al. (80)	D, AE, D+AE, C	D = 37	D = 45.0 (4.7)	D = 36.1(4.1)	6 mos.	18 mos.	WT, BP, TC, HDL-C, LDL-C, TG, HbA1C, INSULIN, GLUCOSE
		AE = 37	AE = 46.4(4.5)	AE = 36.0(3.7)			
		D+AE = 40	D+AE = 46.3(3.8)	D+AE = 35.7(4.1)			
		C = 40	C = 45.3(4.9)	C = 36.0(5.4)			
		79% women					
		Healthy with 1 or 2 biological parents with type 2 diabetes					
		Minority-NR					

[a]Values are mean (SD) unless otherwise stated.
[1]Adhered to exercise protocol.
[2]Did not adhere to exercise protocol.
[3]Post weight loss.
Abbreviations: AE = aerobic exercise, D = diet, D+AE = diet plus aerobic exercise, RE = resistance exercise, D+RE = diet plus resistance exercise, D+AE+RE = diet plus aerobic plus resistance exercise, C = control, BC = body composition, BMI = body mass index, BP = blood pressure, DBP = diastolic blood pressure, DXA = dual energy absorptiometry, MRI = magnetic resonance imaging, BIA = bioelectric impedance, WT = weight, WC = waist circumference, TC = total cholesterol, HDL = high density lipoprotein cholesterol, LDL = low density lipoprotein cholesterol, TG = triglycerides, NR = not reported, NA = not assessed.

Table 2. Intervention Characteristics.

Study	Completion Rate	Diet intervention	Diet compliance	Exercise intervention	Exercise compliance	Follow-up Intervention
Long-term trials						
Anderssen et al. (75)	D = 95% AE = 91% D+AE = 97% C = 100%	Diet counseling at baseline (participant and spouse), 3 and 9 mos.(participant only). Dietary advice was individualized according to participant dietary history and coronary heart disease risk factor profile. Energy restriction recommended for overweight participants. Level of energy restriction was not described.	Food-frequency questionnaire data indicated significantly greater reductions in energy intake in the D (−2268 kJ/day) and D+AE (−2003 kJ/day) compared with the AE (−497 kJ/day) and C groups (−589 kJ/day).	Aerobics, circuit training, and walk/jog. Group supervised format. 3 d/wk,60-80% peak HR, 60 min.	AE and D+AE groups attended 57% and 63% of scheduled sessions, respectively.	NA
Dengel et al. (81)	D = 58.8% D+AE = 62.2% C = 57.7%	Participants reduced energy intake by ~500 kcal/day following an American Heart Association meal plan diet. Weekly behavioral sessions were held over the 10 mo. trial.	RD monitored adherence to the diet by analyzing weekly food records; however, food record data was NR.	Supervised stationary cycling and walking/ jogging, both outdoors and on a treadmill, 3 days/wk., 75-80% max VO_2, 40 min.	Significant increase in VO_2 max in D+AE, not in D or C.	NA
Foster-Schubert et al. (76)	D = 89% AE = 91% D+AE = 92% C = 92%	Used modified versions of the dietary components of both the LookAhead and Diabetes Prevention trial. Total daily energy intake goals of 1,200 to 2,000 kcal/day (<30% fat) were prescribed based on baseline body weight. Weekly group behavioral counseling sessions were held during the first 6 mos. During mos. 7–12 participants attended 2 meetings/mo.; 1 meeting face-to-face and 1 meeting by phone or email.	No significant change in energy intake assessed by food-frequency questionnaire in any intervention group.	Treadmill, cycle ergometer or other aerobic machines, supervised on 3 of 5 days/wk. 70–85% max HR, 45 min.	AE and D+AE groups averaged 80% and 85% of the exercise goal of 225 min/wk., respectively.	NA
Pritchard et al. (78)	NR by group Overall = 88%	Personalized diet plan to achieve a negative energy balance of ~500 kcal/day and included monthly behavioral counseling sessions	A combination of food records and recall data showed significantly decreased energy intake in the diet only group with no significant change in either the aerobic exercise or control groups.	Self-selected unsupervised activity. 71% walked/jogged. 3 days/wk, 65–75% max HR, 30 min.	Self-report exercise frequency = 3–7 sessions/wk. Significant increase in energy expenditure assessed by activity diary.	NA
Racette et al. (5)	D = 90% AE = 79% C = 77%	Reductions in energy intake of 16% over the initial 3 mos. and 20% over the remaining 9 mos. To educate participants on appropriate portion sizes, meals were provided by a metabolic kitchen over 5 consecutive days at week 3 and after the 3 mo. time point. Behavioral counseling sessions were held weekly for the first 6 mos. and less frequently thereafter	Average reduction in energy intake over the 12 mo. intervention based on doubly labeled water was ~12%.	Choice of exercise at research facility, health club, home or outdoors. HR monitored all sessions. Frequency and duration prescribed to achieve 20% energy deficit comparable with deficit in D group.	Completed 5.8 sessions/wk. Average energy expenditure 317 kcal/session.	NA

Table 2. Cont.

Study	Completion Rate	Diet intervention	Diet compliance	Exercise intervention	Exercise compliance	Follow-up Intervention
Wood et al. (82)	D = 82% D+AE = 90% C = 91%	Diet, supervised by a registered dietician, that approximated the goals of the National Cholesterol Education Program Step 1 diet; i.e. ~55% carbohydrate,30% fat, and dietary cholesterol below 300 mg/day. Group behavioral counseling sessions were conducted weekly during the first 3 mos., every other week for the next 3 mos., and monthly, thereafter.	Food record data food showed reduced energy intake in both men and women in the D and D+AE groups compared with C.	Supervised brisk walking and jogging, 3 day/wk., 60–80% max HR, 25 min/day initially, ramped to 45 min/day by study mo. 4.	Significant increase in VO_2 max in D+AE, not in D or C.	NA
Follow-up trials						
Andreou et al.(83)	Weight loss D = 100% D+AE = 100% Follow-up D = 76% D+AE = 75%	Meal plan diet ~1,500 kcal/day (50% carbohydrate, 30% fat, 20% protein). 6 behavioral sessions.	NR	Outdoor walking/ jogging. Prescribed 3 or more days/wk., vigorous, 20 min/day, or 5 or more days/wk., moderate, 30 min/day or, 5 or more day/wk. any combination achieving at least 600 MET-min/wk. Unsupervised.	NR	No specific intervention during follow-up.
Hunter et al.(84)	Of 208 randomized, 121 (59%) met weight loss requirement (BMI 25 kg/m^2). 97 of 121 (80% of those meeting weight loss requirement and 47% of those randomized complete follow-up testing.	Diet (~800 kcal/day) food provided by metabolic kitchen. Energy restriction was maintained until BMI 25 kg/m^2 was achieved.	NR	All exercise supervised	Compliance was required to remain in the study during the weight loss phase.	Exercise during follow-up was prescribed at 2 days/ wk. Compliance not required to remain in the study. Divided sample into exercise adherers (≥60% of scheduled exercise sessions) and non-adherers (<60% of scheduled sessions) for analysis. Participants were provided instructions on eating a balanced diet focusing on low-density food.
				AE: 3 days/wk., 80% max HR, ramped from 20–40 min/ session by wk. 8.		
				RE: ramped to 2 sets of 10 exercises, 80% 1-RM by wk. 4		
Melanson et al. 2004 (91)	Weight loss AE = 44.7% D+AE = 65.1% Follow-up AE = 40.4% D+AE = 51.2%	Energy reduced diet at ~ 500 kcal/day below maintenance requirements. Included 2-4 meal replacements/day(bars, shakes, soups). Weekly behavioral counseling with a dietician and exercise professional	Data from food records indicated significantly greater reductions in energy intake in the D+AE (−621 kcal/day) compared with the AE group (−42 kcal/day)	Unsupervised outdoor walking, 5 days/wk. at a "moderate" pace. Duration individualized to achieve ~300 kcal/ session by wk. 4, increasing to 500 kcal/session by the end of the study	NR	Participants were asked to continue their assigned intervention (AE or D+AE) over follow-up period. Participants returned to the clinic every 2 wks. for assessment of resting HR, BP, and WT. Participants were not given instructions, advice or encouragement in regards to weight management.

Table 2. Cont.

Study	Completion Rate	Diet intervention	Diet compliance	Exercise intervention	Exercise compliance	Follow-up Intervention
Melanson et al. 2006 (92)	Weight loss AE = 84% D+AE(cereal) = 70% D+AE(no cereal) = 71% Follow-up AE = 82% D+AE(cereal) = 66% D+AE(no cereal) = 65%	Energy reduced diet at ~ 500 kcal/day below maintenance requirements. The diet of one group contained a fiber-rich whole-grams cereal. During the weight loss phase, participants were asked to eat 2 meals/day containing cereal. Participants attended weekly behavioral counseling with an exercise professional and a registered dietician.	Energy intake from food records was 16.3%, 30% and 23% below baseline values in the AE, D+AE(cereal) and the D+AE(no cereal) groups, r espectively	Unsupervised outdoor walking, 5 days/wk. at a "moderate" pace. Duration individualized to achieve ~ 300 kcal/session by wk. 4, increasing to 500 kcal/session by the end of the study	NR	Participants asked to continue their assigned intervention (AE or D+AE) over follow-up period. Participants returned to the clinic every 2 wks. for assessment of resting HR, BP, and WT. Participants were not given instructions, advice or encouragement in regards to weight management. D+AE (cereal) group reduced cereal intake to 1 meal/day
Molenar et al.(85)	Weight loss D = 87% D+AE = 79% C = 53% Follow-up D = 76% D+AE = 75% C = 47%	Prescribed 7 individual sessions with dietician over 6 mos. Based on 3-day food records, meal plan prescribed to achieve and sustain a 5%–10% weight loss.	88% in D group and 89% in D+AE group visited dietician. D group completed average 4.5 sessions, D+AE group competed 4.1 sessions.	Prescribed 6 sessions with physiotherapist. Individualized attainable goals to increase daily activity were prescribed at session 1, support for activity provided at additional sessions.	87% of participants in the D+AE group visited the physiotherapist. Completed an average of 5.0 sessions.	No specific intervention during follow-up
Neumark-Sztainer et al. (86)	Weight loss D = 90% D+AE = 100% Follow-up D = 52% D+AE = 62%	Prescribed meal plan at ~1,000 kcal/day with weekly behavioral counseling.	NR	Prescribed 15 min of running/walking, 5 times/wk. and 10 min of exercise 6 times/wk. Instruction and supervision provided for 1 hr./wk.	Participants exercised or walked 2–3 times/wk. for ~15–20 min. Compliance by self-report was 34%.	Behavioral sessions every 2 wks. for 2 mos., and 1 per/wk. for 3 mos.
Skender et al.(77)	Weight loss D = 69% AE = 70% D+AE = 64% Follow-up D = 36% AE = 58% D+AE = 50%	Prescribed meal plan with 30% fat, 50% carbohydrate, and 20% protein designed not to exceed a weight loss of 1 kg/wk Group behavioral counseling over 12 mos.: 12 wkly session, bi-weekly for 3 sessions, 3 monthly sessions	NR	Prescribed brisk walking, goal of 3-5 45-min sessions per wk at a perceived intensity that was vigorous but never strenuous	NR	No specific intervention during follow-up
Snel et al. (87)	Weight loss D = 100% D+AE = 100% Follow-up D = NR D+AE = NR	VLCD ~450 kcal/day. Weekly behavioral counseling	100% of VLCD sachets provided were used	Minimum 4 days/wk. cycle ergometer at home, 30 min at 70% VO_2 max, and 1 hr. in hospital training supervised by physiotherapist. Sessions monitored by HR	Home-averaged 5.3 sessions/wk. at 35.7 min/session. Participants attended 97% of in-hospital sessions	Regular diet ~1,800 kcal/day. Resumed diabetes medication and usual care by their physician
Svendsen et al.(93)	Weight loss Overall = 98% Follow-up D = 92% D+AE+RE = 96% C = 76%	EI was restricted to 4.2 MJ/d (1.6 MJ/d formula diet +2.6 MJ/d freely chosen food).	EI from baseline to end of follow-up was reduced in both the D (−1079 kJ/day) and D+AE+RE group (−1471 kJ/day) and increased in C (+281 kJ/d).	Exercise was supervised and included 3–60 to 90 min sessions/wk. of combined AE (cycle ergometer at ≥70% VO_2 max) and RE at ≥65% maximal lifting capacity.	From baseline to end of follow up $V0_2$ max was reduced in C (−13.4%) and increased in D (+4%) and D+AE+RE (1%).	Participants were on their own but were encouraged to continue exercise and monitor EI to maintain weight loss

Table 2. Cont.

Study	Completion Rate	Diet intervention	Diet compliance	Exercise intervention	Exercise compliance	Follow-up Intervention
Van Aggel-Leijssen et al.(88)	Weight loss Overall = 93% Follow-up D = 75% D+AE = 70%	6-wks VLCD (2.1MJ). Wks 7-10 decreased formula diet increased food of choice. Wks. 7–8, 1.4MJ/d formula+3.5 MJ choice. Wks. 9–10, 0.7 MJ formula +4.9 MJ choice food Weekly meetings	NR	Cycle ergometer, outdoor walk/jog. 4 day/wk., 40% VO_2 max, 60 min. Supervised 3 of 4 sessions/wk.	During follow-up, attended 57% of sessions. Estimated energy expenditure 335 kcal/session. No change in $V0_2$ max.	Asked to maintain weight at post weight loss level. D+ AE group asked to continue exercise.
Volpe et al.(79)	NR	EI designed to achieve weight loss of 0.5 to 1.0 kg/wk. Weekly meetings or 3 mos., bi-weekly meetings for 3 mos.	No change in EI assessed by food records over the weight loss period.	Supervised exercise on a Nordic Track. 5 days/wk, 30 min/ session, intensity NR.	NR	Provided Nordic Tack for home use. Minimal contact with investigators.
Wadden et al.(89)	Weight loss NR Follow-up Overall = 78%	Diet was a 16 wk. VLCD (~925 kcal/day) followed by a conventional energy restricted diet (1,200 to 1,500 kcal/day) for 31 wks. with behavioral counseling; weekly for 28 wks., bi-weekly for 20 wks.	AE groups were prescribed 3 supervised sessions step aerobics/wk. over the first 28 wks. and 2 supervised sessions/wk. over wks. 29–48.	AE groups were prescribed 3 supervised sessions step aerobics/wk. over the first 28 wks. and 2 supervised sessions/wk. over wks. 29–48.	55% of participants reported exercise in the follow-up period. Walking 2.8 times/ wk., total of 13 min/wk.	No specific intervention during follow-up.
			RE was 3 supervised sessions of 10 exercises that progressed in resistance when more than 14 repetitions could be performed on 2 consecutive sets.	RE was 3 supervised sessions of 10 exercises that progressed in resistance when more than 14 repetitions could be performed on 2 consecutive sets		
Wang et al. (90)	Weight Loss NR Follow-up D = 73% D+AE: low intensity = 92% D+AE: high intensity = 85%	Food provided by metabolic kitchen. Energy deficit adjust to ~11,760 kJ/wk.(~1680 kJ/d). Deficits for D only from reduction in EI, D+AE groups deficit from decreased EI (~10,080 kJ/wk., and EEEx(~1680 kJ/wk).	Mean daily caloric intake was 100.1% of provided calorie level.	Supervised treadmill exercise 3 days/wk. Low intensity, 45–50% HRR, 55 min High intensity, 70–75% HRR, 30 min	Attended 85% of sessions. No change in VO_2 max in any group.	No specific intervention during follow-up.
Wing et al. (80)	Weight loss D = 95% AE = 89% D+AE = 78% C = 80% Follow-up D = 95% AE = 84% D+AE = 80% C = 78%	EI of 800–1,000 kcal/day for the first 8 wks. of the intervention which was gradually adjusted to reach 1,200–1,500 kcal/day at wk. 16. Weekly behavioral counseling.	EI during the intervention was significantly lower in the D group compared with the AE, D+AE and C groups.	Increased PA to 1,500 kcal/wk. through brisk walking (3 miles/ day). 2 supervised group walks available during wks. 1–10, 1 supervised walk thereafter.	At 6 mos. over 75% of participants achieved the 1,500 kcal/wk. goal.	Bi-weekly group meetings and 2–6-wk refresher courses in yr. 2.

Abbreviations: AE = aerobic exercise, RE = resistance exercise, C = control, D = diet, D+AE = diet plus aerobic exercise, D+RE = diet plus resistance exercise, D+AE+RE = diet plus aerobic plus resistance exercise, EI = energy intake, HR = heart rate, HRR = heart rate reserve, NR = not reported, NA = not assessed, VLCD = very low calorie diet.

80% of the exercise goal of 225 min/wk., while Wing et al [80] reported 75% of participants achieved the prescribed exercise goal by the end of the active intervention. Pritchard et al [78] found that participants completed between 3–7 exercise session/wk., thus met their exercise goals. Participants in the Racette et al [5] trial completed and average of 5.8 exercise sessions/wk. with an average exercise energy expenditure of 317 kcal/session assessed by heart rate/oxygen consumption regression.

Intervention during follow-up. Three trials which compared diet with aerobic exercise included assessments after a follow-up period [77,79,80]. Volpe et al [79] provided participants with a Nordic Track exercise machine for home use during the follow-up period and had minimal contact with participants. Wing et al [80] provided bi-weekly group meetings over the first 6 months and two 6-week refresher courses during the final year of follow-up. Skender et al [77] provided no specific intervention during the follow-up period.

Outcomes assessed. In addition to body weight, two of the five trials with long-term comparisons assessed waist circumference [75,76], three assessed body composition by DXA [5,76,78] and one trial assessed blood pressure, total, HDL, and LDL cholesterol and triglycerides [75]. One trial with assessments after a follow-up period assessed waist circumference and body composition by under-water weight [79] 2 trials assessed blood pressure, total, HDL, and LDL cholesterol and triglycerides [79,80] while one trial assessed HbA_{1c}, glucose and insulin [80].

Participant characteristics - Diet vs. Aerobic Exercise

Age. Three of the five trials with long-term comparisons reported participant age by intervention group [5,76,78]. The median (range) age for diet groups was 55.6 yrs. (42.3–58.1 yrs.) aerobic exercise groups was 58.1 yrs. (44.9–58.8 yrs.) [5,76,78]. In the long-term trial by Anderssen et al [75] the mean age of the total sample was 40 yrs., while the age range in the trial by Skender et al [77] which provided both long-term and follow-up data was 25–45 yrs. Volpe et al [79] reported a mean age of 44.3 and 43.2 yrs. in the diet and aerobic exercise groups, respectively while the mean age in the trial by Wing et al [80] was 45.0 and 46.4 yrs, respectively.

Sex. One of the five trials with long-term comparisons included only women [76] and one trial included only men [78], while three trials included both men and women. The median (range) percent of women in these trials was 47% (9.6%–62%) [5,75,77]. The median (range) percent women in trials with assessments after a follow-up period was 51% (47%–79%) [77,79,80]. Only Volpe et al presented separate results for men and women [79].

BMI. Four of the five trials with long-term comparisons reported baseline BMI by intervention group ([5,75,76,78]. The median (range) BMI for diet groups was 29.3 kg/m^2 (27.2–31.1 kg/m^2) and aerobic exercise groups was 28.9 kg/m^2 (27.2–30.7 kg/m^2). Two of the three trials with assessments after a follow-up period reported baseline BMI. BMI was 30.9 kg/m^2 [79] and 36.1 kg/m^2 [80] in the diet groups and 30.5 kg/m^2 [79] and 36 kg/m^2 [80] in the aerobic exercise groups in these trials.

Minority representation'. Two of the five trials with long-term comparisons provided information regarding minority participation [5,76]. Foster-Schubert et al [76] included 15% minorities while minority representation was 10.2% in the trial by Racette et al [5]. None of the trials which included assessments after a follow-up period provided information on minority participation.

Physical activity level. Four of the five trials with long-term comparison that provided information on baseline level of physical activity recruited sedentary participants [5,75–77]. Two of the three trials with assessments after a follow-up period that included information on baseline physical activity also recruited sedentary participants [77,79].

Health status. With the exception of the trial by Anderssen et al [75] all trials with long-term comparisons recruited apparently healthy individuals. Anderssen et al [75] recruited participants with high diastolic blood pressure, high total cholesterol and triglycerides, and low HDL cholesterol. Trials with assessments after a follow-up period recruited healthy participants [77,79,80]; however; participants recruited by Wing et al [80] had one or two biological parents with DM2.

Results-Diet vs. Aerobic Exercise

Long term trials

Results for all trials with a diet vs. aerobic exercise comparison are presented in Table 3.

Body weight. The median (range) weight loss for the five trials that provided long-term comparisons was 7.2% (4.2–10.7%) for diet groups and 2.4% (0.3%–8.4%) for aerobic exercise groups [5,75–78]. Weight loss was significantly greater in the diet compared with the aerobic exercise groups in two trials [76,78], non-significant in two trials [5,77] and statistical significance of the between group difference was not reported in one trial [75].

Waist circumference. Waist circumference was reduced by 3.7 cm in the diet group and 1.9 cm in the aerobic exercise group (significance not reported) in the one long-term trial reporting this variable [75].

Fat mass. Three long-term trials assessed change in fat mass [5,76,78]. The median (range) change in fat mass was −6.1 kg (−3.5 to −6.2 kg) in diet and −1.8 (−2.2 to −5.5 kg) aerobic exercise groups. The reduction in fat mass was significantly greater in diet than aerobic exercise groups in two of the three trials [76,78]. However, Racette et al [5] reported no significant difference between the change in fat mass in the diet group (−6.2 kg) compared with the aerobic exercise group (−5.5 kg).

Fat-free mass. Three long-term trials reported change in fat-free mass [5,76,78]. The median (range) change in fat-free mass was −1.7 kg (−0.8 kg to −2.5 kg) in the diet group and −0.6 kg (−0.9 kg to +0.3 kg) in the aerobic exercise groups. The reduction in fat-free mass was significantly greater in the diet compared with the aerobic exercise group in two of the three trials [76,78]. Racette et al [5] reported no significant differences for change in fat-free mass between the diet (−1.7 kg) and aerobic exercise (−0.9 kg) groups.

Chronic disease risk factors. One long-term trial assessed change in chronic disease risk factors[75]; however, the significance of the between group differences were not reported. Anderssen et al [75] reported similar reductions in total cholesterol (diet = −0.23 mmol/l; aerobic exercise = −0.24 mmol/l), LDL-cholesterol (diet = −0.16 mmol/l; aerobic exercise = −0.13 mmol/l) and triglycerides (−0.23 mmol/l; aerobic exercise = −0.24 mmol/l), and similar increases in HDL-cholesterol (diet = 0.05 mmol/l; aerobic exercise = 0.04 mmol/l) in both the diet and aerobic exercise groups. Systolic (diet = −6.4 mmHg; aerobic exercise = −2.2 mmHg) and diastolic blood pressure (diet = −3.4 mmHg; −2.7 mmHg) were reduced in both the diet and aerobic exercise group.

Trials with follow-up assessments

Body weight. Three trials provided data on weight change following active weight loss and follow-up periods of 6 months [79], 12 months [77] and 18 months [80]. Skender et al [77] observed no significant difference in weight loss between the diet (−6.9% and aerobic exercise groups (−3.0%) at the completion of the active intervention; however, after a 12 month follow-up period with no active intervention the diet group regained 113% of lost weight while the aerobic exercise group regained only 7% of the initial weight loss. Wing et al [80] reported weight loss of 9.1% in the diet group and 2.1% in the aerobic exercise group following the active intervention that was reduced to a 2.1% weight loss in the diet group and 1% weight gain in the aerobic exercise group at the 18 month follow-up. Thus, the diet and aerobic exercise groups regained 77% and 148% of their lost weight, respectively. Statistical significance of between group changes was not presented. Volpe et al [79] presented weight data only in figures. Small changes in weight were observed both during the active intervention and follow-up periods, with no significant difference between the diet and aerobic exercise groups for either men or women.

Waist circumference. Volpe et al [79] reported small decreases in waist circumference in the diet (−0.6 cm) and aerobic exercise groups (−2.4 cm) on completion of the active intervention which were essentially maintained in the aerobic exercise group (−2.6 cm) but not in the diet group (+0.4 cm) at 18

Table 3. Comparison of change in weight, body composition, and chronic disease risk factors in response diet compared with aerobic exercise.

Study	Variable	Baseline - end of active intervention		Baseline -end follow-up		During follow-up	
		D	AE	D	AE	D	AE
Long-term trials							
Anderssen et al. (75)	WT (kg/%)	−4.0/−4.2	−0.9/−1.0 ^{nr}	na	na	na	na
	WC (cm)	−3.7	−1.9 ^{nr}	na	na	na	na
	TC (mmol/l)	−0.23	+0.20 ^{nr}	na	na	na	na
	LDL-C(mmol/l)	−0.16	−0.13 ^{nr}	na	na	na	na
	HDL-C(mmol/l)	+0.05	+0.04 ^{nr}	na	na	na	na
	TG (mmol/l)	−0.23	−0.24 ^{nr}	na	na	na	na
	SBP (mmHg)	−6.4	−2.2 ^{nr}	na	na	na	na
	DBP (mmHg)	−3.4	−2.7 ^{nr}	na	na	na	na
Foster-Schubert et al. (76)	WT (kg/%)	−7.1/−8.5	−2.0/-2.4 *	na	na	na	na
	WC (cm)	−4.5	−2.0 *	na	na	na	na
	Fat mass (kg)	−6.1	−2.1 *	na	na	na	na
	Fat-free mass (kg)	−0.8	+0.4 *	na	na	na	na
Pritchard et al.(78)	WT (kg/%)	−6.3/−7.2	−2.6/−3.0 *	na	na	na	na
	Fat mass (kg)	−3.5	−1.8 *	na	na	na	na
	Fat-free mass (kg)	−2.5	−0.6 *	na	na	na	na
Racette et al. (5)	WT (kg/%)	−8/−10.2	−6.4/−8.4 ^{ns}	na	na	na	na
	Fat mass (kg)	−6.2	−5.5 ^{ns}	na	na	na	na
	Fat-free mass (kg)	−1.7	−0.9 ^{ns}	na	na	na	na
Follow-up trials							
Skender et al. (77)	WT (kg/%)	−6.8/−6.9	−2.9/−3.1 ^{ns}	+0.9/0.9	−2.7/2.9 ^{ns}	7.7/7.8	+0.2/0.2 ^{nr}
Volpe et al. (79)	WT (kg)	Figures only					
Men	WC (cm)	0	−1.2 ^{ns}	−0.1	−1.2 ^{ns}	−0.1	0.00 ^{nr}
	Fat mass (kg)	−0.9	−1.6 ^{ns}	+0.2	+0.2 ^{ns}	+1.1	+1.8 ^{nr}
	Fat-free mass (kg)	−1	+0.3 ^{ns}	−1.4	+0.2 ^{ns}	−0.4	−0.1 ^{nr}
	TC (mmol/l)	+0.25	−0.16 ^{ns}	+0.09	−0.18 ^{ns}	−0.16	−.02 ^{nr}
	LDL-C (mmol/l)	+0.09	+0.08 ^{ns}	+ 0.21	+0.37 ^{ns}	+0.12	+0.29 ^{nr}
	HDL-C (mmol/l)	−0.28	−0.24 ^{ns}	−0.18	−0.13 ^{ns}	+0.10	+0.11 ^{nr}
	TG (mmol/l)	−0.19	−0.32 ^{ns}	+0.07	−0.20 ^{ns}	+0.26	+0.10 ^{nr}
	SBP (mmHg)	−18	−15.3 ^{ns}	−13.3	−14.3 ^{ns}	+4.7	+1.0 ^{nr}
	DBP (mmHg)	−8.4	−7.7 ^{ns}	−9.3	−7.9 ^{ns}	−0.9	−0.20 ^{nr}
Women	WT (kg)	Figures only					
	WC (cm)	−1.1	−3.6 ^{ns}	+0.9	−3.9 ^{ns}	+2.0	−0.30 ^{nr}
	Fat mass (kg)	−0.3	−0.5 ^{ns}	−0.4	−1.0 ^{ns}	−0.10	−0.50 ^{nr}

Table 3. Cont.

Study	Variable	Baseline - end of active intervention		Baseline -end follow-up		During follow-up	
		D	AE	D	AE	D	AE
	Fat-free mass (kg)	+0.3	+0.1 ns	+2.1	+0.9 ns	+1.8	+0.80 nr
	TC (mmol/l)	−0.13	+0.6 ns	+0.26	+0.3 ns	+0.39	+0.30 nr
	LDL-C (mmol/l)	+0.29	+0.24 ns	+0.15	+0.44 ns	−0.14	+0.20 nr
	HDL-C (mmol/l)	−0.37	−0.21 ns	−0.24	−0.13 ns	+0.13	+0.80 nr
	TG (mmol/l)	−0.9	−0.9 ns	+0.1	+0.03 ns	+1.0	+0.93 nr
	SBP (mmHg)	−3.7	−0.9 ns	−1.5	+3.0 ns	+2.2	+3.9 nr
	DBP (mmHg)	+1	+0.6 ns	−2.6	+6.3 ns	−3.6	+5.7nr
Wing et al. (80)	WT (kg/%)	−9.1/−9.1	−2.1/−2.1 nr	−2.1/−2.1	+1.0/1.0 nr	+7.0/7.0	+3.1/3.1 nr
	TC (mmol/l)	−0.49	+0.12 nr	−0.12	+0.33 nr	+0.37	+0.21 nr
	LDL-C (mmol/l)	−0.32	+0.03 nr	−0.16	+0.22 nr	+0.16	+0.19 nr
	HDL-C (mmol/l)	−0.1	+0.02 nr	+0.02	+0.05 nr	+0.12	+0.03 nr
	TG (mmol/l)	−0.3	+0.12 nr	+0.19	+0.33 nr	+0.49	+0.21 nr
	Glucose (mmol/l)	−0.2	0.00 nr	+0.3	+0.40 nr	+0.50	+0.40 nr
	Insulin (pmol/l)	−24	−4.0 nr	+20.0	+43.0 nr	+44.0	+47.0 nr
	HbA_{1c} (%)	+0.1	+0.10 nr	−0.10	−0.10 nr	−0.20	−0.20 nr
	SBP (mmHg)	−10.2	−2.4 nr	−0.8	+0.9 nr	+9.4	+3.3 nr
	DBP (mmHg)	−6.2	−1.7 nr	+3.0	+2.0 nr	+9.2	+3.7 nr

Abbreviations: D = diet, AE = aerobic exercise, WT = body weight, WC = waist circumference, TC = total cholesterol, LDL = low density lipoprotein cholesterol, HDL = high density lipoprotein cholesterol, TG = triglycerides, na = not assessed, ns = between group difference for change non- significant, nr = between group difference for change not reported.

*between group difference for change significant at $p<0.05$ or greater.

months. Sex differences for change in waist circumference were not apparent [79].

Fat mass/fat free mass. One trial assessed fat and fat-free mass following active weight loss and after a follow-up period. Volpe et al [79] observed no significant between group difference for change in fat mass at the completion of the active intervention (diet = −0.6 kg, aerobic exercise = −1.1 kg) or from baseline to the end of the follow-up period (diet = −0.1 kg, aerobic exercise = −0.7 kg). Similar results were observed for change in fat-free mass. No significant between group differences for change in fat-free mass were observed during the active intervention (diet = −0.4 kg, aerobic exercise = +0.2 kg) or from baseline to the end of the follow-up period (diet = +0.4 kg, aerobic exercise = +0.6 kg). No sex differences for change in fat mass or fat-free mass were observed [79].

Chronic disease risk factors. Volpe et al [79] reported no significant between group differences for change in total, HDL or LDL cholesterol, triglycerides, diastolic or systolic blood pressure in either men or women following completion of the active intervention (6 months), or at follow-up (6 months). At completion of the active intervention (6 months), Wing et al [80] reported significant within group reductions in the diet group in total, HDL and LDL cholesterol, systolic and diastolic blood pressure, fasting insulin and fasting glucose. Triglycerides and HbA_{1C} were not changed significantly. There were no significant changes in any of these variables in the aerobic exercise group following completion of the active intervention. At follow-up (24 months) the within group change from baseline for the diet group in total, HDL and LDL cholesterol, triglycerides and systolic blood pressure, and fasting insulin were not statistically significant. In the diet group fasting glucose and diastolic blood pressure increased significantly while HbA_{1C} was significantly decreased from baseline. With the exception of within group increases in fasting glucose and total cholesterol, there were no significant changes from baseline to the end of follow-up in the aerobic exercise group in any of the chronic disease risk factors assessed. The significance of between group changes at the end of the active intervention or follow-up were not reported [80].

Diet vs. Diet+Aerobic Exercise

Fifteen trials, which represent 75% of the trials selected for this review, provided a comparison of long-term weight loss [75–77,81,82] or weight loss with assessments after a period of follow-up achieved by diet alone or diet+aerobic exercise [77,79,80,83–90]. Both study and participant characteristics are presented in Tables 1 and 2.

Study characteristics – Diet vs. Diet+Aerobic Exercise

Sample size. The median (range) sample size for diet groups with long-term comparison was 67 (42-118) and diet+aerobic exercise groups was 65 (37-117) [75-77,81,82]. The median (range) sample size for diet groups in trials with follow-up assessments was 30 (13-95) and diet+aerobic exercise groups was 32 (14-111) [77,79,80,83-90].

Trial duration. The duration of the active intervention in four of the five trials with long-term comparisons was 12 months [75–77,82]. Dengel et al [81] used a 10 month active intervention. The median (range) duration of the active weight loss intervention in trials with follow-up assessments was 5.8 months (3–12 months). The median (range) duration of the follow-up periods were 8 months (3-18 months) following completion of the active intervention [77,79,80,83–90].

Completion rate. The median (range) completion rate for long-term comparisons was 82% (59%–95%) for diet groups and 90% (62–97%) for diet+aerobic exercise groups [75–77,81,82]. The completion rate for the active intervention for trials with follow-up assessments was not reported in two trials [79,89] and not reported by intervention group in trials by Hunter et al [84] and Van Aggel-Leijssen [88] where the completion rates for the total sample were 59% and 93%, respectively. The median (range) completion rate at the end of the active intervention for the seven trials reporting this information was 92.5% (69–100%) for diet groups and 89.5% (64–100%) for diet+aerobic exercise groups [77,80,83,85–87,90]. Completion rates at follow-up were not reported in two trials [79,87], and not reported by intervention group in one trial where the overall completion rate at follow-up was 60% [89]. The median (range) completion rate at follow-up for the eight trials reporting this information was 75.5% (36–95%) for diet groups and 72.5% (50–80%) for diet+aerobic exercise groups [77,80,83–86,88,90].

Diet. All long-term trials employed an energy restricted meal plan diet with behavioral counseling during the active intervention [75–77,81,82]. Several trials with follow-up assessments also employed energy restricted meal plans with behavioral counseling during the active weight loss intervention [77,79,80,83,85,86]. However, trials with follow-up assessments also provided meals from a metabolic kitchen [84,90] or used a very low calorie diet with behavioral counseling during active weight loss [87–89].

Compliance with diet protocol. Three trials including long-term comparisons provided information on compliance with the prescribed diet [75,76,82]. Anderssen et al [75] using a food-frequency questionnaire and Wood et al [82] using food records both reported decreased energy intake in the diet and diet+aerobic exercise groups compared with control. Foster-Schubert et al [76] found no significant changes in energy intake assessed by food-frequency questionnaire in either the diet or diet+aerobic exercise groups which was attributed to the imprecision of this measure of energy intake. However, relative fat intake (% of total daily energy intake) decreased 18% and 20% in the diet and die+aerobic exercise groups, respectively. Five trials will follow-up assessments provided information on compliance with the dietary intervention during weight loss [79,80,85,87,90]. Molenar et al [85] reported that 88% of participants attended ~4 of the 7 behavioral sessions prescribed by the intervention. Snel et al [87] reported that participants consumed 100% of VLCD sachets provided while Wang et al [90] reported participants mean energy intake assessed by food records was 100.1% of the calorie level from food provided by a metabolic kitchen. Wing et al [80] reported significantly lower energy intake assessed by food-frequency questionnaire in both diet and diet+aerobic exercise groups compared with control. Volpe et al [79] found no change in energy intake in diet or diet+aerobic exercise groups, assessed by 3-day food records, over the weight loss intervention.

Aerobic exercise mode/supervision. Modes employed in long-term trials included brisk walking/jogging [75,77,81,82] and treadmill or cycle ergometer exercise [76,81]. Exercise was supervised in three trials [75,81,82], unsupervised in one trial [77] and partially supervised in one trial [76]. Aerobic exercise modes in trials with follow-up assessments included outdoor walking/jogging [77,80,83,86] treadmill walking/jogging [88,90] cycle ergometer [87,88], Nordic Track exercise machine [79] and step aerobics [89]. Exercise was supervised in four trials [79,84,89,90], partially supervised in four trials [80,86–88], and unsupervised in two trials [77,83]. Molenar et al [85] provide no specific information regarding any aspect of the exercise intervention.

Aerobic exercise frequency. Exercise in long-term trials was prescribed at 3 days per week in 3 trials [75,81,82], 5 days/

wk. in one trial [76] and 3–5 days/wk. in one trial [77]. Trials with follow-up assessments prescribed exercise at 3 days/wk. [80,84,89,90] 4 days/wk. [87,88], 5 days/wk. [79,86] and 3–5 days/wk. [77,83].

Aerobic exercise intensity. Exercise intensity in long-term trials was prescribed at between 60–85% of peak or maximum heart rate in three trials [75,76,82], 75–80% VO_2 max in one trial [81], and at a self-assessed "vigorous but never strenuous" level on one trial [77]. Trials with follow-up assessments prescribed exercise intensity at 80% maximal heart rate [84], 40% [88] and 70% maximal oxygen uptake [87], and 45–50% or 70–75% heart-rate-reserve [90]. Trials described exercise intensity as "vigorous but not strenuous" [77] and "moderate" or "vigorous" [83]. Exercise intensity was not specified in four trials that included follow-up assessments [79,80,86,89].

Aerobic exercise duration. One long-term trial prescribed 40 min/session [81], three trials prescribed 45 min/session [76,77,82] and one trial 60 min/session [75]. Seven trials with follow-up assessments prescribed exercise duration by time [77,79,84,86–88,90]. The median (range) exercise duration in these trials was 35 min (25–60 min). Wadden et al [89] prescribed exercise duration to expend 300–400 kcal/session. Wing et al [80] prescribed waking at 3 miles/day while exercise duration was not specified in the trial by Andreou et al [83].

Compliance with exercise protocol. Four of the five long-term trials provided data on compliance with the exercise intervention [75,76,81,82]. Anderssen et al [75] reported the diet+aerobic exercise group attended 63% of scheduled exercise sessions. Participants in the diet+aerobic exercise group in the Foster-Schubert [76] trial averaged 85% of the exercise goal of 225 min/wk. Both Dengel et al [81] and Wood et al [82] reported significant increases in maximal oxygen consumption in the diet+ aerobic exercise, but not in diet or control groups. Seven of the eleven trials with follow-up assessments provided information on compliance with the exercise intervention [80,84–88,90]. Hunter et al [84] compared trial outcomes between participants who adhered (82%) or did not adhere (18%) to the aerobic exercise protocol during the follow-up period. Participants in the trial by Neumark et al [86] competed approximately 50% of assigned exercise sessions while Snel et al [87] and Wang et al [90] reported participants attended 97% and 85% of supervised exercise sessions, respectively. Van Aggel-Leijssen et al [88] found no change in aerobic capacity in the diet+aerobic exercise group over the course of the active intervention. Moelanar et al [85] asked participants to attend 6 sessions with a physiotherapist and reported that 87% of participants attended an average of 5 sessions.

Intervention during follow-up. Five of the 11 trials that compared diet with diet+exercise included no specific intervention during the follow-up period [77,83,85,89,90]. Volpe et al [79] provided participants with a Nordic Track exercise machine for home use during the follow-up period and had minimal contact with participants. Wing et al [80] and Neumark-Sztainer et al [86] provided continued behavioral sessions at a reduced frequency as compared with the active weight loss intervention. Hunter et al [84] and Van Aggel-Leijssen et al [88] asked participants to continue with the intervention assigned during weight loss. Participants in the trial by Snel et al [87] resumed their medications for DM2 and received usual care from their physician.

Outcomes assessed. In addition to body weight, two of the five trials with long-term comparisons assessed waist circumference [75,76], and three assessed body composition, two by underwater weight [81,82] and one by DXA [76]. Two trials assessed blood pressure, total, HDL, and LDL cholesterol and triglycerides [75,82]. Five trials with follow-up assessments assessed waist circumference [79,83,85–87] and 6 trials assessed body composition, three by underwater weight [79,88,89], two by bioelectric impedance [83,87] and one by DXA and magnetic resonance imaging [84]. Three trials assessed blood lipids (total, HDL, LDL cholesterol and triglycerides), 2 of which also assessed blood pressure [79,80] and glucose, insulin and HbA_{1c} [80,87].

Participant characteristics – Diet vs. Diet+Aerobic Exercise

Age. Two of the five trials with long-term comparisons reported participant age by intervention group [76,81]. The mean age in the diet groups was 61.0 yrs. and 58.1 yrs. and diet+aerobic exercise groups was 57.1 and 58 yrs. in the trials of Dengel et al. [81]and Foster-Schubert et al. [76],respectively. In the long-term trial by Anderssen et al [75] the mean age of the total sample was 40 yrs., while the age range in the trial by Skender et al [77], which provided both long-term and follow-up data was 25–45 yrs. Wood et al [82] reported a total sample mean age of 40.3 yrs. for men and 39.1 yrs. for women. Eight of the 11 trials with follow-up assessments reported participant age by participant group [79,80,83–85,87–89]. The median (range) age in the diet groups was 40.8 yrs (29–59 yrs.) and diet+aerobic exercise groups was 41.2 (31–56) yrs. Neumark-Stzainer et al [86] and Skender et al [77] reported participant age ranges of 25–50 yrs., and 25–40 yrs., respectively. The mean sample age in the trial by Wang et al [90] was 58.6 yrs.

Sex. One of the five trials with long-term comparisons included only women [76] and one trial included only men [81], while three trials included both men and women [75,77,82]. The median (range) percent of women in these trials was 47% (9.6%–49%) [75,77,82]. Five trials with follow-up assessments included only women [83,84,86,89,90],one trial included only men [88], while five trials included both men and women [77,79,80,85,87]. The median (range) percent of women in these five trials was 47% (40–79%). Only 1 long-term trial [82] and one trial with follow-up assessments [79] presented results for men and women separately.

BMI. Three of the five trials with long-term comparisons reported participant BMI by intervention group [75,76,81]. The median (range) BMI was 30.1 kg/m^2 (29.5–31.1 kg/m^2) for the diet groups and 30.1 kg/m^2 (28.6–31.0 kg/m^2) for the diet+ aerobic exercise groups. Wood et al [82] reported a mean sample BMI of 30.7 kg/m^2 for men and 27.9 kg/m^2 for women while Skender et al [77] did not report baseline BMI. Seven of the 11 trials with follow-up assessments reported baseline BMI by intervention group [79,83,85,87–90] one trial reported mean BMI for the complete sample [86] one trial reported baseline percent body fat [90] and two trials did not report baseline BMI [77,84]. The median (range) BMI for diet groups was 32.0 kg/m^2 (30.9–37.9 kg/m^2) and diet+aerobic exercise groups was 32.6 kg/ m^2 (29.1–37.3 kg/m^2). Neumark-Sztainer et al [86] reported a baseline BMI of 30.3 kg/m^2 in the complete sample. Wang et al [90] recruited participants with baseline percent body fat of 43%, 42.3% and 43.1% in the diet, diet+low intensity aerobic exercise and diet+high intensity exercise groups, respectively.

Minority representation. The percent minority representation was presented in two of the five long-term trials. The sample of Dengel et al [81] included no minorities while the sample of Foster-Schubert et al [76] included 15% minorities. The median (range) percent of minority representation in the five trials with follow-up assessments that provided this information was 34% (0–70%) ([84,86,87,89,90].

Table 4. Comparison of change in weight, body composition, and chronic disease risk factors in response to diet compared with diet plus aerobic exercise.

Study	Variable	Baseline - end of active intervention		Baseline - end follow-up		During follow-up	
		D	D+AE	D	D+AE	D	D+AE
Long-term trials							
Anderssen et al. (75)	WT (kg/%)	−4/−4.2	−5.6/−6.2 ^{nr}	na	na	na	na
	WC (cm)	−3.7	−5.7 ^{nr}	na	na	na	na
	TC (mmol/l)	−0.23	−0.48 ^{nr}	na	na	na	na
	LDL-C (mmol/l)	−0.18	−0.39 ^{nr}	na	na	na	na
	HDL-C (mmol/l)	+0.05	+0.13 ^{nr}	na	na	na	na
	TG (mmol/l)	−0.23	−0.58 ^{nr}	na	na	na	na
	SBP (mmHg)	−6.4	−5.9 ^{nr}	na	na	na	na
	DBP (mmHg)	−3.4	−5.2 ^{nr}	na	na	na	na
Dengel et al. (81)	WT (kg/%)	−9.3/−10.1	−8.1/−8.6 ^{ns}	na	na	na	na
	Fat mass (kg)	−6.8	−6.7 ^{ns}	na	na	na	na
	Fat-free mass (kg)	−2.1	−1.3 ^{ns}	na	na	na	na
Foster-Schubert et al. (76)	WT (%)	−7.1/−8.5	−8.9/−10.8 *	na	na	na	na
	WC (cm)	−4.5	−7.5 *	na	na	na	na
	Fat mass (kg)	−6.1	−8.2 *	na	na	na	na
	Fat-free mass (kg)	−0.8	−0.4 ^{ns}	na	na	na	na
Wood et al. (82)	WT (kg/%)	−5.1/−5.2	−8.7/−8.8 *	na	na	na	na
Men	Fat mass (kg)	−4.3	−7.8 *	na	na	na	na
	TC (mmol/l)	−0.42	−0.38 ^{ns}	na	na	na	na
	LDL-C (mmol/l)	−0.39	−0.27 ^{ns}	na	na	na	na
	HDL-C (mmol/l)	+0.02	+0.14 *	na	na	na	na
	TG (mmol/l)	−0.12	−0.48 *	na	na	na	na
	SBP (mmHg)	−4.1	−5.4 ^{ns}	na	na	na	na
	DBP(mmHg)	−2.4	−4.9 ^{ns}	na	na	na	na
Women	WT (%)	−4.1/−5.5	−5.1/−6.8 *	na	na	na	na
	Fat mass (kg)	−4.0	−5.5 ^{ns}	na	na	na	na
	TC (mmol/l)	−0.39	−0.28 ^{ns}	na	na	na	na
	LDL-C (mmol/l)	−0.28	−0.29 ^{ns}	na	na	na	na
	HDL-C (mmol/l)	−0.15	+0.02 *	na	na	na	na
	TG (mmol/l)	+0.09	−0.02 ^{ns}	na	na	na	na
	SBP (mmHg)	−4.1	−3.6 ^{ns}	na	na	na	na
	DBP (mmHg)	−2.2	−2.0 ^{ns}	na	na	na	na
Follow-up trials							

Table 4. Cont.

Study	Variable	Baseline - end of active intervention		Baseline - end follow-up		During follow-up	
		D	D+AE	D	D+AE	D	D+AE
Andreou et al. (83)	WT (kg/%)	−6.1/−7.5	−15.5/−19.5 nr	−8.4/−10.3	−17.3/−21.7 nr	−2.3/−2.8	−1.8/−2.2 nr
	WC (cm)	−5.5	−11.2 nr	−8.0	−14.2 nr	−2.5	−3.0 nr
	%fat	−0.5	−8.2 nr	−1.2	−10.0 nr	−0.7	−1.8 nr
Hunter et al.(84)	WT (kg/%)	na	na	na	na	+6.4/9.8	Adhere =3.1/4.9% *
	WT(kg/%)	na	na	na	na	+6.4/9.8	Non-Adhere =7.1/10.9 ns
	WC (cm)	na	na	na	na	+5.5	Adhere =1.9 ns
	WC (cm)	na	na	na	na	+5.5	Non-Adhere=+7.9 ns
	% Fat	na	na	na	na	+5.3	Adhere=3.4 *
	% Fat	na	na	na	na	5.3	Non-Adhere =6.4 ns
	Visceral fat (cm^2)	na	na	na	na	+12.4 **	Adhere=0.8 ns within
	Visceral fat (cm^2)	na	na	na	na	+12.4 **	Non-Adhere =25.5 **
Molenar et al. (85)	WT (kg/%)	−2.2/−2.3	−3.0/−3.2 ns	−2/−2.1	−3.1/−3.3 ns	−0.2/−0.2	+0.1/0.1 nr
	WC (cm)	−2.1	−3.7 ns	−2.1	−4.2 ns	0.0	−0.5 nr
Neumark-Sztainer et al. (86)	WT (kg/%[a])	−3.8	−3.6 ns	−3.9	−4.6 ns	−0.1	−1.0 nr
	WC (cm)	−7.4	−8.5 ns	na	na	na	na
Skender et al. (77)	WT (kg/%)	− 6.8/−6.9	−8.9/−8.9 ns	+0.9/0.9	−2.2/−2.2%	+7.7/7.8 ns	+6.7/6.7 nr
Snel et al. (87)	WT (kg/%)	−24/−21.2	−28.0/−24.6 *	−10/−8.8	−16.0/−14.0 *	14/12.4	+12/12.2 nr
	WC (cm)	−19	−25.0 *	−8	−16.0 *	+11	+9.0 nr
	Fat mass (kg)	−16.7	−21.9 nr	−5.7	−10.0 nr	+11.0	+11.9 nr
	TC (mmol/l)	−0.6	−0.9 nr	−0.6	−1.1 nr	0.0	−0.2 nr
	LDL-C (mmol/l)	−0.7	−0.6 ns	−1.1	−0.9 ns	−0.2	−0.3 nr
	HDL-C (mmol/l)	0	+0.1 ns	+0.2	0.0ns	+0.2	+0.1nr
	TG (mmol/l)	−0.8	−1.3 ns	+0.5	−0.6 ns	+0.2	+0.7nr
	Glucose (mmol/l)	−4.4	−4.3 ns	+1.0	−1.7 ns	+5.4	+2.6 nr
	Insulin (mU/l)	−11	−16.0 *	−7	−12.0 *	+4	+4.0 nr
	HbA_{1c} (%)	−1.1	−1.5 ns	+0.4	−0.3ns	+1.5	+1.2 nr
	SBP (mmHg)	−21	−13.0 ns	−4.0	+1.0 ns	+17	+14 nr
	DBP (mmHg)	−9	−6.0 ns	+2.0	+1.0 ns	+11.0	+7.0 nr
Van Aggel-Leijssen et al.(88)	WT (kg/%)	−15.4/−14.9	−14.8/−14.4 ns	−8.3/−8.0	−5.9/−5.8 ns	7.1/6.9	+8.9/8.6 nr
	Fat mass (kg)	−12.6	−12.5ns	−7.9	−6.7 ns	+4.7	+5.8 nr
	Fat-free mass (kg)	−2.1	−2.1 ns	−0.3	−0.8 ns	+1.8	+1.3 nr
Volpe et al. (79)	WT (kg)	Figures only					
Men	WC (cm)	0	−4.9 *	−0.1	−1.9 ns	−0.1	+3.0 nr

Table 4. Cont.

Study	Variable	Baseline - end of active intervention		Baseline - end follow-up		During follow-up	
		D	D+AE	D	D+AE	D	D+AE
	Fat mass (kg)	−0.9	−4.5 ^{ns}	+0.2	−2.8 ^{ns}	+1.1	+1.7 ^{nr}
	Fat-free mass (kg)	−1	−0.3 ^{ns}	−1.4	+0.1 ^{ns}	−0.4	+0.4 ^{nr}
	TC (mmol/l)	0.25	−0.27 ^{ns}	+0.09	−0.04 ^{ns}	−0.16	+0.11 ^{nr}
	LDL-C (mmol/l)	0.09	+ 0.02 ^{ns}	+ 0.21	+ 0.25 ^{ns}	+0.12	+0.23 ^{nr}
	HDL-C (mmol/l)	−0.28	−0.22 ^{ns}	−0.18	−0.13^{ns}	+0.10	+0.90 ^{nr}
	TG (mmol/l)	−0.19	−0.24 ^{ns}	+0.07	−0.20 ^{ns}	+0.26	+0.04 ^{nr}
	SBP (mmHg)	−18	−11.8 ^{ns}	−13.3	−15.6 ^{ns}	+4.7	−3.8 ^{nr}
	DBP (mmHg)	−8.4	−9.7 ^{ns}	−9.3	−12.3 ^{ns}	−0.9	− 2.6 ^{nr}
Women	WT (kg)	Figures only					
	WC (cm)	−1.1	+0.1 ^{ns}	+0.9	−2.1^{ns}	+2	−2.2 ^{nr}
	Fat mass (kg)	−0.3	−4.2 *	−0.4	−1.9 ^{ns}	−0.1	+2.3 ^{nr}
	Fat-free mass (kg)	+0.3	+1.5 ^{ns}	+1.2	+1.1 ^{ns}	+0.9	−0.4 ^{nr}
	TC (mmol/l)	−0.13	−0.7 ^{ns}	+0.26	−0.21 ^{ns}	+0.39	−0.14 ^{nr}
	LDL-C (mmol/l)	0.29	+0.38 ^{ns}	+0.15	−0.10 ^{ns}	−0.14	−0.24 ^{nr}
	HDL-C (mmol/l)	−0.37	−0.26 ^{ns}	−0.24	−0.23 ^{ns}	+0.13	+0.03 ^{nr}
	TG (mmol/l)	−0.9	−0.34 ^{ns}	+0.1	−0.26 ^{ns}	+1.0	+0.08 ^{nr}
	SBP (mmHg)	−3.7	−4.3 ^{ns}	−1.5	+1.2 ^{ns}	+2.2	+5.5 ^{nr}
	DBP (mmHg)	+1	−4.3 ^{ns}	−2.6	+1.2 ^{ns}	−3.6	+5.5 ^{nr}
Wadden et al. (89)	WT (kg/%)	−15.3/−16.3	−13.5/−13.9 ^{ns}	−6.9/−7.7	−8.5/−8.6 ^{ns}	+8.4/8.6	+5.0/5.3 ^{nr}
Wang et al. (90)	WT (kg/%)	−12.8/−14	LI = −13.1/−14.8 ^{ns}	−8.1/−8.0	LI = −6.8/−7.7 ^{ns}	+4.7/6	+6.3/7.1 ^{nr}
		−12.8/14	HI = −10.8/−11.0^{ns}	−8.1/−8.0	HI = −7.0/−7.8 ^{ns}	+5.8/6.2	+3.1/3.2 ^{nr}
Wing et al. (80)	WT (kg/%)	−9.1/−9.1	−10.3/−10.4 ^{nr}	−2.1/−2.1	−2.1/−2.5 ^{nr}	+7.0/7.0	+8.2/7.9 ^{nr}
	TC (mmol/l)	−0.49	−0.33 ^{nr}	−0.12	+0.09 ^{nr}	+0.37	+0.42 ^{nr}
	LDL-C (mmol/l)	−0.32	−0.13 ^{nr}	−0.16	+0.12 ^{nr}	+0.16	+0.25 ^{nr}
	HDL-C (mmol/l)	−0.1	−0.06 ^{nr}	+0.02	+0.05 ^{nr}	+0.12	+0.11 ^{nr}
	TG (mmol/l)	−0.3	−0.69 ^{nr}	+0.19	−0.28 ^{nr}	+0.21	+0.41 ^{nr}
	Glucose (mmol/l)	−0.2	−0.20 ^{nr}	+0.30	+0.50 ^{nr}	+0.50	+0.70 ^{nr}
	Insulin (pmol/l)	−24	−37.0 ^{nr}	+20.0	−12.0 ^{nr}	+44.0	+25.0 ^{nr}
	HbA_{1c} (%)	0.1	+0.03 ^{nr}	−0.10	+0.04 ^{nr}	−0.20	+0.01 ^{nr}
	SBP (mmHg)	−10.2	−12.3 ^{nr}	−0.8	−4.8 ^{nr}	+9.4	+7.5 ^{nr}
	DBP (mmHg)	−6.2	−6.9 ^{nr}	+3.0	−0.2 ^{nr}	+9.2	+6.7 ^{nr}

Abbreviations: D = diet, D+AE = diet plus aerobic exercise, WT = body weight, WC = waist circumference, TC = total cholesterol, LDL = low density lipoprotein cholesterol, HDL = high density lipoprotein cholesterol, TG = triglycerides, na = not assessed, ns = between group difference for change non- significant, nr = between group difference for change not reported.

[a]baseline weight not reported.

*between group difference for change significant at $p < 0.05$ or greater.

**within group change significant at $p < 0.05$ or greater.

Physical activity level. All five trials with long-term comparison recruited sedentary participants [75–77,81,82]. Two of the three trials with assessments after a follow-up period that included information on baseline physical activity also recruited sedentary participants [77,79].

Health status. With the exception of the trial by Anderssen et al [75] all trials with long-term comparisons recruited apparently healthy individuals. Anderssen et al [75] recruited participants with high diastolic blood pressure, high total cholesterol and triglycerides, and low HDL cholesterol. Trials will assessments after a follow-up period recruited healthy participants with the exception of Snel et al [87] who recruited participants with DM2 who were insulin dependent and Wing et al [80] who recruited healthy participants with one or two biological parents with DM2.

Results: Diet vs. Diet+Aerobic Exercise

Long-term trials

Results for all trials with a diet vs. diet+aerobic exercise comparison are presented in Table 4.

Body weight. The median (range) for weight loss was 6.9% (4.2–10.1%) in diet groups and 8.8% (6.2–11.5%) in diet+aerobic exercise groups. Weight loss was greater in the diet+aerobic exercise group compared with the diet only group in four of five trials. However, between group differences were statistically significant in only two [76,82] of the four trials providing this information. Wood et al [82] reported significantly greater weight loss in the diet+aerobic exercise group compared with the diet group in both men and women.

Waist circumference. Two long-term trials assessed change in waist circumference. Anderssen et al [75] reported decreased waist circumference in both the diet (−3.7 cm) and diet+aerobic exercise groups (−5.7 cm); however statistical significant of the between group difference was not reported. Foster-Schubert et al [76] reported significantly greater reductions in waist circumference in the diet+aerobic exercise (−7.0 cm) compared with the diet only group (−4.5 cm).

Fat mass/fat-free mass. Fat mass was assessed in three long-term trials [76,81,82]. Dengel et al [81] found no significant difference in change in fat mass between diet (−2.1 kg) and diet+aerobic exercise (−1.3 kg) groups. However, both Foster-Schubert et al [76] (diet = −6.1 kg; diet+aerobic exercise = −8.2 kg) and Wood et al [82] in men (diet = −4.3 kg; diet+aerobic exercise = −7.8 kg) observed significantly greater loss of fat mass in diet+aerobic exercise compared with diet only groups. Wood et al [82] observed no significant between group difference for change in fat mass in women (diet = −4.0 kg, diet+aerobic exercise = −5.5 kg). Dengel et al [81] reported decreased fat-free mass in both the diet (−2.1 kg) and diet+aerobic exercise groups (−1.3 kg) with no significant between group difference. Foster-Schubert et al [76] also reported decreased fat-free mass in both the diet (−0.8 kg) and diet+aerobic exercise groups (−0.4 kg) with no significant between group difference. Wood et al [82] did not present data on fat-free mass.

Chronic disease risk factors. Two long-term trials compared change in chronic disease risk factors between diet and diet+aerobic exercise groups [75,82]. Anderssen et al [75] reported decreases in both systolic (diet = −6.4 mmHg; diet+aerobic exercise = −5.9 mmHg) and diastolic blood pressure (diet = −3.4 mmHg; diet+aerobic exercise = −5.2 mmHg) in diet and diet+aerobic exercise groups. The statistical significance of the between group differences was not reported. Wood et al [82] reported decreased systolic and diastolic blood pressure in both diet and diet+aerobic exercise groups. The difference for change between groups was not significant. Anderssen et al [75] reported larger decreases in total cholesterol (diet = −0.23 mmol/l, diet+aerobic exercise = −0.48 mmol), LDL cholesterol (diet = −0.18 mmol/l; diet+aerobic exercise = −0.39 mmol/l) and trigylcerides (diet = −0.23 mmol/l; diet+aerobic exercise = −0.58 mmol/l) and larger increases in HDL cholesterol (diet = +0.5 mmol/l; diet+aerobic exercise = +0.13 mmol/l) in the diet+exercise compared to the diet group; however, statistical significance of the between group differences was not reported. Wood et al [82] found no significant difference for change in either total or LDL cholesterol between diet and diet+aerobic exercise groups for either men or women. The increase in HDL cholesterol was significantly greater in the diet+aerobic exercise groups (men = +0.14 mmol/l; women = +0.2 mmol/l) compared with the diet group (men = +0.2 mmol/l; women = −0.15 mmol/l) in both men and women. Among men, the decrease in triglycerides was significantly greater in the diet+aerobic exercise group (−0.48 mmol/l) compared with the diet group (−0.12 mmol). No between group differences were shown for change in triglycerides in women (diet = +0.9 mmol; diet+aerobic exercise = −0.2 mmol/l).

Trials with follow-up assessments

Body weight. Eight of the 11 trials that assessed weight change, both after an active intervention and a follow-up period, reported or provided numerical data with which percent weight change could be calculated [77,80,83,85,87–90]. The median (range) for weight loss from baseline to completion of the weight loss intervention in these 8 trials was 11.6% (2.3–21.2%) in diet groups and 13.6% (3.2–24.6%) in diet+aerobic exercise groups. Weight loss was greater in diet+aerobic exercise compared with diet only groups in six trials [77,79,80,83,85,87]; however, the between group differences were statistically significant in only one trial, in women but not men [79]. Six of these 8 trials reported clinically significant (≥5%) weight loss at the completion of the active intervention in both the diet and diet+aerobic exercise groups [77,80,87–90].

The median (range) percent weight loss from baseline to the completion of follow-up was 7.9% (+0.9 to −10.3%) in diet groups and 6.8% (−2.5 to −21.7%) in diet+aerobic exercise groups. Weight loss was greater in the diet+aerobic exercise compared with diet only groups in 7 of 9 trials providing this data [77,79,80,83,85–87,89,90]; however, between group differences were not statistically significant in the 7 trials that reported the significance for between group differences [77,79,85–87,89,90]. Weight change from baseline to the completion of follow-up did not differ by sex in the one follow-up trial reporting this data [79].

Four of the 6 trials that reported ≥5% weight loss in both the diet and diet+aerobic exercise groups at the end of the active intervention continued to observe ≥5% weight loss in both groups at follow-up [87–90]. Among the 6 trials reporting clinically significant weight loss on completion of the weight loss intervention, the median (range) of percent of lost weight regained at follow-up was 57.5% (37–113%) for diet groups and 52.5% (35–75%) for diet+aerobic exercise groups [77,80,87–90].

Hunter et al [84] reassessed body weight in a sample of initially overweight and obese women one-year following completion of a weight loss intervention by diet (800 kcal/day,food from metabolic kitchen) or diet+aerobic exercise. During weight loss, supervised aerobic exercise (treadmill) was prescribed at 3 days/week and ramped to 40 min/session at 80% maximal heart rate by week eight. Compliance with the exercise protocol was required to remain in the study. The weight loss intervention was continued until participants reached a BMI of 25 kg/m^2 (mean 154 days) at which time they were asked to continue with their original group assignment with supervised exercise frequency reduced to two days/week for exercise groups over the next 12 months. All groups were given instruction on following a balanced diet that focused on consumption of low-density foods. Exercise during the follow-up period was not required to remain in the study, thus two groups were formed; participants who adhered (≥60% of scheduled sessions) and those who did not adhere (<60% of scheduled sessions). Results indicated that body weight increased significantly during the one-year follow-up, with a significant group by time interaction. The increase in weight from the end of weight loss was significantly less in participants who adhered to aerobic exercise (+4.9%) compared with those who failed to adhere (+10.9%) or in the diet group (+9.9%).

Waist circumference. Four trials with follow up assessment reported change in waist circumference [79,83,85,87]. The median (range) change in waist circumference from baseline to the end of the active intervention was −2.1 cm (0 to −19 cm) for diet groups and −4.9 cm (+0.1 to −25 cm) for diet+aerobic exercise groups. Volpe et al [79] reported statistically significant between group differences for change for waist circumference, in men (diet = 0 cm; diet+aerobic exercise = −4.9 cm) but not in women (diet = +0.1, diet+aerobic exercise = +0.9 cm). Andreou et al [83] reported larger decreases in waist circumference in the diet+aerobic exercise (−11.2 cm) compared to the diet group (−5.5 cm); however, the statistical significance of the between group difference was not reported.

The median (range) change in waist circumference from baseline to the completion of follow-up was −2.1 cm (+0.9 cm to −8.0 cm) for diet groups and −4.2 cm (−1.9 to −16.0 cm) in diet+aerobic exercise groups [79,83,85,87]. No significant between group differences were noted. Andreou et al [83] reported larger decreases in waist circumference in the diet+aerobic exercise (−14.2 cm) compared to the diet group (−8.0 cm). The statistical significance of the between group difference was not reported.

Waist circumference was unchanged or slightly decreased during the follow-up period in two trials ([83,85] and increased in two trials [79,87]. Participants in the trial by Snel et al [87] regained a large portion of the losses in waist circumference over the follow-up period (diet = 58%; diet+aerobic exercise = 36%). Volpe et al [79] reported that men in the diet+aerobic exericise group who had a significant reduction in waist circumference during the active intervention (−4.9 cm) regained 61% of the loss during follow-up. Hunter et al [84], using the previously described study protocol, found that waist circumference increased significantly during a one-year follow-up, with a significant group by time interaction. The increase in waist circumference from the end of weight loss was significantly less in participants who adhered to aerobic exercise (+1.9 cm) compared with those who failed to adhere (+7.9 cm) or in the diet group (+5.5 cm).

Fat mass/% fat. Four trials with follow-up assessments reported change in fat mass or % fat over the active intervention [79,83,87,88]. The median (range) change in fat mass was −13.2 kg (−0.6 to −16.7 kg) for the diet groups and −12.7 kg (−4.3 to −21.8 kg) for diet+aerobic exercise groups [79,87,88]. Between group differences for change in fat mass were statistically significant only in women in the trial reported by Volpe et al [79] (diet = −0.3 kg; diet+aerobic exercise = −4.2 kg). Andreou et al [83] reported greater loss of percent body fat in the diet+aerobic exercise group (−8.2%) compared with the diet group (−0.5%); however statistical significance of the between group difference was not reported.

The median (range) change in fat mass from baseline to the completion of follow-up was −5.7 kg (−0.1 kg to −7.9 kg) for diet groups and −6.7 kg (−2.4 to −10 kg) in the diet+aerobic exercise groups [79,87,88]. Andreou et al [83] reported significantly greater loss of percent body fat in the diet+aerobic exercise group (−10.0%) compared with the diet group (−1.2%).

Fat mass increased in both diet and diet+aerobic exercise groups during the follow-up period in three trials [79,87,88]; however Andreou et al [83] showed small continued decreases in percent body fat (diet = −0.7%; diet+aerobic exercise = −1.8%) during follow-up. Snel et al [87] reported participants regained 66% and 54% of their fat mass loss in the diet and diet+aerobic exercise groups, respectively over a follow-up of 14 months. Van Aggel-Leijssen [88] reported participants in the diet group regained 40% of their fat mass loss while participants in the diet+aerobic exercise group regained 47% of lost fat mass over 40 wks. Volpe et al [79] showed significant loss of fat mass during the active intervention only in the diet+aerobic exercise group. Over the follow-up period (6 months) men in the diet+aerobic exercise group regained 38% of fat mass loss while women regained 55% of their fat mass loss. Hunter et al [84],using the previously described study protocol, found that the increase in percent body fat from the end of weight loss was significantly less in participants who adhered to aerobic exercise (+3.4%) compared with those who failed to adhere (+ 6.4%) or in the diet group (+5.3%). Intra-abdominal adipose tissue increased significantly from the end of weight loss in both the diet group (+24.8%) and the group non-adherent to the aerobic exercise protocol (+54.4%) but not in the group who adhered to aerobic exercise (1.6%).

Fat-free mass/%lean mass. There were no significant between group differences for change in fat-free mass from baseline to completion of the weight loss intervention or from baseline to the end of follow-up in the two trials that reported this outcome [79,88]. Andreou et al [83] showed a non-significant increase in percent lean body mass in the diet only group (+0.5%) and a significant increase in percent lean body mass in the diet+ aerobic exercise group (8.2%) over the active intervention (18 wks.). At follow-up, 18 weeks after completing the active intervention, Andreou et al [83] found a significant between group difference in change from baseline for percent lean body mass which was reduced in the diet group (−1.1%) and increased in the diet+aerobic exercise group (+10%). Volpe et al [79] reported no significant difference for change in fat-free mass between diet and diet+aerobic exercise groups following completion of the weight loss intervention or from baseline to the end of follow-up in either men or women.

Chronic Disease Risk Factors. Three trials reported chronic disease risk factors [79,80,87]. At completion of the active intervention (6 months), Wing et al [80] reported significant within group reductions in total, HDL and LDL cholesterol, systolic and diastolic blood pressure, fasting insulin and fasting glucose in the diet only group. Triglycerides and HbA_{1C} were not changed significantly. In the diet+aerobic exercise group there were significant reductions in total cholesterol, triglycerides, systolic blood and diastolic blood pressure, triglycerides, glucose, and insulin. HDL cholesterol, LDL cholesterol and HbA_{1C} were not significantly changed. At follow-up (24 months) the within group change from baseline for the diet group in total, HDL and LDL cholesterol, triglycerides and systolic blood pressure, and fasting insulin were not statistically significant. In the diet group fasting glucose and diastolic blood pressure increased significantly while HbA_{1C} was significantly decreased from baseline. For the diet+ aerobic exercise group, there were no significant within group changes from baseline in total, HDL and LDL cholesterol, triglycerides, systolic and diastolic blood pressure, and fasting insulin. Both glucose and fasting insulin were significantly increased from baseline. Thus, risk factor changes associated with the active intervention were not maintained at follow-up. The statistical significance of between group changes at the end of the active intervention or follow-up were not reported [80]. Snel et al [87] in a sample of obese patients with insulin dependent DM2 reported that significant reductions in systolic and diastolic blood pressure, triglycerides, LDL cholesterol, glucose and HbA_{1c} observed in the diet only group following completion of the active intervention (4 months) were no longer significant at follow-up (18 months). In the diet group, insulin was significantly reduced at both 4 and 18 months, HDL cholesterol was significantly increased only at 18 months, while total cholesterol was not significantly altered at either 4 or 18 months. In the diet+aerobic exercise group, significant reductions in systolic and diastolic blood pressure, triglycerides, glucose and HbA_{1c} observed at 4 month were no longer significant at 18 months. Insulin, total and LDL cholesterol were significantly reduced from baseline at both 4 and 18 months, while HDL cholesterol was significantly increased only at 18 months. Volpe et al [79] reported no significant changes in systolic blood or diastolic blood pressure, total, HDL or LDL cholesterol, or triglycerides in either the diet or diet+aerobic exercise groups after completion of the active intervention (6 months) or at follow-up (12 months) in either men or women.

Aerobic Exercise vs. Diet+Aerobic Exercise

Seven trials, which represent 35% of the trials selected for this review, provided a comparison of long-term weight loss [75–77] or weight loss with assessments after a period of follow-up achieved by aerobic exercise or diet+aerobic exercise [77,79,80,91,92]. The trial by Skender et al [77] provides data for both a long-term intervention (12 months) and a follow-up (12 months). Study and participant characteristics are presented in Tables 1 and 2.

Study characteristics

Sample size. In long-term trials, Anderssen et al [75] included 49 and 65 participants in the aerobic and diet+aerobic exercise groups, respectively, while Foster-Schubert et al [76] included 117 participants in both the aerobic exercise and diet+ aerobic exercise groups. The median (range) sample size for the five trials that included follow-up assessments was 43 (34–47) for aerobic exercise groups and 42 (28–46) for diet+aerobic exercise groups [77,79,80,84,91,92].

Trial Duration. Both long-term trials were 12 month in duration [75,76]. Two trials with follow-up assessments used 12 week active interventions with 12 week follow-up periods [91,92]. Both Volpe et al [79] and Wing et al [80] used 6 month active interventions. Volpe et al [79] reassessed participants after 6 months while Wing et al [80] completed follow-up assessments 18 months after completion of the active intervention. Skender et al [77] assessed participants after a 12 month active intervention and a 12 month follow-up period.

Completion rate. The long-term trial by Anderssen et al [75] reported a completion rate of 91% and 97% for the aerobic exercise and diet+aerobic exercise groups, respectively. Foster-Schubert et al [76] reported completion rates of 91% in the aerobic exercise group and 92% in the diet+aerobic exercise group. Four of the five trials that included follow-up assessments reported completion rates by intervention group [77,80,91,92]. The median (range) completion rate for the aerobic exercise groups over the active interventions was 77% (44.7–89%) for the aerobic exercise groups and 67.8% (65.1–78%) for the diet+ aerobic exercise groups. The median (range) completion rate at follow-up was 69% (40.4–82%) for aerobic exercise groups and 58.4% (51.2–80%) in the diet+aerobic exercise groups.

Diet. Long-term trials and trials with follow-up assessments generally employed energy restricted meal plan diets with behavioral counseling. Melanson et al [91] included 2 to 4 meal replacements/day, while Melanson et al [92]used 2 meals/day of a high fiber cereal in one intervention group.

Compliance with diet protocol. Anderssen et al [75] found greater reductions in energy intake assessed by food-frequency questionnaire in the diet+aerobic exercise group while Foster-Schubert et al [76] reported no change in energy intake assessed by food frequency questionnaire for either the aerobic exercise or diet+aerobic exercise groups. Four of the five trials with follow-up assessments reported dietary compliance. Trials by Melanson et al [91,92] and Wing et al [80] showed greater reductions in energy intake assessed by food records in the diet+aerobic exercise groups compared with the aerobic exercise groups. Volpe et al [79] found no change in energy intake assessed by food records in either the aerobic exercise or diet+aerobic exercise groups.

Aerobic exercise mode/supervision. Modes employed in long-term trials comparing aerobic exercise with diet+aerobic exercise included brisk walking/jogging [75], and treadmill or cycle ergometer exercise [76]. Anderssen et al [75] provided supervised exercise while exercise was partially supervised in the trial by Foster-Schubert et al [76]. Aerobic exercise modes in trials with follow-up assessments included outdoor walking/jogging [77,80,91,92] and the Nordic Track exercise machine [79]. Exercise was unsupervised in three trials [77,91,92],partially supervised in one trial [80] and supervised in one trial [79].

Aerobic exercise frequency. Exercise frequency in long-term trials was 3 days/wk. [75,79] or 5 days/wk. [76]. Exercise frequency was 5 days/wk. in three trials [79,91,92], 3 days/wk. in one trial [80] and 3–5 days/wk. in one trial [77] that included follow-up assessments.

Aerobic exercise intensity. Anderssen et al [75] prescribed exercise intensity at 60–80% of peak heart rate while Foster-Schubert et al [76] prescribed 75%–85% of maximal VO_2. Both trials by Melanson et al [91,92] prescribed walking at a "moderate" pace while Skender et al [77] prescribed walking that was "vigorous but never strenuous". Exercise intensity was not specified in two trials [79,80].

Aerobic exercise duration. Anderssen et al [75] prescribed 60 minutes/day while Foster-Schubert et al [76] prescribed 45 min/day. Two trials with follow-up assessments prescribed individualized exercise duration designed to expend ~500 kcal/ session by completion of the intervention [91,92]. Volpe et al [79] prescribed 30 minutes/day, Skender et al [77] prescribed 45 min/ day, and Wing et al [80] prescribed walking at 3 miles/day.

Compliance with exercise protocol. Anderssen et al [75] reported that participants in the aerobic exercise group and diet+ aerobic exercise groups attended 57% and 63% of scheduled exercise sessions, respectively. Foster-Schubert et al [76] found that participants in the aerobic exercise and diet+aerobic exercise groups achieved 80% and 85% of the weekly exercise goal (225 min/wk), respectively. Only one trial with follow-up assessments included information on exercise compliance [80]. Wing et al [80] reported that 75% of participants met the exercise goal by the end of the active intervention.

Intervention during follow-up. Both trials by Melanson et al [91,92] asked participants to continue with the intervention assigned at baseline. Volpe et al [79] provided a Nordic Track exercise machine for home use but provided minimal investigator contact. Wing et al [80] provided continued behavioral sessions at a reduced frequency as compared with the active weight loss intervention

Outcomes assessed. In addition to body weight, four trials with comparisons of aerobic exercise and diet+aerobic exercise assessed waist circumference [75,76,79,91],and three trials assessed body composition, one by underwater weight [79], one by DXA [76] and one by air displacement [91]. Four trials assessed blood lipids (total, HDL, LDL cholesterol and triglycerides [75,79,80,91], 3 of which also assessed blood pressure [75,79,80] and one trial also assessed glucose, insulin and HbA_{1c} [80].

Participant characteristics – Aerobic Exercise vs. Diet+ Aerobic Exercise

Age. In the long-term trial by Anderssen et al [75] the mean age of the total sample was 40 yrs., while the age range in the trial by Skender et al [77], which provided both long-term and follow-up data was 25–45 yrs. Foster-Schubert et al [76] reported a mean age of 58.1 yrs. and 58.0 yrs., in the aerobic exercise and diet+ aerobic exercise groups, respectively. Three of the five trials with follow up assessments reported mean age by intervention group [79,80,92]. The median (range) age was 43.5 yrs. (42.6–46.4 yrs.) in the aerobic exercise groups and 45.0 yrs. (42.1–46.3 yrs.) in the diet+aerobic exercise groups. Melanson et al 2004 [91] reported a mean age of the complete sample of 42.6 years.

Sex. The long-term trials by Foster-Schubert et al [76] and Anderssen et al [75] included 100% and 9.6% women, respectively. The median (range) percent women was 79% (47–88%) in the five trials that included follow-up assessments [77,79,80,91,92]. Only Volpe et al [79] reported separate results for men and women.

BMI. The mean BMI in the long-term trial by Anderssen et al [75] was 28.6 kg/m^2 in both the aerobic exercise and diet+aerobic exercise groups. Foster-Schubert et al [76] reported a mean BMI of 30.7 kg/m^2 in the aerobic exercise group and 31.0 kg/m^2 in the diet+aerobic exercise group. Four of the 5 trials with follow-up assessments provided BMI by intervention group [79,80,91,92]. The median (range) BMI was 30.8 kg/m^2 (30.5–36.0 kg/m^2) in aerobic exercise groups and 31.3 kg/m^2 (30.5–35.7 kg/m^2) in diet+aerobic exercise groups.

Minority representation. The minority representation in the one long-term trial reporting this information was 15% [76]. The minority representation in the one trial with follow-up assessments that presented this information was 24.9% [92].

Physical activity level. Both long-term trials [75,76] and the 4 of 5 trials with follow-up assessments recruited sedentary participants [77,79,91,92].

Health status. One long-term trial recruited healthy participants [76] while the other recruited participants with high BMI, and elevated diastolic blood pressure, total cholesterol and triglycerides [75]. All trials with follow-up assessments recruited healthy participants [77,79,80,91,92]; however, Wing et al [80] recruited participants with 1 or 2 biological parents with DM2.

Results – Aerobic Exercise vs. Diet+Aerobic Exercise

Results for all trials with an aerobic exercise vs. diet+aerobic exercise comparison are presented in Table 5.

Long-term trials

Body weight. Anderssen et al [75] reported decreased body weight in both the aerobic exercise (−1.0%) and diet+aerobic exercise groups (−6.2%); however the statistical significance of the between group difference was not reported. Foster-Schubert et al [76] reported significantly greater weight loss in the diet+aerobic exercise (−10.8%) compared with the aerobic exercise group (−2.4%).

Waist circumference. Anderssen et al [75] reported decreased waist circumference in both the aerobic exercise (−1.9 cm) and diet+aerobic exercise groups (−5.7 cm); however statistical significance of the between group difference was not reported. Foster-Schubert et al [76] reported significantly greater reductions in waist circumference in the diet+aerobic exercise (−7.0 cm) compared with the aerobic exercise group (−2.1 cm).

Fat/fat-free mass. Foster-Schubert et al [76] reported significant between group differences for both change in fat mass (aerobic exercise = −2.1 kg, diet+aerobic exercise = −8.2 kg) and fat-free mass (aerobic exercise = +0.3 kg, diet+aerobic exercise = −0.4 kg).

Chronic disease risk factors. Anderssen et al [75] reported decreases in both systolic (aerobic exercise = −2.2 mmHg; diet+ aerobic exercise = −5.9 mmHg) and diastolic blood pressure (aerobic exercise = −2.7 mmHg; diet+aerobic exercise = −5.2 mmHg) in diet and diet+aerobic exercise groups. Larger decreases in total cholesterol (aerobic exercise = −0.20 mmol/l, diet+aerobic exercise = −0.48 mmol), LDL cholesterol (aerobic exercise = −0.13 mmol/l; diet+aerobic exercise = −0.39 mmol/l) and trigylcerides (aerobic exercise = −0.24 mmol/l; diet+ aerobic exercise = −0.58 mmol/l) were observed in diet+aerobic exercise groups compared to aerobic exercise alone. The increase in HDL cholesterol was greater in the diet+aerobic exercise (+0.13 mmol/l) compared with aerobic exercise only (+0.04 mmol/l). Anderssen et al [75] did not report the statistical significance of the between group differences.

Trials with follow-up assessments

Body weight. Four of the 5 trials that assessed weight change, both after an active intervention and a follow-up period, reported or provided numerical data with which percent weight change could be calculated [77,80,91,92]. The median (range) for weight loss from baseline to the completion of the weight loss intervention was 2% (0.1–3%) in aerobic exercise groups and 7.8% (3.2–24.6%) in diet+aerobic exercise groups. Weight loss in the diet+ aerobic exercise groups was significantly greater than aerobic exercise groups in the 3 trials providing this information [77,91,92]. No trials reported weight loss ≥5% in the aerobic exercise group while weight loss ≥5% was observed in all diet+ aerobic exercise groups. Volpe et al [79] presented weight loss data only in figures. In women, weight loss was significantly greater in the diet+aerobic exercise compared with the aerobic exercise group; however, no significant between group differences in weight loss were observed for men.

The median (range) percent weight loss from baseline to the completion of follow-up was 1.5% (0.5–2.9%) in aerobic exercise groups and 5.7% (2.2–7.1%) in diet+aerobic exercise groups in the 4 trials reporting this information [77,80,91,92]. Weight loss was significantly greater in the diet+aerobic exercise compared with aerobic exercise only groups in 2 [91,92] of 4 trials providing this data [77,79,91,92]. Volpe et al [79] found no significant between group differences for weight loss from baseline to the completion of follow-up in men or women. It is interesting to note that the 2 trials reporting significantly greater weight loss from baseline to the end of follow-up in the diet+aerobic exercise compared with aerobic exercise group included only a 12 week follow-up after 12 weeks of weight loss [91,92].

Four trials provided numerical data on weight change during follow-up [77,80,91,92]. Two trials reported by Melanson et al [91,92] with relatively short duration of follow-up (12 wks.)

Table 5. Comparison of change in weight, body composition, and chronic disease risk factors in response to aerobic exercise compared with diet plus aerobic exercise.

Study	Variable	Baseline -end of active intervention		Baseline-end follow-up		During follow-up	
		AE	D+AE	AE	D+AE	AE	D+AE
Long-term trials							
Anderssen et al. (75)	WT (kg/%)	−0.9/−1.0	−5.6/−6.2^{nr}	na	na	na	na
	WC (cm)	−1.9	−5.7 ^{nr}	na	na	na	na
	TC (mmol/l)	−0.2	−0.48 ^{nr}	na	na	na	na
	LDL-C (mmol/l)	−0.13	−0.39 ^{nr}	na	na	na	na
	HDL-C (mmol/l)	0.04	+0.13 ^{nr}	na	na	na	na
	TG (mmol/l)	−0.24	−0.58 ^{nr}	na	na	na	na
	SBP (mmHg)	−2.2	−5.9 ^{nr}	na	na	na	na
	DBP (mmHg)	−2.7	−5.2 ^{nr}	na	na	na	na
Foster-Schubert et al. (76)	WT (kg/%)	−2/−2.4	−8.9/−10.8 *	na	na	na	na
	WC (cm)	−2	−7.5 *	na	na	na	na
	Fat mass (kg)	−2.1	−8.2 *	na	na	na	na
	Fat-free mass (kg)	+0.3	−0.4 *	na	na	na	na
Follow-up trials							
Melanson et al. 2004 (91)	WT (kg/%)	−0.1/−0.1	−6.9/−7.8 *	−0.4/−0.5	−7.1/−7.9 *	−0.3/−0.4	−0.20/−0.01 ^{nr}
	WC (cm)	−1	−5.3 *	−1.8	−5.1 *	−0.8	+0.20 ^{nr}
	Fat mass (kg)	−0.6	−6.3 *	−1.7	−7.6 *	−1.1	−1.3 ^{nr}
	Fat-free mass (kg)	+0.7	−0.5 ^{ns}	+1.5	+0.50 ^{ns}	+0.8	+1.0 ^{nr}
	TC (mmol/l)	−0.04	−0.96 ^{nr}	−0.13	−0.34 ^{nr}	−0.09	+0.62 ^{nr}
	LDL-C (mmol/l)	−0.02	−0.22 ^{nr}	−0.07	−0.17 ^{nr}	−0.05	+0.05 ^{nr}
	HDL-C (mmol/l)	−0.07	−0.05 ^{nr}	−0.14	+0.008 ^{nr}	−0.07	+0.058 ^{nr}
	TG (mmol/l)	0.38	−0.34 ^{nr}	−0.22	−0.43 ^{nr}	−0.60	−0.90 ^{nr}
Melanson et al. 2006 (92)	WT (kg/%)	−1.6/1.9%	−4.7/−5.4 (no cereal) *	−1.75/2	−5.7/−6.6 (no cereal) *	−0.15/−0.1	−1.0/−1.2 ^{nr}
			−5.0/−6.0 (cereal) *		−6.2/−6.2% (cereal) *		−1.2/0.2 ^{nr}
Skender et al. (77)	WT (kg/%)	−2.9/−3.1	−8.9/−8.9 ^{ns}	−2.7/−2.9	−2.2/−2.2 ^{ns}	0.2/0.2	6.7/6.7
Volpe et al. (79)	WT (kg)	Figures only					
Men	WC (cm)	−1.2	−4.7 ^{ns}	−1.2	−1.9 ^{ns}	−0.1	+2.8 ^{nr}
	Fat mass (kg)	−1.6	−5.8 *	0.4	+2.0 ^{ns}	−2.8	+3.0 ^{nr}
	Fat-free mass (kg)	+0.3	−0.3 ^{ns}	+0.20	+0.1 ^{ns}	−0.1	+0.4 ^{nr}
	TC (mmol/l)	−0.16	−0.27 ^{ns}	−0.18	−0.04 ^{ns}	−0.02	+0.23 ^{nr}
	LDL-C (mmol/l)	+0.08	+0.02 ^{ns}	+0.37	+0.15 ^{ns}	+0.29	+0.13 ^{nr}
	HDL-C (mmol/l)	−0.24	−0.22 ^{ns}	−0.18	−0.13 ^{ns}	+0.06	+0.90 ^{nr}
	TG (mmol/l)	−0.32	−0.24 ^{ns}	+0.07	−0.20 ^{ns}	+0.39	−0.04 ^{nr}

Table 5. Cont.

Study	Variable	Baseline -end of active intervention		Baseline-end follow-up		During follow-up	
		AE	D+AE	AE	D+AE	AE	D+AE
	SBP (mmHg)	−15.3	−11.8 ^{ns}	−14.4	−15.6 ^{ns}	+0.90	−4.8 ^{nr}
	DBP (mmHg)	−7.7	−9.7 ^{ns}	−7.9	−12.3^{ns}	−0.20	−2.6 ^{nr}
Women	WT (kg)	Figures only					
	WC (cm)	−3.6	+0.10 ^{ns}	−3.9	−2.1 ^{ns}	−0.30	−2.2 ^{nr}
	Fat mass (kg)	−0.5	−4.2 *	−1	−1.9 *	−0.5	+2.3 ^{nr}
	Fat-free mass (kg)	+0.1	+1.5 ^{ns}	+0.9	+1.1 ^{ns}	+0.80	−0.40 ^{nr}
	TC (mmol/l)	+0.06	−0.07 ^{ns}	+0.03	−0.18 ^{ns}	−0.03	−0.11 ^{nr}
	LDL-C (mmol/l)	+0.22	+0.38 ^{ns}	+0.15	+0.10 ^{ns}	−0.07	−0.28 ^{nr}
	HDL-C (mmol/l)	−0.21	−0.26 ^{ns}	−0.13	−0.23 ^{ns}	+0.80	+0.03 ^{nr}
	TG (mmol/l)	−0.06	−0.34 ^{ns}	+0.03	−0.16 ^{ns}	+0.09	+0.18 ^{nr}
	SBP (mmHg)	−0.9	−3.1 ^{ns}	+3.0	+2.1 ^{ns}	+3.90	+5.20 ^{nr}
	DBP (mmHg)	0.6	−4.30^{ns}	+6.3	+1.2 ^{ns}	+5.7	+5.5 ^{nr}
Wing et al. (80)	WT (kg/%)	−2.1/−2.1	−10.3/−10.4 ^{nr}	1/1	−2.5/−2.5 ^{nr}	3.1/3.1	+7.8/+7.9 ^{nr}
	TC (mmol/l)	+0.12	−0.33 ^{nr}	+0.33	+0.09 ^{nr}	+0.21	+0.42 ^{nr}
	LDL-C (mmol/l)	+0.03	−0.13 ^{nr}	+0.22	+0.12 ^{nr}	+0.19	+0.25 ^{nr}
	HDL−C (mmol/l)	+0.02	+0.02 ^{nr}	+0.05	+0.02 ^{nr}	+0.03	0.00 ^{nr}
	TG (mmol/l)	+0.12	−0.69 ^{nr}	+0.33	−0.28 ^{nr}	+0.21	+0.41 ^{nr}
	Glucose (mmol/l)	0	−0.20 ^{nr}	+0.40	+0.50 ^{nr}	+0.40	+0.70 ^{nr}
	Insulin (pmol/l)	−4	−37.0 ^{nr}	+43.0	−12.0 ^{nr}	+47.0	+0.25 ^{nr}
	HbA_{1c} (%)	+0.1	+0.03 ^{nr}	−0.10	+0.04 ^{nr}	−0.20	+0.01 ^{nr}
	SBP (mmHg)	−2.4	−12.3 ^{nr}	+0.9	−4.8 ^{nr}	+3.30	+7.5 ^{nr}
	DBP (mmHg)	−1.7	−6.9 ^{nr}	+2.0	−0.2 ^{nr}	+3.7	+6.7 ^{nr}

AE = aerobic exercise, D+AE = diet plus aerobic exercise, WT = body weight, WC = waist circumference, TC = total cholesterol, LDL = low density lipoprotein cholesterol, HDL = high density lipoprotein cholesterol, TG = triglycerides, na = not assessed, ns = between group difference for change non- significant, nr = between group difference for change not reported.
*between group difference for change significant at $p < 0.05$ or greater.

Table 6. Comparison of change in weight, body composition, and chronic disease risk factors in response to combinations of diet, aerobic and resistance exercise.

Study	Variable	Baseline - end of active intervention		Baseline - end Follow-up		During follow-up	
		D	**D+RE**	**D**	**D+RE**	**D**	**D+RE**
Hunter et al. (84)	WT (kg/%)	na	na	na	na	+6.4/9.8	Adhere = +3.9/5.9 *
	WT(kg/%)	na	na	na	na	+6.4/9.8	Non-Adhere = +6.2/9.5 ^{ns}
	WC (cm)	na	na	na	na	+5.5	Adhere = +2.9 ^{ns}
	WC (cm)	na	na	na	na	+5.5	Non-Adhere = +5.3 ^{ns}
	% Fat	na	na	na	na	+5.3	Adhere = +4.4 *
	% Fat	na	na	na	na	+5.3	Non-Adhere = +5.8 ^{ns}
	Visceral fat (cm^2)	na	na	na	na	+12.4 **	Adhere = −0.4 ^{ns} within
	Visceral fat (cm^2)	na	na	na	na	+12.4 **	Non-Adhere = +10.4 ^{ns} within
Wadden et al. (89)	WT (kg/%)	−15.3/−16.3	−17.3/−17.3 ^{ns}	−6.9/−7.7	−10.1/−10.0 ^{ns}	+8.4/8.6	+7.2/7.3 ^{nr}
		D+AE	**D+RE**	**D+AE**	**D+RE**	**D+AE**	**D+RE**
Hunter et al. (84)	WT (kg/%)	na	na	na	na	Adhere = +3.1/4.9%	Adhere = +3.9/5.9 ^{ns}
	WT(kg/%)	na	na	na	na	Non-Adhere = +7.1/10.9	Non-Adhere = +6.2/9.5 ^{ns}
	WC (cm)	na	na	na	na	Adhere = +1.9	Adhere = +2.9 ^{ns}
	WC (cm)	na	na	na	na	Non-Adhere = +7.9	Non-Adhere = +5.3 ^{ns}
	% Fat	na	na	na	na	Adhere = +3.4	Adhere = +4.4 *
	% Fat	na	na	na	na	Non-Adhere = +6.4	Non-Adhere = +5.8 ^{ns}
	Visceral fat (cm^2)	na	na	na	na	Adhere = +0.8 ^{ns} within	Adhere = −0.4 ^{ns} within
	Visceral fat (cm^2)	na	na	na	na	Non-Adhere = +25.5 **	Non-Adhere = +10.4 ^{ns} within
Wadden et al. (89)	WT (kg/%)	−13.5/−13.9	−17.3/−17.3 ^{ns}	−8.5/−8.6	−10.1/−10.0 ^{ns}	+5/5.3	+7.2/7.3 ^{nr}
		D	**D+AE+RE**	**D**	**D+AE+RE**	**D**	**D+AE+RE**
Wadden et al. (89)	WT (kg/%)	−15.3/−16.3	−16.6/−17.6 ^{ns}	−6.9/−7.7	+8.6/8.6 ^{ns}	+8.4/8.6	+8.0/9.0 ^{nr}
		D+AE	**D+AE+RE**	**D+AE**	**D+AE+RE**	**D+AE**	**D+AE+RE**
Wadden et al. (89)	WT (kg/%)	−13.5/13.9	−16.6/−17.6 ^{ns}	−8.5/8.6	+8.6/8.6 ^{ns}	+5/5.3	+8.0/9.0 ^{nr}
		D+RE	**D+AE+RE**	**D+RE**	**D+AE+RE**	**D+RE**	**D+AE+RE**
Wadden et al. (89)	WT (kg/%)	−17.3/−17.3	−16.6/−17.6 ^{ns}	−10.1/−10.0	+8.6/8.6 ^{ns}	+7.2/7.3	+8.0/9.0 ^{nr}

D = diet, D+AE = diet plus aerobic exercise, D+RE = diet plus resistance exercise, D+AE+RE = diet plus aerobic plus resistance exercise, WT = body weight, WC = waist circumference, na = not assessed, ns = between group difference for change non- significant, nr = between group difference for change not reported.

*between group difference for change significant at $p<0.05$ or greater.

**within group change significant at $p<0.05$ or greater.

reported small continued weight loss (~1 kg) during the follow-up period in both aerobic exercise and diet+aerobic exercise groups. Skender et al [77] reported the percent of lost weight regained at follow-up was 7% in the aerobic exercise group and 75% in the diet+aerobic exercise group. In the trial by Wing et al [80] the percentage of lost weight regained at follow-up was 55% and 76% for the aerobic exercise and diet+aerobic exercise groups, respectively.

Waist circumference. Two trials reported change in waist circumference [79,91]. Melanson et al [91] reported significantly greater reductions in waist circumference from baseline to the completion of weight loss intervention (12 wks.) in the diet+aerobic exercise (−5.3 cm) compared with the aerobic exercise group (−1.0 cm) which were maintained or slightly enhanced at a 24 wk. follow-up (diet+aerobic exercise = −5.1 cm; aerobic exercise = −1.8 cm). Volpe et al [79] found no significant between group difference for change in waist circumference in either men (aerobic exercise = −1.2 cm, diet+aerobic exercise = −4.7 cm) or women (aerobic exercise = −3.6 cm, diet+aerobic exercise = +0.1 cm) at the end of the active intervention (6 mos.) or follow-up at 12 mos. (men: aerobic exercise = −1.2 cm, diet+aerobic exercise = −1.9 cm, (women: aerobic exercise = −3.9 cm, diet+aerobic exercise = −2.1 cm).

Fat mass/fat-free mass. Two trials reported change in fat and fat-free mass [79,91]. Melanson et al [91] reported significantly greater reductions in fat mass in the diet+aerobic exercise (−6.3 kg) compared with the aerobic exercise group (−0.6 kg) from baseline to the end of a 12 wk. weight loss intervention which were maintained or slightly enhanced at a 24 wk. follow-up (diet+aerobic exercise = −7.6 kg; aerobic exercise = −1.7 kg). Volpe et al [79] reported significantly greater decreases in fat mass in the diet+aerobic exercise compared with the aerobic exercise group for both men (aerobic exercise = −1.6 kg, diet+aerobic exercise = −5.8 kg) and women (aerobic exercise = −0.5 kg, diet+aerobic exercise = −4.2 kg) at the completion of the 6 month intervention. However, these differences were not shown at the 12 mo. follow-up in either men (aerobic exercise = +0.4 kg, diet+aerobic exercise = −2.8 kg) or women (aerobic exercise = −1.0 kg, diet+aerobic exercise = −1.9 kg).

Melanson et al [91] observed no significant changes in fat-free mass over the 12 week active intervention in either the aerobic exercise or diet+aerobic exercise groups. However, at follow-up, fat-free mass was significantly increased in the aerobic exercise group (+1.5 kg) but not in the diet+aerobic exercise group (+0.5 kg), with no significant between group differences. Volpe et al [79] observed small non-significant increases in fat-free on completion of the active intervention and at follow up in both men and women, with no significant between group differences.

Chronic Disease Risk Factors. Three trials reported chronic disease risk factors [79,80,91]. At completion of the active intervention (6 months), Wing et al [80] reported no significant within group changes in the aerobic exercise group in total, HDL and LDL cholesterol, triglycerides, systolic and diastolic blood pressure, fasting insulin, fasting glucose or HbA_{1C}. At the 24 month follow-up significant increases in total cholesterol, glucose and insulin were observed, with no significant changes in any of the other risk factors. In the diet+aerobic exercise group there were significant reductions in total cholesterol, triglycerides, systolic blood and diastolic blood pressure, glucose, and insulin at 6 months. However, at follow-up (24 months) no significant changes were observed in any of these parameters and HbA_{1C}, and fasting glucose were both significantly increased over baseline. Thus, risk factor changes associated with the active intervention were not maintained at follow-up. The statistical significance of between group for change at the end of the active intervention or follow-up were not reported [80]. Volpe et al [79] reported no significant changes in systolic blood or diastolic blood pressure, total, HDL or LDL cholesterol, or triglycerides in either the aerobic exercise or diet+aerobic exercise groups after completion of the active intervention (6 months) or at follow-up (12 months) in either men or women. Melanson et al [91] did not report the statistical significance for between group changes; however, reductions in total and LDL cholesterol observed during the active intervention were maintained or enhanced in the aerobic exercise but not in the diet+aerobic exercise group.

Additional diet/diet+exercise comparisons

Trials by Hunter et al [84], Wadden et al [89] and Svendsen et al [93] provided comparisons of various combinations of diet, aerobic and resistance exercise (Table 6).

Hunter et al [84] reassessed weight, waist circumference, and body composition (DXA, computed tomography) in a sample of initially overweight and obese women one-year following completion of a weight loss intervention by diet, diet+resistance exercise or diet+aerobic exercise. The basic study design and descriptions and results of the diet and aerobic training components of this trial were presented previously. Here we present results for diet vs. diet+resistance training and diet+aerobic vs. diet+resistance training. Supervised resistance exercise was ramped to 2 sets of 10 exercises at 80% of one repetition maximum, 3 days/week by week four. During the weight loss phase compliance with the exercise protocol was required to remain in the study. The weight loss intervention was continued until participants reached a BMI of 25 kg/m^2 (mean 154 days) at which time they were asked to continue with their original group assignment with supervised exercise frequency reduced to two days/week for exercise groups over the next 12 months. All groups were given instruction on following a balanced diet that focused on consumption of low-density foods. Exercise during the follow-up period was not required, thus two groups were formed; participants who adhered (≥60% of scheduled sessions) and those who did not adhere (<60% of scheduled sessions) to the exercise protocols. Results indicated that body weight increased significantly during the one-year follow-up, with a significant group by time interaction. No significant between group differences for change in any outcomes were observed in participants who adhered to either the aerobic or resistance exercise protocols. However, participants who adhered to the aerobic (+4.9%) or resistance exercise (+5.9%) gained significantly less weight than any of the other 3 groups (aerobic non-adhere = +10.9%; resistance non-adhere = +9.5%; no exericise = 9.8%). Similar results were observed for change in % fat in that participants who adhered to either aerobic or resistance exercise showed smaller increases in % fat than the other 3 groups. Waist circumference increased in all groups with no significant between group differences. In addition, the change in visceral fat in groups who were adherent to exercise was non-significant (aerobic = +1.6%; resistance = −0.9%) while significant increases in visceral fat were observed in the two non-adherence groups (aerobic = +54.4%; resistance = +29.4%) and the no exercise group (+24.8%). Thus, irrespective of the mode of weight loss, increases in weight, % fat and visceral fat were minimized only in those who continued with either aerobic or resistance exercise.

Wadden et al [89] reported results for weight change from a 1-year follow-up in a sample of overweight/obese women (age ~41 yrs; BMI ~36 kg/m^2) who completed a weight loss intervention [89] employing combinations of diet, aerobic and resistance exercise. Participants were randomized to 4 conditions (diet: n = 29, diet+aerobic exercise: n = 31, diet+resistance exercise: n = 31 and diet + aerobic+resistance exercise: n = 29) for a 48 week weight loss phase and followed-up at 1-year during which time there was no intervention. Diet was a 16 week VLCD (~925 kcal/day) followed by a conventional energy restricted diet (1,200 to 1,500 kcal/day) for 31 weeks with behavioral counseling; weekly for 28 weeks, bi-weekly for 20 weeks. Participants in aerobic exercise groups were prescribed 3 supervised sessions of step aerobics/wk. over the first 28 weeks and 2 supervised sessions/wk. over weeks 29–48. Participants in resistance exercise groups were prescribed 3 supervised sessions of 10 exercises that progressed in resistance when more than 14 repetitions could be performed on two consecutive sets. Weight loss over the first 48 weeks was significant in all intervention groups (diet = −16.3%, diet + aerobic exercise = −13.9%, diet+resistance exercise = −17.3%, diet+aerobic+resistance exercise = −17.6%) with no significant between group differences. Weight loss at 1-year follow-up was also significant in all intervention groups (diet = −7.7%, diet + aerobic exercise = −8.6%, diet+resistance exercise = −10.0%, diet+aerobic+resistance exercise = −8.6%) with no significant between group differences. All intervention groups regained similar amounts of weight following weight loss (diet = +8.4 kg, 54.9% of lost weight, diet + aerobic exercise = +5.0 kg, 37% of lost weight, diet+resistance exercise = +7.2 kg, 41.6% of lost weight, diet+aerobic+resistance exercise = +8 kg, 48.2% of lost weight). Weight loss in 27 participants who reported exercising regularly in the 4 months preceding the one year follow-up (12.1 kg) was significantly greater than 22 participants who reported no regular exercise (6.1 kg). Weight regain over the follow-up period was also significantly less in exercisers (5.5 kg) compared with non-exercisers (8.4 kg).

Svendsen et al. [93] randomly assigned overweight and obese post-menopausal women (mean age = ~54 yrs.) to one of three groups: diet, diet+aerobic+resistance exercise, or a no intervention control: n = 21). Participants were assessed 24 weeks following completion of a 12 week weight loss intervention. During the weight loss phase energy intake was restricted to 4.2 MJ/d (1.6 MJ/d formula diet +2.6 MJ/d freely chosen food). Exercise was supervised and included 3–60 to 90 minute session per week of combined aerobic (cycle ergometer at ≥70% VO_2 max) and resistance exercise at ≥65% maximal lifting capacity). During the 24-week follow-up, participants did not participate in any intervention but were encouraged to continue exercise and monitor energy intake to maintain weight loss. Main outcome data were presented in figures only. Both the diet and diet+aerobic+resistance exercise groups showed significant reductions in weight and fat mass at both 12 and 24 weeks (~8 kg) compared with control with little or no regain in weight or fat mass in either group over the follow-up period. However, fat-free mass was significantly reduced in the diet only group compared with diet+aerobic+resistance exercise and control groups at both 12 and 24 weeks. Participant in the diet+aerobic+resistance exercise group that were self-reported participating in exercise during the follow-up period based on self-report showed significantly greater reductions in weight (exerciser = 10.9 kg; non-exerciser = 6.6 kg) and fat mass (exerciser = 10.0 kg, non-exerciser = 5.4 kg) compared with non-exercisers in this group. Total and LDL cholesterol decreased significantly during weight loss in both the diet and diet+aerobic+resistance exercise groups compared with controls; however, these changes were not maintained at the 24 week follow-up. Triglycerides decreased significantly during weight loss in both active intervention groups compared with control. Unlike total and LDL cholesterol, the change in triglycerides was maintained at 24 weeks. HDL cholesterol was unchanged in any intervention group at 12 weeks. At 24 weeks HDL cholesterol was significantly higher in both active intervention groups compared with control.

Risk of bias. The risk of bias is presented in Table 7. The description of the procedures for random sequence generation were unclear in 15 of 20 (75%) of trials included in this review [5,75,77–80,82–86,88–90,93]. Three trials adequately described randomization procedures and were considered low risk of bias [76,91,92]. Randomization bias was high in two trials; one trail allowed participants who refused their random assignment to select their intervention group [81], and one trial employed a "pseudo randomized" process [87]. No trials described procedures for allocation concealment. The blinding of participants and personnel is not feasible in a diet/diet+ exercise trial. While blinding of personnel performing outcome assessments is feasible, these procedures were employed in only one trial [76]. The risk of attrition bias was high in five trials where the study sample represented approximately 60% or less (range 48–61%) of those randomized at baseline [77,81,86,89,91]. The most important other source of potential bias was inadequate statistical power. Only 3 of 20 trials (15%) reported adequate statistical power to detect between group differences for change in body weight [76,79,83]; however, one trial did not specifically indicate that the reported power was based on the body weight outcome [79]. Nine of the 17 trials (~53%) that did not report statistical power were conducted in small samples (~20 participants/group or less) and thus likely to be inadequately powered to detect between group differences [5,77,78,84,86–88,90,91].

Discussion

Summary of evidence

In this paper we systematically reviewed 20 randomized trials to address the question: Does the method of weight loss, i.e., energy restriction, exercise (aerobic or resistance), and the various combinations effect long-term changes in weight, body composition or chronic disease risk factors in overweight or obese adults?

Diet vs. Aerobic Exercise. Long-term weight loss tended to be greater with diet compared with aerobic exercise with ad libitum eating. This observation is in agreement with results from other reviews which have shown only modest weight loss with aerobic exercise [69,70,94–96]. However, most trials of aerobic exercise for weight loss are limited in that the energy expenditure of exercise is neither rigorously controlled or accurately measured, and the level of prescribed exercise is insufficient to produce significant weight loss [97]. With the exception of the trial by Racette et al. [5], long-term trials included in this review prescribed insufficient levels of exercise and observed weight loss of ~3% or less in exercise only groups. In contrast, Racette et al. [5] prescribed exercise energy expenditure (~1,900 kcal/wk) to match the energy deficit induced by diet and observed clinically significant weight loss in the aerobic exercise group (−8.4%) that was not significantly different from weight loss in the diet only group (−10.4%). The results of Racette et al [5] are in agreement with those from short-term trials (12-14 wks) which have shown clinically significant weight loss (6.0–7.7%) with equivalent energy deficits induced by either diet or aerobic exercise of 500–700 kcal/day [4,98] and longer term trials (10–16 months) which have shown weight loss induced by exercise alone (≥2000 kcal/wk) ranging from 4.3–5.7% [6,7]. The results of the long-term trial of Racette et al [5], and from other short and long-term trials in the literature [4,6,7,98], suggest that clinically significant weight loss can be achieved with aerobic exercise alone when exercise energy

Table 7. Study Risk of bias.

Study	Random Sequence Generation (selection bias)	Allocation concealment (selection bias)	Blinding participants and personnel (performance bias)	Blinding of outcome assessment (detection bias)	Incomplete outcome data (attrition bias)	Selective reporting (reporting bias)	Other bias
Anderssen et al. (75)	Unclear	NR	NA	NR	Low risk	Low risk	Unclear
Andreou et al. (83)	Unclear	NR	NA	NR	Low risk	Low risk	Low risk
Dengel et al. (81)	High risk	NR	NA	NR	High risk	Low risk	Unclear
Foster-Schubert et al. (76)	Low risk	NR	NA	Low risk	Low risk	Low risk	Low risk
Hunter et al. (84)	Unclear	NR	NA	NR	Low risk	Low risk	High risk
Melanson et al. 2004 (91)	Low risk	NR	NA	NR	High risk	Low risk	High risk
Melanson et al. 2006 (92)	Low risk	NR	NA	NR	Low risk	Low risk	Unclear
Molenar et al. (85)	Unclear	NR	NA	NR	Low risk	Low risk	Low risk
Neumark-Sztainer et al. (86)	Unclear	NR	NA	NR	High risk	Low risk	High risk
Pritchard et al. (78)	Unclear	NR	NA	NR	Low risk	Low risk	High risk
Racette et al. (5)	Unclear	NR	NA	NR	Low risk	Low risk	High risk
Snel et al. (87)	High risk	NR	NA	NR	Low risk	Low risk	High risk
Skender et al. (77)	Unclear	NR	NA	NR	High risk	Low risk	High risk
Svendsen et al. (93)	Unclear	NR	NA	NR	Low risk	Low risk	Unclear
Van Aggel-Leijssen et al. (88)	Unclear	NR	NA	NR	Low risk	Low risk	High risk
Vople et al. (79)	Unclear	NR	NA	NR	Unclear	Low risk	Low risk
Wadden et al. (89)	Unclear	NR	NA	NR	High risk	Low risk	Unclear
Wang et al. (90)	Unclear	NR	NA	NR	Low risk	Low risk	High risk
Wing et al. (80)	Unclear	NR	NA	NR	Low risk	Low risk	Unclear
Wood et al. (82)	Unclear	NR	NA	NR	Low risk	Low risk	Unclear

NR = not reported, NA = not applicable.

deficits are similar in magnitude to those induced by energy restriction.

Similar to changes in body weight, reductions in both fat mass and waist circumference in long-term trials tended to be greater in the diet only compared with the exercise only groups. Fat-free mass in long-term trials tended to be preserved in exercise groups, which may be a function of the minimal levels of weight loss observed in the aerobic exercise groups [5,76]. However, in our recently completed 10 month aerobic exercise trial (5 days/wk., 400 or 600 kcal/day) we showed fat-free mass was unchanged in the 400 kcal/day group and increased slightly (1.1%) in the 600 kcal/day group despite weight loss of 4.3% and 5.7% in the 400 and 600 kcal/day groups, respectively [6]. In this review, we identified only 1 long-term trial that compared changes in chronic disease risk factors between diet and aerobic exercise. Although statistical significance of between group changes was not reported, there were no obvious between group differences for changes in risk factors including total, LDL and HDL cholesterol, triglycerides and blood pressure [75].

Results from trials investigating differences in weight regain following weight loss by diet or aerobic exercise were mixed [77,79,80]. Trials, with follow-up periods ranging from 6 to 18 months, reported less weight regain in the aerobic exercise compared with the diet group [77], less weight regain in the diet compared with the aerobic exercise group [80], and no between group differences in weight regain between diet and aerobic exercise groups [79]. Only one of these trials included an intervention during the follow-up period consisting of behavioral group meetings at a reduced frequency from the active intervention [80]. Results from these trials are difficult to interpret in terms of assessing the impact of differences in weight loss method (diet or aerobic exercise) on weight change during follow-up, as weight loss at the end of the active intervention was minimal in the aerobic exercise groups (~2.6%) compared with weight loss in the diet only groups (~8%). Thus, without clinically significant weight loss in the aerobic exercise groups, the impact of weight loss by this mode on subsequent weight regain, and or subsequent changes in body composition cannot be evaluated. Results from the 2 trials that evaluated the effect of diet or aerobic exercise interventions on chronic disease risk factors at follow-up were also mixed [79,80]. One trial observed no significant changes in risk factors in either diet or aerobic exercise groups on completion of the active intervention or at follow-up [79], while one trial reported beneficial changes in risk factors on completion of the active intervention in the diet group which were not maintained at follow-up [80]. The limited available data suggest no sex differences in weight, body composition or chronic disease risk factors in response to diet or aerobic exercise interventions [79].

Diet vs. Diet+Aerobic exercise. Adding aerobic exercise to an energy restricted diet tended to result in slightly greater long-term weight loss than energy restricted diet alone. Although weight loss was significantly greater in the diet+aerobic exercise group in 2 of the 4 trials presenting this data, the additional weight loss achieved when adding aerobic exercise to an energy restricted diet was quite small, i.e., ~2.2% [76,82]. These findings are in general agreement with a previous meta-analysis by Wu et al [66] who reported greater long-term weight loss with interventions including diet+aerobic exercise compared with diet alone with small between group differences (pooled mean difference = 1.14 kg). As previously discussed, the exercise prescribed and/or actually completed in these trials (i.e. ~155 min/wk) was likely insufficient to elicit significant additional weight loss [75,76,81,82]. Significantly greater long-term weight loss with diet+aerobic exercise compared to diet alone has been shown in both men and women [82].

Reductions in both fat mass and waist circumference were greater in diet+aerobic exercise compared with diet only groups; however, as observed with body weight, the between group differences in both fat mass and waist circumference, even when statistically significant, were small (waist circumference = 2.0–3.0 cm, fat mass = 0.1–2.7 kg) [76,81,82]. Reductions in fat-free mass were smaller in diet+aerobic exercise compared with the diet only groups; however, no significant between group differences were noted. However, other reviews [95,96] and results from short-term [99–101] and longer duration trials [6] have suggested that aerobic exercise combined with an energy restricted diet preserves fat-free mass during weight loss. One trial reported greater reductions in fat mass with diet+aerobic exercise compared with in men, but not in women [82].

We identified only 2 long-term trials that compared changes in chronic disease risk factors between diet and diet+aerobic exercise [75,82]. Although statistical significance of between group changes was not reported, Anderssen et al [75] showed beneficial changes in total, LDL, and HDL cholesterol, triglycerides, and blood pressure that were of greater magnitude in the diet+aerobic exercise compared with the diet only group. Wood et al [82] observed significantly greater increases in HDL-cholesterol and reductions in triglycerides in men and greater increases in HDL-cholesterol in women in the diet+aerobic exercise compared with diet only groups. Thus, we found limited evidence to suggest a difference for change in chronic disease risk factors when weight loss is achieved with diet alone or a combination of diet+aerobic exercise.

Results from trials investigating differences in weight regain following weight loss by diet or diet+aerobic exercise do not suggest an obvious benefit for weight loss by either weight loss method [77,80,83,85,87–90]. In agreement with the long-term trials described previously, weight loss was generally greater following completion of the active intervention in the diet+aerobic exercise (~14%) compared with the diet only groups (~12%). However, during the follow-up period, which ranged from 18 weeks to 12 months, the percentage of lost weight that was regained was similar in both the diet (~58%) and diet+aerobic exercise groups (~53%). Weight regain was similar in the diet and diet+aerobic exercise groups in the 2 trials that included an intervention during follow-up. One trial by [80] included behavioral group meetings at a reduced frequency from the active intervention and one trial included low intensity exercise (40% VO_2 max); however compliance with exercise was low (57%) [88]. Wadden et al [89] did not prescribe exercise during follow-up; however, noted that weight regain was significantly reduced in participants who self-reported exercise during follow-up compared with those who did not, irrespective of group assignment (diet or diet+aerobic exercise). The finding of no difference in weight regain with weight loss by diet or diet+aerobic exercise is in agreement with those of several previous reviews [65–67,70].

Results for the change in waist circumference between diet and diet+aerobic exercise were mixed. Greater reductions in waist circumference were observed in diet+aerobic exercise groups on completion of the active intervention in some [83,87] but not all trials [79]. One trial with a short follow-up period (18 wks) showed continued decreases in waist circumference during follow-up in both diet and diet+aerobic exercise groups [83], while in 2 trials the reductions in waist circumference observed at the end of the active intervention were eliminated at the completion of the follow–up period [79,87]. One trial reported a significantly greater decrease in waist circumference in a diet+aerobic exercise group compared with diet at completion of the active intervention in men, but not in women; however, the sex differences was not observed at follow-up [79]. Results for changes in fat mass or percent body fat between diet and diet+aerobic exercise were also mixed with some [79,83,87], but not all trials [88] reporting greater decreases in fat mass/percent fat with diet+aerobic exercise compared with diet alone. The decrease in fat mass in the diet+aerobic exercise groups was significantly greater than diet alone in women but not men at the end of the acive intervention, but not at follow-up in the one trial reporting this data [79]. Fat mass/percent fat increased during the follow-up period in both diet and diet+aerobic exercise with no between group differences in these trials with the exception of the one trial with a short follow-up period (18 wks.) where fat mass decreased slightly in both intervention groups [83]. There were no between group differences for change in fat-free mass either at the end of the active intervention or at follow-up in the 2 trials reporting this variable [79,88]. We found no evidence for differences between diet and diet+aerobic exercise for changes in chronic disease risk factors or any sex differences at the end of an active intervention or at follow-up in the 3 trials presenting risk factor data [79,80,87]. One trial observed significant reductions in total cholesterol, triglycerides, blood pressure, glucose and insulin at the completion of the active intervention in the diet only group that were not maintained at follow-up [80].

Aerobic exercise vs. Diet+aerobic exercise. As discussed previously, trials which have included aerobic exercise groups have generally prescribed aerobic exercise that is insufficient to elicit significant weight loss. The 2 long-term trials comparing aerobic exercise with diet+aerobic exercise prescribed ~185 min/wk and observed weight loss in the aerobic exercise groups of ≤2.4% over 12 months, which was considerably less than the weight loss observed in the diet+aerobic exercise groups (~6% and ~11%) over the same time frame [75,76]. Likewise, reductions in waist circumference were also larger in diet+aerobic exercise compared aerobic exercise only groups [75,76]. In the one trial that assessed changes in body composition, reductions in fat mass were significantly greater in the diet+aerobic exercise compared with the aerobic exercise only group while fat-free mass maintained in the aerobic exercise group and decreased in the diet+aerobic exercise groups [76]. The results of the one long-term trial that assessed chronic disease risk factors suggested greater reductions in total and LDL cholesterol, triglycerides, and blood pressure and greater increases in HDL cholesterol in the diet+aerobic exercise compared with the aerobic exercise group [75].

Results for trials investigating weight regain following weight loss by aerobic exercise or diet+aerobic exercise were mixed [77,80,91,92]. Two trials with a relatively short active intervention (12 wks.) and follow-up period (12 wks.) both observed significantly greater weight loss in the diet+aerobic exercise compared with the aerobic exercise only group at the end of the active intervention and at follow-up [91,92]. The two trials with longer duration follow-up periods (12 &18 mos.) reported no differences between aerobic exercise and diet+aerobic exercise groups for weight change at the end of the active intervention or at follow-up with both groups regaining most of their lost weight during follow-up [77,80]. Only the trial by Wing et al [80] included an intervention during the follow-up period. Similar to changes in body weight, the reductions in waist circumference and fat mass were significantly greater in the diet+aerobic exercise compared with aerobic exercise at the end of the active intervention and at follow-up when the intervention (12 wks.) and follow-up periods (12 wks.) were relatively short [91]. However, the trials with longer duration interventions and follow-up found no between group difference for change in waist circumference at either time point [79]. Greater reductions in fat mass at the end of the active intervention were shown in both men and women in the diet+ aerobic compared with the aerobic exercise group, that were maintained at follow-up in men but not in women [79]. No trials showed any between group differences for change in fat-free mass at the end of the active intervention or at follow-up [79,91]. As previously discussed, weight loss (range 0.1% to 3.1%) as well as changes in body composition in the aerobic exercise groups in all these trials was minimal, making it impossible to evaluate the effect of weight loss by aerobic exercise on subsequent weight regain. Results from the 3 trials that compared change in risk factors between aerobic exercise and diet + aerobic exercise were mixed [79,80,91]. One trial with a relatively short active intervention (12 wks.) and follow-up period (12 wks.) observed significantly greater reductions in total and LDL-cholesterol and triglycerides but not in HDL-cholesterol in the diet+aerobic exercise compared with the aerobic exercise group both at the end of the active intervention and at follow-up[91]. However, trials with longer active intervention (6 mos.) and follow-up periods (6 or 18 mos.) observed both no change in lipid parameters or blood pressure at the end of the active intervention or at follow-up [79] or greater changes in these parameters at the end of the active intervention in the diet+aerobic exercise compared with aerobic exercise groups in both men and women, that were not maintained at follow-up.

Other comparisons. A limited number of trials have compared the effect of aerobic and resistance training, or combinations of diet with aerobic and resistance training on weight loss [84,89,93]. No advantage in weight loss either at the completion of the active intervention or at follow-up was shown for any of these intervention combinations.

Limitations in the available literature

We identified several important limitations in the literature relative to addressing our primary question regarding the effect of the method of weight loss, i.e., energy restriction, exercise (aerobic or resistance), and the various combinations on long-term changes in weight, body composition or chronic disease risk factors in overweight or obese adults. The literature is limited by a lack of randomized trials that have addressed this question. For this review, we intended to evaluate trials with at least a 6 month active weight loss intervention followed by at least 12 months of active or passive weight maintenance. However, we were able to identify only 3 randomized trials that satisfied these criteria [77,80,89]. These trials were not statistically powered to address the question of interest and 2 of these trials reported on a final sample that represented ≤60% of participants randomized at baseline [77,89]. Expanding our inclusion criteria to include randomized trials with active interventions and follow-up periods of any duration identified only 6 long-term trials (>6 mos.) and 14 trials with a follow-up period after weight loss. However, 43% of the weight loss/follow-up trials had follow-up periods of 6 months or less.

The available literature is also limited by the fact that the aerobic exercise that was prescribed, either alone, or in combination with a diet, was insufficient to produce significant weight loss. This is particularly problematic when evaluating the effect of the method of weight loss on weight regain, as greater weight loss following an active intervention is associated with greater weight loss at follow-up [12,102]. Thus, the effect of exercise on long-term weight loss, or weight regain when exercise is prescribed during weight loss and/or during follow-up has not been adequately evaluated. Additional limitations include lack of data by sex or minority status, and lack of trials including resistance exercise. For example, of the 20 trials included in this review, 35% were conducted on all female samples, and 45% in samples that were predominantly female. Only 2 trials, one long-term (12-mos.) [82] and one follow-up (6 mos. weight loss, 6 mos. follow-up) [79] provided results separately by sex [79,82]. Results of these trials suggest potential sex differences for change in weight and body composition which warrant additional investigation. Sixty percent of trials either failed to report minority representation or included no minorities, and only 3 trials evaluated the impact of resistance training either in combination with diet [84,89] or in combination with diet and aerobic exercise [89,93].

Limitations of this review

Our conclusions should be cautiously interpreted as they are based on both data from a limited number of randomized trials, several with a high risk of one or more forms of bias. In addition, we did not contact authors to obtain missing data; however the author of one trial [78] was contacted for clarification regarding the statistical significance of one between group difference for data presented in a table.

Conclusions

The present systematic review found limited evidence to suggest better long-term weight loss and more favorable long-term changes in body composition and chronic disease risk factors when diet is combined with aerobic exercise compared with either diet or aerobic exercise alone. However, no advantage for minimizing weight regain or changes in body composition or chronic disease risk factors following weight loss was shown for any weight loss mode. As previously discussed, the available literature on this topic is extremely limited and suffers numerous methodological shortcomings. Therefore, we recommend additional randomized trials to specifically evaluate the impact of mode of weight loss on changes in weight, body composition and chronic disease risk factors following both active weight loss and maintenance that include the following: 1) adequate statistical power to detect clinically significant differences in these outcomes both overall and by sex; 2) weight loss and maintenance phases of ≥6 months and ≥12 months, respectively; 3) supervised, verified exercise during weight loss of sufficient energy expenditure to achieve weight loss similar to that achieved in comparison groups (i.e. diet only or diet+exercise). 4) maintenance periods with and without prescribed exercise; and 5) resistance training.

Author Contributions

Conceived and designed the experiments: JED. Analyzed the data: ANS KL EAW LTP JJH SDH. Wrote the paper: RAW JED.

References

1. Donato K, Pi-Sunyer F, Becker D, Bouchard C, Carleton R, et al. (1998) Executive summary of the clinical guidelines on the identification, evaluation, and treatment of overweight and obesity in adults. Archives of Internal Medicine 158: 1855–1867.
2. Meckling KA, O'Sullivan C, Saari D (2004) Comparison of a low-fat diet to a low-carbohydrate diet on weight loss, body composition, and risk factors for diabetes and cardiovascular disease in free-living, overweight men and women. J Clin Endocrinol Metab 89: 2717–2723.
3. Rosenkilde M, Auerbach P, Reichkendler MH, Ploug T, Stallknecht BM, et al. (2012) Body fat loss and compensatory mechanisms in response to different doses of aerobic exercise—a randomized controlled trial in overweight sedentary males. Am J Physiol Regul Integr Comp Physiol 303: R571–579.
4. Ross R, Dagnone D, Jones PJH, Smith H, Paddags A, et al. (2000) Reduction in obesity and related comorbid conditions after diet-induced weight loss or exercise -induced weight loss in men: A randomized, controlled trial. Annals of Internal Medicine 133: 92–103.
5. Racette SB, Weiss EP, Villareal DT, Arif H, Steger-May K, et al. (2006) One year of caloric restriction in humans: feasibility and effects on body composition and abdominal adipose tissue. J Gerontol A Biol Sci Med Sci 61: 943–950.
6. Donnelly JE, Honas JJ, Smith BK, Mayo MS, Gibson CA, et al. (2013) Aerobic exercise alone results in clinically significant weight loss for men and women: midwest exercise trial 2. Obesity (Silver Spring) 21: E219–228.
7. Donnelly JE, Hill JO, Jacobsen DJ, Potteiger JA, Sullivan D, K., et al. (2003) Effects of a 16-month randomized controlled exercise trial on body weight and composition in young, overweight men and women. Archives of Internal Medicine 163: 1343–1350.
8. Ogden CL, Carroll MD, Kit BK, Flegal KM (2014) Prevalence of childhood and adult obesity in the United States, 2011–2012. Jama 311: 806–814.
9. Weiss EC, Galuska DA, Kettel Khan L, Gillespie C, Serdula M, K. (2007) Weight regain in U.S. adults who experienced substantial weight loss, 1999-2002. American Journal of Preventive Medicine 33: 34–40.
10. Phelan S, Wing RR, Loria CM, Y K, Lewis CE (2010) Prevlance and predictors of weight-loss maintenance in a biracial cohort: Results from the Coronary Artery Riks Development in Young Adults Study. American Journal of Preventive Medicine 39: 546–554.
11. Delany JP, Kelley DE, Hames KC, Jakicic JM, Goodpaster BH (2014) Effect of physical activity on weight loss, energy expenditure, and energy intake during diet induced weight loss. Obesity (Silver Spring) 22: 363–370.
12. Barte JCM, ter Bogt NCW, Bogers RP, Teixeira PJ, Blissmer B, et al. (2010) Maintenance of weight loss after lifestyle interventions for overweight and obesity, a systematic review. Obesity Reviews doi: 10.111/j.1467-789X2010.00740.x
13. Kraschnewski JL, Boan K, Esposito J, Sherwood NE, Lehman EB, et al. (2010) Long-term weight loss maintenance in the United states. International Journal of Obesity 34: 1644–1654.
14. Anderson JW, Konz EC, Frederich RC, Wood CL (2001) Long-term weight-loss maintenance: a meta-analysis of US studies. Am J Clin Nutr 74: 579–584.
15. Pavlou KN, Krey S, Steffee WP (1989) Exercise as an adjunct to weight loss and maintenance in moderately obese subjects. American Journal of Clinical Nutrition 49 1115–1123
16. Martins C, Kulseng B, King NA, Holst JJ, Blundell JE (2010) The effects of exercise-induced weight loss on appetite-related peptides and motivation to eat. J Clin Endocrinol Metab 95: 1609–1616.
17. Maclean PS, Bergouignan A, Cornier MA, Jackman MR (2011) Biology's response to dieting: the impetus for weight regain. Am J Physiol Regul Integr Comp Physiol 301: R581–600.
18. Sumithran P, Proietto J (2013) The defence of body weight: a physiological basis for weight regain after weight loss. Clin Sci (Lond) 124: 231–241.
19. Strohacker K, McCaffery JM, MacLean PS, Wing RR (2014) Adaptations of leptin, ghrelin or insulin during weight loss as predictors of weight regain: a review of current literature. Int J Obes (Lond) 28: 388–396.
20. Reed JL, Chaput JP, Tremblay A, Doucet E (2013) The maintenance of energy balance is compromised after weight loss. Can J Diabetes 37: 121–127.
21. Ochner CN, Barrios DM, Lee CD, Pi-Sunyer FX (2013) Biological mechanisms that promote weight regain following weight loss in obese humans. Physiol Behav 120C: 106–113.
22. Schwartz A, Kuk JL, Lamothe G, Doucet E (2012) Greater than predicted decrease in resting energy expenditure and weight loss: results from a systematic review. Obesity (Silver Spring) 20: 2307–2310.
23. Martin CK, Das SK, Lindblad L, Racette SB, McCrory MA, et al. (2011) Effect of calorie restriction on the free-living physical activity levels of nonobese humans: results of three randomized trials. J Appl Physiol (1985) 110: 956–963.
24. Camps SG, Verhoef SP, Westerterp KR (2013) Weight loss, weight maintenance, and adaptive thermogenesis. Am J Clin Nutr 97: 990–994.
25. Filozof CM, Murua C, Sanchez MP, Brailovsky C, Perman M, et al. (2000) Low plasma leptin concentration and low rates of fat oxidation in weight-stable post-obese subjects. Obes Res 8: 205–210.
26. Weiss EP, Villareal DT, Racette SB, Steger-May K, Premachandra BN, et al. (2008) Caloric restriction but not exercise-induced reductions in fat mass decrease plasma triiodothyronine concentrations: a randomized controlled trial. Rejuvenation Res 11: 605–609.
27. Kozlowska L, Rosolowska-Huszcz D (2004) Leptin, thyrotropin, and thyroid hormones in obese/overweight women before and after two levels of energy deficit. Endocrine 24: 147–153.
28. Wadden TA, Mason G, Foster GD, Stunkard AJ, Prange AJ (1990) Effects of a very low calorie diet on weight, thyroid hormones and mood. Int J Obes 14: 249–258.
29. Tomiyama AJ, Mann T, Vinas D, Hunger JM, Dejager J, et al. (2010) Low calorie dieting increases cortisol. Psychosom Med 72: 357–364.

30. Johnstone AM, Faber P, Andrew R, Gibney ER, Elia M, et al. (2004) Influence of short-term dietary weight loss on cortisol secretion and metabolism in obese men. Eur J Endocrinol 150: 185–194.
31. Cummings DE, Weigle DS, Frayo RS, Breen PA, Ma MK, et al. (2002) Plasma ghrelin levels after diet-induced weight loss or gastric bypass surgery. N Engl J Med 346: 1623–1630.
32. Sumithran P, Prendergast LA, Delbridge E, Purcell K, Shulkes A, et al. (2011) Long-term persistence of hormonal adaptations to weight loss. N Engl J Med 365: 1597–1604.
33. Pfluger PT, Kampe J, Castaneda TR, Vahl T, D'Alessio DA, et al. (2007) Effect of human body weight changes on circulating levels of peptide YY and peptide YY3-36. J Clin Endocrinol Metab 92: 583–588.
34. Essah PA, Levy JR, Sistrun SN, Kelly SM, Nestler JE (2010) Effect of weight loss by a low-fat diet and a low-carbohydrate diet on peptide YY levels. Int J Obes (Lond) 34: 1239–1242.
35. Reinehr T, de Sousa G, Niklowitz P, Roth CL (2007) Amylin and its relation to insulin and lipids in obese children before and after weight loss. Obesity (Silver Spring) 15: 2006–2011.
36. Rissanen P, Franssila-Kallunki A, Rissanen A (2001) Cardiac parasympathetic activity is increased by weight loss in healthy obese women. Obes Res 9: 637–643.
37. Straznicky NE, Lambert EA, Lambert GW, Masuo K, Esler MD, et al. (2005) Effects of dietary weight loss on sympathetic activity and cardiac risk factors associated with the metabolic syndrome. J Clin Endocrinol Metab 90: 5998–6005.
38. Straznicky NE, Lambert GW, Lambert EA (2010) Neuroadrenergic dysfunction in obesity: an overview of the effects of weight loss. Curr Opin Lipidol 21: 21–30.
39. Rosenbaum M, Hirsch J, Gallagher DA, Leibel RL (2008) Long-term persistence of adaptive thermogenesis in subjects who have maintained a reduced body weight. American Journal of Clinical Nutrition 88: 906–912.
40. Doucet E, St Pierre S, Almeras N, Mauriege P, Richard D, et al. (2000) Changes in energy expenditure and substrate oxidation resulting from weight loss in obese men and women: is there an important contribution of leptin? J Clin Endocrinol Metab 85: 1550–1556.
41. Bray GA (1969) Effect of caloric restriction on energy expenditure in obese patients. Lancet 2: 397–398.
42. Doucet E, St-Pierre J, Almeas N, Despres JP, Bouchard C, et al. (2001) Evidence for the existence of adaptive thermogenesis during weight loss. British Journal of Nutrition 85: 715–723.
43. Redman LM, Heilbronn LK, Martin CK, de Jonge L, Williamson DA, et al. (2009) Metabolic and behavioral compensations in response to caloric restriction: implications for the maintenance of weight loss. PLoS One 4: e4377.
44. Weinsier RL, Nagy TR, Hunter GR, Darnell BE, Hensrud DD, et al. (2000) Do adaptive changes in metabolic rate favor weight regain in weight-reduced individuals? An examination of the set-point hheory. American Journal of Clinical Nutrition 72: 1088–1094.
45. Das SK, Roberts SB, McCrory MA, Hsu LK, S.A S, et al. (2003) Long-term changes in energy expenditure and body composition after massive weight loss induced by gastric bypass surgery. American Journal of Clinical Nutrition 78: 22–30.
46. Slentz CA, Duscha BD, Johnson JL, Ketchem K, Aiken LR, et al. (2004) Effect of the amount of exercise on body weight, body composition, and measures of central obesity: STRRIDE-A randomized controlled trial. Archives of Internal Medicine 164: 31–39.
47. Wilmore JH, Stanforth PR, Hudspeth LA, Gagnon J, Daw EW, et al. (1998) Alterations in resting metabolic rate as a consequence of 20 wk of endurance training: the heritage family study. American Journal of Clinical Nutrition 68: 66–71.
48. Potteiger JA, Kirk EP, Jacobsen DJ, Donnelly JE (2008) Changes in resting metabolic rate and substrate oxidation after 16 months of exericse training in overweight adults. International Journal of Sport Nutrition and Exercise Metabolism 18: 79–95.
49. Schwartz A, Doucet E (2010) Relative changes in resting energy expenditure during weight loss: a systematic review. Obes Rev 11: 531–547.
50. Hopkins M, Gibbons C, Caudwell P, Hellstrom PM, Naslund E, et al. (2014) The adaptive metabolic response to exercise-induced weight loss influences both energy expenditure and energy intake. Eur J Clin Nutr.
51. Leibel RL, Rosenbaum M, Hirsch J (1995) Changes in energy expenditure resulting from altered body weight. The New England Journal of Medicine 332: 621–628.
52. Bonomi AG, Soenen S, Goris AH, Westerterp KR (2013) Weight-loss induced changes in physical activity and activity energy expenditure in overweight and obese subjects before and after energy restriction. PLoS One 8: e59641.
53. Long SJ, Hart K, Morgan LM (2002) The ability of habitual exercise to influence appetite and food intake in response to high-and low-energy preloads in man. British Journal of Nutrition 87: 517–523.
54. Martins C, Truby H, Morgan LM (2007) Short-term appetite control in response to a 6-week exercise programme in sedentary volunteers. British Journal of Nutrition 98: 834–842.
55. van Walleghen EL, Orr JS, Gentile CL, Davy KP, Davy BM (2007) Habitual physical activity differentially affects acute and short-term energy intake regulation in young and older adults. International Journal of Obesity 31: 1277–1285.
56. King NA, Caudwell PP, Hopkins M, Stubbs JR, Naslund E, et al. (2009) Dual-process action of exercise on appetite control: increase in oreigeneic drive but improvement in meal-induced satiety American Journal of Clinical Nutrition 90: 921–927.
57. Martins C, Kulseng B, Rehfeld JF, King NA, Blundell JE (2013) Effect of chronic exercise on appetite control in overweight and obese individuals. Med Sci Sports Exerc 45: 805–812.
58. Mayer J, Roy P, Mitra KP (1956) Relation between caloric intake, body weight, and physical work: studies in an industrial male population in West Bengal. American Journal of Clinical Nutrition 4: 169–175.
59. Murgatroyd PR, Goldberg GR, Leahy FE, Gilsenan MB, Prentice AM (1999) Efffects of inactivity and diet compositon on human energy balance. International Journal of Obesity 23: 1269–1275.
60. King NA, Tremblay A, Blundell JE (1997) Effects of exercise on appetite control: implications for energy balance. Medicine and Science in Sports and Exercise 29: 1076–1089.
61. Stubbs RJ, Hughes DA, Johnstone AM, Horgan GW, King N, et al. (2004) A decrease in physical activity affects appetite, energy, and nutrient balance in lean men feeding ad libitum. Am J Clin Nutr 79: 62–69.
62. Broom DR, Batterham RL, King JA, Stensel DJ (2009) Influence of resistance and aerobic exercise on hunger, circulating levels of acylated ghrelin, and peptice YY in healthy males. American Journal of Physiology 296.
63. Hagobian TA, Braun B (2010) Physical activity and hormonal regulation of appetite: Sex differences and weight control. Exercise and Sport Science Reviews 38: 25–30.
64. Cornier MA, Melanson EL, Salzberg AK, Bechtell JL, Tregellas JR (2012) The effects of exercise on the neuronal response to food cues. Physiol Behav 105: 1028–1034.
65. Curioni CC, Lourenco PM (2005) Long-term weight loss after diet and exercise: a systematic review. Int J Obes (Lond) 29: 1168–1174.
66. Wu T, Gao X, Chen M, van Dam RM (2009) Long-term effectiveness of diet-plus-exercise interventions vs. diet-only interventions for weight loss: a meta-analysis. Obes Rev 10: 313–323.
67. Franz MJ, VanWormer JJ, Grain AL, Boucher JL, Histon T, et al. (2007) Weight-loss outcomes: A systematic review and meta-analysis of weight-loss clinical trials with a minimum 1-year follow-up. Journal of the American Dietetic Association 107: 1755–1767.
68. Fogelholm M, Kukkonen-Harjula K (2000) Does physical activity prevent weight gain - a systematic review. Obesity Reviews 1: 95–111.
69. Catenacci VA, Wyatt HR (2007) The role of physical activity in producing and maintaining weight loss. Nat Clin Pract Endocrinol Metab 3: 518–529.
70. Miller WC, Koceja DM, Hamilton EJ (1997) A meta-analysis of the past 25 years of weight loss research using diet, exercise or diet plus exercise intervention. International Journal of Obesity 21: 941–947.
71. Liberati A, Altman DG, Tetzlaff J, Mulrow C, Gotzce PC, et al. (2009) The PRISMA statement for reporting systematic reviews and meta-analyses of studies that evaluate health care interventions: explanation and elaboration. Journal of Clinical Epidemiology 62: e1–e34.
72. Moher D, Liberati A, Tetzlaff J, Altman DG (2009) Preferred reporting items for systematic reviews and meta-analyses: the PRISMA statement. PLoS Med 6: e1000097.
73. Harris PA, Taylor R, Thielke R, Payne J, Gonzalez N, et al. (2009) Research electronic data capture (REDCap)—a metadata-driven methodology and workflow process for providing translational research informatics support. J Biomed Inform 42: 377–381.
74. Higgins JPT, Green S, editors (updated March 2011) Cochrane Handbook for Systematic Reviews of Interventions: The Cochrane Collaboration. Available: www.cochrane-handbook.org/ p.
75. Anderssen SA, Haaland A, Hjermann I, Urdal P, Gjesdal K, et al. (1995) Oslo diet and exercise study: a one-year randomized intervention trial. Effect on hemostatic variables and other coronary rish factors. Nutrition Metabolism and Cadiovascular Disease 5: 189–200.
76. Foster-Schubert KE, Alfano CM, Duggan CR, Xiao L, Campbell KL, et al. (2012) Effect of diet and exercise, alone or combined, on weight and body composition in overweight-to-obese postmenopausal women. Obesity (Silver Spring) 20: 1628–1638.
77. Skender ML, Goodrick GK, Del Junco DJ, Reeves RS, Darnell L, et al. (1996) Comparison of 2-year weight loss trends in behavioral treatments of obesity: Diet, exercise, and combination of interventions. Journal of the American Dietetic Association 96: 342–346.
78. Pritchard JE, Nowson CA, Wark JD (1997) A worksite program for overweight middle-aged men achieves lesser weight loss with exercise than with dietary change. J Am Diet Assoc 97: 37–42.
79. Volpe SL, Kobusingye H, Bailur S, Stanek E (2008) Effect of diet and exercise on body composition, energy intake and leptin levels in overweight women and men. J Am Coll Nutr 27: 195–208.
80. Wing RR, Venditti E, Jakicic JM, Polley BA, Lang W (1998) Lifestyle Intervention In Overweight Individuals With a Family History Of Diabetes. Diabetes Care 21: 350–359.
81. Dengel DR, Hagberg JM, Coon PJ, al e (1994) Effects of weight loss by diet alone or combined with aerobic exercise on body composition in older obese men. Metabolism - Clinican & Experimental 43: 867–871.

82. Wood PD, Stefanick ML, Williams PT, Haskell WL (1991) The effects on plasma lipoproteins of a prudent weight-reducing diet, with or without exercise, in overweight men and women. N Engl J Med 325: 461–466.
83. Andreou E, Philippou C, Papandreou D (2011) Effects of an intervention and maintenance weight loss diet with and without exercise on anthropometric indices in overweight and obese healthy women. Ann Nutr Metab 59: 187–192.
84. Hunter GR, Brock DW, Byrne NM, Chandler-Laney PC, Del Corral P, et al. (2010) Exercise training prevents regain of visceral fat for 1 year following weight loss. Obesity 18: 690–695.
85. Molenaar EA, van Ameijden EJ, Vergouwe Y, Grobbee DE, Numans ME (2010) Effect of nutritional counselling and nutritional plus exercise counselling in overweight adults: a randomized trial in multidisciplinary primary care practice. Fam Pract 27: 143–150.
86. Neumark-Sztainer D, Kaufmann NA, Berry EM (1995) Physical activity within a community-based weight control program: program evaluation and predictors of success. Public Health Rev 23: 237–251.
87. Snel M, van Diepen JA, Stijnen T, Pijl H, Romijn JA, et al. (2011) Immediate and long-term effects of addition of exercise to a 16-week very low calorie diet on low-grade inflammation in obese, insulin-dependent type 2 diabetic patients. Food Chem Toxicol 49: 3104–3111.
88. Van Aggel-Leijssen DP, Saris WHM, Hul GB, van Baak MA (2002) Long-term effects of low-intensity exercise training on fat metabolism in weight-reduced obese men. Metabolism 51: 1003–1010.
89. Wadden TA, Vogt RA, Foster GD, Anderson DA (1998) Exercise and the maintenance of weight loss: 1-year follow-up of a controlled clinical trial. Journal of Consulting and Clinical Psychology 66: 429–433.
90. Wang X, Lyles MF, You T, Berry MJ, Rejeski WJ, et al. (2008) Weight regain is related to decreases in physical activity during weight loss. Medicine and Science in Sports and Exercise 40: 1781–1788.
91. Melanson KJ, Dell'Olio J, Carpenter MR, Angelopoulos TJ (2004) Changes in multiple health outcomes at 12 and 24 weeks resulting from 12 weeks of exercise counseling with or without dietary counseling in obese adults. Nutrition 20: 849–856.
92. Melanson KJ, Angelopoulos TJ, Nguyen VT, Martini M, Zukley L, et al. (2006) Consumption of whole-grain cereals during weight loss: effects on dietary quality, dietary fiber, magnesium, vitamin B-6, and obesity. J Am Diet Assoc 106: 1380–1388; quiz 1389–1390.
93. Svendsen OL, Hassager C, Christiansen C (1994) Six months' follow-up on exercise added to a short-term diet in overweight postmenopausal women—effects on body composition, resting metabolic rate, cardiovascular risk factors and bone. Int J Obes Relat Metab Disord 18: 692–698.
94. Wing RR (1999) Physical activity in the treatment of the adulthood overweight and obesity: current evidence and research issues. Med Sci Sports Exerc 31: S547–552.
95. Garrow JS, Summerbell CD (1995) Meta-analysis: effect of exercise, with or without dieting, on the body compostion of overweight subjects. European Journal of Clinical Nutrition 49: 1–10.
96. Weinheimer EM, Sands LP, Campbell WW (2010) A systematic review of the separate and combined effects of energy restriction and exercise on fat-free mass in middle-aged and older adults: implications for sarcopenic obesity. Nutr Rev 68: 375–388.
97. Donnelly JE, Blair SN, Jakicic JM, Manore MM, Rankin JW, et al. (2009) Appropriate physical activity intervention strategies for weight loss and prevention of weight regain for adults. Medicine & Science in Sports & Exercise 41: 459–471.
98. Ross R, Janssen I, Dawson J, Kungl AM, Kuk JL, et al. (2004) Exercise-induced reduction in obesity and insulin resistance in women: a randomized controlled trial. Obes Res 12: 789–798.
99. Janssen I, Fortier A, Hudson R, Ross R (2002) Effects of an energy-restrictive diet with or without exercise on abdominal fat, intermuscular fat, and metabolic risk factors in obese women. Diabetes Care 25: 431–438.
100. Janssen I, Ross R (1999) Effects of sex on the change in visceral, subcutaneous adipose tissue and skeletal muscle in response to weight loss. International Journal of Obesity 23: 1035–1046.
101. Rice B, Janssen I, Hudson R, Ross R (1999) Effects of aerobic or resistance exercise and/or diet on glucose tolerance and plasma insulin levels in obese men. Diabetes Care 22: 684–691.
102. Astrup A, Rossner S (2000) Lessons from obesity management programmes: greater initial weight loss improves long-term maintenance. Obes Rev 1: 17–19.

9

Effects of Moderate Aerobic Exercise Training on Hemorheological and Laboratory Parameters in Ischemic Heart Disease Patients

Barbara Sandor[1], Alexandra Nagy[2], Andras Toth[1], Miklos Rabai[1], Bela Mezey[1], Arpad Csatho[2], Istvan Czuriga[1], Kalman Toth[1], Eszter Szabados[1]*

1 1st Department of Medicine, University of Pecs, School of Medicine, Pecs, Hungary, **2** Department of Behavioural Sciences, University of Pecs, School of Medicine, Pecs, Hungary

Abstract

Background and Design: In this study we set out to determine the effects of long-term physical training on hemorheological, laboratory parameters, exercise tolerability, psychological factors in cardiac patients participating in an ambulatory rehabilitation program.

Methods: Before physical training, patients were examined by echocardiography, tested on treadmill by the Bruce protocol, and blood was drawn for laboratory tests. The enrolled 79 ischemic heart disease patients joined a 24-week cardiac rehabilitation training program. Blood was drawn to measure hematocrit (Hct), plasma and whole blood viscosity (PV, WBV), red blood cell (RBC) aggregation and deformability. Hemorheological, clinical chemistry and psychological measurements were repeated 12 and 24 weeks later, and a treadmill test was performed at the end of the program.

Results: After 12 weeks Hct, PV, WBV and RBC aggregation were significantly decreased, RBC deformability exhibited a significant increase ($p<0.05$). Laboratory parameters (triglyceride, uric acid, hsCRP and fibrinogen) were significantly decreased ($p<0.05$). After 24 weeks the significant results were still observed. By the end of the study, IL-6 and TNF-α levels displayed decreasing trends ($p<0.06$). There was a significant improvement in MET ($p<0.001$), and the BMI decrease was also significant ($p<0.05$). The vital exhaustion parameters measured on the fatigue impact scale indicated a significant improvement in two areas of the daily activities ($p<0.05$).

Conclusions: Regular physical training improved the exercise tolerability of patients with ischemic heart disease. Previous publications have demonstrated that decreases in Hct and PV may reduce cardiovascular risk, while a decrease in RBC aggregation and an increase in deformability improve the capillary flow. Positive changes in laboratory parameters and body weight may indicate better oxidative and inflammatory circumstances and an improved metabolic state. The psychological findings point to an improvement in the quality of life.

Editor: Paula A. da Costa Martins, Maastricht University Faculty of Health, Medicine, and Life Sciences, Netherlands

Funding: The authors have no funding or support to report.

Competing Interests: The authors have declared that no competing interests exist.

* Email: szabados.eszter@pte.hu

Introduction

In the past few decades, mortality due to coronary artery disease (CAD) has decreased substantially in the industrialized countries thanks to the improved medical care, but it remains the leading cause of death worldwide. In addition to the optimal pharmacological therapies and modern revascularization procedures, a number of preventive strategies have been created with a view to the further reduction of the morbidity and mortality of CAD [1].

The recent guidelines of the European Society of Cardiology (ESC) and the American Heart Association/American College of Cardiology (AHA/ACC) indicate that physical activity has a pivotal role in the primary prevention in healthy subjects [1], and moreover it reduces the all-cause and cardiovascular (CV) mortality too [1,2,3,4,5,6,7]. Moderate aerobic exercise training in patients with CAD improves myocardial perfusion, muscular endurance and psychosocial well-being leading to enhanced flexibility, ameliorated symptoms, better cardiorespiratory fitness and a reduced CV risk [1]. Training from 2.5 to 5 hours a week can result in a 20–30% CV and all-cause mortality risk reduction. In summary, moderate physical activity reduces the CV risk in a dose-dependent manner in both male and female healthy subjects, and even in patients with known CAD [1]. Physical activity conducted by physiotherapists and supervised by a cardiologist in a cardiac rehabilitation (CR) program is an excellent possibility for secondary prevention, where effective risk factor management can be achieved through long-term life style changes [1].

Impaired hemorheological parameters, including reduced erythrocyte deformability and increased erythrocyte aggregation, may have a deleterious effect on the vascular system leading to the development of various CV, cerebrovascular and peripheral arterial diseases [8,9,10,11,12]. Whereas publications from the last 25 years have clearly revealed a relationship between hemorheological factors and physical training, those studies involved healthy volunteers or a small numbers of CV patients participating in short-term (10–12 weeks) exercise training. Furthermore, the possible connections between hemorheology and long-term, moderate aerobic physical activity have not been investigated in a relatively large population with ischemic heart disease.

Our study had the aim of determining the beneficial effects of aerobic physical training on ischemic heart disease patients participating in a long-term (24 weeks) ambulatory CR program.

Methods

79 non-smoker patients with stable ischemic heart disease (39 males and 40 females, mean age: 65.3±5.68 years) were selected for the study; their co-morbidities are presented in Table 1. The patients received their medication in accordance with current guidelines for the secondary prevention of CAD [13] and with their co-morbidities (Table 2). Modifications in either agent or dose were not made during the trial. Patients with an ejection fraction <40%, and MET <5 or a significant ST depression during a treadmill-based exercise tolerance test using the Bruce protocol were excluded from the study [14,15]. ST depression was accepted significant in thoracic leads by 1 mm and in limb leads by 2 mm. There were neither arrhythmias nor AV blocks detected among our patients.

The investigation was approved by the Regional Ethics Committee (licence number: 4378) of the University of Pecs and written informed consent was signed by all subjects.

Study design

At baseline, the following measurements were performed: psychological tests, resting electrocardiography (ECG), resting echocardiography (Table 3), treadmill-based exercise tolerance testing using the Bruce protocol, clinical chemistry (fasting total cholesterol, triglyceride, high-density lipoprotein (HDL), low-density lipoprotein (LDL), uric acid, hsCRP, fasting glucose, total plasma protein, albumin, blood cell counts, fibrinogen, cytokines (TNF-α and IL-6) and hemorheological measurements (Hct, whole blood viscosity (WBV), the ratio Hct/WBV, plasma viscosity (PV), red blood cell aggregation and red blood cell deformability).

The patients participated in a 24-weeks physical training program lasting for 1 hour 3 times weekly, designed and conducted by a physiotherapist and supervised by a cardiologist. After 12 weeks, the hemorheological measurements, clinical chemistry (except cytokines) and psychological tests were repeated. At the end of the 24 weeks, the resting ECG measurements, the treadmill tests with the Bruce protocol, the clinical chemistry, the hemorheological measurements and the psychological tests were repeated.

Aerobic exercise training program

The present aerobic exercise training program was preceded and ended with blood pressure and pulse measurements. The patients began with warm-up exercises (breathing exercises, and stretching of the large joints) for 5–10 minutes. In the second phase, they participated in a moderate-intensity training. Intensity was defined as 50–70% of peak VO_2 (starting at 50% and gradually increasing to 70% of VO_{2max}). The intensity was assessed by the Borg scale (13–15/20) [16] and pulse measurements. The training involved static (exercises with medicine ball, half-squats, toe raisis, body flexions) and dynamic (walking, jogging, ball games e.g. basketball, football) exercise elements. The aerobic phase lasted 35–40 minutes. Finally, relaxation exercises were performed (stretching and breathing exercises) for 10 minutes.

Blood collecting

Blood samples were obtained from the antecubital vein at baseline, after 12 weeks and after 24 weeks. The blood was collected into two lithium heparin-coated (12 ml), one clot activator-coated and gel-containing (5 ml), one potassium EDTA-coated (3 ml) and one sodium fluoride and potassium oxalate-coated (2 ml) Vacutainer tube with a 21-gauge Eclipse Blood Collection butterfly needle set, using a minimal tourniquet.

Hemorheological measurements

Hemorheological measurements were performed within 2 hours after blood sampling. Hct was measured by using a micro-Hct centrifuge (Haemofuge Heraeus Instr., Germany). WBV and PV were determined at a shear rate of 90 s^{-1} with a Hevimet 40 capillary viscometer (Hemorex Ltd., Budapest, Hungary). Plasma was prepared by a 10-minute centrifugation of whole blood at 1500 g. Measurements were made at 37°C. The ratio Hct/WBV was utilized to characterize RBC oxygen transport effectiveness [11].

Red blood cell aggregation was measured with LORCA (Laser-assisted Optical Rotational Cell Analyzer; R&R Mechatronics, Hoorn, The Netherlands) [17,18] aggregometer, using blood samples with standard 40% Hct. RBC aggregation index (AI) was

Table 1. Characteristics of the study population.

population characteristic		number of patients	%
ischemic heart disease	myocardial infarction	32/79	40.51
	previous CABG	35/79	44.3
	previous PCI	18/79	22.78
	proven by coronary angiography or coronary CT	18/79	22.78
hypertension		71/79	89.87
diabetes mellitus		24/79	30.38

Table 2. Medication during the 24 week long physical training.

medication	number of patients	%
cholesterol lowering drugs	70/79	88.61
antiplatelet drugs	79/79	100
β-blocker	59/79	74.68
RAAS inhibitor	65/79	82.28

determined at 37°C via syllectometry (i.e., laser backscatter versus time). The RBC disaggregation threshold (γ), i.e., the minimal shear rate needed to prevent RBC aggregation or to breakdown existing RBC aggregates, was determined using a re-iteration procedure. Measurements were made at 37°C.

Erythrocyte deformability was characterized with a LORCA ektacytometer [19] at 37°C, which provided nine values of elongation index (EI) in the shear stress range from 0.3 to 30 Pa. The deformability results were analyzed by means of the Lineweaver-Burke nonlinear equation, with calculation of the maximal EI (EI_{max}) at infinite shear, and the shear stress value ($SS_{1/2}$) required for half of this maximal elongation [20]. For deformability measurements, blood samples were suspended in a highly viscous (32.6 mPas) polyvinylpyrrolidone solution.

Cytokine measurements

Cytokines were determined with an automated chemiluminescence immunoassay system (Immulite 1000, Siemens). For TNF-α, a solid-phase chemiluminescent immunometric assay (cat. no. LKNF1), and for IL-6, a solid-phase chemiluminescent sequential immunometric assay (cat. no. LK6P1) was used. Master calibration and bi-level cytokine controls were applied during the runs.

Psychological surveys

In order to examine the effects of the 24-week physical training on the patients' subjective experience with fatigue, we applied the Fatigue Impact Scale (FIS) [21,22]. The FIS consists of 40 items which evaluate the impact of fatigue on three aspects of daily life: physical (10 items), cognitive (10 items) and psychosocial (20 items) functions. In addition, we monitored patients' depression severity by the short version of the Beck Depression Inventory (9 items).

Statistics

Data are shown as means ± SD. Differences were evaluated by a one-way repeated ANOVA statistical test (Tamhane post-hoc test) after using the Kolmogorov–Smirnov test to check on the normality of the data distribution. Multivariate linear regression and stepwise analyses of the data were performed with regard to differences between the baseline and the 24-week MET values for whole blood and plasma viscosity, LORCA aggregation index, LORCA erythrocyte deformability at 5,33 Pa shear stress and BMI.

A sample size and power analysis was performed for the overall population using PS program version 3.1.2. For the sample size of $n = 79$ patients needed to detect a true difference of $\delta = 1.94$ in MET with 92.6% power, where type I error probability is $\alpha = 0.05$.

The psychological data revealed a significant deviation from the normal distribution, and; the nonparametric Friedman test was therefore applied to analyze potential changes in psychological functioning. The analyses of the psychological data was restricted to those patients who had no missing surveys and gave no indication of moderate to severe depression at any of the three measurements. Five patients indicated moderate to severe depression during the rehabilitation period, and six of them had missing surveys. These patients were excluded from the psychological data analyses, which included 68 patients' data (86% of the total sample).

Significance level was defined as $p<0.05$. SPSS statistical software, version 11.0.1. was used to conduct descriptive analyses and to describe the sample.

Results

As concerns the hemorheological results, the Hct displayed a decreasing tendency during the investigated period, while the WBV exhibited a significant reduction ($p<0.05$), resulting in a significantly increased Hct/WBV ratio ($p<0.05$). The PV was significantly decreased after 12 weeks and remained significantly lower relative to the baseline at the end of the program ($p<0.001$) (Table 4). The red blood cell aggregation parameters of LORCA aggregometer likewise demonstrated significant reductions. The LORCA parameter (AI) decreased significantly during the 24-week training program ($p<0.05$) (Table 5), while the LORCA EIs of erythrocyte deformability increased significantly ($p<0.001$), supported by the Lineweaver-Burke nonlinear equation analyses showing a significantly higher EI_{max} and a significantly lower $SS_{1/2}$ (Table 6).

Table 3. Results of the echocardiographycal measurements at baseline.

echocardiographical parameters	
ejection fraction (%)	59.92±8.41
left ventricle end-systolic diameter (mm)	50.09±6.7
left ventricle end-diastolic diameter (mm)	31.71±5,51

N = 79, values are means ± SD.

Table 4. Changes in certain hemorheological parameters (hematocrit (Hct), whole blood viscosity (WBV), plasma viscosity (PV) and the Hct/WBV ratio) after the 12- and 24-week ambulatory exercise training of ischemic heart disease patients.

hemorheological parameters	mean ± SD	p value
hematocrit (%)	44.18±4.56 vs. 42.98±6.0 vs. 42.13±7.7	0.11
whole blood viscosity (mPas)	4.35±0.59 vs. 4.26±0.62 vs. 4.08±0.77	0.03
plasma viscosity (mPas)	1.27±0.22 vs. 1.18±0.2 vs. 1.14±0.23	0.001
Hct/WBV (1/mPas)	10.2±0.63 vs. 10.25±1.18 vs. 10.33±1.7	0.04

N = 79; values are baseline, 12 week and 24 week means ± SD. Levels of significance and p values are also shown.

The clinical chemistry parameters relating to uric acid, triglycerides, hsCRP and fibrinogen decreased significantly during the training period (Table 7).

The cytokine measurements did not indicate a significant decrease ($p<0.05$), but only a falling trend as compared with the baseline values (Table 7).

As expected, the functional capacity described by the MET significantly improved ($p<0.001$), and the treadmill time also increased significantly, by 17.4% ($p<0.001$), during the training program. Moreover, the patients lost weight, with the body mass index (BMI) undergoing a significant decrease during the trial ($p< 0.001$), however lean body mass index calculated by the Hume formula [23], showed a slight but not significant increase at the end of the 24 week (Table 8).

For the Δ values between the baseline and 24-week measurements were calculated from every parameter showing a significant difference to the baseline. The Δ parameters, which were in positive or negative correlation to the MET were used for the multivariate linear regression analyses: five independent variables were investigated in association with the difference in MET (ΔMET was regarded as the dependent variable). Regression analysis showed that the predictive model provided a good fit to the data with a significant F value (F(5), $p<0.001$), and the five predictors explained 76% of the difference in MET values ($R^2 = 0.76$). The results in Table 9 indicated that the change in red blood cell aggregation index (LORCA) (standardized $\beta = -0.337$), WBV (standardized $\beta = 0.406$) and red blood cell deformability at 5,33 Pa shear stress (standardized $\beta = -0.197$) values were significant independent variables of the regression model and the most strongly related to the variation of the MET values. Furthermore, the analyses revealed a strong independent predictive association between the ΔAI (LORCA), ΔWBV as well as Δdeformability and the dependent variables.

Although gender specific subgroup analyses was made regarding hemorheological, laboratory chemistry and exercise tolerance parameters, but no differences were observed. Data are not shown.

In the course of the study, there was no drop out, and no noteworthy CV event or unplanned hospitalization occurred. Analysis of the FIS data revealed a significant decline in the symptoms of fatigue in the physical [$chi^2(2) = 6.12$, $p<0.05$], the psycho-social [$chi^2(2) = 7.09$, $p<0.05$] and in the cognitive domain [$chi^2(2) = 8.85$, $p<0.05$]. More specifically, patients' perception of their physical, cognitive, and social functional limitations caused by fatigue declined significantly over the course of the physical training period.

Discussion

The fundamental problem of CAD patients can not be solved completely via revascularization techniques (percutaneous coronary intervention or a coronary artery bypass graft), effective and long-term lifestyle changes are at least as vital as other therapeutic procedures [24]. Recent studies such as EuroAction [25] and GOSPEL [26] have indicated that regular long-term physical activity results in more benefit than short-term training programs as regards the prognosis of cardiac patients. A physical training program is strongly recommended by the ESC and the AHA/ACC as well [1,2,3].

Aerobic exercise training is defined as a sub-category of physical activity in which planned, structured, and repetitive bodily movements are performed to maintain or improve physical fitness [1]. According to the recommendations of ESC guidelines regarding physical activity and CAD prevention [1,2], patients with previous acute myocardial infarction, CABG, PCI, stable angina pectoris, or stable chronic heart failure should undergo exercise training (I (A) strong evidence) [27], which should be performed at least 30 minutes long (preferably 45–60 minutes) and 3–5 times weekly, in form of an aerobic exercise training (I (B) evidence) [1,2], at 70–85% of the peak heart rate [2] or 40–60% of heart rate reserve [2] or 10/20–14/20 of the Borg Scale [16].

It is a long revealed fact that impaired hemorheological factors are CV risk factors, and the improvement of these could result in lower CV risk and mortality [8–12]. The triphasic association of hemorheology and physical exercise is as well identified by now. Still, the possible connections between hemorheology and long-term aerobic physical training in a relatively large ischemic heart disease population have not been investigated previously. A systematic literature search in PubMed with the keywords

Table 5. Changes in erythrocyte aggregation measured with LORCA aggregometers and with standard 40% Hct after the 12- and 24-week ambulatory exercise training of ischemic heart disease patients.

hemorheological parameters	mean ± SD	p value
LORCA AI	65.26±5.9 vs. 64.04±6.9 vs. 63.9±5.4	0.01
LORCA γ (1/s)	128.6±37.4 vs. 116.17±41.4 vs. 123.1±37.9	0.07

N = 79; values are baseline, 12 week and 24 week means ± SD. Levels of significance and p values are also shown.

Table 6. Changes in erythrocyte deformability parameters EI_{max} and $SS_{1/2}$ calculated by the Lineweaver-Burke nonlinear equation after the 12- and 24-week ambulatory exercise training of ischemic heart disease patients.

hemorheological parameters	mean ± SD	p value
EI_{max}	0.669±0.16 vs. 0.674±0.01 vs. 0.673±0.1	0.04
$SS_{1/2}$ (mPas)	2.104±0.57 vs. 1.831±0.2 vs. 1.769±0.4	0.0004

N = 79; values are baseline, 12 week and 24 week means ± SD. Levels of significance and p values are also shown.

hemorheology, physical activity, physical exercise, cardiovascular diseases and atherosclerosis, identified only 14 nonrandomized controlled studies from the past 25 years in which original data were used to determine changes in hemorheological parameters, mostly in healthy volunteers and athletes (9 publications), but also partially in patients with CV diseases (5 publications), participating in short-term (10–12 weeks) exercise training [28] (Tables S1 in File S1, Table S2 in File S2, Table S3 in File S3). Investigations involving healthy volunteers have proven that short-term physical activity has acute effects on the hemorheological parameters, including increases in Hct and WBV due to the fluid shift, water loss and release of sequestered red blood cells from the spleen [29–31]. In contrast, long-term training causes autohemodilution, resulting in reduction of PV and WBV [29]. On the other hand, the findings of red blood cell aggregation and deformability studies are not concordant. Some investigations dealing with long-term physical activity performed by healthy volunteers, suggested the deterioration of rheological factors [32–34], whereas others reached the opposite conclusion [35–37]. These discrepancies might be explained by differences in training periods (short,- or long-term), study designs [29,31,35], methods [32,33,36,37], the selected populations [31,33,34] and the exercise performed (cycling vs. running) [29,31].

Only few studies have focused on the effects of exercise on hemorheological factors in CV patients [28]. Several investigations have shown that acute training evokes increases in PV and fibrinogen [38]. *Levine et al.* were unable to demonstrate any hemorheological effects after a 10-week CR training [39], but *Church et al.* reported reductions in WBV and PV after a 12-week CR program [40]. In our present study, we investigated whether we could demonstrate any hemorheological changes in ischemic heart disease patients participating in a 24-week ambulatory CR training program. The results pointed to a slight decrease in Hct, while significant decreases were observed in WBV and PV, resulting in a significantly increased Hct/WBV ratio. The red blood cell aggregation indices and the measured deformability parameters were also significantly enhanced at the end of the training program.

Although the blood flow of the coronary vessel system is primarily determined by hemodynamic factors (i.e. continuous changes in flow, extravascular pressure, perfusion pressure and shear rate during a cardiac cycle), under certain conditions (e.g. a flow decrease caused by vessel stenosis, especially in ischemic heart disease patients) the role of rheological parameters becomes important. The observed beneficial changes in the macrorheological parameters presented in this investigation (e.g. Hct and viscosity) presumably reduce the CV risk of ischemic heart disease patients [11,12,41,42].

In addition to the positive findings among macrorheological parameters, microrheological changes could also have a pivotal role in the development of better physical fitness. The diameter of the narrowest capillaries in the body (3–5 μm), found in the myocardium, is appreciably less than the resting diameter of a normal red blood cell (7–8 μm), which highlights the importance of the microrheological parameters (e.g. erythrocyte aggregation and deformability). Decreased red blood cell aggregation and improved deformability observed in our trial support capillary flow, especially in patients suffering from ischemic heart disease. In the background of increased deformability we could assume recently published data, which have stated that aerobic training with low lactate levels (as aerobic exercise) could enhance RBC deformability [43], which together with an increased Hct/WBV ratio indicate a better RBC oxygen transport effectiveness leads to a better oxygen supply of the myocardiocytes, and the working

Table 7. Changes in clinical chemistry after the 12- and 24-week ambulatory exercise training of ischemic heart disease patients.

clinical chemistry	mean ± SD	p value
glucose (mmol/l)	5.16±2.9 vs. 5.19±1.7 vs. 4.80±2.0	0.48
uric acid (umol/l)	336.39±55.85 vs. 327.17±82.68 vs. 312.88±95.1	0.006
total cholesterol (mmol/l)	4.99±1.1 vs. 4.87±1.3 vs. 4.61±1.4	0.17
HDL (mmol/l)	1.40±0.3 vs. 1.39±0.4 vs. 1.33±0.5	0.53
LDL (mmol/l)	2.57±0.7 vs. 2.50±0.8 vs. 2.46±0.9	0.69
triglyceride (mmol/l)	1.70±0.8 vs. 1.56±0.7 vs. 1.46±0.8	0.017
hsCRP (mg/l)	6.02±2.3 vs. 2.98±2.4 vs. 3.04±2.5	0.0008
fibrinogen (g/l)	3.28±1.3 vs. 3.03±0.5 vs. 3.15±0.8	0.03
IL 6 (pg/ml)	3.95±1.87 vs. 1.88±1.24	0.06
TNF α (pg/ml)	11.53±5.9 vs. 10.21±2.95	0.11

N = 79; values are baseline, 12 week and 24 week means ± SD. Levels of significance and p values are also shown.

Table 8. Changes in exercise tolerability parameters (MET and treadmill time) and BMI as well as lean body mass index after the 24-week ambulatory exercise training of ischemic heart disease patients.

treadmill	mean ± SD	p value
MET	7.93±2.4 vs. 9.87±5.7	<0.001
treadmill time (min)	7.68±2.17 vs. 9.02±2.18	0.001
BMI (kg/m^2)	28.16±5.53 vs. 25.45±4.1	<0.001
lean body mass index (kg)	51.71±6.6 vs. 52.78±9.4	0.09

N = 79; values are baseline and 24 week means ± SD. Levels of significance and p values are also shown.

muscles (43, 44). According to a lately observed phenomenon, cerebral and muscle tissue oxygenation indicis (TOI) measured by NIRS are positively correlated with Hct/WBV ratio in sickle-cell patients (SC and SS patients) comparing to healthy volunteers, which could also support our findings [45]. Thus, our results may suggest that cardiac patients could achieve a condition of "hemorheological fitness" characterized by improved tissue perfusion, better oxygen delivery and lower vascular resistance [28,43,44,45] by participating in a physical training program for 24 weeks.

Furthermore, all hemorheological alterations may also contribute to the better exercise tolerability proved by the treadmill test parameter MET and the treadmill time. Moreover, the multivariate linear regression analyses showed that changes in red blood cell deformability, aggregation and WBV are independent predictors of the positive changes in MET. These results are in accordance with the above mentioned findings about improving RBC deformability and Hct/WBV ratio since they have a pivotal role in the enhancement of capillary blood flow, as well as in the oxygen supply of the myocardiocytes and the working muscles during exercise [43,44,45]. Beneath better physical tolerance, the improvement of MET by 1 value could reduce the risk of all-cause and CV mortality by 13% and 15%, respectively [46,47].

Of the clinical chemistry indicators, uric acid, triglyceride, hsCRP and fibrinogen underwent significant decreases during our study. Although we are aware that these biomarkers are considered to display only low specificity in a CV risk assessment and are easily influenced by common inflammatory diseases, our data suggest that regular long-term physical activity might exert a favorable effect on the inflammation status of patients with CAD. Further overproduction of proinflammatory cytokines such as IL-6 or TNF-α could be a marker of chronic inflammation leading to provoked and accelerated atherosclerosis [48,49], with a higher risk of CV events and mortality [50]. Our data demonstrated an almost significant decreases in IL-6 and TNF-α levels, suggesting that a longer training program might be required to achieve significant reductions in these parameters.

Interestingly, no significant change was observed in the fasting glucose. Our findings in case of glucose levels are supported by recent publication; authors did not observed any effect on the glycemic control caused by exercise training in 16 aged, female patients with type 2 diabetes mellitus neither with weekly 2 times for 60 minutes nor with weekly 4 times for 30 minutes [51]. Although the same paper described the beneficial hemorheological effects (decreased RBC aggregation and increased RBC deformability) of the mentioned training protocol [51].

However total cholesterol and LDL cholesterol levels did not change during the trial, triglyceride and uric acid levels decreased significantly by the end of the training program. It is well known that hypertriglyceridemia is a significant independent CV risk factor [52,53] and a recently published metaanalysis concluded that an elevated serum uric acid level should be considered as a risk factor for CV mortality [54]. The significant reductions in triglyceride and uric acid levels in our study may reflect a better metabolic state evoked by regular physical activity.

Beside laboratory parameters, both overweight and obesity are associated with an elevated risk of death in CAD and of all-cause mortality [55–57]. The BMI was significantly decreased by the end of the 24-week exercise training in our study. Although the results of the multivariate linear regression model indicated that the positive change in functional capacity is not influenced by the reduction in BMI. Accordingly, the better physical exercise tolerance can not be explained merely by the decreases in BMI and obesity. The beneficial effects of the physical activity generally on all the measured CV risk factors, including the hemorheological factors, must also be involved.

Moreover, CAD is often accompanied by an increased subjective feeling of fatigue (i.e. a feeling of physical tiredness and a lack of energy) and this might have a serious detrimental impact on a wide variety of everyday functions, including physical, mental and social functioning [58]. Our psychological results

Table 9. Results of the multivariate linear regression analyses after the 24-week ambulatory exercise training of ischemic heart disease patients; N = 79.

predictor (pre and post data)	standardized β	p value (p<0.05)
Δ whole blood viscosity (4.35 vs. 4.08)	0.406	0.001
Δ plasma viscosity (1.27 vs. 1.14)	−0.025	0.84
Δ LORCA aggregation index (66.67 vs. 62.25)	−0.337	0.011
Δ BMI (28.16 vs. 25.45)	−0.197	0,08
Δ elongation index (5.33Pa) (0.490 vs. 0.510)	−0.157	0.015

showed a significant amelioration as concerns the FIS physical and psycho-social aspects, indicating an improvement in the quality of life among our ischemic heart disease patients.

Our study was designed as a self-control study, as our working group have already proved the worsening of the hemorheological factors in patients with stable CAD, even if these patients have received correct drug therapy, but have not attended at any CR program [41,42]. Kesmarky et al. have observed significant deterioration in WBV and Hct as well as in fibrinogen levels, along with an increase of PV, 6 months after a percutaneous coronary angioplasty [41]. In accordance, Marton et al. described the same significant increase in WBV, Hct and PV in ischemic heart disease patients 1 year after their myocardial infarction [42].

Conclusions

Our study has revealed new data regarding the effects of a long-term ambulatory CR training program on stable CAD patients. Besides the anticipated improvement in functional capacity and the reduction in BMI, the regular, moderate-intensity, long-term physical activity led to favorable hemorheological changes, decreased level of inflammation and improvements in certain metabolic parameters, such as the triglyceride and uric acid contents, suggesting that these parameters may play important part in the positive effects of regular physical activity in patients with CAD.

Supporting Information

Table S1 Publications relating to hemorheological alterations induced by acute exercise training programs in healthy volunteers.

Table S2 Publications relating to hemorheological alterations induced by short-term exercise training programs in healthy volunteers.

Table S3 Publications relating to hemorheological alterations induced by long-term exercise training programs in patients with cardiovascular diseases.

Author Contributions

Conceived and designed the experiments: BS AN BM AC KT ES. Performed the experiments: BS AN AT MR BM AC. Analyzed the data: BS AN AC. Contributed reagents/materials/analysis tools: IC KT ES. Wrote the paper: BS MR AC IC KT ES.

References

1. Piepoli MF, Corra U, Benzer W, Bjarnason-Wehrens B, Dendale P, et al. (2010) Secondary prevention through cardiac rehabilitation: physical activity counselling and exercise training. Eur Heart J 31: 1967–1976.
2. Perk J, De Backer G, Gohlke H, Graham I, Reiner Z, et al. (2012) European Guidelines on cardiovascular disease prevention in clinical practice (version 2012). Eur Heart J 33: 1635–1701.
3. Eckel RH, Jakicic JM, Ard JD, de Jesus JM, Houston Miller N, et al. (2013) 2013 AHA/ACC Guideline on Lifestyle Management to Reduce Cardiovascular Risk: A Report of the American College of Cardiology/American Heart Association Task Force on Practice Guidelines. Circ. Epub ahead of print 12 Nov DOI: 10.1161/01.cir.0000437740.48606.d1
4. Van de Werf F, Bax J, Betriu A, Blomstrom-Lundqvist C, Crea F, et al. (2008) Management of Acute Myocardial Infarction in patients presenting with ST-segment elevation. The Task Force on the Management of Acute Myocardial Infarction of the European Society of Cardiology. Eur Heart J 29: 2909–2945.
5. Bassand JP, Hamm CW, Ardissino D, Boersma E, Budaj A, et al. (2007) Guidelines for the diagnosis and treatment of non-ST-segment elevation acute coronary syndromes. Task Force for Diagnosis and Treatment of Non-ST-Segment Elevation Acute Coronary Syndromes of European Society of Cardiology. Eur Heart J 28: 1598–1660.
6. Antman EM, Hand M, Armstrong PW, Bates ER, Green LA, et al. (2008) 2007 focused update of the ACC/AHA 2004 Guidelines for the Management of Patients With ST-Elevation Myocardial Infarction: a report of the American College of Cardiology/American Heart Association Task Force on Practice Guidelines (Writing Group to Review New Evidence and Update the ACC/AHA 2004 Guidelines for the Management of Patients With ST-Elevation Myocardial Infarction). J Am Coll Cardiol 51: 210–247.
7. Anderson JL, Adams CD, Antman EM, Bridges CR, Califf RM, et al. (2007) ACC/AHA 2007 guidelines for the management of patients with unstable angina/non-ST-elevation myocardial infarction: a report of the American College of Cardiology/American Heart Association Task Force on Practice Guidelines (Writing Committee to Revise the 2002 Guidelines for the Management of Patients With Unstable Angina/Non-ST-Elevation Myocardial Infarction): developed in collaboration with the American College of Emergency Physicians, American College of Physicians, Society for Academic Emergency Medicine, Society for Cardiovascular Angiography and Interventions, and Society of Thoracic Surgeons. J Am Coll Cardiol 50: 1–157.
8. Carter C, McGee D, Reed D, Yano K, Stemmermann G (1983) Hematocrit and the risk of coronary heart disease: The Honolulu heart program. Am Heart J 105: 674–679.
9. Kannel WB, D'Agostino RB, Belanger AJ (1987) Fibrinogen, cigarette smoking, and risk of cardiovascular disease: insights from the Framingham study. Am Heart J 113: 1006–1010.
10. Lowe GD, Smith WCS, Tunstall-Pedoe HD, Crombie IK, Lennieet SE, et al. (1988) Cardiovascular risk and haemorheology - results from the Scottish heart health study and the MONICA project, Glasgow. Clin Hemorheol Microcirc 8: 517–524.
11. Baskurt OK (2007) Mechanisms of blood rheology alterations. In: Baskurt OK, Hardeman MR, Rampling MW, Meiselman HJ, editors. Handbook of Hemorheology and Hemodynamics. Amsterdam: IOS Press. pp.170–190.
12. Toth K, Kesmarky G (2007) Clinical significance of hemorheological alterations. In: Baskurt OK, Hardeman MR, Rampling MW, Meiselman HJ, editors. Handbook of Hemorheology and Hemodynamics. Amsterdam: IOS Press. pp. 392–433.
13. Montalescot G, Sechtem U, Achenbach S, Andreotti F, Arden C, et al. (2013) 2013 ESC guidelines on the management of stable coronary artery disease. The Task Force on the management of stable coronary artery disease of the European Society of Cardiology. Eur Heart J 34: 2949–3003.
14. Dickstein K, Cohen-Solal A, Filippatos G, McMurray JJ, Ponikowski P, et al. (2008) ESC Guidelines for the diagnosis and treatment of acute and chronic heart failure 2008: the Task Force for the Diagnosis and Treatment of Acute and Chronic Heart Failure 2008 of the European Society of Cardiology. Developed in collaboration with the Heart Failure Association of the ESC (HFA) and endorsed by the European Society of Intensive Care Medicine (ESICM). Eur Heart J 29: 2388–2442.
15. Hunt SA, Abraham WT, Chin MH, Feldman AM, Francis GS, et al. (2005) American College of Cardiology, American Heart Association Task Force on Practice Guidelines, American College of Chest Physicians, International Society for Heart, Lung Transplantation, Heart Rhythm Society. ACC/AHA guideline update for the diagnosis and management of chronic heart failure in the adult: summary article: a report of the American College of Cardiology/American Heart Association Task Force on Practice Guidelines. Circ 112: 1825–1852.
16. Borg G (1970) Perceived exertion as an indicator of somatic stress. Scandinavian journal of rehabilitation medicine. 2: 92–98.
17. Ziljstra WG (1958) Syllectometry, a new method for studying rouleaux formation of red blood cells. Acta Phys Pharm Neerl 7: 153–154.
18. Bauersachs RM, Wenby RB, Meiselman HJ (1989) Determination of specific red blood cell aggregation indices via an automated system. Clin Hemorheol Microcirc 9: 1–25.
19. Dobbe JG, Streekstra GJ, Hardeman MR, Ince C, Grimbergen CA (2002) The measurement of the distribution of red blood cell deformability using an automated rheoscope. Cytometry 50: 313–325.
20. Baskurt OK, Meiselman HJ (2013) Data reduction methods for ektacytometry in clinical hemorheology. Clin Hemorheol Microcirc 54: 99–107.
21. Ekman I, Ehrenberg A (2002) Fatigue in chronic heart failure—does gender make a difference? Eur J Cardiovasc Nurs 1: 77–82.
22. Fisk JD, Ritvo PG, Ross L, Haase DA, Marrie TJ, et al. (1994) Measuring the functional impact of fatigue: initial validation of the fatigue impact scale. Clin Infect Dis 18: S79–S83.
23. Hume R (1966) Prediction of lean body mass from height and weight. J Clin Pathol 19: 389–91.
24. Ford ES, Ajani UA, Croft JB, Critchley JA, Labarthe DR, et al. (2007) Explaining the decrease in U.S. deaths from coronary disease, 1980–2000. N Engl J Med 356: 2388–2398.

25. Wood DA, Kotseva K, Connolly S, Jennings C, Mead A, et al. (2008) Nurse-coordinated multidisciplinary, family-based cardiovascular disease prevention programme (EUROACTION) for patients with coronary heart disease and asymptomatic individuals at high risk of cardiovascular disease: a paired, cluster-randomised controlled trial. Lancet 371: 1999–2012.
26. Giannuzzi P, Temporelli PL, Marchioli R, Maggioni AP, Balestroni G, et al. (2008) Global secondary prevention strategies to limit event recurrence after myocardial infarction: results of the GOSPEL study, a multicenter, randomized controlled trial from the Italian Cardiac Rehabilitation Network. Arch Intern Med 168: 2194–2204.
27. Taylor RS, Brown A, Ebrahim S, Jolliffe J, Noorani H, et al. (2004) Exercise-based rehabilitation for patients with coronary heart disease: systematic review and meta-analysis of randomized controlled trials. Am J Med 116: 682–692.
28. Connes P, Simmonds MJ, Brun JF, Baskurt OK (2013) Exercise hemorheology: Classical data, recent findings and unresolved issues. Clin Hemorheol Microcirc 53: 187–199.
29. Brun JF, Khaled S, Raynaud E, Bouix D, Micallef JP, et al. (1998) The triphasic effects of exercise on blood rheology: Which relevance to physiology and pathophysiology? Clin Hemorheol Microcirc 19: 89–104.
30. Connes P (2010) Hemorheology and exercise: Effects of warm environments and potential consequences for sickle cell trait carriers. Scand J Med Sci Sports 20: S48–S52.
31. Ernst E (1987) Influence of regular physical activity on blood rheology. Eur Heart J 8: 59–62.
32. Kilic-Toprak E, Ardic F, Erken G, Unver-Kocak F, Kucukatay V, et al. (2012) Hemorheological responses to progressive resistance exercise training in healthy young males. Med Sci Monit 18: CR351–CR360.
33. Cakir-Atabek H, Atsak P, Gunduz N, Bor-Kucukatay M (2009) Effects of resistance training intensity on deformability and aggregation of red blood cells. Clin Hemorheol Microcirc 41: 251–261.
34. Tripette J, Hardy-Dessources MD, Beltan E, Sanouiller A, Bangou J, et al. (2011) Endurance running trial in tropical environment: A blood rheological study. Clin Hemorheol Microcirc 47: 261–268.
35. Yalcin O, Erman A, Muratli S, Bor-Kucukatay M, Baskurt OK (2003) Time course of hemorheological alterations after heavy anaerobic exercise in untrained human subjects. J Appl Physiol 94: 997–1002.
36. Connes P, Bouix D, Py G, Prefaut C, Mercier J, et al. (2004) Opposite effects of in vitro lactate on erythrocyte deformability in athletes and untrained subjects. Clin Hemorheol Microcirc 31: 311–318.
37. Connes P, Caillaud C, Py G, Mercier J, Hue O, et al. (2007) Maximal exercise and lactate do not change red blood cell aggregation in well trained athletes. Clin Hemorheol Microcirc 36: 319–326.
38. Lee KW, Blann AD, Ingram J, Jolly K, Lip GY, et al. (2005) Incremental shuttle walking is associated with activation of haemostatic and haemorheological markers in patients with coronary artery disease: The Birmingham rehabilitation uptake maximization study (BRUM). Heart 91: 1413–1417.
39. Levine GN, O'Malley C, Balady GJ (1995) Exercise training and blood viscosity in patients with ischemic heart disease. Am J Cardiol 76: 80–81.
40. Church TS, Lavie CJ, Milani RV, Kirby GS (2002) Improvements in blood rheology after cardiac rehabilitation and exercise training in patients with coronary heart disease. Am Heart J 143: 349–355.
41. Késmárky G, Tóth K, Vajda G, Habon L, Halmosi R, et al. (2001) Hemorheological and oxygen free radical associated alterations during and after percutaneous transluminal coronary angioplasty. Clin Hemorheol Microcirc 24: 33–41.
42. Marton Zs, Horvath B, Alexy T, Kesmarky G, Gyevnar Z, et al. (2003) Follow-up of hemorheological parameters and platelet aggregation in patients with acute coronary syndromes. Clin Hemorheol Microcirc 29: 81–94.
43. Brun JF, Varlet-Marie E, Romaina AJ, Guiraudou M, Raynaud de Mauverger E (2013) Exercise hemorheology: Moving from old simplistic paradigms to a more complex picture. Clin Hemorheol Microcirc 55: 15–27.
44. Smith MM, Lucas AR, Hamlin RR, Devor ST (2013) Associations among hemorheological factors and maximal oxygen consumption. Is there a role for blood viscosity in explaining athletic performance? Clin Hemorheol Microcirc (Epub ahead of pront) DOI:10.3233/CH-131708
45. Waltz X, Hardy-Dessourcesa MD, Lemonne N, Mougenel D, Lalanne-Mistrih ML, et al. (2014) Is there a relationship between the hematocrit-to-viscosity ratio and microvascular oxygenation in brain and muscle? Clin Hemorheol Microcirc (Epub ahead of print) DOI 10.3233/CH-131742
46. Kodama S, Saito K, Tanaka S, Maki M, Yachi Y, et al. (2009) Cardiorespiratory fitness as a quantitative predictor of all-cause mortality and cardiovascular events in healthy men and women: a meta-analysis. JAMA 301: 2024–2035.
47. Aktas MK, Ozduran V, Pothier CE, Lang R, Lauer MS (2004) Global risk scores and exercise testing for predicting all-cause mortality in a preventive medicine program. JAMA 292: 1462–1468.
48. Ross R (1999) Atherosclerosis-an inflammatory disease. N Engl J Med 340: 115–126.
49. Lowe GD, Welsh P, Rumley A (2011) Inflammatory cytokines and cardiovascular risk. In: Preedy VR and Hunter JR, editors. Cytokines. Jersey: St. Helier Science Publishers. pp. 235–250.
50. IL6R Genetics Consortium Emerging Risk Factors Collaboration (2012) Interleukin-6 receptor pathways in coronary heart disease: a collaborative meta-analysis of 82 studies. Lancet 79: 1205–1215.
51. Simmonds MJ, Minahan CL, Serre KR, Gass GC, Marshall-Gradisnik SM, et al. (2012) Preliminary findings in the heart rate variability and haemorheology response to varied frequency and duration of walking in women 65–74 yr with type 2 diabetes. Clin Hemorheol Microcirc 51: 87–99.
52. Sarwar N, Danesh J, Eiriksdottir G, Sigurdsson G, Wareham N, et al. (2007) Triglycerides and the risk of coronary heart disease: 10,158 incident cases among 262,525 participants in 29 Western prospective studies. Circ 115: 450–458.
53. Nordestgaard BG, Benn M, Schnohr P, Tybjaerg-Hansen A (2007) Nonfasting triglycerides and risk of myocardial infarction, ischemic heart disease, and death in men and women. JAMA 298: 299–308.
54. Zhao G, Huang L, Song M, Song Y (2013) Baseline serum uric acid level as a predictor of cardiovascular disease related mortality and all-cause mortality: A meta-analysis of prospective studies. Atherosclerosis 231: 61–68.
55. Whitlock G, Lewington S, Sherliker P, Clarke R, Emberson J, et al. (2009) Body-mass index and cause-specific mortality in 900 000 adults: collaborative analyses of 57 prospective studies. Lancet 373: 1083–1096.
56. Berrington de Gonzalez A, Hartge P, Cerhan JR, Flint AJ, Hannan L, et al. (2010) Body-mass index and mortality among 1.46 million white adults. N Engl J Med 363: 2211–2219.
57. Zheng W, McLerran DF, Rolland B, Zhang X, Inoue M, et al. (2011) Association between body-mass index and risk of death in more than 1 million Asians. N Engl J Med 364: 719–729.
58. Cossette S, Frasure-Smith N, Lesperance F (2001) Clinical implications of a reduction in psychological distress on cardiac prognosis in patients participating in a psychosocial intervention program. Psychosom Med 63: 257–266.

10

Association between Serum Irisin Levels and Non-Alcoholic Fatty Liver Disease in Health Screen Examinees

Eun Sung Choi[1], Mi Kyung Kim[1], Min Kyung Song[2], Jeong Min Kim[1], Eun Soo Kim[1], Woo Jin Chung[1], Kyung Sik Park[1], Kwang Bum Cho[1], Jae Seok Hwang[1], Byoung Kuk Jang[1,3]*

1 Department of Internal Medicine, Keimyung University School of Medicine, Daegu, South Korea, **2** Department of Food Science and Nutrition, Graduate School, Keimyung University, Daegu, South Korea, **3** Institute for Cancer Research, Keimyung University, Daegu, South Korea

Abstract

Irisin is a recently found myokine that aids obesity control and improves glucose homeostasis by acting on white adipose tissue cells and increases total energy consumption. The aim of this study was to evaluate serum irisin levels in patients with non-alcoholic fatty liver disease (NAFLD) and to compare these levels with those of normal controls. Among 595 health screen examinees who had visited our institute between January 2013 to March 2013, 355 patients (84 NAFLD patients and 271 normal controls) were enrolled depending on whether they gave written informed consents and their history of alcohol intake, blood tests, and abdominal ultrasonographic findings. Age; sex; laboratory test parameters; homeostasis model assessment-insulin resistance; and levels of leptin, adiponectin, and irisin were assessed. Serum irisin levels (ng/ml) were significantly higher in the NAFLD group than in normal controls (63.4±32.6 vs. 43.0±29.7, $p<0.001$) and higher in the mild fatty liver group than in the moderate-to-severe fatty liver group (68.3±38.2 vs. 56.6±21.2, $p<0.001$). Additionally, serum irisin levels were not different between the non-obese and obese groups (48.4±34.2 vs. 45.8±22.9, $p=0.492$); however, the levels were significantly lowest in normal controls and highest in the mild fatty liver group in the non-obese (44.9±31.7 vs. 73.1±48.5 vs 59.7±18.0, $p<0.001$) and obese groups (35.0±17.0 vs. 62.9±21.2 vs. 54.6±23.3, $p<0.001$). Serum irisin levels were significantly higher in NAFLD patients, which is not consistent with the results of previously published studies. Therefore, more studies are needed to confirm the role of irisin in NAFLD.

Editor: Yanqiao Zhang, Northeast Ohio Medical University, United States of America

Funding: This work was supported by the research promoting grant from the Keimyung University Dongsan Medical Center in 2012. The funders had no role in study design, data collection and analysis, decision to publish, or preparation of the manuscript.

Competing Interests: The authors have declared that no competing interests exist.

* Email: jangha106@dsmc.or.kr

Introduction

Non-alcoholic fatty liver disease (NAFLD) involves a spectrum of hepatic diseases from hepatic steatosis to steatohepatitis and cirrhosis. While the percentage of NAFLD patients who progress to cirrhosis is low (5%), NAFLD is the most common cause of chronic liver disease because of the rapidly increasing prevalence of obesity [1]. The liver stores energy as glycogen and stores digested triglycerides in the form of fatty acids. Under stressful conditions such as obesity, excessive nutrition, and drug-induced liver injury, hepatocytes collect excess lipids; the prolonged storage of lipids leads to NAFLD [2].

NAFLD can be improved through weight reduction and exercise, without medical therapy [3]; however, the mechanism of improvement remains unknown even though many studies have been conducted to address this issue. Recently, irisin, a newly found myokine, has been recognized as an important factor in disease improvement. Irisin that is secreted in muscles during or after exercise expedites energy homeostasis and metabolism, improving obesity and glucose intolerance [3–5]. A laboratory study found that irisin induces white adipose cells to consume fat and product energy, and ultimately aids weight reduction and glucose intolerance [6]. Recent studies have shown that in patients with fatty liver disease, serum irisin levels are lower than that of healthy individuals [7].

Therefore, in this study, we examined serum irisin levels in NAFLD patients and healthy individuals and determined whether serum irisin levels are lower in NAFLD patients.

Materials and Methods

Between January 2013 and March 2013, we performed a prospective analysis of 595 health screen examinees who visited the Keimyung University Dongsan Medical Center in Daegu, Korea. Viral hepatitis patients with positive serologic markers for hepatitis B or C, liver cirrhosis, malignant tumor, or other hepatobiliary diseases were excluded. One interviewer investigated the history of weekly alcohol intake, and 355 subjects who consumed <140 g of alcohol in case of women and <210 g of alcohol in case of men, each week, were enrolled. Among them, 84 examinees were diagnosed with NAFLD, and 271 examinees were designated as the normal controls. The diagnosis of NAFLD is based on a history of no or little weekly alcohol intake (<140 g for women and <210 g for men), the presence of hepatic steatosis by imaging, and the ruling out of other hepatic diseases [8]. We assessed several parameters such as age, sex, body measurements, and laboratory test parameters; abdominal ultrasonography was performed to verify the presence of steatosis and assess the degree of steatosis. We mainly used abdominal ultrasonography as the imaging tool, and a radiology expert carried out and registered the ultrasonographic results. Additionally, we analyzed serum irisin, leptin, and adiponectin levels with the ELISA kit (R&D, Minneapolis, MN, USA). We triple-checked these parameters and used mean values for analysis. We used the homeostasis model assessment-insulin resistance (HOMA-IR) value as the indicator of insulin resistance calculated using the following formula: fasting blood glucose (mg/dL) × insulin (mU/L)/(18×22.5) [9]. Furthermore, we examined liver function parameters and serum cholesterol levels, body mass index (BMI), abdominal circumference, thigh circumference, waist circumference, and hip circumference. We calculated BMI using the following formula: subject's weight (kg)/height $(m)^2$. We applied the term "obese group" to subjects whose BMI was>25, and "non-obese group" to subjects whose BMI was <25, according to the World Health Organization.

Based on abdominal ultrasonography results, subjects were categorized as the control group, mild fatty liver group, and moderate-to-severe fatty liver group. We compared the demographic characteristics, body measurements, body composition, and laboratory study results between the groups. The grade of steatosis was assessed by a single radiologist. The normal liver parenchyma has echogenicity equal to or slightly greater than that of the renal cortex. In fatty liver disease, the liver shows higher echogenicity than the renal cortex because of fatty infiltration. In mild fatty liver disease, only the echogenicity increases; in moderate fatty liver disease, the walls of the portal vein branches are indistinct; and in severe fatty liver disease, the diaphragmatic outline is indistinct [8]. We applied the term "mild fatty liver group" to subjects whose ultrasonographic finding was consistent with mild fatty liver, and "moderate-to-severe fatty liver group" to subjects whose ultrasonographic findings were consistent with moderate and severe fatty liver. Metabolic syndrome was diagnosed when three or more of the following criteria were met: 1) abdominal circumference ≥90 cm for men and ≥85 cm for women, 2) triglyceride (TG) level ≥150 mg/dL, 3) decreased high-density lipoprotein (HDL) at <40 mg/dL for men and < 50 mg/dL for women, 4) blood pressure ≥130/85 mmHg, and 5) fasting blood sugar (FBS) level ≥150 mg/dL, or history of diabetes mellitus (DM)[9].

Ethics statement

The study protocol was approved by the institutional review board of Keimyung University Dongsan Hospital (IRB Number 12-221).

Statistical analysis

Statistical analyses were performed with SPSS software version 18.0 for Windows (IBM, NY, USA). Continuous variables are expressed as mean ± SD. Categorical data were compared using the χ^2 test. The Mann-Whitney U test and Kruskal-Wallis test were used to compare differences in continuous variables between each group. The correlation of irisin levels with other parameters was analyzed using Spearman correlation analysis. For all analyses, a *p* value ≤0.05 was considered to indicate statistical significance.

Results

Characteristics of study participants

Comparative data of the study groups are presented in Table 1. The mean age of the NAFLD group was significantly higher than that of the control group ($p = 0.004$), and the proportion of women was significantly higher in the control group ($p<0.001$). As expected, the mean BMI was significantly higher in the NAFLD group ($p<0.001$). Furthermore, there were statistically significant differences in FBS, insulin, HOMA, leptin, adiponectin, total cholesterol, TG, HDL, low-density lipoprotein (LDL), C-reactive protein (CRP), aspartate aminotransferase (AST), and alanine aminotransferase (ALT) levels between the two groups.

Serum irisin levels according to the study group

The serum irisin level in the NAFLD group was significantly higher than that of the control group ($p<0.001$) (Table 1). According to the severity of steatosis, the serum irisin level was highest in the mild fatty liver group and lowest in the control group ($p<0.001$) (Figure 1, Table 2). Furthermore, other parameters such as serum levels of FBS, insulin, HOMA, leptin, total cholesterol, TG, LDL, CRP, AST, and ALT; systolic blood pressure; and diastolic systolic blood pressure were significantly higher in the moderate-to-severe fatty liver group than the mild fatty liver group and normal controls (Table 2). The adiponectin and HDL levels were significantly lower in the NAFLD group than the control group, especially in the moderate-to-severe fatty liver group ($p<0.001$). The waist and hip circumferences were higher in the NAFLD group, especially in the severe fatty liver group ($p< 0.001$) (Table 2).

Serum irisin levels according to the presence of obesity

Serum irisin levels (ng/ml) were not different between the non-obese and obese groups (48.4±34.2 vs. 45.8±22.9, $p = 0.492$) (Table 3). According to the severity of steatosis, the serum irisin level was lowest in normal controls and highest in the mild fatty liver group in the non-obese group (44.9±31.7 vs. 73.1±48.5 vs. 59.7±18.0, $p<0.001$). In the obese group (52 healthy controls and 46 NAFLD patients), the results were similar (35.0±17.0 vs. 62.9±21.2 vs. 54.6±23.3, $p<0.001$) (Figure 2, Table S1). According to the presence of obesity, in the control group, the serum irisin levels were significantly higher in the non-obese group than in the obese group (44.9±31.7 vs. 35.0±17.0, $p = 0.030$). On the other hand, in the NAFLD group including both the mild fatty liver group and the moderate-to-severe fatty liver group, the serum irisin level tended to be higher in the non-obese group than the obese group; however, the difference did not reach statistical significance (73.1±48.5 vs. 62.9±21.2, $p = 0.365$ and 59.7±18.0 vs. 54.6±23.3, $p = 0.505$) (Figure 2).

Serum irisin levels according to the presence of type 2 DM

Among the study subjects, there were 10 type 2 DM patients. When DM patients were excluded from the control group, serum irisin levels were still significantly higher in the NAFLD group than in the control group (63.4±32.6 vs. 43.0±29.9, $p<0.001$).

Serum irisin levels according to the presence of metabolic syndrome

There were 37 study subjects with metabolic syndrome: 17 (6.3%) in the control group and 20 (23.8%) in the NAFLD group. There was no difference in serum irisin levels between the subjects with and without metabolic syndrome (45.5±19.3 vs. 47.9±32.5,

Table 1. Baseline characteristics of the subjects according to the study group.

	Control Group (n = 271)	NAFLD Group (n = 84)	*p* value
Age (yr)	44.4±9.9	48.0±9.8	0.004
Sex (Female)	215	46	<0.001
DM(n)	6	4	0.256
Metabolic syndrome(n)	17	20	<0.001
Irisin (ng/ml)	43.0±29.7	63.4±32.6	<0.001
BMI (kg/m^2)	22.4±2.7	25.7±3.0	<0.001
FBS (mmol/L)	83.8±12.9	92.9±22.6	<0.001
Insulin (mIU/L)	3.5±2.4	6.4±4.1	<0.001
Homa	0.8±0.9	1.9±3.8	<0.001
Leptin (ng/ml)	2.2±1.5	3.3±3.0	0.002
Adiponectin (μg/ml)	6.2±3.9	3.6±2.5	<0.001
Systolic BP (mmHg)	115.8±17.7	124.5±14.9	<0.001
Diastolic BP (mmHg)	71.6±11.8	77.7±9.6	<0.001
Total cholesterol (mmol/L)	186.5±32.8	196.2±33.3	0.009
TG (mmol/L)	86.0±47.3	146.1±82.8	<0.001
HDL (mmol/L)	53.8±11.1	46.5±8.1	<0.001
LDL (mmol/L)	149.9±37.2	178.9±42.6	<0.001
CRP (mg/dL)	0.1±0.2	0.2±0.5	<0.001
AST (IU/L)	20.6±6.9	26.3±13.2	<0.001
ALT (IU/L)	17.4±8.1	33.4±24.9	<0.001
Waist (cm)	82.9±50.8	88.6±8.7	<0.001
Hip girth (cm)	90.6±7.6	96.0±6.9	<0.001
Weekly hours of exercise (min)	38.6±35.1	50.3±41.1	0.035

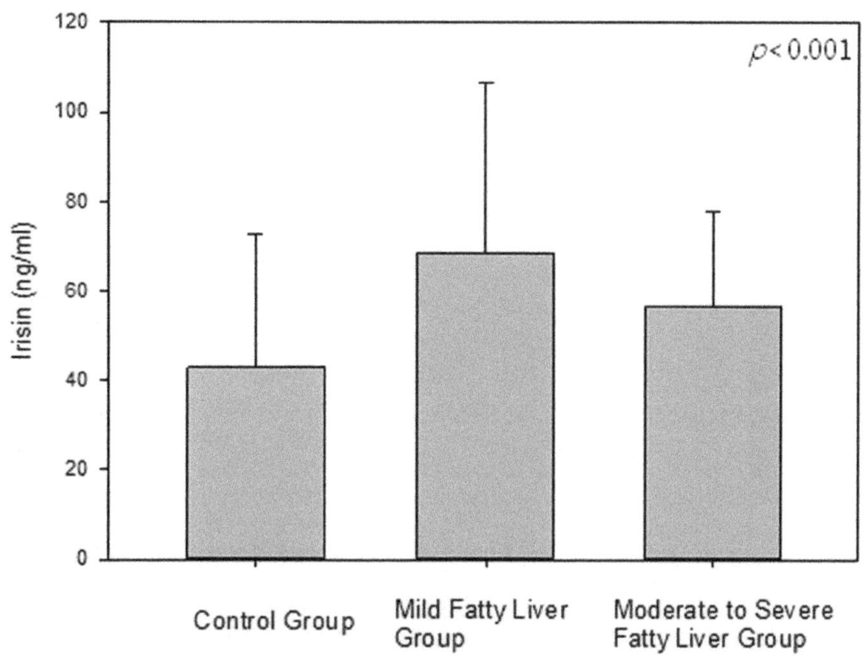

Figure 1. Serum irisin level in the control group and NAFLD group.

Table 2. Baseline characteristics of the subject according to steatosis severity.

	Control Group (n = 271)	Mild Fatty Liver Group (n = 47)	Moderate to Severe Fatty Liver Group (n = 37)	*p* value
Age (yr)	44.4±9.9	47.1±9.1	49.2±10.6	0.012
Sex (Female)	215	29	17	<0.001
Irisin (ng/ml)	43.0±29.7	68.3±38.2	56.6±21.3	<0.001
BMI (kg/m²)	22.4±2.7	24.9±2.5	26.6±3.5	<0.001
FBS (mmol/L)	83.8±12.9	90.8±18.2	95.7±27.3	<0.001
Insulin (mIU/L)	3.5±2.4	5.9±3.7	6.9±4.4	<0.001
Homa	0.8±0.9	1.3±0.9	2.6±5.7	<0.001
Leptin (ng/ml)	2.2±1.5	3.3±3.3	3.3±2.6	0.009
Adiponectin (µg/ml)	6.2±3.9	3.7±2.6	3.4±2.5	<0.001
Systolic BP (mmHg)	115.8±17.7	122.2±16.2	127.3±12.7	<0.001
Diastolic BP (mmHg)	71.6±11.8	76.3±10.5	79.4±8.0	<0.001
Total cholesterol (mmol/L)	186.5±32.8	196.2±30.0	196.3±37.5	0.032
TG (mmol/L)	86.0±47.3	140.9±93.7	152.7±67.2	<0.001
HDL (mmol/L)	53.8±11.1	47.6±8.7	45.0±7.1	<0.001
LDL (mmol/L)	149.9±37.2	176.8±43.0	181.8±42.5	<0.001
CRP (mg/dL)	0.1±0.2	0.1±0.1	0.3±0.8	<0.001
AST (IU/L)	20.6±6.9	23.2±12.1	30.3±13.6	<0.001
ALT (IU/L)	17.4±8.1	26.4±22.5	42.3±25.4	<0.001
Waist (cm)	82.9±50.8	87.0±7.7	90.6±9.6	<0.001
Hip girth (cm)	90.6±7.6	95.0±6.3	97.3±7.5	<0.001
Weekly hours of exercise (min)	38.6±35.1	47.4±29.2	55.0±55.8	0.107

$p = 0.663$). Even after the metabolic syndrome patients were excluded from the control group, serum irisin levels were still significantly higher in the NAFLD group than the control group (63.4±32.6 vs. 43.7±30.3, $p<0.001$)

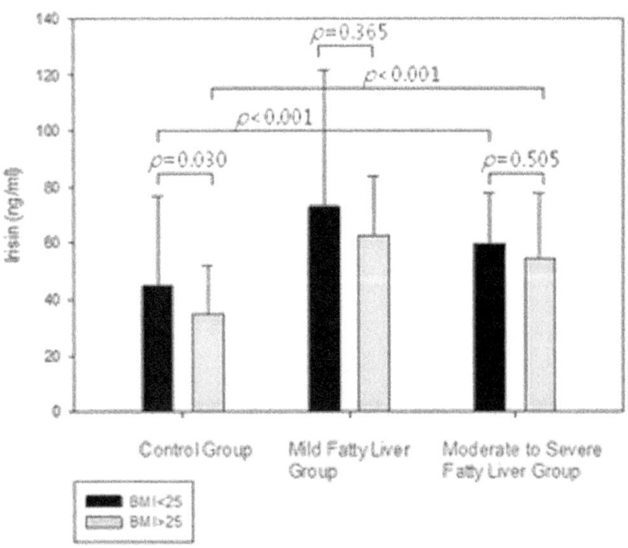

Figure 2. Serum irisin level of subjects according to obesity status.

Serum irisin levels according to the amount of exercise

The serum irisin level was not correlated with the quantity of exercise ($r = -0.083$, $p = 0.254$) (Table 4). Based on the weekly hours of exercise, we divided the subjects into three groups: the subjects in Group 1 (n = 195) did not exercise; those in Group 2 (n = 93) performed 1-h aerobic exercise weekly; and those in Group 3 (n = 67) performed>1-h aerobic exercise weekly. Serum irisin levels showed a slight decrease as the level of exercise increased (Group 1, 48.6±24.9; Group 2, 46.6±41.9; and Group 3, 46.5±32.4; $p = 0.055$). In Group 1, there were 42 NAFLD subjects (21.5%) and 44 obese subjects (22.6%). In Group 2, there were 20 NAFLD subjects (21.5%) and 28 obese subjects (30.1%). In Group 3, there were 22 NAFLD subjects (32.8%) and 26 obese subjects (38.8%).

Serum irisin levels according to the sex

Serum irisin levels tended to be higher in men than in women; however, there was no statistically significant difference between both sexes (52.9±32.7 vs. 45.8±30.9, $p = 0.063$). However, in both sex groups, there were significant differences between the sub-groups of NAFLD. In the male group, the serum irisin level was highest in the mild fatty liver group and lowest in the control group (49.5±38.2 vs. 62.9±23.6 vs. 53.5±18.7, $p = 0.008$). In the female group, the results were similar (41.3±26.9 vs. 71.6±45.1 vs. 60.5±24.3, $p<0.001$) (Figure 3, Table S2).

Association between the serum irisin level and other parameters

The correlation analysis revealed that the serum level of irisin correlated with that of insulin ($r = 0.204$, $p<0.001$) and HOMA-

Table 3. Baseline characteristics of the subject according to the obesity status.

	Non-obese Group (n = 257)	Obese Group (n = 98)	*p* value
Age (yr)	43.9±9.7	48.6±10.0	<0.001
Sex (Female)	205	56	<0.001
DM (n)	345	10	0.472
Metabolic syndrome (n)	318	37	<0.001
NAFLD (n)	271	84	<0.001
Irisin (ng/ml)	48.4±34.2	45.8±22.9	0.492
FBS (mmol/L)	83.6±11.3	92.0±23.6	0.001
insulin (mIU/L)	3.4±1.9	6.1±4.5	<0.001
Homa	0.7±0.5	1.8±3.8	0.005
Leptin (ng/ml)	2.1±1.5	3.3±2.8	<0.001
Adiponectin (μg/ml)	5.9±3.8	4.4±3.2	<0.001
Systolic BP (mmHg)	114.7±15.5	126.2±19.6	<0.001
Diastolic BP (mmHg)	71.2±10.7	77.6±12.4	<0.001
Total cholesterol (mmol/L)	185.5±32.4	197.7±33.4	0.002
TG (mmol/L)	90.1±54.7	126.8±74.9	<0.001
HDL (mmol/L)	53.6±11.2	47.9±8.8	<0.001
LDL (mmol/L)	149.9±37.4	175.0±42.5	<0.001
CRP (mg/dL)	0.1±0.3	0.1±0.3	0.188
AST (IU/L)	20.8±7.9	25.1±11.3	0.001
ALT (IU/L)	18.5±12.5	28.2±20.1	<0.001
Waist (cm)	79.7±7.3	87.9±9.5	<0.001
Hip girth (cm)	90.4±7.7	95.8±6.8	<0.001
Weekly hours of exercise (min)	38.6±35.1	50.3±41.1	0.008

Table 4. Correlations between serum irisin levels and other study parameters.

	r	r^2	%	*p* value
BMI (kg/m^2)	0.068	0.004624	0.4624	0.201
FBS (mmol/L)	0.054	0.002916	0.2916	0.313
Insulin (mIU/L)	0.204	0.041616	4.1616	<0.001
Homa	0.205	0.042025	4.2025	<0.001
Leptin (ng/ml)	−0.026	0.000676	0.0676	0.632
Adiponectin (μg/ml)	−0.086	0.007396	0.7396	0.109
Systolic BP (mmHg)	0.076	0.005776	0.5776	0.155
Diastolic BP (mmHg)	0.067	0.004489	0.4489	0.212
Total cholesterol (mmol/L)	−0.030	0.0009	0.09	0.580
TG (mmol/L)	0.086	0.007396	0.7396	0.107
HDL (mmol/L)	−0.055	0.003025	0.3025	0.307
LDL (mmol/L)	0.002	0.000004	0.0004	0.969
CRP (mg/dL)	0.065	0.004225	0.4225	0.221
AST (IU/L)	0.013	0.000169	0.0169	0.803
ALT (IU/L)	0.149	0.022201	2.2201	0.005
Waist (cm)	0.147	0.021609	2.1609	0.005
Hip girth (cm)	0.102	0.010404	1.0404	0.057
Weekly hours of exercise (min)	−0.083	0.006889	0.6889	0.254

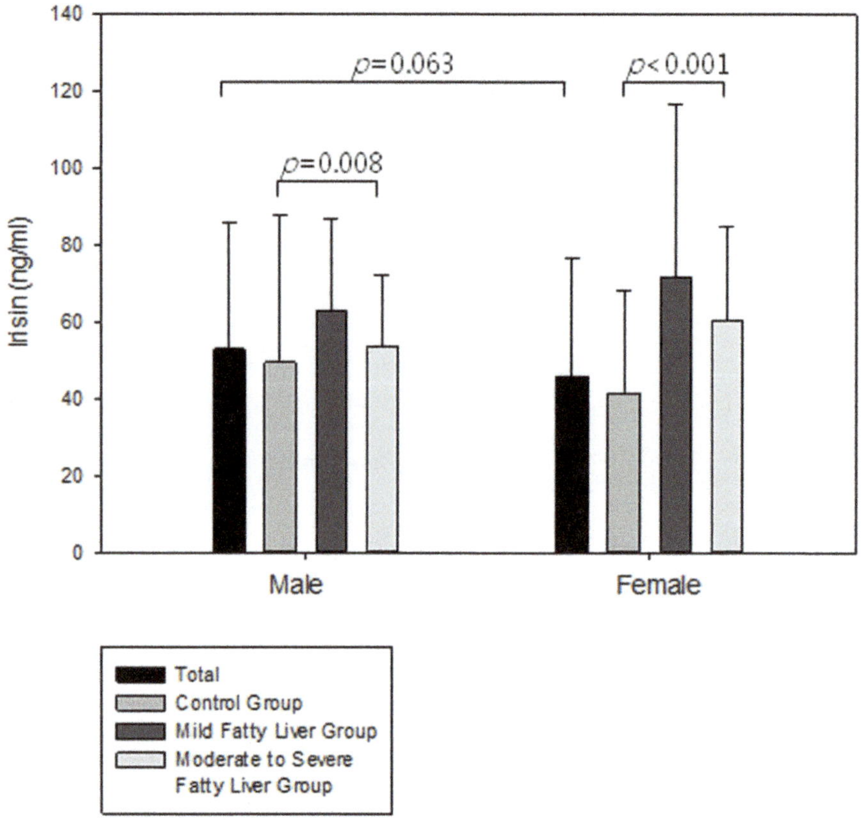

Figure 3. Serum irisin level according to sex.

IR (r = 0.205, $p<0.001$). However, when we analyzed the correlation in the control group, the mild fatty liver group and the moderate-to-severe fatty liver group separately, the serum level of irisin did not significantly correlate with that of insulin (r = 0.100, $p = 0.100$ vs. r = 0.186, $p = 0.210$ vs. r = −0.145, $p = 0.413$) and HOMA-IR (r = 0.092, $p = 0.130$ vs. r = 0.172, $p = 0.247$ vs. r = −0.079, $p = 0.657$). The serum irisin level did not correlate with other parameters such as leptin, adiponectin, triglyceride, AST, and ALT levels (Table 4).

Discussion

Exercise is known to be beneficial in humans because it activates the transcriptional coactivator PGC1α in muscles and stimulates the expression of Fndc5, a membrane protein that is cleaved and secreted as irisin [4]. Irisin was firstly recognized as a muscle-derived glycosylated polypeptide in 2012 by Bostrom et al. [4]. Irisin acts on white adipose cells, which stimulate UCP1 expression and brown fat progress [4]. Huh et al. reported that the amount of muscle is the primary predictor of the serum level of irisin. Serum irisin levels increase in response to acute exercise and decrease after surgically induced weight loss and with decrease in body mass [3].

Polyzos et al. published a recent study that evaluated serum irisin levels in patients with NAFLD and controls; serum irisin levels were significantly lower in obese controls and NAFLD patients than in lean controls. Their results indicate that irisin may be independently and positively associated with the presence of portal inflammation [7].

However, in the present study, serum irisin levels in the obese group were increased, which was consistent with the results of a previous study, but were inconsistent with those of another study on NAFLD subjects. In our analysis, serum irisin levels did not decrease in NAFLD patients; instead, the serum irisin level in the NAFLD group was higher than that of the control group. Furthermore, the serum irisin level was higher in the mild NAFLD group than the severe NAFLD group. Zhang et al. reported that serum irisin levels were low in obese adults with NAFLD and reduced gradually with the increase in intrahepatic triglyceride levels [10]. However, they did not evaluate serum irisin levels in normal controls. In that respect, our results also reveal a gradual decrease in the serum irisin level according to the severity of steatosis. Therefore, we hypothesized that the serum irisin level increases as a defense mechanism in the early stage of NAFLD and then, decreases with the progression of NAFLD.

Although the mean BMI was higher in the NAFLD group, the serum irisin level was not different between the non-obese and obese groups. However, in the non-obese and obese groups, the serum irisin level was highest in the mild fatty liver group and lowest in the control group. Among the normal controls, the serum irisin level was lower in the obese group. In the mild fatty liver group and moderate-to-severe fatty liver group, there was no statistically significant difference in the serum irisin level between the obese and non-obese subjects; however, it tended to be lower in the obese group (Figure 2, Table S1). Consequently, we speculate that the increase of serum irisin in NAFLD patients is an independent process, not associated with BMI.

Liu et al. reported that serum irisin was significantly lower in type 2 DM subjects than in non-diabetic controls [11]. However, in the present study, the number of patients with type 2 DM was too small to analyze the relationship between serum irisin level and type 2 DM.

Park et al. reported that serum irisin levels were significantly higher in subjects with metabolic syndrome. They concluded that irisin is associated with metabolic syndrome independently from obesity. This association can be mediated not only by higher BMI or adiposity, but also by other mechanisms yet to be fully identified, including the direct effects on risk factors for metabolic syndrome [12]. However, although our data did not show a significant difference in serum irisin level between the metabolic syndrome group and normal control group, the number of subjects with metabolic syndrome was too low to reach a definite conclusion.

Our results showed that the quantity of exercise was not positively correlated with serum irisin levels. In fact, some authors recently reported that the regulation of irisin by exercise has been shown only in small sized cohorts, and the timing of irisin increase after exercise was uncertain [13,14]. Kraemer et al. found temporarily elevated serum irisin levels in response to exercise, only during the first hour [15]. Hecksteden et al. failed to find an increase in serum irisin levels in healthy subjects after aerobic exercise [16]. In the present study, serum irisin levels showed a slight tendency to decrease with exercise; however, statistical significance was not reached. It is worth noting that there were more NAFLD patients and obese subjects in the exercise groups than in the non-exercise group. It is possible that the subjects who had NAFLD or were obese exercised more intensely than the healthy non-obese subjects before they were enrolled in the present study. Therefore, multiple complicated mechanisms may be involved in the relationship between serum irisin level and the quantity of exercise.

In the present study, serum irisin levels tended to be higher in men than in women. However, the number of women (n = 261) included in our study was much higher than the number of men (n = 94). Therefore, we analyzed the characteristics of subjects per sex. The proportion of NAFLD patients in the male group was 40.4% (38/94) and that of the female group was 17.6% (46/261). This factor may have influenced the higher irisin level in the male group. Nevertheless, there were significant differences between the subgroups of NAFLD in both sex groups (Figure 3, Table S2).

The serum irisin level is known to be lower in patients with fatty liver disease than in healthy individuals. However, recently published studies assert that serum irisin is not associated with BMI, age, and other biological parameters [14,16] and that it is somewhat inversely associated. Our results would support these findings. One hypothesis from Silja et al. is that human Fndc5 is a transcribed pseudo-gene that has lost the ability to be effectively translated into full-length Fndc5 protein. Therefore, unlike in mice, the role of irisin is lost in humans [17].

Although our study included a relatively large number of subjects, it has several limitations. Data regarding the amount of alcohol intake and the weekly hours of exercise were obtained by personal history taking; therefore, data may have been underestimated or overestimated. We were unable to evaluate the intensity of exercise and the amount of muscle by imaging modality such as dual-energy X-ray absorptiometry or computed tomography. Finally, this study was limited by its cross-sectional design.

Conclusion

In conclusion, although irisin is an interesting newly discovered protein, very little is known about it. It may be too premature to speculate an association between serum irisin levels and NAFLD. Our results showed that serum irisin levels were higher in NAFLD patients, which is not consistent with the results of previously published studies. Future studies will be required to ascertain the precise mechanisms regulating the effects of irisin on energy expenditure.

Acknowledgments

This work was supported by the research promoting grant from the Keimyung University Dongsan Medical Center in 2012.

Author Contributions

Conceived and designed the experiments: MKK BKJ. Performed the experiments: BKJ MKK MKS. Analyzed the data: ESC BKJ WJC JSH. Contributed reagents/materials/analysis tools: ESC JMK ESK KSP KBC. Wrote the paper: ESC BKJ.

References

1. Angulo P (2002) Nonalcoholic fatty liver disease. The New England journal of medicine 346: 1221–1231.
2. Sahini N, Borlak J (2014) Recent insights into the molecular pathophysiology of lipid droplet formation in hepatocytes. Progress in lipid research 54: 86–112.
3. Huh JY, Panagiotou G, Mougios V, Brinkoetter M, Vamvini MT, et al. (2012) FNDC5 and irisin in humans: I. Predictors of circulating concentrations in serum and plasma and II. mRNA expression and circulating concentrations in response to weight loss and exercise. Metabolism 61: 1725–1738.
4. Bostrom P, Wu J, Jedrychowski MP, Korde A, Ye L, et al. (2012) A PGC1-alpha-dependent myokine that drives brown-fat-like development of white fat and thermogenesis. Nature 481: 463–468.
5. Moon HS, Dincer F, Mantzoros CS (2013) Pharmacological concentrations of irisin increase cell proliferation without influencing markers of neurite outgrowth and synaptogenesis in mouse H19-7 hippocampal cell lines. Metabolism: clinical and experimental 62: 1131–1136.
6. Polyzos SA, Kountouras J, Shields K, Mantzoros CS (2013) Irisin: a renaissance in metabolism? Metabolism: clinical and experimental 62: 1037–1044.
7. Polyzos SA, Kountouras J, Anastasilakis AD, Geladari EV, Mantzoros CS (2014) Irisin in patients with nonalcoholic fatty liver disease. Metabolism: clinical and experimental 63: 207–217.
8. Chang Y, Jung HS, Yun KE, Cho J, Cho YK, et al. (2013) Cohort study of non-alcoholic fatty liver disease, NAFLD fibrosis score, and the risk of incident diabetes in a Korean population. The American journal of gastroenterology 108: 1861–1868.
9. Kassi E, Pervanidou P, Kaltsas G, Chrousos G (2011) Metabolic syndrome: definitions and controversies. BMC medicine 9: 48.
10. Zhang HJ, Zhang XF, Ma ZM, Pan LL, Chen Z, et al. (2013) Irisin is inversely associated with intrahepatic triglyceride contents in obese adults. Journal of hepatology 59: 557–562.
11. Liu JJ, Wong MD, Toy WC, Tan CS, Liu S, et al. (2013) Lower circulating irisin is associated with type 2 diabetes mellitus. Journal of diabetes and its complications 27: 365–369.
12. Hee Park K, Zaichenko L, Brinkoetter M, Thakkar B, Sahin-Efe A, et al. (2013) Circulating irisin in relation to insulin resistance and the metabolic syndrome. The Journal of clinical endocrinology and metabolism 98: 4899–4907.

13. Bostrom PA, Fernandez-Real JM, Mantzoros C (2014) Irisin in humans: recent advances and questions for future research. Metabolism: clinical and experimental 63: 178–180.
14. Sanchis-Gomar F, Alis R, Pareja-Galeano H, Sola E, Victor VM, et al. (2014) Circulating irisin levels are not correlated with BMI, age, and other biological parameters in obese and diabetic patients. Endocrine 2014 Feb 8.
15. Kraemer RR, Shockett P, Webb ND, Shah U, Castracane VD (2014) A transient elevated irisin blood concentration in response to prolonged, moderate aerobic exercise in young men and women. Hormone and metabolic research 46: 150–154.
16. Sanchis-Gomar F, Alis R, Pareja-Galeano H, Romagnoli M, Perez-Quilis C (2014) Inconsistency in Circulating Irisin Levels: What is Really Happening? Hormone and metabolic research 2014 Jan 23.
17. Raschke S, Elsen M, Gassenhuber H, Sommerfeld M, Schwahn U, et al. (2013) Evidence against a beneficial effect of irisin in humans. PloS one 8:e73680.

11

Aerobic Exercise for Parkinson's Disease: A Systematic Review and Meta-Analysis of Randomized Controlled Trials

Hai-Feng Shu, Tao Yang, Si-Xun Yu, Hai-Dong Huang, Ling-Li Jiang, Jian-Wen Gu, Yong-Qin Kuang*

Department of Neurosurgery, General Hospital of the People's Liberation Army Chengdu Military Region, Chengdu, Sichuan, China

Abstract

Background: Although some trials assessed the effectiveness of aerobic exercise for Parkinson's disease (PD), the role of aerobic exercise in the management of PD remained controversial.

Objective: The purpose of this systematic review is to evaluate the evidence about whether aerobic exercise is effective for PD.

Methods: Seven electronic databases, up to December 2013, were searched to identify relevant studies. Two reviewers independently extracted data and assessed methodological quality based on PEDro scale. Standardised mean difference (SMD) and 95% confidence intervals (CI) of random-effects model were calculated. And heterogeneity was assessed based on the I^2 statistic.

Results: 18 randomized controlled trials (RCTs) with 901 patients were eligible. The aggregated results suggested that aerobic exercise should show superior effects in improving motor actions (SMD, −0.57; 95% CI −0.94 to −0.19; p = 0.003), balance (SMD, 2.02; 95% CI 0.45 to 3.59; p = 0.01), and gait (SMD, 0.33; 95% CI 0.17 to 0.49; p<0.0001) in patients with PD, but not in quality of life (SMD, 0.11; 95% CI −0.23 to 0.46; p = 0.52). And there was no valid evidence on follow-up effects of aerobic exercise for PD.

Conclusion: Aerobic exercise showed immediate beneficial effects in improving motor action, balance, and gait in patients with PD. However, given no evidence on follow-up effects, large-scale RCTs with long follow-up are warrant to confirm the current findings.

Editor: Alfonso Fasano, University of Toronto, Italy

Funding: This work was supported by National Natural Science Foundation of China (No. 81100975, 81371430), China Postdoctoral Science Foundation (No. 2012T50850), Research Foundation of General Hospital of Chengdu Military Region (No. 424121H3), and Science Foundation of Health Office of Sichuan Province (No. 42412D16). The funders had no role in study design, data collection and analysis, decision to publish, or preparation of the manuscript.

Competing Interests: The authors have declared that no competing interests exist.

* Email: yongqinkuangdr@163.com

Introduction

Parkinson's disease (PD) is a relatively progressive and neurodegenerative movement disorder that is characterized by many motor and non-motor symptoms such as resting tremor, bradykinesia, balance decrements, gait disruption, and reduced quality of life [1]. It is estimated that PD affects approximately 340,000 adults in the United States and this number would be probably doubled by the year of 2030 [2]. Although the causes of PD are still under investigation, its incidence obviously increases among people aged more than 50 years old [3]. In China, for example, PD prevalence is 1.70% in people aged more than 65 years old [4].

In recent years, aerobic exercise is widely used in assisting pharmacological treatments of PD. It may promote brain health by reducing inflammation, suppressing oxidative stress, and stabilizing calcium homeostasis [5]. Studies in healthy older rodents have shown that regular aerobic exercise triggered plasticity-related changes in the central nervous system, including synaptogenesis, enhanced glucose utilization, angiogenesis, and neurogenesis [6]. Other studies have shown that aerobic exercise, such as treadmill training, dancing, etc, may be beneficial in improving balance, gait, physical function, and quality of life in individuals with PD [7–9].

Some systematic reviews and meta-analyses supported that exercise therapies were effective in improving both motor and non-motor impairments of patients with PD [10,11], but no review has addressed the specific effectiveness of aerobic exercise for PD. In the previous reviews, it is difficult to extract accurate information regarding the contribution of aerobic exercises in patients with PD because multiple exercise therapies were often involved.

Therefore, this systematic review aims to evaluate the evidence about whether aerobic exercise is effective for patients with PD. And we conducted meta-analyses of randomized controlled trials

Table 1. Characteristics of randomized controlled trials of aerobic exercise for PD.

First author, year, country	Hoehn and Yahr stage	Mean duration of PD (year)	Sample size, mean age (year)	Duration (week)	Follow-up (week)	Main outcome assessments	Experimental group intervention	Control group intervention
Thaut, 1996, US	NR	7	37, 71	3	—	Gait	Walking (30 min/9sessions)	1) Walking plus rhythmic auditory stimulation (30 min/9sessions); 2) Usual care
Miyai, 2000, Japan	2.5–3	4.2	10, 68	4	—	UPDRS, Gait	Body-weight-supported treadmill (45 min/12sessions)	Physical therapy (45 min/12sessions)
Miyai, 2002, Japan	2.5–3	4.3	20, 70	4	24	UPDRS, Gait	Body-weight-supported treadmill (45 min/12sessions)	Physical therapy (45 min/12sessions)
Protas, 2005, US	2–3	7.6	18, 72	8	—	Gait	Gait and step training (60 min/ 24sessions)	Usual care
Burini, 2006, Italy	2–3	11	26, 64	7	—	UPDRS, Gait, PDQ-39	Aerobic exercise (45 min/20sessions)	Qigong (50 min/20sessions)
Cakit, 2007, Turkey	2–3	5.6	31, 72	8	—	Gait, BBT	Treadmill training	Usual care
Fisher, 2008, US	1–2	1	30, 63	8	—	UPDRS, Gait	Body-weight-supported treadmill (45 min/24sessions)	1) Traditional physical therapy (45 min/ 24sessions) 2) Education (60 min/6sessions)
Hackney, 2008, US	1.5–3	7.1	33, 64	13	—	UPDRS, BBS, Gait	Tai Chi (60 min/20sessions)	No intervention
Frazzitta, 2009, Italy	3	13	40, 71	4	—	UPDRS, Gait	Treadmill training associated with auditory and visual cues (20 min/ 28sessions)	Auditory and visual cues
Hackney, 2009, US	1–3	7.3	48, 67	13	—	UPDRS, BBS, Gait	1) Tango; 2) Waltz/Foxtrot (60 min/20sessions)	No intervention
Sage, 2009, Canada	NR	3.5	36, 66	12	—	UPDRS, Gait	Aerobic exercise (30 min/36sessions)	1) Sensory attention focused exercise (40–60 min/ 30–34sessions); 2) Waiting list
Reuter, 2011,Germany	2–3	5.5	90, 63	24	—	UPDRS, Gait, PDQ-39	1) Nordic walking (70 min/72sessions); 2) Walking (70 min/72sessions)	Flexibility and relaxation (70 min/72sessions)
Canning, 2012,Australia	1–2	5.5	20, 62	6	6	UPDRS, Gait, PDQ-39	Home-based treadmill training (30–40 min/24sessions)	Usual care
Li, 2012, US	1–4	7	195, 69	24	—	UPDRS, Gait	Tai Chi (60 min/48sessions)	1)Stretching; 2)Resistance training (60 min/ 48sessions)
Picelli, 2012, Italy	3–4	7.5	34, 68	4	4	UPDRS, Gait, BBS	Robot-assisted gait training (40 min/12sessions)	Physical therapy
Schenkman, 2012, US	1–3	4.5	121, 64	64	—	UPDRS, FRT, PDQ-39	Aerobic exercise (45–60 min/320–448sessions)	1)Flexibility/balance/function exercise; 2) Home-based exercise (45–60 min/320–448sessions)
Shulman, 2013, US	1–3	6.2	67, 66	12	—	UPDRS, Gait	1) Higher-intensity treadmill (30 min/36sessions); 2) Lower-intensity treadmill (50 min/ 36sessions)	Stretching and resistance
Amano, 2013, US	2–3	8	45, 66	16	—	UPDRS, Gait	Tai Chi (60 min/32–48sessions)	1) Qigong (60 min/32–48sessions); 2) No exercise

PD: Parkinson's disease; NR: No reported; UPDRS: Unified Parkinson's Disease Rating Scale; PDQ39: Parkinson's Disease Questionnaire 39; BBT: Berg Balance Test; BBS: Berg Balance Scale; FRT: Functional Reach Test.

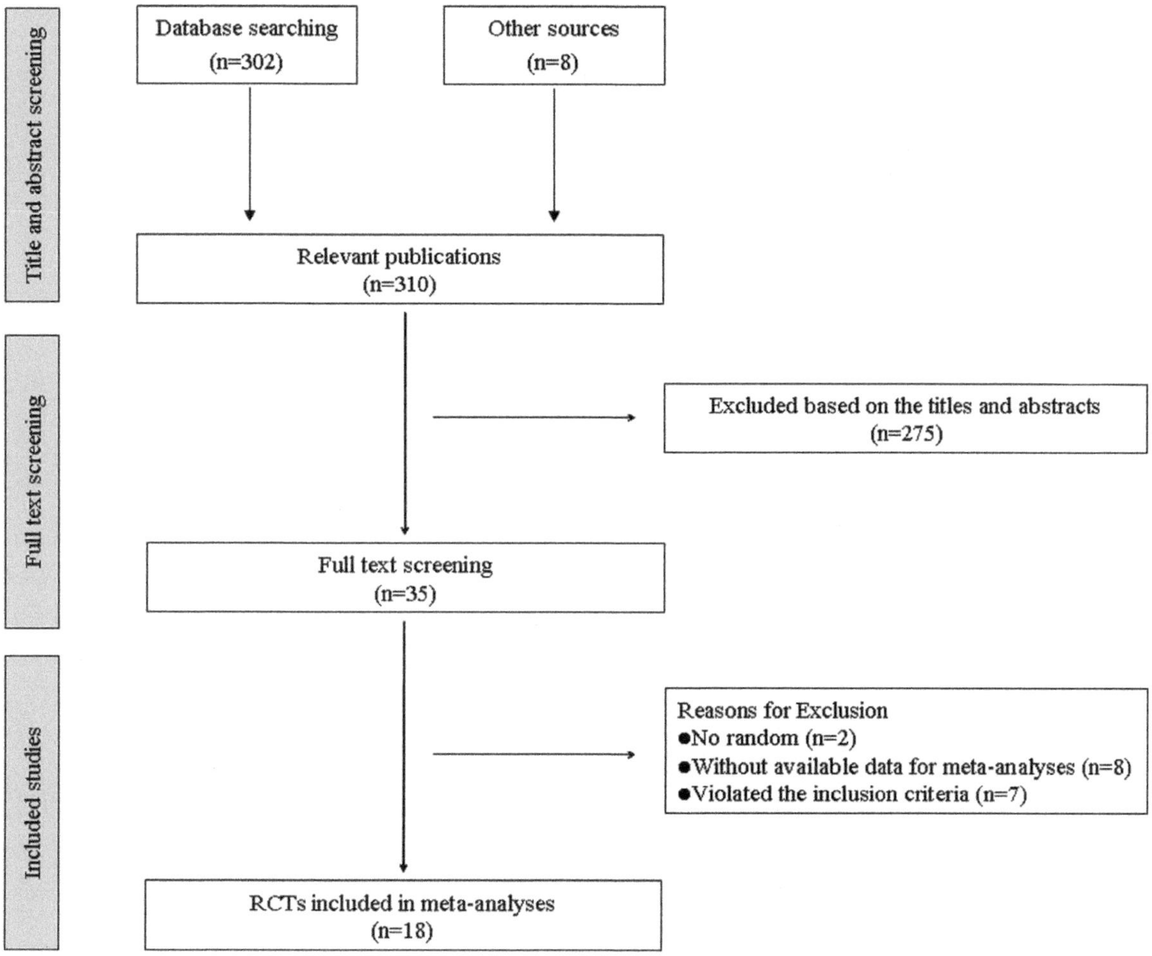

Figure 1. Flow chart for this meta-analysis. RCTs: randomized controlled trials.

(RCTs) focusing specifically on balance, gait, and quality of life in patients with PD.

Methods

Search Strategy

The following electronic databases were searched from their inception to December 2013: PubMed, EMBASE, OVID-MEDLINE, Cochrane Library, CNKI (China Knowledge Resource Integrated Database), Weipu Database for Chinese Technical Periodicals, and Wan Fang Data. The following keywords were used in combinations: Parkinson, Parkinson's disease, Parkinsonism, exercise, physical activity, and physical therapy. Literature was also identified by citation tracking using reference lists from papers and internet searching. In order to include unpublished studies in our review, dissertations and trial registrations were also searched, and we contacted experts in this field. Two authors (HFS and TY) undertook the initial literature search and identified eligible studies. If it was unclear as to whether the study met the inclusion criteria, advice was sought from a third author and any disagreement was settled down by a consensus after discussion.

Study Selection

The studies that met the following criteria were included: (1) RCTs of aerobic exercise for PD; (2) the target population was aged 20–85 years and confirmed diagnosis of PD; (3) the main intervention should be aerobic exercise and the exercise should be specifically suitable for the challenges and difficulties presented by PD; (4) the effect of aerobic exercise intervention was compared with any comparator, including other forms of exercise or physical activity; (5) the outcomes included at least one of the following: balance, gait, or health-related quality of life; (6) RCTs should contain available data for the meta-analysis; (7) the paper was available in either English or Chinese.

A study was excluded if: (1) the effect of a non-aerobic exercise intervention was evaluated (such as resistance training, behavioral interventions, music therapy, cueing strategies.); (2) the paper did not report outcomes for the first assessment period (cross-over studies only) so as to prevent any bias of carry over or order effects.

Data Extraction

Two reviewers (HFS and SXY) independently extracted data onto predefined criteria in Table 1. We contacted primary authors when relevant information was not reported. Differences were settled by discussion with reference to the original article. For crossover studies, we considered the risk for carryover effects to be prohibitive, so we selected only the first phase of the study. First

Table 2. PEDro scale of quality for eligible randomized controlled trials.

Study	Eligibility criteria	Random allocation	Concealed allocation	Similar at baseline	Subjects blinded	Therapists blinded	Assessors blinded	<15% dropouts	Intention-to-treat analysis	Between-group comparisons	Point measures and variability data	Total
Thaut, 1996 US	1	1	0	1	0	0	0	1	1	1	1	6
Miyai, 2000, Japan	1	1	0	1	0	0	0	1	1	1	1	6
Miyai, 2002, Japan	1	1	0	1	0	0	0	0	0	1	1	4
Protasa, 2005, US	1	1	0	1	0	0	1	1	1	1	1	7
Burini, 2006, Italy	1	1	1	1	0	0	1	0	0	1	1	6
Cakit, 2007, Turkey	1	1	0	1	0	0	1	0	0	1	1	5
Fisher, 2008, US	1	1	1	1	0	0	1	1	1	1	1	8
Hackney, 2008, US	1	1	0	1	0	0	1	0	0	1	1	5
Frazzitta, 2009, Italy	1	1	0	1	0	0	0	1	1	1	1	6
Hackney, 2009, US	1	1	0	1	0	0	1	0	0	1	1	5
Sage, 2009, Canada	1	1	0	1	0	0	1	1	0	1	1	6
Reuter, 2011,Germany	1	1	0	1	0	0	1	1	1	1	1	7
Canning, 2012,Australia	1	1	1	1	0	0	1	1	1	1	1	8
Li, 2012, US	1	1	0	1	0	0	1	1	1	1	1	7
Picelli, 2012, Italy	1	1	0	1	0	0	1	1	0	1	1	6
Schenkman, 2012, US	1	1	1	1	0	0	1	0	0	1	1	6
Shulman, 2013, US	1	1	0	1	0	0	1	0	0	1	1	5
Amano, 2013, US	1	1	0	1	0	0	1	1	1	1	1	7

Criteria (2–11) were used to calculate the total PEDro score. Each criterion was scored as either 1 or 0 according to whether the criteria was met or not, respectively.

	Experimental			Control				Std. Mean Difference	
Study or Subgroup	**Mean**	**SD**	**Total**	**Mean**	**SD**	**Total**	**Weight**	**IV, Random, 95% CI**	**Year**
1.1.1 UPDRS I									
Miyai 2000	-0.3	0.33	5	0	0.33	5	2.2%	-0.82 [-2.14, 0.50]	2000
Miyai 2002	-0.3	0.47	12	-0.2	0.18	12	3.9%	-0.27 [-1.08, 0.53]	2002
Fisher 2008	0	2.15	10	0.3	0.99	10	3.6%	-0.17 [-1.05, 0.71]	2008
Subtotal (95% CI)			**27**			**27**	**9.7%**	**-0.33 [-0.87, 0.22]**	
Heterogeneity: Tau² = 0.00; Chi² = 0.67, df = 2 (P = 0.71); I² = 0%									
Test for overall effect: Z = 1.18 (P = 0.24)									
1.1.2 UPDRS II									
Miyai 2000	-2	1.48	5	-0.4	1.59	5	2.1%	-0.94 [-2.29, 0.41]	2000
Miyai 2002	-2.9	1.75	12	-1.1	1.39	12	3.7%	-1.10 [-1.97, -0.23]	2002
Fisher 2008	0.6	3.98	10	-0.9	4.28	10	3.6%	0.35 [-0.54, 1.23]	2008
Schenkman 2012	-0.7	4.54	41	-0.93	4.64	80	6.3%	0.05 [-0.33, 0.43]	2012
Subtotal (95% CI)			**68**			**107**	**15.7%**	**-0.31 [-0.97, 0.35]**	
Heterogeneity: Tau² = 0.27; Chi² = 8.15, df = 3 (P = 0.04); I² = 63%									
Test for overall effect: Z = 0.92 (P = 0.36)									
1.1.3 UPDRS III									
Miyai 2000	-3.2	1.48	5	-0.6	1.59	5	1.8%	-1.53 [-3.04, -0.02]	2000
Miyai 2002	-3	1.37	12	-1.3	1.53	12	3.6%	-1.13 [-2.00, -0.26]	2002
Fisher 2008	-2.8	10.63	10	-2.7	8.91	10	3.6%	-0.01 [-0.89, 0.87]	2008
Hackney 2008	-1.5	6.6	17	4.3	5.6	16	4.4%	-0.92 [-1.64, -0.20]	2008
Hackney 2009	-2.15	3.03	31	5	2.74	17	4.1%	-2.40 [-3.17, -1.62]	2009
Sage 2009	-1.8	7.96	13	1.2	8.54	15	4.2%	-0.35 [-1.10, 0.40]	2009
Frazzitta 2009	-7.1	5.34	20	-5.8	5.26	20	4.9%	-0.24 [-0.86, 0.38]	2009
Schenkman 2012	-2.5	8.54	41	-1.16	9.11	80	6.3%	-0.15 [-0.53, 0.23]	2012
Picelli 2012	-6.31	7.22	17	0.13	8.46	17	4.5%	-0.80 [-1.50, -0.10]	2012
Li 2012	-6.42	5.46	65	-3.23	6.92	130	6.7%	-0.49 [-0.79, -0.19]	2012
Canning 2012	2.4	5.1	10	2.3	4.9	10	3.6%	0.02 [-0.86, 0.90]	2012
Amano 2013	0.57	6.9	27	-2.25	6.26	18	5.0%	0.42 [-0.19, 1.02]	2013
Subtotal (95% CI)			**268**			**350**	**52.7%**	**-0.57 [-0.94, -0.19]**	
Heterogeneity: Tau² = 0.29; Chi² = 44.17, df = 11 (P < 0.00001); I² = 75%									
Test for overall effect: Z = 2.98 (P = 0.003)									
1.1.4 UPDRS IV									
Miyai 2000	-0.4	0.5	5	-0.3	0.39	5	2.4%	-0.20 [-1.45, 1.04]	2000
Miyai 2002	0	0.33	12	0.2	0.18	12	3.8%	-0.73 [-1.56, 0.10]	2002
Subtotal (95% CI)			**17**			**17**	**6.2%**	**-0.56 [-1.26, 0.13]**	
Heterogeneity: Tau² = 0.00; Chi² = 0.47, df = 1 (P = 0.49); I² = 0%									
Test for overall effect: Z = 1.60 (P = 0.11)									
1.1.5 UPDRS tot									
Miyai 2000	-6	3.29	5	-1.1	3.51	5	1.9%	-1.30 [-2.74, 0.14]	2000
Miyai 2002	-5.5	5.35	12	-2.5	2.91	12	3.8%	-0.67 [-1.50, 0.15]	2002
Fisher 2008	-2.1	15.32	10	-3.2	11.05	10	3.6%	0.08 [-0.80, 0.96]	2008
Schenkman 2012	-3.2	12.24	41	-2.39	12.95	80	6.3%	-0.06 [-0.44, 0.31]	2012
Subtotal (95% CI)			**68**			**107**	**15.7%**	**-0.28 [-0.73, 0.18]**	
Heterogeneity: Tau² = 0.07; Chi² = 4.39, df = 3 (P = 0.22); I² = 32%									
Test for overall effect: Z = 1.19 (P = 0.23)									
Total (95% CI)			**448**			**608**	**100.0%**	**-0.45 [-0.68, -0.22]**	
Heterogeneity: Tau² = 0.18; Chi² = 62.98, df = 24 (P < 0.0001); I² = 62%									
Test for overall effect: Z = 3.86 (P = 0.0001)									
Test for subgroup differences: Chi² = 1.38, df = 4 (P = 0.85), I² = 0%									

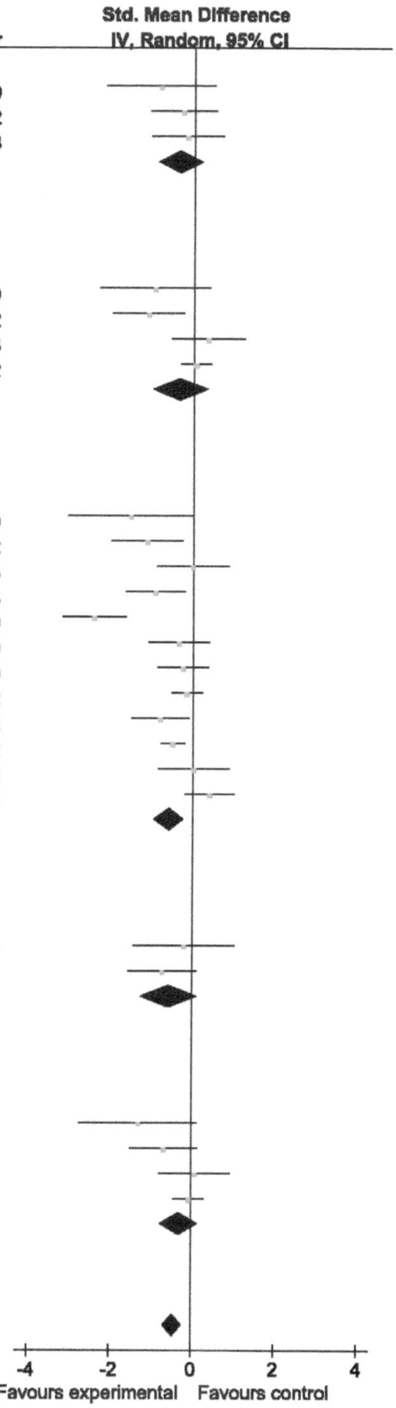

Figure 2. Forest plot showing the effect of aerobic exercise on unified Parkinson's disease rating scale (UPDRS).

author, country, and year of the study were extracted as general study information. Population data, outcome assessments, interventions, and length of follow-up were taken to analyze the study characteristics.

Quality Assessment

The methodological quality of RCTs was assessed independently by two reviewers (SXY and HDH) with PEDro scale, which is based on the Delphi list and has been reported to have a fair-to-good reliability for RCTs of the physiotherapy in systematic reviews [12,13]. The PEDro score ranged from 0 to 10 points. A cut point of 6 on the PEDro scale was used to indicate high-quality studies as this had been reported to be sufficient to determine high quality versus low quality in previous studies [12]. Disagreements were resolved by discussion between the reviewers, with the information of the primary author being sought if necessary. The PEDro scores were all settled down by consensus.

Study or Subgroup	Experimental Mean	SD	Total	Control Mean	SD	Total	Weight	Std. Mean Difference IV, Random, 95% CI	Year
Cakit 2007	7.09	1.27	27	-1.42	0.23	27	16.5%	9.19 [7.31, 11.07]	2007
Hackney 2008	3.3	3	17	-0.5	2.1	16	20.5%	1.42 [0.65, 2.20]	2008
Hackney 2009	-1	5.33	31	-1.2	2.46	17	21.0%	0.04 [-0.55, 0.63]	2009
Picelli 2012	5.56	3.39	17	-0.06	5.57	17	20.6%	1.19 [0.45, 1.93]	2012
Schenkman 2012	0.2	2.94	41	0.8	2.88	80	21.4%	-0.21 [-0.58, 0.17]	2012
Total (95% CI)			133			157	100.0%	2.02 [0.45, 3.59]	

Heterogeneity: Tau² = 2.96; Chi² = 106.58, df = 4 (P < 0.00001); I² = 96%
Test for overall effect: Z = 2.52 (P = 0.01)

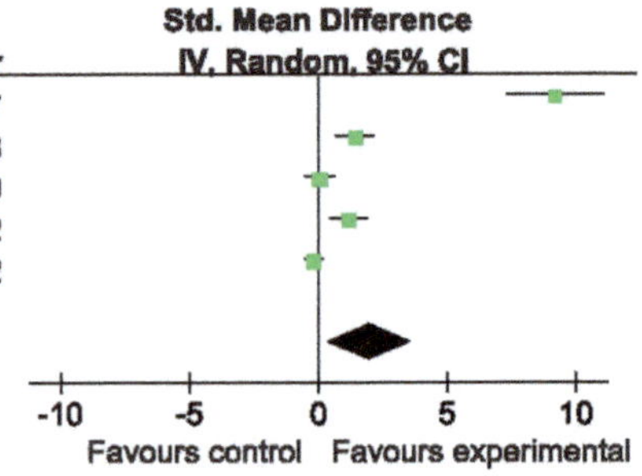

Figure 3. Forest plot showing the effect of aerobic exercise on balance in patients with Parkinson's disease.

Data Analysis

Meta-analysis was conducted with Cochrane Collaboration software (Review Manager Version 5.1). For continuous data, standardized mean difference (SMD) and 95% confidence intervals (CI) of random-effects model were calculated for all eligible trials. Heterogeneity across studies was tested based on the I^2 statistic, a quantitative measure of inconsistency across studies, and studies with $I^2<40\%$ was considered to have low heterogeneity, I^2 of 40% to 75% was considered moderate heterogeneity, and $I^2>75\%$ was considered high heterogeneity. Trials, including 2 similar intervention or control groups, had the groups combined with computational formula provided by the Cochrane handbook to create a single pair-wise comparison. Detailed subgroup analyses were conducted based on different outcomes and outcome measures.

Results

Study Selection

Searching identified 310 records, of which 35 documents were retrieved from the screening of titles and abstracts. At last, 18 trials published between 1996 and 2013 were included in our meta-analysis [7–9,14–28]. 17 literatures were eliminated for the reasons that 2 of them failed to randomize [29,30], 8 without available data for the meta-analyses [31–38], and 7 violated the inclusion criteria [39–45]. Detailed selection process was showed in Figure 1. In course of document screening, no divergent views were found between the reviewers.

Study Characteristics

Participants. There were 901 patients in the 18 eligible RCTs. Mean and standard deviation (SD) of age for all participants was 67±3.3 years, and the PD duration was 6.4±2.7 years. Most trials recruited participants with mild-to-moderate PD, including 14 with Hoehn and Yahr stage I to III [7,8,15–22,24,26–28] and 2 with Hoehn and Yahr stage I to IV [9,25].

Interventions. All the eligible literatures reported aerobic exercise interventions including treadmill training, Tai Chi, walking, dancing, etc. The interventions in control group were various, such as no intervention, usual care, stretching, resistance exercises, physical therapy, and other exercise. The intervention time spanned from 3 weeks to 16 months. Detailed characteristics of the included trials were summarized in Table 1.

Methodological Quality

The quality of the included studies was summarized in Table 2. The total scores for the methodological quality ranged from 4 to 8 points. No studies reported subjects-blinding and therapists-blinding, which were the common failing for the non-pharmacological clinical trials. However, most of them (78%) performed assessors-blinding [7–9,17–21,23–28]. Although all trials adopted random assignment of patients, only 4 used adequate method of allocation concealment [8,18,20,26]. The expulsion of 7 studies was definitely higher than 15% [7,16,18,19,21,26,27]. As for the intention-to-treat analysis, 9 trials were failed for cancelling the dropout data in the last results [7,16,18,19,21,23,25–27]. For the remaining items on PEDro scale, the eligible studies showed a high methodological quality.

Quantitative Data Synthesis

Unified Parkinson's disease rating scale (UPDRS). UPDRS, as the most common marker in the clinical study of PD, was employed in most eligible RCTs. The aggregated result showed a statistically significant benefit in favor of aerobic exercise for PD in UPDRS III (SMD, −0.57; 95% CI −0.94 to −0.19; p = 0.003; Figure 2) [7–9,15,16,20–23,25,26,28]. But it was not associated with significant improvements in UPDRS I (SMD, −0.33; 95% CI −0.87 to 0.22; p = 0.24; Figure 2) [15,16,20], UPDRS II (SMD, −0.31; 95% CI −0.97 to 0.35; p = 0.36; Figure 2) [15,16,20,26], UPDRS IV (SMD, −0.56; 95% CI −1.26 to 0.13; p = 0.11; Figure 2) [15,16], nor UPDRS tot (SMD, −0.28; 95% CI −0.73 to 0.18; p = 0.23; Figure 2) [15,16,20,26]. This suggested that aerobic exercise could positively improve motor actions in patients with PD.

Balance. 5 studies assessed equilibrium function of patients with PD. Nearly half of trials showed favorable effects of aerobic exercise in improving balance in patients with PD, and the aggregated result also supported it (SMD, 2.02; 95% CI 0.45 to 3.59; p = 0.01; Figure 3) [7,19,21,25,26].

Gait. Aerobic exercise showed superior effects in improving gait in patients with PD (SMD, 0.33; 95% CI 0.17 to 0.49; p< 0.0001; Figure 4). 6-minute walking test, stride/step length, gait velocity, cadence, and time up and go were analyzed in eligible studies. The aggregated results suggested that aerobic exercise should show significant effects compared with control therapies in 6-minute walking test (SMD, 0.72; 95% CI 0.08 to 1.36; p = 0.03; Figure 4) [7,8,21,22,27], stride/step length (SMD, 0.31; 95% CI 0.08 to 0.53; p = 0.008; Figure 4) [7–9,17,21–23,28], gait velocity (SMD, 0.35; 95% CI 0.10 to 0.60; p = 0.005; Figure 4) [7–9,14,15,17,20–24,28], and time up and go (SMD, 0.42; 95% CI 0.08 to 0.76; p = 0.02; Figure 4) [7,9,21,23,25]. However, none of the trials indicated the evidence in favor of aerobic exercise for PD in the assessment of the cadence (SMD, −0.18; 95% CI −0.52 to 0.15; p = 0.28; Figure 4) [14,17,20,23,28].

Quality of life. Four trials reported beneficial effects of aerobic exercise for PD in the quality of life, but there was no difference between aerobic exercise and control therapies

	Experimental			Control				Std. Mean Difference	
Study or Subgroup	Mean	SD	Total	Mean	SD	Total	Weight	IV, Random, 95% CI	Year
1.1.1 6MWT									
Burini 2006	35	65.83	13	-11	71.8	13	2.4%	0.65 [-0.15, 1.44]	2006
Hackney 2008	44.4	65.9	17	0.8	43.4	16	2.7%	0.76 [0.05, 1.47]	2008
Frazzitta 2009	130	121.02	20	57	80.73	20	3.0%	0.70 [0.06, 1.34]	2009
Hackney 2009	53.75	21.46	31	-7.5	33.65	17	2.5%	2.29 [1.53, 3.05]	2009
Canning 2012	13.3	28.8	10	18.1	39.3	10	2.1%	-0.13 [-1.01, 0.74]	2012
Shulman 2013	118.07	100.91	45	106.9	86.25	22	3.6%	0.11 [-0.40, 0.62]	2013
Subtotal (95% CI)			**136**			**98**	**16.2%**	**0.72 [0.08, 1.36]**	
Heterogeneity: Tau² = 0.50; Chi² = 25.20, df = 5 (P = 0.0001); I² = 80%									
Test for overall effect: Z = 2.22 (P = 0.03)									
1.1.2 Stride/Step length									
Protasa 2005	4.6	15.4	9	0.2	13.06	9	1.9%	0.29 [-0.64, 1.22]	2005
Fisher 2008	0.04	0.1	10	0.03	0.12	10	2.1%	0.09 [-0.79, 0.96]	2008
Hackney 2008	-0.1	22.8	17	0	6.6	16	2.8%	-0.01 [-0.69, 0.68]	2008
Sage 2009	4.6	11.43	13	0.3	12.22	15	2.5%	0.35 [-0.40, 1.10]	2009
Hackney 2009	0.05	0.07	31	-0.02	0.09	17	3.1%	0.89 [0.27, 1.51]	2009
Canning 2012	-0.17	0.73	10	-0.07	0.73	10	2.1%	-0.13 [-1.01, 0.75]	2012
Li 2012	10.3	21.91	65	1.1	20.8	130	4.7%	0.43 [0.13, 0.73]	2012
Amano 2013	0	0.11	27	0.01	0.12	18	3.2%	-0.09 [-0.68, 0.51]	2013
Subtotal (95% CI)			**182**			**225**	**22.5%**	**0.31 [0.08, 0.53]**	
Heterogeneity: Tau² = 0.01; Chi² = 7.72, df = 7 (P = 0.36); I² = 9%									
Test for overall effect: Z = 2.66 (P = 0.008)									
1.1.3 Gait velocity									
Thaut 1996	4	11.69	26	-3.4	17.26	11	2.7%	0.54 [-0.18, 1.25]	1996
Miyai 2000	-1.7	0.89	5	-0.6	0.99	5	1.1%	-1.06 [-2.43, 0.32]	2000
Protasa 2005	0.17	0.38	9	0.01	0.25	9	1.9%	0.47 [-0.47, 1.41]	2005
Fisher 2008	0.06	0.21	10	0.02	0.19	10	2.1%	0.19 [-0.69, 1.07]	2008
Hackney 2008	0.01	20.8	17	0.1	10.8	16	2.8%	-0.01 [-0.69, 0.68]	2008
Sage 2009	9.4	23.44	13	-0.4	23.74	15	2.5%	0.40 [-0.35, 1.15]	2009
Hackney 2009	0.05	0.06	31	0.02	0.1	17	3.2%	0.39 [-0.21, 0.98]	2009
Frazzitta 2009	0.4	0.29	20	0.3	0.18	20	3.0%	0.41 [-0.22, 1.03]	2009
Reuter 2011	1.2	1.02	60	0	1.01	30	3.8%	1.17 [0.70, 1.64]	2011
Li 2012	10.5	23.28	65	2.7	25.5	130	4.7%	0.31 [0.01, 0.61]	2012
Canning 2012	0.09	0.12	10	0.06	0.09	10	2.1%	0.27 [-0.61, 1.15]	2012
Amano 2013	0.01	0.26	27	0.03	0.25	18	3.2%	-0.08 [-0.67, 0.52]	2013
Subtotal (95% CI)			**293**			**291**	**33.1%**	**0.35 [0.10, 0.60]**	
Heterogeneity: Tau² = 0.07; Chi² = 19.09, df = 11 (P = 0.06); I² = 42%									
Test for overall effect: Z = 2.79 (P = 0.005)									
1.1.4 Cadence									
Thaut 1996	-0.4	8.79	26	8.1	12.99	11	2.6%	-0.82 [-1.55, -0.09]	1996
Protasa 2005	7.5	8.48	9	6.6	15.49	9	2.0%	0.07 [-0.86, 0.99]	2005
Fisher 2008	0.19	10.47	10	0.76	9.8	10	2.1%	-0.05 [-0.93, 0.82]	2008
Sage 2009	1.4	10.24	13	0	9.48	15	2.6%	0.14 [-0.61, 0.88]	2009
Amano 2013	-0.11	12.67	27	1.5	10.19	18	3.2%	-0.13 [-0.73, 0.46]	2013
Subtotal (95% CI)			**85**			**63**	**12.4%**	**-0.18 [-0.52, 0.15]**	
Heterogeneity: Tau² = 0.00; Chi² = 4.00, df = 4 (P = 0.41); I² = 0%									
Test for overall effect: Z = 1.08 (P = 0.28)									
1.1.5 Time up and go									
Hackney 2008	1	0.1	17	0.1	1.1	16	2.6%	1.14 [0.40, 1.89]	2008
Hackney 2009	1	5.33	31	-2	2.4	17	3.1%	0.65 [0.04, 1.26]	2009
Sage 2009	0.7	2.63	13	0	2.54	15	2.5%	0.26 [-0.48, 1.01]	2009
Li 2012	1.44	1.77	17	0.49	6.75	17	2.8%	0.19 [-0.49, 0.86]	2012
Picelli 2012	1.05	3.07	65	0.51	3.29	130	4.7%	0.17 [-0.13, 0.47]	2012
Subtotal (95% CI)			**143**			**195**	**15.8%**	**0.42 [0.08, 0.76]**	
Heterogeneity: Tau² = 0.06; Chi² = 7.01, df = 4 (P = 0.14); I² = 43%									
Test for overall effect: Z = 2.41 (P = 0.02)									
Total (95% CI)			**839**			**872**	**100.0%**	**0.33 [0.17, 0.49]**	
Heterogeneity: Tau² = 0.12; Chi² = 77.67, df = 35 (P < 0.0001); I² = 55%									
Test for overall effect: Z = 4.09 (P < 0.0001)									
Test for subgroup differences: Chi² = 10.26, df = 4 (P = 0.04), I² = 61.0%									

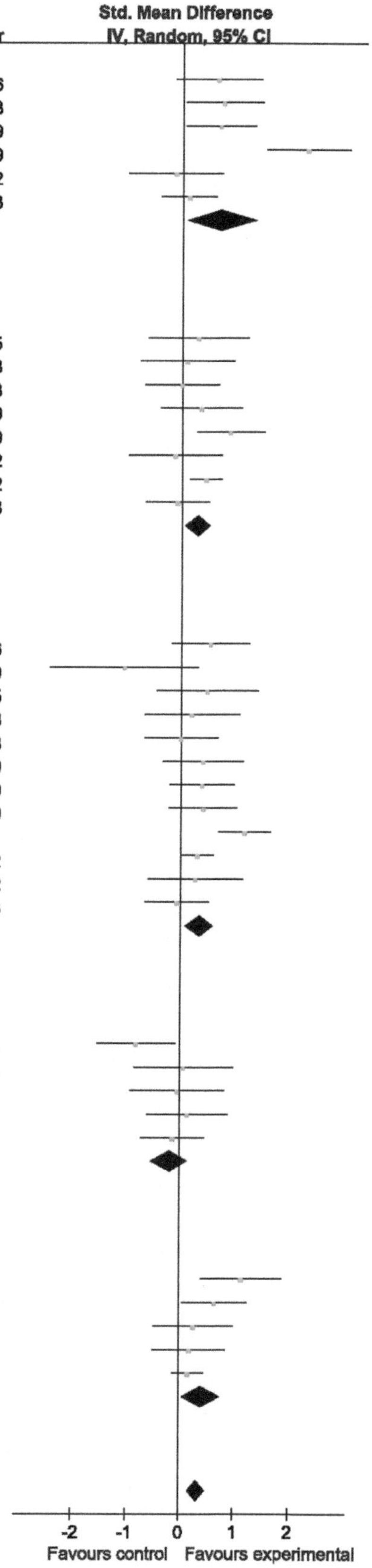

Figure 4. Forest plot showing the effect of aerobic exercise on gait in patients with Parkinson's disease.

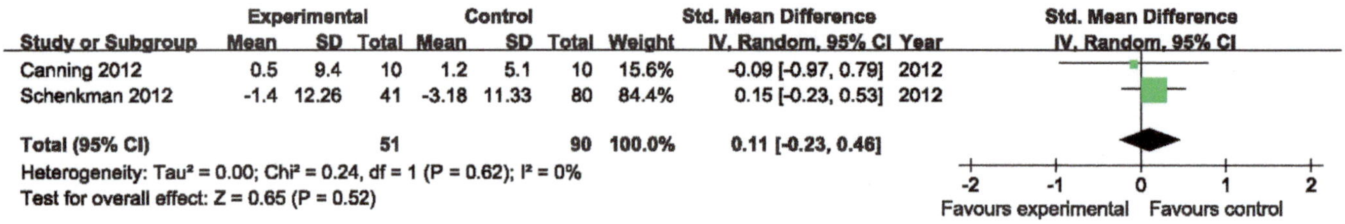

Figure 5. Forest plot showing the effect of aerobic exercise on quality of life in patients with Parkinson's disease.

[8,18,24,26]. And the synthetical effect size did not either show superior effects of aerobic exercise (SMD, 0.11; 95% CI −0.23 to 0.46; p = 0.52; Figure 5) [8,26].

Follow-up Effect

3 trials reported the follow-up effects of aerobic exercise for PD. The follow-up duration ranged from 4 weeks to 24 weeks. 1 study showed persistency effects of aerobic exercise in the number of steps for the 10-m walk [16], 1 in quality of life [8], and 1 in balance, gait, and motor action [25].

Adverse Events

Only two studies reported non-serious adverse events during the aerobic exercise training period. Two patients experienced hypotension in hot weather, four fell due to obstacles, five twisted ankles during cross-country walking, and one complained of pain in Reuter's study [24]. The other study reported one non-injurious fall and two complaints of soreness or pain during aerobic exercise intervention [26].

Discussion

This is the first systematic review to evaluate the effectiveness of aerobic exercise for PD. Our meta-analyses suggested that aerobic exercise significantly improve motor action, balance, and gait including gait velocity, stride/step length, and walking ability in patients with PD. Currently, there was no sufficient evidence to support or refute the value of aerobic exercise in improving quality of life in patients with PD compared with other therapies. And there was no valid evidence on follow-up effects of aerobic exercise for PD.

In our systematic review, most eligible trials showed moderate methodological quality based on PEDro score, which suggested that our findings were believable. We analyzed the 18 RCTs of aerobic exercise, including treadmill training, dancing, walking, and Tai Chi for PD conditions. Our aggregated results supported that aerobic exercise showed superior effects in improving motor action, balance, and gait in patients with PD. It was similar to related systematic reviews. Herman's systematic review suggested that treadmill training should play an important role in improving gait and mobility in patients with PD [46]. But it was only a qualitative review, and any strictly qualitative approach may be problematic since it can be more subjective than meta-analyses. Mehrholz's review also concluded that treadmill training was likely to improve gait hypokinesia and showed better safety [47]. Comparing with these reviews, larger new eligible RCTs (the last searching December 2013), more electronic databases (especially including 3 Chinese databases), and detailed subgroup meta-analyses (motor action, balance, gait and quality of life) strengthened our confidence in our systematic review.

In our review, two parts of analyses (UPDRS II and quality of life) came to the same conclusion that there was no sufficient evidence to support or refute the value of aerobic exercise in improving quality of life in patients with PD compared with other therapies. Some related systematic reviews drew a different conclusion that the evidence supported exercise as being beneficial with regards to health-related quality of life for patients with PD [48,49], but the evidence was gained through the utilization of various exercise therapies. The reviews, focusing on aerobic exercise for PD, only suggested that treadmill training potentially improve quality of life in patients with PD [46,47]. Modestly, our review included meta-analyses with larger data, but more trials were warranted to prove it.

PD is a complex disease that can compromise physical performance. Depending on the symptom severity, PD can present many obstacles to traditional exercise programming. Tough movement can be difficult for PD patients to perform. Recently, more studies have reported that intensive exercise achieved optimal results in the rehabilitation of patients with PD [50]. In these studies, intensity of exercise interventions depends on frequency and duration of exercises, number of repetitions, and complexity of exercises. A treatment is generally considered intensive when involving 2 to 4 hours of exercises per week, for 6 to 14 weeks. And larger studies reported the effect of intensive exercise in improving cell proliferation and neuronal differentiation [50–52]. In our review, almost 80% of aerobic exercises are intensive exercise. And the intensive aerobic exercise showed superior effects in improving motor action, balance, and gait of patients with PD.

Based on maximal heart rate or metabolic equivalents, the recent studies have showed that lower-intensity treadmill training yields more improvements in gait velocity than higher-intensity treadmill training for PD patients [27]. But Fisher's study led to different conclusion in gait of early PD undergoing high-intensity body weight-supported treadmill training [20]. The different conclusions may be rooted in the variation in types of treadmill training, duration and amount of exercises, patient characteristics, and main outcome measures. However, the physical activity guidelines reported by the U.S. Department of Health and Human Services suggested that moderate intensity physical activity could generate multiple health benefits [53]. Considering the disease characteristics and safety of exercise interventions, moderate or light intensity exercises should be considered beneficial and adoptive for individuals with PD [54–56]. In our review, the Hohen and Yahr stage of participants mainly arranged from I to III. So the exploration of these RCTs suggested that low to moderate intensity aerobic exercise, such as treadmill training, Tai Chi, dancing, etc, would benefit mild to moderate staged PD patients. However, the evidence is not conclusive. Future research should further investigate intensity level of aerobic exercise to check and monitor its effectiveness based on maximal heart rate or metabolic equivalents.

There were some limitations in our review. The large span of the durations (from 3 weeks to 64 weeks) in aerobic exercise interventions could influence our analysis. So it is difficult to conduct subgroup analyses on the different durations of aerobic exercise and determine the optimal size of aerobic exercise for PD. And there was insufficient data for the follow-up effect of aerobic exercise for PD, which is important for final decision of the clinicians. In addition, we could not get rid of the publication bias due to retrieval of documents in English and Chinese databases only.

Conclusions

This systematic review shows the positive evidence that aerobic exercise has immediate beneficial effects in improving motor action, balance, and gait in patients with PD. However, this is not sufficient to reach any definitive conclusion because there are very few studies with a follow-up evaluation. Large-scale RCTs with long follow-up are warrant to confirm the current findings of aerobic exercise for PD.

Author Contributions

Conceived and designed the experiments: HFS JWG YQK. Performed the experiments: HFS TY SXY HDH. Analyzed the data: HFS SXY LLJ. Contributed reagents/materials/analysis tools: HFS TY SXY HDH. Wrote the paper: HFS YQK.

References

1. Jankovic J (2008) Parkinson's disease: clinical features and diagnosis. J Neurol Neurosurg Psychiatry 79: 368–376.
2. Dorsey ER, Constantinescu R, Thompson JP, Biglan KM, Holloway RG, et al. (2007) Projected number of people with Parkinson disease in the most populous nations, 2005 through 2030. Neurology 68: 384–386.
3. Van Den Eeden SK, Tanner CM, Bemstein AL, Fross RD, Leimpeter A, et al. (2003) Incidence of Parkinson's disease: variation by age, gender, and race/ethnicity. Am J Epidemiol 157: 1015–1022.
4. Zhang ZX, Roman GC, Hong Z, Wu CB, Qu QM, et al. (2005) Parkinson's disease in China: prevalence in Beijing, Xian, and Shanghai. Lancet 365: 595–597.
5. Cotman CW, Berchtold NC, Christie LA (2007) Exercise builds brain health: key roles of growth factor cascades and inflammation. Trends Neurosci 30: 464–472.
6. Hirsch MA, Farley BG (2009) Exercise and neuroplasticity in persons living with Parkinson's disease. Eur J Phys Rehabil Med 45: 215–229.
7. Hackney ME, Earhart GM (2009) Effects of dance on movement control in Parkinson's disease: a comparison of Argentine tango and American ballroom. J Rehabil Med 41: 475–481.
8. Canning CG, Allen NE, Dean CM, Goh L, Fung VS (2012) Home-based treadmill training for individuals with Parkinson's disease: a randomized controlled pilot trial. Clinl Rehabil 26: 817–826.
9. Li F, Harmer P, Fitzgerald K, Eckstrom E, Stock R, et al. (2012) Tai Chi and Postural Stability in Patients with Parkinson's Disease. N Engl J Med 366: 511–519.
10. de Dreu MJ, van der Wilk AS, Poppe E, Kwakkel G, van Wegen EE (2012) Rehabilitation, exercise therapy and music in patients with Parkinson's disease: a meta-analysis of the effects of music-based movement therapy on walking ability, balance and quality of life. Parkinsonism Relat Disord 18 (Suppl 1): 114–119.
11. Goodwin VA, Richards SH, Taylor RS, Taylor AH, Campbell JL (2008) The effectiveness of exercise interventions for people with Parkinson's disease: a systematic review and meta-analysis. Mov Disord 23: 631–640.
12. Maher CG, Sherrington C, Herbert RD, Moseley AM, Elkins M (2003) Reliability of the PEDro scale for rating quality of randomized controlled trials. Phys Ther 83:713–721.
13. Macedo LG, Elkins MR, Maher CG, Moseley AM, Herbert RD, et al. (2010) There was evidence of convergent and construct validity of Physiotherapy Evidence Database quality scale for physiotherapy trials. J Clin Epidemiol 63:920–925.
14. Thaut MH, McIntosh GC, Rice RR, Miller RA, Rathbun J, et al. (1996) Rhythmic auditory stimulation in gait training for Parkinson's disease patients. Mov Disord 11:193–200. Available: http://www.ncbi.nlm.nih.gov/pubmed/8684391.
15. Miyai I, Fujimoto Y, Ueda Y, Yamamoto H, Nozaki S, et al. (2000) Treadmill training with body weight support: Its effect on Parkinson's disease. Arch Phys Med Rehabil 81: 849–852.
16. Miyai I, Fujimoto Y, Yamamoto H, Ueda Y, Saito T, et al. (2002) Long-term effect of body weight–supported treadmill training in Parkinson's disease: a randomized controlled trial. Arch Phys Med Rehabil 83: 1370–1373.
17. Protas EJ, Mitchell K, Williams A, Qureshy H, Caroline K, et al. (2005) Gait and step training to reduce falls in Parkinson's disease. NeuroRehabilitation 20:183–190.
18. Burini D, Farabollini B, Iacucci S, Rimatori C, Riccardi G, et al. (2006) A randomised controlled cross-over trial of aerobic training versus Qigong in advanced Parkinson's disease. Eura Medicophys 42:231–238.
19. Cakit BD, Saracoglu M, Genc H, Erdem HR, Inan L (2007) The effects of incremental speed-dependent treadmill training on postural instability and fear of falling in Parkinson's disease. Clin Rehabil 21:698–705.
20. Fisher BE, Wu AD, Salem GJ, Song J, Lin CH, et al. (2008) The effect of exercise training in improving motor performance and corticomotor excitability in people with early Parkinson's disease. Arch Phys Med Rehabil 89: 1221–1229.
21. Hackney ME, Earhart GM (2008) Tai Chi improves balance and mobility in people with Parkinson disease. Gait Posture; 28: 456–460.
22. Frazzitta G, Maestri R, Uccellini D, Bertotti G, Abelli P (2009) Rehabilitation treatment of gait in patients with Parkinson's disease with freezing: a comparison between two physical therapy protocols using visual and auditory cues with or without treadmill training. Mov Disord 24: 1139–1143.
23. Sage MD, Almeida QJ (2009) Symptom and gait changes after sensory attention focused exercise vs aerobic training in Parkinson's disease. Mov Disord 24: 1132–1138.
24. Reuter I, Mehnert S, Leone P, Kaps M, Oechsner M, et al. (2011) Effects of a Flexibility and Relaxation Programme, Walking, and Nordic Walking on Parkinson's Disease. J Aging Res. doi:10.4061/2011/232473
25. Picelli A, Melotti C, Origano F, Waldner A, Gimigliano R, et al. (2012) Does robotic gait training improve balance in Parkinson's disease? a randomized controlled trial. Parkinsonism Relat Disord18: 990–993.
26. Schenkman M, Hall DA, Barón AE, Schwartz RS, Mettler P, et al. (2012) Exercise for people in early-or mid-stage Parkinson disease: a 16-month randomized controlled trial. Phys Ther 92:1395–1410.
27. Shulman LM, Katzel LI, Ivey FM, Sorkin JD, Favors K, et al. (2013) Randomized Clinical Trial of 3 Types of Physical Exercise for Patients with Parkinson Disease. JAMA Neurol. 70: 183–190.
28. Amano S, Nocera JR, Vallabhajosula S, Juncos JL, Gregor RJ, et al. (2013) The effect of Tai Chi exercise on gait initiation and gait performance in persons with Parkinson's disease. Parkinsonism Relat Disord 19: 955–960.
29. Visser JE, Oude Nijhuis LB, Janssen L, Bastiaanse CM, Borm GF, et al. (2010) Dynamic posturography in Parkinson's disease: diagnostic utility of the "first trial effect". Neuroscience 168:387–394.
30. Bridgewater KJ, Sharpe MH (1998) Trunk muscle performance in early Parkinson's disease. Phys Ther 78:566–576.
31. Lee KS, Lee WH, Hwang S (2011) Modified constraint-induced movement therapy improves fine and gross motor performance of the upper limb in Parkinson disease. Am J Phys Med Rehabil 90:380–386.
32. Lopane G, Contin M, Scaglione C, Albani F, Baruzzi A, et al. (2010) The effect of a clinically practical exercise on levodopa bioavailability and motor response in patients with Parkinson disease. Clin Neuropharmacol 33:254–256.
33. Mak MK, Hui-Chan CW (2008) Cued task-specific training is better than exercise in improving sit-to-stand in patients with Parkinson's disease: A randomized controlled trial. Mov Disord 23:501–509.
34. Bloomer RJ, Schilling BK, Karlage RE, Ledoux MS, Pfeiffer RF, et al. (2008) Effect of resistance training on blood oxidative stress in Parkinson disease. Med Sci Sports Exerc 40:1385–1389.
35. Schmitz-Hübsch T, Pyfer D, Kielwein K, Fimmers R, Klockgether T, et al. (2006) Qigong exercise for the symptoms of Parkinson's disease: a randomized, controlled pilot study. Mov Disord 21:543–548.
36. Kurtais Y, Kutlay S, Tur BS, Gok H, Akbostanci C (2008) Does treadmill training improve lower-extremity tasks in Parkinson disease? A randomized controlled trial. Clin J Sport Med 18:289–291.
37. Lehman DA, Toole T, Lofaid D, Hirsch MA (2005) Training with verbal instructional cues results in near-term improvement of gait in people with Parkinson disease. J Neurol Phys Ther 29:2–8.
38. Lopane G, Contin M, Scaglione C, Albani F, Baruzzi A, et al. (2010) The effect of a clinically practical exercise on levodopa bioavailability and motor response in patients with Parkinson disease. Clin Neuropharmacol 33:254–256.
39. Combs SA, Diehl MD, Chrzastowski C, Didrick N, McCoin B, et al. (2013) Community-based group exercise for persons with Parkinson disease: a randomized controlled trial. NeuroRehabilitation 32:117–124.
40. Pelosin E, Avanzino L, Bove M, Stramesi P, Nieuwboer A, et al. (2010) Action observation improves freezing of gait in patients with Parkinson's disease. Neurorehabil Neural Repair 24:746–752.

41. Frazzitta G, Bertotti G, Riboldazzi G, Turla M, Uccellini D, et al. (2012) Effectiveness of intensive inpatient rehabilitation treatment on disease progression in parkinsonian patients: a randomized controlled trial with 1-year follow-up. Neurorehabil Neural Repair 26: 144–150.
42. Yousefi B, Tadibi V, Khoei AF, Montazeri A (2009) Exercise therapy, quality of life, and activities of daily living in patients with Parkinson disease: a small scale quasi-randomised trial. Trials doi:10.1186/1745-6215-10-67
43. Ashburn A, Fazakarley L, Ballinger C, Pickering R, McLellan LD, et al. (2007) A randomised controlled trial of a home based exercise programme to reduce the risk of falling among people with Parkinson's disease. J Neurol Neurosurg Psychiatry 78: 678–684.
44. Ellis T, de Goede CJ, Feldman RG, Wolters EC, Kwakkel G, et al. (2005) Efficacy of a physical therapy program in patients with Parkinson's disease: a randomized controlled trial. Arch Phys Med Rehabil 86: 626–632.
45. Nadeau A, Pourcher E, Corbeil P (2013) Effects of 24 weeks of treadmill training on gait performance in Parkinson disease. Med Sci Sports Exerc (In press).
46. Herman T, Giladi N, Hausdorff JM (2009) Treadmill training for the treatment of gait disturbances in people with Parkinson's disease: a mini-review. J Neural Transm 116:307–318.
47. Mehrholz J, Friis R, Kugler J, Twork S, Storch A, et al. (2010) Treadmill training for patients with Parkinson's disease. Cochrane Database Syst Rev 1, Art. No.: CD007830. doi: 10.1002/14651858.CD007830.pub2
48. Goodwin VA, Richards SH, Taylor RS, Taylor AH, Campbell JL (2008) The effectiveness of exercise interventions for people with Parkinson's disease; a systematic review and meta-analysis. Mov Disord 23:631–640.
49. Roy IS, Roy SS (2012) A systematic review on various models of exercise on people with Parkinson disease. JAHSP 10:1–10.
50. Frazzitta G, Balbi P, Maestri R, Bertotti G, Boveri N, et al. (2013) The beneficial role of intensive exercise on Parkinson disease progression. Am J Phys Med Rehabil 92:523–532.
51. Petzinger GM, Fisher BE, McEwen S, Beeler JA, Walsh JP, et al. (2013) Exercise-enhanced neuroplasticity targeting motor and cognitive circuitry in Parkinson's disease. Lancet Neurol 12:716–726.
52. van Praag H, Shubert T, Zhao C, Gage FH (2005) Exercise enhances learning and hippocampal neurogenesis in aged mice. J Neurosci 25:8680–8685.
53. Physical Activity Guidelines Advisory Committee (2008) Physical activity guidelines advisory committee report, 2008. Washington, DC: US Department of Health and Human Services, 2008.
54. US Department of Health and Human Services (2008) 2008 physical activity guidelines for Americans. Be active, healthy, and happy.
55. Nelson ME, Rejeski WJ, Blair SN, Duncan PW, Judge JO, et al. (2007) Physical activity and public health in older adults: recommendation from the American College of Sports Medicine and the American Heart Association. Med Sci Sports Exerc 39:1435–1445.
56. Hall EE, Ekkekakis P, Petruzzello SJ (2002) The affective beneficence of vigorous exercise revisited. Br J Health Psychol 7:47–66.

12

The Relationship between the Blood Pressure Responses to Exercise following Training and Detraining Periods

Emily A. Moker[1], Lori A. Bateman[2], William E. Kraus[2], Linda S. Pescatello[1]*

1 Department of Kinesiology, University of Connecticut, Storrs, CT, United States of America, 2 Division of Cardiology, Department of Medicine, Duke University Medical Center, Durham, NC, United States of America

Abstract

Background: Exercise training lowers blood pressure (BP), while BP increases and returns to pre-training values with detraining. Yet, there is considerable variability in these BP responses. We examined the relationship between the BP responses after 6 months of training followed by 2 weeks of detraining among the same people.

Methodology/Principal Findings: Subjects (n = 75) (X±SD, 50.2±10.6 yr) were sedentary, obese, and had prehypertension. They completed an aerobic (n = 34); resistance (n = 28); or aerobic + resistance or concurrent (n = 13) exercise training program. We calculated a metabolic syndrome *z* score (MetSz). Subjects were classified as BP responders (BP decreased) or non-responders (BP increased) to training and detraining. Linear and multivariable regression tested the BP response. Chi Square tested the frequency of responders and non-responders. The systolic BP (SBP, $r = -0.474$) and diastolic (DBP, $r = -0.540$) response to training negatively correlated with detraining ($p < 0.01$), independent of modality ($p > 0.05$). Exercise responders reduced SBP 11.5±7.8 (n = 29) and DBP 9.8±6.2 mmHg (n = 31); non-responders increased SBP 7.9.±10.9 (n = 46) and DBP 4.9±7.1 mmHg (n = 44) ($p < 0.001$). We found 65.5% of SBP training responders were SBP detraining non-responders; while 60.9% of SBP training non-responders were SBP detraining responders ($p = 0.034$). Similarly, 80.6% of DBP training responders were DBP detraining non-responders; while 59.1% of DBP training non-responders were DBP detraining responders ($p < 0.001$). The SBP detraining response ($r = -0.521$), resting SBP ($r = -0.444$), and MetSz ($r = 0.288$) explained 44.8% of the SBP training response ($p < 0.001$). The DBP detraining response ($r = -0.553$), resting DBP ($r = -0.450$), and MetSz ($r = 0.463$) explained 60.1% of the DBP training response ($p < 0.001$).

Conclusions/Significance: As expected most subjects that decreased BP after exercise training, increased BP after detraining. An unanticipated finding was most subjects that increased BP after exercise training, decreased BP after detraining. Reasons why the negative effects of exercise training on BP maybe reversed with detraining among some people should be explored further.

Trial Registration Information: ClinicalTrials.gov 1R01HL57354; 2003–2008; NCT00275145

Editor: James M. Wright, University of British Columbia, Canada

Funding: Supported by the Studies of a Targeted Risk Reduction through Defined Exercise (STRRIDE-AT/RT) 1R01HL57354; 2003-2008; NCT00275145. The funders had no role in study design, data collection and analysis, decision to publish, or preparation of the manuscript.

Competing Interests: The authors have declared that no competing interests exist.

* Email: Linda.Pescatello@uconn.edu

Introduction

Hypertension is one of the most important cardiovascular disease (CVD) risk factors [1,2], and is the most common primary diagnosis in the United States [3]. Once blood pressure (BP) becomes higher than normal, there is a rapid progression to established hypertension. For, one in five people with prehypertension develop hypertension within 4 years [4,5]; and most American will acquire hypertension if they live into old age [1].

Aerobic exercise training lowers resting BP 5 to 7 mmHg, while resistance exercise training lowers BP 2 to 3 mmHg among people with hypertension [6]. The BP lowering effects of exercise training occur rapidly within just three exercise sessions, persist with continued training, and diminish to pre-training levels within 2 weeks after training has ceased [7,8]. For these reasons, the American College of Sports Medicine recommends individuals with hypertension engage in moderate intensity, aerobic exercise on most days of the week for 30–60 minutes per day, and moderate intensity, resistance training two to three days per week as a supplement to aerobic exercise training to lower BP [6,9].

Despite the general consensus that exercise training lowers BP, there is considerable individual variability in the BP response to exercise training. We [10] and others [11,12] have shown 20–25% of the people with hypertension do not lower BP following exercise. Furthermore, a percentage of these may adversely respond to exercise training as antihypertensive therapy, increasing BP 10 or more mmHg for reasons that are not clear [13]. We have completed several studies showing that resting BP and the components of the metabolic syndrome (MetS) as defined by the Adult Treatment Panel III [1] account for a clinically meaningful amount of the variability in the BP response to aerobic exercise [14–18]. In another study we showed that these effects may be dependent upon exercise modality [19]. Furthermore, the relationship between the BP response to exercise training and detraining has yet to be examined among the same people.

Therefore, the purpose of this study was to examine the BP responses after 6 months of exercise training followed by a 2 week detraining period among sedentary, middle-aged adults with prehypertension and mild to moderate dyslipidemia from the clinical trial, Studies of a Targeted Risk Reduction through Defined Exercise (STRRIDE-AT/RT) (1R01HL57354; 2003–2008; NCT00275145) [20]. We hypothesized the majority of STRRIDE-AT/RT participants would decrease their BP after 6 months of exercise training and increase their BP to pre-training levels after 2 weeks of detraining. However, there would be considerable variability in the BP responses to training and detraining that would be partially accounted for by resting BP and the MetS.

Methods

This is a sub-study of the Studies of a Targeted Risk Reduction Intervention through Defined Exercise or STRRIDE-AT/RT (1R01HL57354; 2003-2008; NCT00275145)[19–22]. The two primary purposes of STRRIDE-AT/RT were to: 1) investigate the effects of different types and intensities of exercise training regimens on established CVD risk factors; and 2) to study the peripheral biologic mechanisms through which exercise training altered these CVD risk factors. Subjects were recruited from September 1, 2004 to December 31, 2008. We only describe the STRRIDE-AT/RT methods used in this sub-study below. However, the informed consent for this trial are available as Protocol Informed Consent S1.

Subjects

Volunteers were men and women 18–70 years who were exercising ≤ 2 d·wk^{-1} or had a peak oxygen uptake (VO_2peak) $\leq$ 35 mL·kg^{-1}·min^{-1}. Study inclusion criteria were: (a) body mass index (BMI) 25–35 kg·m^{-2}; (b) resting systolic BP (SBP) $<$ 160 mmHg and/or diastolic BP (DBP) $<$90 mmHg; and (c) fasting low density lipoprotein-cholesterol (LDL) 130–190 mg·dL^{-1}; or fasting high density lipoprotein-cholesterol (HDL) $\leq$40 mg·dL^{-1} for men and $\leq$45 mg·dL^{-1} for women. Subjects had no known metabolic, muscular, or coronary heart disease(s) and were not taking any antilipidemic or antihypertensive medications. Prior to participating in the study, individuals were screened by telephone and signed a written informed consent approved by the IRB of the participating institutions, Duke University Medical Center and East Carolina University. This sub-study did not meant the definition of " human subjects research" under Study Design Overview 45.CFR46.102(d) or 45.CFR. 46.102(f) at the University of Connecticut. Therefore, we were not required to file an application for review by the University of Connecticut.

Subjects attended a baseline assessment prior to the start of the 6 month exercise training intervention in which they completed a health screening questionnaire and a series of health fitness and anthropometric measurements. Pre-training measurements were performed at the completion of a 4 month wait list control period during which subjects were asked to maintain their current lifestyle. Subjects were then randomized into one of three exercise training programs: aerobic (AT) (n = 34), resistance (RT) (n = 28), or aerobic exercise and resistance concurrently (AT+RT) (n = 13). Measurements were performed again following the 6 month exercise training intervention. To be included in this sub-study, STRRIDE-AT/RT subjects had to have obtained BP measurements before (i.e, at the completion of the wait list control period) and after exercise training and the 2 week detraining period.

Exercise Training Intervention

Aerobic. The AT group performed a peak cardiopulmonary graded exercise test before exercise training to determine the AT intensity. After a ramp period of 1 month, subjects exercised 3 d·wk^{-1} at 65–80% VO_2peak on average 130$\pm$22.7 min·wk^{-1} for 5 months expending the caloric equivalent to walking or jogging 20 mi·wk^{-1}. To ensure attainment of the proper AT intensity, subjects wore a heart rate monitor (Polar Electro, Inc., Woodbury, NY) at each session that was uploaded weekly. Subjects were instructed to use the treadmill as the primary mode to train, however, the bicycle ergometer, elliptical, and stair climber were other options.

Resistance. The RT group began with one set of 8 to 12 repetitions per set of eight exercises (four upper and four lower) targeting major groups for the first 2 weeks followed by two sets during weeks three and four until they reached the intended three sets during week five. Subjects exercised at 70–85% of their one repetition maximum 3 d·wk^{-1} for 5 months using Cybex weight machines (Cybex International Inc; Medway, MA). The Duke University Medical Center RT group used only Cybex machines, while the East Carolina University RT group used Cybex weight machines to perform the upper and lower body exercises, abdominal crunch exercises were also incorporated, and at week 14 subjects transitioned to free weights for the upper body exercises. Subjects who were able to perform three sets of 12 repetitions in two consecutive sessions increased resistance in 5 lb increments.

Aerobic and Resistance. The AT+RT group performed the identical training program as the AT and RT groups in combination.

Exercise Supervision. All training sessions were closely monitored. East Carolina University provided direct supervision, while Duke University Medical Center had direct supervision and/or used the FitLinxx Strength Training Partner (FitLinxx; Norwalk, CT). FitLinxx Strength Training Partneris a computer system designed to electronically track workouts and automatically send training results to the FitLinxx server.

Anthropometric Assessments. Height was measured to the nearest quarter cm and weight to the nearest 0.1 kg on a digital scale (Scale 5005; Scale Tronix Inc, Wheaton, IL) to calculate body mass index (BMI, kg·m^{-2}). Waist circumference (WC) was taken around the abdominal waist at the iliac crest. Each measurement was taken twice to the nearest 0.1 cm and averaged.

Blood Pressure. A trained research nurse measured BP by auscultation on the non-dominant arm before and after training and detraining. Subjects sat quietly in the laboratory for 60 minutes with feet flat on the floor in the relaxed position. Two BP measurements were obtained 20–30 minutes apart and then averaged by a nurse trained in standard procedures. [23] Mean arterial pressure (MAP) was calculated as: DBP+0.33* (SBP-DBP).

Fasting Blood Sample Determinations. Subjects fasted for 12 hours. Total cholesterol, LDL, HDL, triglycerides (TG), glucose, and insulin were analyzed from fasting plasma using the nuclear magnetic resonance spectroscopy technique (LipoScience; Raliegh, NC).

Metabolic Syndrome Classification. Presence of the metabolic syndrome (MetS) was defined as having three or more of the following: triglycerides (TG) ≥150 mg·dL[1], BP ≥130/85 mmHg, glucose ≥100 mg·dL^{-1}, WC ≥102 cm for men and ≥88 cm for women, and/or HDL <40 mg·dL^{-1} for men and <50 mg·dL^{-1} for women [24].

The MetS z-score was a continuous standardized calculation of the five MetS components: HDL, TG, glucose, WC, and MAP [19]. Individual subject data, current ATP III criteria [24], and standard deviations (SD) from the entire STRRIDE-AT/RT cohort at baseline were used to calculate the MetS z-score. The equations used to calculate the MetS z score were: {z Score = [(40-HDL)/6.2]+[(TG-150)/66.2]+[(glucose-100)/10.4]+[(WC-102)/9.3]+[(MAP-100)/8.7]} for men; and {z Score = [(50-HDL)/11.8]+[(TG-150)/66.2]+[(glucose-100)/10.4]+[(WC-88)/9.2]+[(MAP-100)/8.7]} for women [19].

Cardiopulmonary Graded Exercise Test. All subjects completed a cardiopulmonary graded exercise test on a treadmill with a 12-lead electrocardiograph and had expired gas measured using a TrueMax 2400 Metabolic Cart (ParvoMEdics; Sandy, UT). The test protocol included 2 minute stages with the workload increasing by one metabolic equivalent per stage. VO_2peak was determined by averaging the two consecutive highest 15 second readings. A respiratory exchange ratio ≥1.10 was the criteria used to terminate the test.

Statistical Analysis

Descriptive statistics (mean±SD) were calculated for all variables. Repeated measures analysis of covariance was used to test the change in BP, MetS z score, and other individual components of the MetS after exercise training (i.e., after versus before training) and after detraining (i.e., after 2 weeks of detraining versus after training) by exercise groups (AT, RT, AT+RT) with gender as a fixed factor. Pre-training BMI and the MetS z score, and the change in VO_2peak after training were covariates. Bonferroni post-hoc tests were used to test for BP differences among groups. Chi-Square was used to test the frequencies of individuals who decreased (i.e., responders, BP change <0 mmHg) or increased (i.e., non-responders, BP change ≥0 mmHg) BP after exercise training and detraining. Simple linear and multivariable regressions were performed to test for correlates of the BP response to exercise training with a variance inflation factor <2 used to indicate covariance among the independent variables was low [10].

There is considerable inter- and intra-variability in the response of cardiometabolic risk factors to exercise [12,13]. Therefore, we used chi-square to test the frequencies of subjects whose BP decreased (i.e., responders, BP change <0 mmHg) or increased (i.e., non-responders, BP change ≥0 mmHg) and MetS profile improved (i.e., number of MetS components decreased) or became worse (i.e., number of MetS components increased) by summing the response of the individual components of the MetS after versus before exercise training. The MetS profile components used for these determinations were MAP, WC, HDL, triglycerides, and glucose to be consistent with the MetS z score equations [19]. All statistical analyses were performed with the Statistical Package for Social Science (SPSS) version 19.0 for Macintosh (IBM, Armok, NY) with $p<0.05$ established as the level of statistical significance.

Results

Subjects

The sub-study population consisted of 75 sedentary, middle aged, obese men (n = 38) and women (n = 37) with prehypertension, mild to moderate dyslipidemia, and normal fasting glucose (Table 1). In addition, 29.3% of the total sample had the MetS [24]; while 34.5% of SBP training responders, 26.1% of SBP training non-responders, 35.5% of DBP training responders, and 25.0% of DBP training non-responders had the MetS with no difference in prevalence between BP responders and non-responders ($p>0.05$). SBP training responders had a higher BMI (p = 0.025) and resting BP (p = 0.003) and lower glucose levels (p = 0.031) and VO_2peak (p = 0.051) than SBP non-responders. DBP training responders had a higher resting BP compared to DBP non-responders (p = 0.025). All other characteristics were not different between SBP and DBP training responders and non-responders ($p>0.05$).

The Blood Pressure Responses to Exercise Training and Detraining

Overall and by Exercise Modality. The change in SBP (0.4±10.6 mmHg) and DBP (−0.8±7.0 mmHg) after training was not different among the total sample ($p>0.05$); and the change in SBP/DBP was also not different among exercise groups, i.e., AT (n = 34) 1.9±10.8/0.1±6.0 mmHg, RT (n = 28) 2.5±8.3/−0.8±5.5 mmHg, and AT+/RT (n = 13) −4.0±10.1/−2.4±9.1 mmHg, respectively ($p>0.05$). The change in SBP (0.3±11.7 mmHg) and DBP (0.9±8.7 mmHg) after detraining was not different among the total sample ($p>0.05$); and the change in SBP/DBP was also not different among exercise groups, i.e., AT −1.4±11.0/−2.3±8.2 mmHg, RT 0.6±10.2/1.4±7.8 mmHg, and AT+RT 3.1±11.3/3.9±8.3 mmHg, respectively ($p>0.05$).

Responders versus Non-responders. Training responders decreased SBP (n = 29) by −11.5±7.8 mmHg and DBP (n = 31) by −9.8±6.2 mmHg; whereas non-responders increased SBP (n = 46) by 7.9±10.9 mmHg and DBP (n = 44) 4.9±13.5 after training ($p<0.001$). Furthermore, the SBP and DBP response differed between training responders and non-responders ($p<0.001$). Detraining responders tended to decrease SBP (n = 46) by −3.1±12.9 mmHg (p = 0.109) and decreased DBP (n = 44) by −3.4±7.5 mmHg (p = 0.005); whereas detraining non-responders tended to increase (n = 29) SBP by 6.5±16.7 mmHg (p = 0.051) and increased DBP (n = 31) by 5.3±12.9 mmHg (p = 0.031) after detraining. In addition, the SBP and DBP response was different between detraining responders and non-responders ($p<0.001$).

We found of the 29 people who were classified as SBP training responders (SBP decreased), 34.5% were SBP detraining responders (SBP decreased) and 65.5% were SBP detraining non-responders (SBP increased). Of 46 people who were classified as SBP training non-responders (SBP increased), 60.9% were SBP detraining responders (SBP decreased) and 39.1% were SBP detraining non-responders (SBP increased) (p = 0.034). Of the 31 people who were classified as DBP training responders (DBP decreased), 19.4% were DBP detraining responders (DBP decreased) and 80.6% were DBP detraining non-responders (DBP increased). Of the 44 people that were classified as DBP training non-responders (DBP increased), 59.1% were DBP detraining responders (DBP decreased) and 40.9% were DBP detraining non-responders (DBP increased) ($p<0.001$). Therefore, the majority of subjects that decreased BP after training (responders), increased BP after detraining (nonresponders); while the majority of subjects that increased BP after training (nonresponders), decreased BP after detraining (responders). Last, 62.1% of SBP training responders were also DBP training responders; whereas 52.2% of SBP detraining responders were also DBP detraining responders.

Predictors of Blood Pressure to Exercise Training. Table 2 displays the correlates of the BP response after training. Factors accounting for 44.8% of the variance in SBP

Table 1. Baseline subject characteristics (Mean±SD) of the total sample and by blood pressure exercise training responders and non-responders.

Variable	Total Sample (n = 75)	SBP		DBP	
		Responder (n = 29)	Non- responder (n = 46)	Responder (n = 31)	Non- responder (n = 44)
Age (yr)	50.2±10.6	52.6±12.0	48.7±9.5	50.2±11.0	50.3±10.4
SBP (mmHg)	120.0±13.7	125.8±14.3†	116.3±12.0	121.7±15.9	118.7±11.9
DBP (mmHg)	79.1±9.2	80.7±9.7	78.1±8.8	81.9±9.7*	77.1±8.4
BMI (kg/m^{-2})	30.5±3.2	31.5±2.7*	29.8±3.3	30.3±2.9	30.6±3.3
WC (cm)	97.0±9.8	97.3±9.8	96.7±9.9	97.5±10.0	96.5±9.7
CHOL (mg·dL^{1})	226.2±31.6	228.7±36.8	224.6±28.2	228.6±31.4	224.5±31.9
HDL (mg·dL^{-1})	52.1±15.0	55.2±14.6	50.2±15.1	51.8±16.6	52.4±13.9
LDL (mg·dL^{-1})	144.2±25.1	143.4±30.5	144.8±21.3	143.9±26.	144.4±24.6
TG (mg·dL^{-1})	153.3±85.7	150.0±68.6	155.4±95.5	171.8±101.2	140.3±71.2
Glucose (mg·dL^{-1})	92.4±11.5	88.8±13.9*	94.7±9.1	89.9±14.3	94.3±8.8
Insulin (mg·dL^{1})	8.9±4.5	9.2±5.7	8.7±3.6	8.5±4.6	9.3±4.5
VO_{2peak} (mL·kg^{-1}·min^{-1})	28.1±6.5	26.3±5.6*	29.3±6.8	29.8±6.9	27.0±6.0

SBP, systolic blood pressure; DBP, diastolic blood pressure; BMI, body mass index; WC, waist circumference; CHOL, total cholesterol; HDL, high density lipoprotein; LDL, low density lipoprotein; VO_{2peak}, peak oxygen uptake; MetS z score; metabolic syndrome z score.
*p<0.05, †p = 0.001, Responder vs non-responder.

response to training were the SBP response to detraining, resting SBP, and the change in the MetS z score after training (p<0.001). Factors accounting for 60.1% of the variance in the DBP to training were the DBP response to detraining, resting DBP, and the change in the MetS z score after training (p<0.001).

The Blood Pressure and Metabolic Syndrome Response to Exercise Training. The MetS z score was not different after exercise training among the total sample (p>0.05) (Table 3). The MetS z score decreased (i.e, improved) among SBP and DBP training responders after training (p<0.001), but was not different among SBP and DBP training non-responders (p>0.05). MAP was not different after exercise training among the total sample (p> 0.05). MAP decreased among SBP and DBP training responders after training, and increased among SBP and DBP training non-responders (p<0.001). WC decreased after training among the total sample (p = 0.005) and SBP training non-responders (p = 0.010). HDL increased after training among DBP training non-responders (p = 0.005). TG decreased after training among the total sample (p = 0.003) and SBP training non-responders (p = 0.025).

We found of the 29 people classified as SBP training responders (SBP decreased), the MetS improved in 31.0% (number of components decreased) and the MetS became worse in 69.0% (number of components increased). Of the 46 people classified as SBP training non-responders (SBP increased), the MetS improved in 52.2% (number of components decreased) and the MetS became worse in 47.8% (number of components increased) (p = 0.059). Of the 31 people who were classified as DBP training responders (DBP decreased), the MetS improved in 29.0% (number of components decreased) and the MetS became worse in 71.0% (number of components increased). Of the 44 people classified as DBP training non-responders (DBP increased), the MetS improved in 54.5% (number of components decreased) and the MetS became worse in 45.5% (number of components increased) (p = 0.025). Thus, for the majority of subjects that decreased BP after training (responders), the number of components of the MetS increased or became worse after training.

Table 2. Correlates of the blood pressure response after versus before 6 months of exercise training.

	Correlates	β	t	Partial r	r^2	p
SBP	Detraining SBP	−.461	−5.149	−.521		<0.001
	Resting SBP	−.379	−4.171	−.444		<0.001
	MetS z score	.235	2.536	.288		0.013
Model Summary				.686	.448	<0.001
DBP	Detraining DBP	−.448	−5.595	−.553		<0.001
	Resting DBP	−.339	−4.245	−.450		<0.001
	MetS z score	.371	4.405	.463		<0.001
Model Summary				.786	.601	<0.001

SBP, systolic blood pressure; DBP, diastolic blood pressure; MetS z score; metabolic syndrome z score.

Table 3. The response (Mean±SD) of the metabolic syndrome z score and the individual components of the metabolic syndrome z score after versus before 6 months of exercise training.

Component	Total Sample (n = 75)	SBP		DBP	
		Responder (n = 29)	Non-responder (n = 46)	Responder (n = 31)	Non-responder (n = 44)
Metabolic Syndrome z score	−0.5±2.0	−1.7±1.9†&	0.3±2.4	−1.4±2.9*&	0.4±1.5
MAP (mmHg)	−0.7±9.5	−8.5±6.1†&	5.1±9.2†	−8.2±7.2†&	4.8±8.5†
WC (cm)	−1.2±3.6*	−1.1±3.4	−2.1±5.1*	−1.8±5.3	−0.6±3.6
HDL (mg·dL^{-1})	1.2±5.5	1.4±7.6	1.5±6.9	−1.9±7.9	2.1±4.6*
TG (mg·dL^{-1})	−20.4±58.2*	−25.7±66.0*‡	−15.6±80.0	−31.5±72.9	−13.8±61.9
Glucose (mg·dL^{-1})	0.9±9.7	−0.1±11.2	1.7±13.7	−1.2±11.8	0.4±10.9

MAP, mean arterial pressure; WC, Waist Circumference; TG, Triglycerides.
*p<0.05, †p<0.001 After versus before exercise.
‡p<0.05, &p<0.001, Responders versus non-responders.

Discussion

The purpose of this STRRIDE-AT/RT sub-study was to examine the relationship between the BP response after 6 months of exercise training followed by a 2 week detraining period among 75 sedentary, middle aged men and women with prehypertension and mild to moderate dyslipidemia, 29.3% of which had the MetS. As hypothesized, the BP response after 6 months of exercise training was negatively correlated with the BP response following 2 weeks of detraining. Furthermore, the majority of SBP (65%) and DBP (80%) exercise training responders BP decreased) were SBP and DBP detraining non-responders (BP increased). An unanticipated finding was the majority of SBP (~61%) and DBP (59%) exercise training non-responders (BP increased) were SBP and DBP detraining responders (BP decreased). The major correlates of the SBP and DBP response to exercise training were the BP response to detraining, resting BP, and the MetS z score, which accounted for 44.8% and 60.1% of the variability in the SBP and DBP response to exercise training, respectively. Last, the BP response to exercise training did not necessarily align with the response of the MetS to exercise training as the majority of subjects that decreased BP after training, experienced an increase in the number of MetS components after training.

The results of this sub-study provide new findings demonstrating that for a majority of middle aged men and women with prehypertension that experienced an adverse BP response to exercise training, these adverse BP effects were reversed following detraining. Furthermore, the BP response to exercise training may not align with the response of other cardiometabolic risk factors to exercise. Our findings are consistent with our reports [10,14,15,17] and those of others [11,12] indicating there is a clinically meaningful proportion of people that do not lower BP following exercise training. Recently, Bouchard et al. [13] consolidated the findings from six large exercise training studies that included STRRIDE-AT/RT to examine the variability in the response of cardiometabolic risk factors to exercise training. They found ~12% of the participants experienced an adverse SBP response increasing SBP>10 mmHg, whereas a similar amount had an excellent response to exercise training decreasing SBP≤ 10 mmHg. Fasting insulin, TG, and HDL exhibited similar patterns of response, and similar to our findings, the response of these cardiometabolic risk factors was often different from the BP response to exercise training.

Insight into reasons for the unexpected finding of why some people experienced an adverse BP response to exercise training that was reversed with detraining may partially reside within the correlates of the BP response to exercise training that we found. The major predictors of the BP response to exercise training were the BP response to detraining, resting BP, and the MetS z score. These findings are consistent with our previous work showing resting BP and the MetS are important predictors of the BP response to exercise among sedentary, middle-aged, overweight men with pre- to Stage 1 hypertension [6,10,15–18]. Hypertension is a contributor to and component of the MetS [25]. Therefore, the mechanisms by which the MetS and its individual components would account for a clinically meaningful proportion of the BP response to exercise training may be partially explained by their apparent common underlying pathophysiology.

Erdogen et al. [26] examined the progression of prehypertension to established hypertension among 98 men and women 30 to 63 years with the MetS and prehypertension over 3 years. They found that the progression of prehypertension to hypertension positively correlated with resting SBP (p = 0.002) and the MetS (p = 0.009) among 98 men and women 30 to 63 years with the MetS and prehypertension over 3 years. Ferriera et al. [27] found apparently healthy individuals between 36 and 42 years with prehypertension at baseline and that had persistent MetS over 6 years exhibited the maladaptive arterial remodeling changes that were related to changes in SBP and DBP. However, these maladaptive arterial changes were reversed in individuals with prehypertension who recovered from the MetS. Collectively, these findings indicate that the MetS and its components should be explored further as clinical characteristics that may eventually be used to distinguish between individuals that respond and do not respond to exercise as antihypertensive therapy.

A limitation of this STRRIDE-AT/RT sub-study was its primary purpose was not the primary purpose of STRRIDE-AT/RT. Thus, our sub-study sample may have been underpowered to detect changes in BP as a result of exercise training as well as BP differences among the exercise training groups. Nonetheless, our sub-study sample was more than adequately powered to examine its primary purpose as the effect size to detect differences in the BP response after versus before 6 months of exercise training between responders and non-responders ranged from medium (0.341) to large (0.741). It is also possible that misclassification of BP responders and non-responders to exercise training and detraining may have occurred due to the inherent variability in BP measurement as well as regression to the mean [13,28]. In order to minimize these biases, the research personnel collecting BP data were well trained clinicians in standard BP measurement protocols [23], each subject served as their own control, and multiple BP measurements were taken and averaged. Furthermore, the coefficient of variation among SBP and DBP before training and detraining approximated 5% indicating acceptable reproducibility.

In conclusion, the BP response after 6 months of exercise training was negatively correlated with the BP response following 2 weeks of detraining. Nonetheless, the majority of BP exercise training responders were BP detraining non-responders; whereas, the majority of BP exercise training non-responders were BP detraining responders. Furthermore, the BP response to exercise training did not necessarily align with the response of the other components of the MetS to exercise training. Further research is needed to elucidate reasons why detraining may reverse the adverse effects of exercise on BP for some individuals that may partially reside in the common underlying pathophysiology of hypertension and the MetS.

Supporting Information

Protocol Informed Consent S1 From the Studies of a Targeted Risk Reduction through Defined Exercise (STRRIDE-AT/RT) (1R01HL57354; 2003–2008; NCT00275145).

Author Contributions

Conceived and designed the experiments: WEK, LAB, LSP. Performed the experiments: WEK, LAB. Analyzed the data: EAM, LSP. Wrote the paper: EAM, LSP. Reviewed and contributed to the final version of the manuscript: EAM, LAB, WEK, LSP.

References

1. Chobanian AV, Bakris GL, Black HR, Cushman WC, Green LA, et al. (2003) Seventh report of the joint national committee on prevention, detection, evaluation, and treatment of high blood pressure. Hypertension 42: 1206–1252.
2. Roger VL, Go AS, Lloyd-Jones DM, Benjamin EJ, Berry JD, et al. (2012) Heart disease and stroke statistics—2012 update: A report from the american heart association. Circulation 125: e2–e220.
3. Wang G, Yan L, Ayala C, George MG, Fang J. (2013) Hypertension-associated expenditures for medication among US adults. Am J Hypertens.
4. Fields LE, Burt VL, Cutler JA, Hughes J, Roccella EJ, et al. (2004) The burden of adult hypertension in the united states 1999 to 2000: A rising tide. Hypertension 44: 398–404.
5. Wang Y, Wang QJ. (2004) The prevalence of prehypertension and hypertension among US adults according to the new joint national committee guidelines: New challenges of the old problem. Arch Intern Med 164: 2126–2134.
6. Pescatello LS, Franklin BA, Fagard R, Farquhar WB, Kelley GA, et al. (2004) American college of sports medicine position stand. exercise and hypertension. Med Sci Sports Exerc 36: 533–553.
7. Meredith IT, Jennings GL, Esler MD, Dewar EM, Bruce AM, et al. (1990) Time-course of the antihypertensive and autonomic effects of regular endurance exercise in human subjects. J Hypertens 8: 859–866.
8. Murray A, Delaney T, Bell C. (2006) Rapid onset and offset of circulatory adaptations to exercise training in men. J Hum Hypertens 20: 193–200.
9. Pescatello LS, Arena R, Riebe DW, Thompson PD, editors. (2013) ACSMâ€s guidelines for exercise testing and prescription. Baltimore, MD: Lippincott Williams & Wilkins.
10. Pescatello LS, Kulikowich JM. (2001) The aftereffects of dynamic exercise on ambulatory blood pressure. Med Sci Sports Exerc 33: 1855–1861.
11. Hagberg JM, Park JJ, Brown MD. (2000) The role of exercise training in the treatment of hypertension: An update. Sports Med 30: 193–206.
12. Bouchard C, Rankinen T. (2001) Individual differences in response to regular physical activity. Med Sci Sports Exerc 33: S446-51; discussion S452–3.
13. Bouchard C, Blair SN, Church TS, Earnest CP, Hagberg JM, et al. (2012) Adverse metabolic response to regular exercise: Is it a rare or common occurrence? PLoS One 7: e37887.
14. Ash GI, Eicherb JD, Pescatello LS. (2013) The promises and challenges of the use of genomics in the prescription of exercise for hypertension: The 2013 update. Curr Hypertens Rev 9: 130–147.
15. Eicher JD, Maresh CM, Tsongalis GJ, Thompson PD, Pescatello LS. (2010) The additive blood pressure lowering effects of exercise intensity on post-exercise hypotension. Am Heart J 160: 513–520.
16. Olson KM, Augeri AL, Seip RL, Tsongalis GJ, Thompson PD, et al. (2012) Correlates of endothelial function and the peak systolic blood pressure response to a graded maximal exercise test. Atherosclerosis 222: 202–207.
17. Pescatello LS, Blanchard BE, Tsongalis GJ, O'Connell AA, Gordish-Dressman H, et al. (2008) A comparison of the genetic and clinical profile of men that respond and do not respond to the immediate antihypertensive effects of aerobic exercise. Appl Clin Genet 1: 7–17.
18. Pescatello LS, Blanchard BE, Van Heest JL, Maresh CM, Gordish-Dressman H, et al. (2008) The metabolic syndrome and the immediate antihypertensive effects of aerobic exercise: A randomized control design. BMC Cardiovasc Disord 8: 12-2261-8-12.
19. Bateman LA, Slentz CA, Willis LH, Shields AT, Piner LW, et al. (2011) Comparison of aerobic versus resistance exercise training effects on metabolic syndrome (from the studies of a targeted risk reduction intervention through defined exercise - STRRIDE-AT/RT). Am J Cardiol 108: 838–844.
20. Kraus WE, Torgan CE, Duscha BD, Norris J, Brown SA, et al. (2001) Studies of a targeted risk reduction intervention through defined exercise (STRRIDE). Med Sci Sports Exerc 33: 1774–1784.
21. Johnson JL, Slentz CA, Houmard JA, Samsa GP, Duscha BD, et al. (2007) Exercise training amount and intensity effects on metabolic syndrome (from studies of a targeted risk reduction intervention through defined exercise). Am J Cardiol 100: 1759–1766.
22. Slentz CA, Houmard JA, Johnson JL, Bateman LA, Tanner CJ, et al. (2007) Inactivity, exercise training and detraining, and plasma lipoproteins. STRRIDE: A randomized, controlled study of exercise intensity and amount. J Appl Physiol 103: 432–442.
23. Pickering TG, Hall JE, Appel LJ, Falkner BE, Graves J, et al. (2005) Recommendations for blood pressure measurement in humans and experimental animals: Part 1: Blood pressure measurement in humans: A statement for professionals from the subcommittee of professional and public education of the american heart association council on high blood pressure research. Circulation 111: 697–716.
24. [Anonymous]. (2001) Third report of the national cholesterol education program (NCEP). expert panel on detection, evaluation, and treatment of high blood cholesterol in adults (adult treatment panel III). executive summary. 2013.
25. Galassi A, Reynolds K, He J. (2006) Metabolic syndrome and risk of cardiovascular disease: A meta-analysis. Am J Med 119: 812–819.
26. Erdogan D, Ozaydin M, Icli A, Gonul E, Yucel H, et al. (2012) Echocardiographic predictors of progression from prehypertension to hypertension. J Hypertens 30: 1639–1645.
27. Ferreira I, Beijers HJ, Schouten F, Smulders YM, Twisk JW, et al. (2012) Clustering of metabolic syndrome traits is associated with maladaptive carotid remodeling and stiffening: A 6-year longitudinal study. Hypertension 60: 542–549.
28. Shepard R. (2003) Regression to the mean A threat to exercise science. Sports Med 33: 575–584.

13

Three Minutes of All-Out Intermittent Exercise per Week Increases Skeletal Muscle Oxidative Capacity and Improves Cardiometabolic Health

Jenna B. Gillen[1], Michael E. Percival[1], Lauren E. Skelly[1], Brian J. Martin[1], Rachel B. Tan[1], Mark A. Tarnopolsky[1,2], Martin J. Gibala[1]*

1 Department of Kinesiology, McMaster University, Hamilton, Ontario, Canada, **2** Department of Pediatrics and Medicine, McMaster University, Hamilton, Ontario, Canada

Abstract

We investigated whether a training protocol that involved 3 min of intense intermittent exercise per week — within a total training time commitment of 30 min including warm up and cool down — could increase skeletal muscle oxidative capacity and markers of health status. Overweight/obese but otherwise healthy men and women (n = 7 each; age = 29±9 y; BMI = 29.8±2.7 kg/m^2) performed 18 training sessions over 6 wk on a cycle ergometer. Each session began with a 2 min warm-up at 50 W, followed by 3×20 s "all-out" sprints against 5.0% body mass (mean power output: ~450–500 W) interspersed with 2 min of recovery at 50 W, followed by a 3 min cool-down at 50 W. Peak oxygen uptake increased by 12% after training (32.6±4.5 vs. 29.1±4.2 ml/kg/min) and resting mean arterial pressure decreased by 7% (78±10 vs. 83±10 mmHg), with no difference between groups (both $p<0.01$, main effects for time). Skeletal muscle biopsy samples obtained before and 72 h after training revealed increased maximal activity of citrate synthase and protein content of cytochrome oxidase 4 ($p<0.01$, main effect), while the maximal activity of β-hydroxy acyl CoA dehydrogenase increased in men only ($p<0.05$). Continuous glucose monitoring measured under standard dietary conditions before and 48–72 h following training revealed lower 24 h average blood glucose concentration in men following training (5.4±0.6 vs. 5.9±0.5 mmol/L, $p<0.05$), but not women (5.5±0.4 vs. 5.5±0.6 mmol/L). This was associated with a greater increase in GLUT4 protein content in men compared to women (138% vs. 23%, $p<0.05$). Short-term interval training using a 10 min protocol that involved only 1 min of hard exercise, 3x/wk, stimulated physiological changes linked to improved health in overweight adults. Despite the small sample size, potential sex-specific adaptations were apparent that warrant further investigation.

Editor: Naoyuki Hayashi, Tokyo Institute of Technology, Japan

Funding: This project was supported by a Natural Sciences and Engineering Research Council (NSERC) operating grant and McMaster University Internally Sponsored Research Grant to MJG. JBG held a NSERC Vanier Canada Graduate Scholarship. MEP was supported by a NSERC Canada Graduate Scholarship (Masters). LES held a NSERC undergraduate student research award and NSERC Canada Graduate Scholarship (Masters). The funders had no role in study design, data collection and analysis, decision to publish, or preparation of the manuscript.

Competing Interests: The authors have declared that no competing interests exist.

* Email: gibalam@mcmaster.ca

Introduction

Interval exercise is characterized by repeated bursts of relatively intense effort, interspersed by periods of rest or lower-intensity exercise for recovery. Short-term interval training protocols can induce physiological remodeling similar to continuous moderate-intensity training, despite reduced time commitment and a relatively small total exercise volume [1]. Recent studies have also shown improvements in various health indices including markers of glycemic control in both healthy individuals [2–4] and people with cardiometabolic disorders including type 2 diabetes [5] after low-volume interval training. These studies have been conducted on relatively small numbers of subjects and involved relatively short training interventions. Nonetheless, the findings have garnered significant interest from a public health perspective, given one of the most commonly cited barriers to regular exercise participation is "lack of time" [6].

A common interval training model is the Wingate Test, which involves a 30 s "all out" burst of cycling on a specialized ergometer. Typically, 4–6 such intervals are performed, separated by ~4–5 min of recovery, with three training sessions performed each week [1]. Despite the very small total amount of exercise, a training session typically lasts ~25 min, given the brief warm-up and cool down that are usually included in addition to the recovery periods. The relative "time efficiency" of Wingate-based training has therefore been questioned [7], considering the ~75 min time commitment per week, which falls within the physical activity guidelines advocated by some public health agencies. While 150 min of moderate-intensity exercise per week is the general recommendation [8,9] some guidelines include 75 min of vigorous physical activity as an alternative [9].

Several recent studies investigated physiological and health-related adaptations to very low-volume interval training protocols that involved a time commitment of ≤15 min per session [10–12]. For example, Metcalfe and colleagues [10] reported that a 10 min training protocol, involving low-intensity cycling except for 2, 20 sec all out sprints, improved cardiorespiratory fitness (VO_2 peak) in previously sedentary adults when performed 3x/wk for 6 wk. The potential for very low-volume interval training protocols to improve VO_2 peak has also been described by Ma et al. [11] and Hazell et al. [12]. Metcalfe et al. [10] also reported that insulin sensitivity based on oral glucose tolerance tests was improved after training in men but not women, highlighting the potential for sex-based differences in the adaptive response. Only one study has examined muscle adaptations to this type of training, with Ma et al. [11] reporting increased protein content of some mitochondrial enzymes after training, although the maximal activity of citrate synthase was unchanged.

The purpose of the present study was to clarify and advance our understanding of the impact of very low-volume interval training on physiological and health related adaptations to very low-volume SIT. Specifically, we examined the impact of a training protocol that involved only 1 minute of intense intermittent exercise within a 10 min time commitment, including warm-up and cool-down. Sedentary but otherwise healthy subjects trained 3x/wk for 6 wk, and needle biopsies were obtained before and after training to examine skeletal muscle remodeling. We also assessed changes in several markers reflective of cardiometabolic health. In light of the findings by Metcalfe et al. [11], a secondary aim was to explore potential sex-based differences in the adaptive response to this type of training. We hypothesized that the training intervention would increase skeletal muscle oxidative capacity, as reflected by the maximal activity and protein content of mitochondrial enzymes, increase VO_2 peak, and reduce resting blood pressure and 24 h mean blood glucose concentration measured using continuous glucose monitoring (CGM) under conditions of controlled activity and feeding. We further hypothesized that reductions in 24 h glucose would be superior in men.

Materials and Methods

The protocol for this study and supporting TREND checklist are available as supporting information; see Checklist S1 and Protocol S1.

Subjects

Fourteen overweight or obese men and women were recruited by poster advertisement from the McMaster University community and took part in the study (Table 1). Subjects were deemed sedentary based on their self-reported habitual physical activity, which consisted of $\leq$2 sessions/wk of structured exercise lasting $\leq$ 30 min. Participants were allocated into the male or female intervention group and matched for age, body mass index and VO_2 peak. The experimental protocol, which consisted of familiarization and baseline testing, a 6 wk training intervention, and post-training measurements, was approved by the Hamilton Integrated Research Ethics Board and all visits took place at McMaster University. All subjects provided written informed consent prior to their participation.

Experimental Protocol

Familiarization and baseline testing. Participants reported to the laboratory on four separate occasions over 14 d for familiarization and baseline testing during May-July 2013. On the first visit, subjects initially sat quietly for 10 min prior to 3 separate measurements of blood pressure using an automatic blood pressure cuff (Contec 08A, Qinhuangdao, China), with the lowest of these values used for analysis as previously reported [13]. Subjects subsequently performed an incremental maximal oxygen uptake (VO_2 peak) test on an electronically braked cycle ergometer (Lode Excalibur Sport V 2.0, Groningen, The Netherlands) as previously described [14,15]. Briefly, following a 2 min warm-up at 50 W, the resistance was increased by 1 W every 2 s until volitional exhaustion or the point at which pedal cadence fell below 50 rpm. A metabolic cart with an on-line gas collection system (Moxus modular oxygen uptake system, AEI Technologies, Pittsburgh, PA) acquired oxygen consumption (VO_2) and carbon dioxide production (VCO_2) data. VO_2 peak was defined as the highest average oxygen consumption over a 30 s period. Approximately 15 min following the VO_2 peak test, participants performed 1–2×20 s all-out sprints on an electronically braked cycle ergometer (Veletron, RacerMate, Seattle, WA, USA) to become acquainted with the interval protocol.

Approximately 5 d after the familiarization session, participants returned to the laboratory and were fitted with a continuous glucose monitor (CGM; CGMS; iPro, Medtronic, Northridge, CA) and chest-worn accelerometer (Actiheart; Camntech, Cambridge, United Kingdom). Subjects were also given a glucose meter (OneTouch UltraMini, Lifescan, Milpitas, CA) with instructions on how to perform capillary blood sampling. Participants received a standardized food parcel, which they were instructed to consume at prescribed meal times over the subsequent 24 h. The diet was individualized for each participant and energy intake was estimated using the Mifflin-St Jeor equation [16]. Mean total energy was 2623±123 and 1886±146 kcal for men and women, respectively, derived from 56±1% carbohydrate, 30±1% fat and 14±1% protein.

Starting at 600 h the day following CGM insertion, participants began consuming the control diet under free-living conditions and CGM data was collected for a 24 h period. Participants obtained capillary blood glucose samples at four points over the 24 h period when blood glucose was expected to be stable (i.e. upon awakening, before lunch, before dinner and before bed) and were automatically stored in the glucose meter provided. Average blood glucose concentration, glucose area under the curve (AUC) and the daily peak glucose concentration (G_{max}) were calculated from CGM data for a 24 h period from 600 to 559 h before and after training. Physical activity was monitored continuously over this 24 h period using a chest-worn device (Actiheart) that simultaneously measured heart rate and activity with an internal accelerometer that senses the frequency and intensity of torso movements to calculate energy expenditure. Following CGM removal at ~1200 h, glucose data were uploaded as previously described [5].

Approximately 2 d later, participants reported to the lab following a 10 h overnight fast. A single resting blood sample was obtained by venipuncture from an antecubital vein. Plasma and serum were separated by centrifugation (10 min at 4000 rpm) and stored at −20°C for subsequent analysis. A resting skeletal muscle biopsy was obtained using procedures we have previously described [17]. Briefly, muscle samples were obtained from the vastus lateralis under local anesthesia (1% lidocaine) using a Bergstrom needle adapted with suction. Samples were sectioned into several pieces, immediately snap frozen in liquid nitrogen and stored at −80°C for later analysis.

Training protocol. At least 5 d following the muscle biopsy, subjects initiated the interval training program, which consisted of 18 supervised sessions over 6 wk during June-August 2013. Training was performed on Monday, Wednesday and Friday each week. Each session consisted of 3×20 s all-out cycling efforts against a load corresponding to 0.05 kg/kg body mass, separated by 2 min of low intensity cycling (50 W), on an electronically braked ergometer (Veletron, RacerMate, Seattle, WA, USA). All

Table 1. Subject Characteristics.

VARIABLE	MEN	WOMEN
Age (y)	29±9	30±10
Height (cm)	176±5	162±8
Weight (kg)	97±8	75±12*
Body Mass Index (kg/m^2)	31±2	29±2
VO2peak (L/min)	3.0±0.5	2.0±0.2*
VO2peak (ml/kg/min)	31±4	28±4
Maximal Workload (W)	262±30	202±23*

Values are means ± S.D. N = 7 for men and women. VO2peak, maximal oxygen uptake.
*Significantly different from men (p≤0.05).

training sessions included a 2 min warm-up and 3 min cool-down at 50 W, for a total time commitment of 10 min. The weekly training protocol therefore involved a total of 3 min of very intense intermittent exercise within a time commitment of 30 min including warm-up, cool-down and the recovery between efforts. Peak and mean power output was recorded for each sprint and an average determined for each session. Heart rate (HR) was measured continuously on the first training session.

Post-testing. Resting blood pressure was measured 24 h after the final training session, before subjects were fitted with the CGM and Actiheart. CGM data was collected for a 24 h period starting ~48 h after the final exercise session and diet was controlled to be the same as baseline. There was no difference in activity counts between the baseline and post-testing CGM period ($P>0.05$). Fasting blood and a resting muscle biopsy sample were obtained 72 h following the last training bout. Approximately 4 d following the biopsy and 1 wk after the final training session, a maximal exercise test was performed using the same procedures as at baseline. All procedures and controls were identical to those employed during baseline testing and took place during July-September 2013. A flow chart of all participants involved in the trial is depicted in Figure 1.

Blood Analysis

Plasma glucose was analyzed using a kit assay (Pointe Scientific, Canton MI, USA) and serum insulin was measured by ELISA according to manufacturer instructions (ALPCO Immunoassays, Salem NH, USA). Insulin resistance was calculated using HOMA-IR [18].

Muscle Analysis

Enzyme activity. One piece of muscle (~25 mg) was homogenized in Lysing Matrix D tubes (MP Biomedicals, Solon, OH, USA) using the FastPrep-24 Tissue and Cell Homogenizer (MP Biomedicals, Solon, OH, USA) for 10×5 s cycles at a speed of 4 m/s with samples placed on ice for 5 min in between cycles. Samples were homogenized in 20 volumes of buffer containing 70 mM sucrose, 220 mM mannitol, 10 mM HEPES supplemented with protease inhibitors (Complete Mini, Roche Applied Science, Laval, PQ, Canada) and used to determine the maximal activity of citrate synthase and 3-β-hydroxyacyl CoA dehydrogenase (β-HAD) as we have previously described [14,19,20]. Protein concentration of homogenates was determined using a commercial assay (BCA Protein Assay, Pierce, Rockford, IL, USA) and enzyme activity is expressed as mmol/kg protein/hr.

Western blotting. A second piece of muscle (~30 mg) was homogenized in RIPA buffer using Lysing Matrix D tubes (MP Biomedicals, Solon, OH, USA) with the FastPrep-24 Tissue and Cell Homogenizer (MP Biomedicals, Solon, OH, USA). Samples were processed for 4×20 s cycles at 4.0 m/s, with samples placed on ice for 5 min in between cycles, followed by 2×20 s cycles at 4.0 m/s, with samples placed on ice for 2 min in between cycles. Western blot analysis was conducted using techniques described previously [14,19]. Briefly, protein concentration of homogenates was determined (BCA Protein Assay) and equal amounts of protein were prepared in 4× Laemmli's buffer and heated to 95°C before being separated by 10% SDS-PAGE and electrotransferred to nitrocellulose membranes. Ponceau S staining was performed following transfer to visualize equal loading and transfer. Following 1 h blocking in 5% fat-free milk Tris-buffered saline 0.1% Tween 20 (TBS-T), membranes were incubated in the primary antibody (glucose transporter 4; Millipore, AB1345 or COXIV; Mitosciences, MS408) overnight at 4°C in 3% fat-free milk TBS-T based on previously optimized conditions. After 3×5 min washes in TBS-T, membranes were incubated in the species-specific secondary antibody diluted (1:10,000) in 3% fat-free milk TBS-T for 1 h at room temperature, washed in TBS-T for 6×5 min, and visualized by chemiluminescence (SuperSignal West Dura, Pierce) using a FluorChem SP Imaging System (Alpha Innotech Corporation, San Leandro, CA, USA). ImageJ software (NIH) was used to quantify the optical density of protein bands. Protein content was expressed as a fold change relative to pre-training for all subjects. α-tubulin (Cell Signaling Technology, #2125), which did not change following training ($p = 0.91$), was used as a loading control.

Statistical Analysis

All data were analyzed using a two-factor analysis of variance (ANOVA), with the between factor group (men, women) and the within factor time (pre-, post-training) using SPSS Statistics software. Significant interactions and main effects were subsequently analyzed using a Tukey's honestly significant difference post hoc test. The level of significance for all analyses was set at $P<0.05$ and all data are presented as means ± S.D for n = 7 in each group, except for the CGM data which represents n = 6 per group.

Results

Descriptive characteristics of training

Adherence to the training sessions was 100%. Mean HR, measured continuously during the first training session and

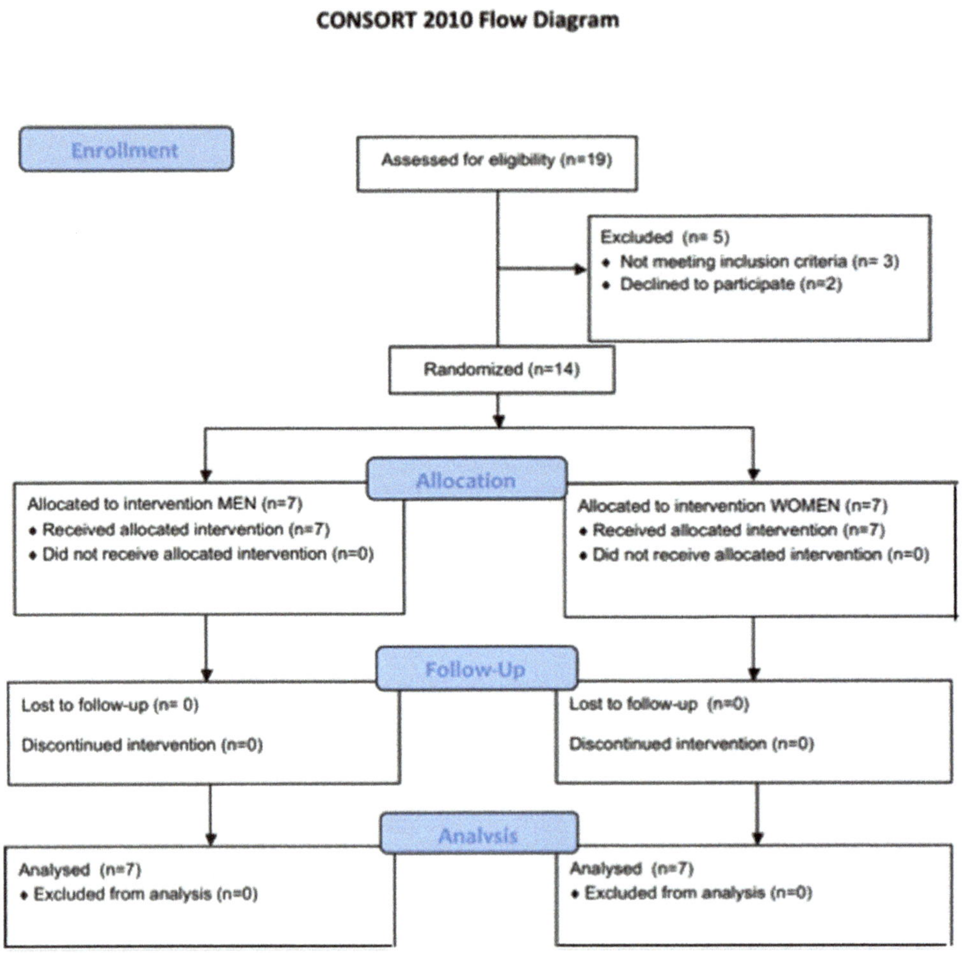

Figure 1. Flow diagram of participants through all phases of the trial.

averaged over the entire 10 min protocol including warm-up and cool-down, was 83±2% of HR_{max}. Relative PPO and MPO measured on the first and last training session did not differ between men and women and increased with training (Table 2, main effect for time, $p<0.01$). The average HR response for all subjects and average MPO for men and women during session 1 is depicted in Figure 2.

Table 2. Markers of Health and Fitness.

	MEN		WOMEN	
VARIABLE	**PRE**	**POST**	**PRE**	**POST**
Body Mass (kg)	77±12	77±13	79±15	79±15
FPG (mmol/L)	5.1±0.3	5.2±0.3	5.0±0.3	5.0±0.3
FPI (uIU/ml)	13.5±7.9	10.7±7.0*	9.6±4.0	7.1±3.0*
HOMA-IR	3.1±1.9	2.5±1.5*	2.1±0.9	1.5±0.6*
Gmax (mmol/L)	8.0±1.3	6.8±1.1*	7.3±0.6	7.6±0.9
Resting SBP (mmHg)	124±8	116±8*	109±11	100±11*
Resting DBP (mmHg)	71±11	67±5	66±9	60±9
Resting MAP (mmHg)	88±8	83±4*	80±10	74±9*
Relative PPO (W/kg FFM)	11.3±4.1	12.2±3.6*	10.0±0.6	11.8±1.1*
Relative MPO (W/kg FFM)	9.0±1.6	10.6±1.5*	9.0±0.5	12.0±0.1*

Values are means ± S.D. N=7 for men and women. *Significantly different than pre-training ($p\leq0.05$).
FPG, fasting plasma glucose; FPI, fasting plasma insulin; Gmax: daily peak glucose concentration.

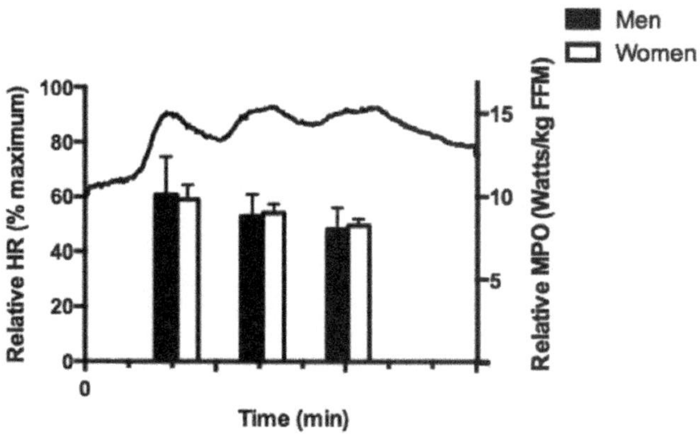

Figure 2. Characterization of the low-volume SIT protocol. Solid line represents average heart rate (HR) response, expressed as a % of maximum, for all subjects during the first training session (left side y-axis). Bar graph represents relative mean power output (MPO) per kilogram fat-free mass (FFM) for men (dark bar) and women (white bar) during the first training session (right side y-axis).

Skeletal muscle adaptations to very low-volume SIT

The maximal activity of citrate synthase increased by ~40% after training (Fig. 3A, main effect for time, $p<0.001$). COXIV protein content also increased after training with no differences between groups (Fig. 3B, main effect for time, $p<0.01$), however β-HAD maximal activity only increased after training in the men (Fig. 3C; interaction between training and sex, $p<0.05$). GLUT4 protein content increased in both men and women following training (Fig. 4A, main effect for time, $p<0.01$), however men increased to a greater extent compared to women (138% vs. 23%, interaction between training and sex, $p<0.05$).

Indices of cardiometabolic health

Very low-volume interval training increased VO_2 peak by 12% in both men and women (Fig. 5, main effect for time, $p<0.001$), which was associated with a 14% increase in maximal workload (Table 1, main effect for time, $p<0.001$). Mean arterial pressure (MAP) was reduced by 6% and 8% in men and women respectively following training (Table 2, main effect for time, $p<0.01$). Systolic blood pressure (SBP) was also reduced following training (Table 2, main effect for time, $P<0.01$), while diastolic blood pressure (DBP) trended towards being lower (Table 2, $p=0.07$). Insulin sensitivity measured by HOMA-IR was improved after training (Table 2, main effect for time, $p<0.05$), owing mainly to a decrease in fasting serum insulin (Table 2, main effect for time, $p\leq0.05$). There was no change in fasting plasma glucose in either group (Table 2, $p>0.05$). CGM revealed a lower 24 h average blood glucose concentration after training in men (5.4 ± 0.6 vs. 5.9 ± 0.5 mmol/L, $p<0.05$) but not women (Fig. 4B,

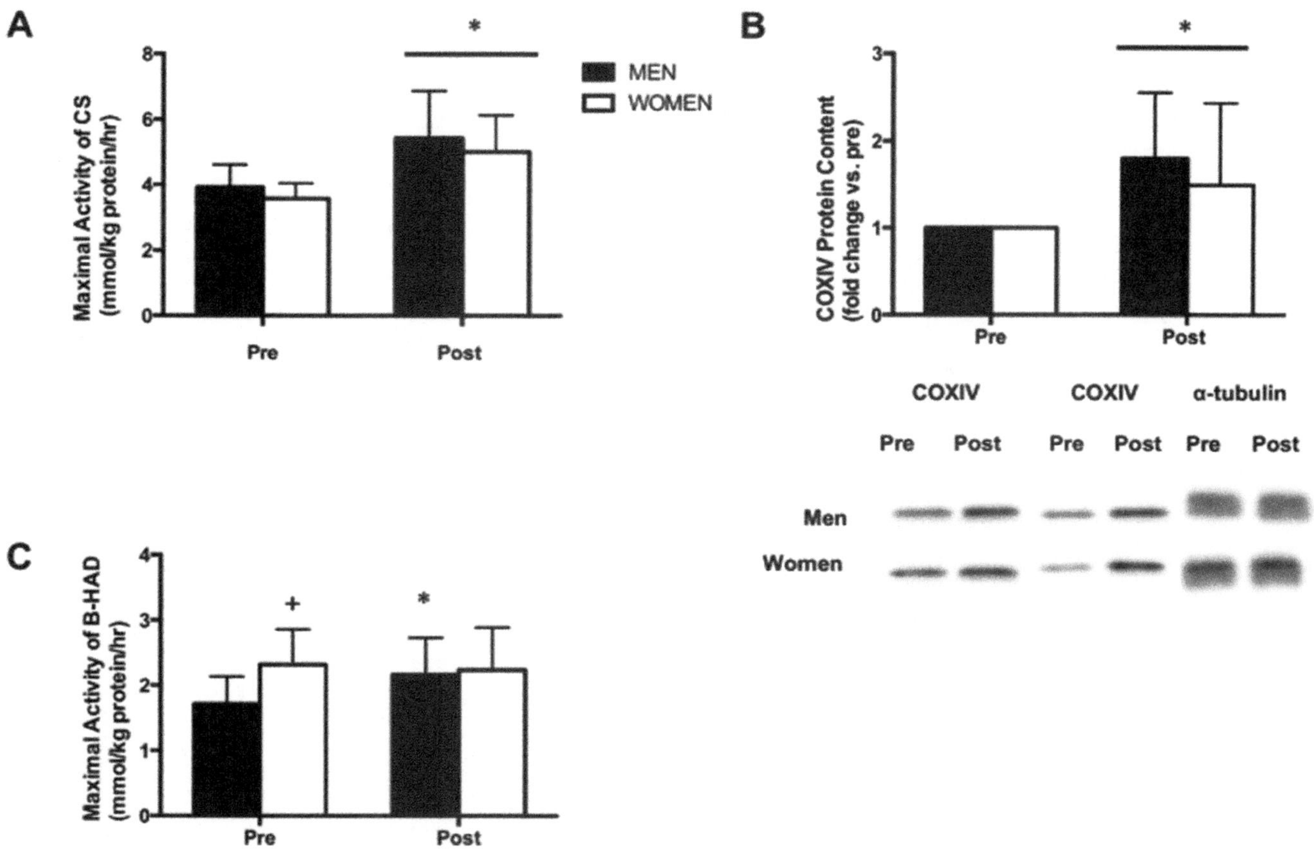

Figure 3. Very low-volume SIT improves skeletal muscle mitochondrial capacity. Measured in muscle biopsy samples obtained from the vastus lateralis before (PRE) and 72 h after (POST) 6-week SIT in men and women. Maximal activity of citrate synthase (A), protein content of COXIV (B) and maximal activity of β-HAD (C). Values are means ± SD (n = 7 per group). Representative Western blots for 2 men and 2 women are shown for COXIV. α-tubulin was used a loading control and representative Western blots are shown. *P<0.05, pre- vs. post-training; +p<0.05, men vs. women at same time point; line denotes a main effect.

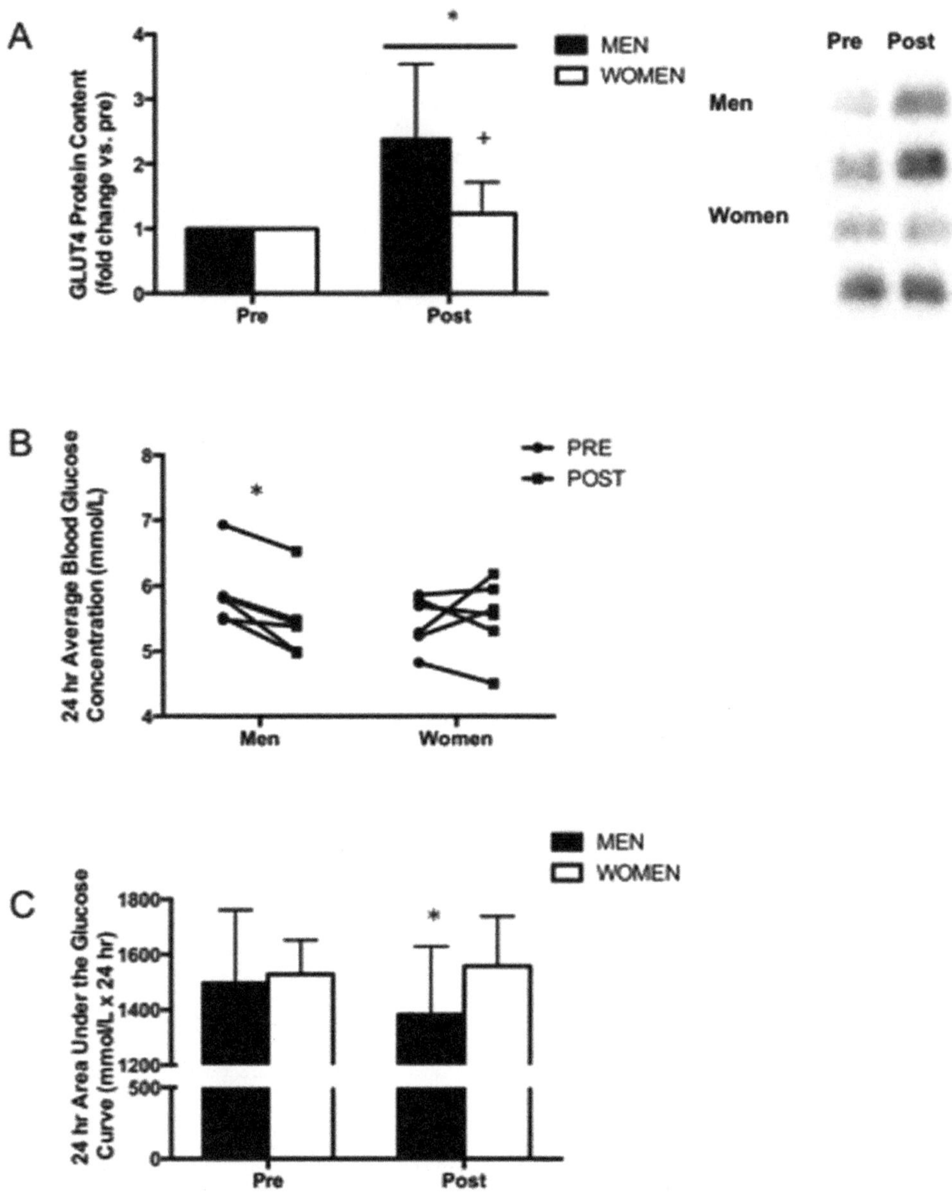

Figure 4. Improved indices of blood glucose control in men following very low-volume SIT. GLUT4 protein content measured in muscle biopsy samples obtained from the vastus lateralis before (PRE) and 72 h after (POST) 6 week SIT in men and women (A). Individual 24 h average blood glucose concentration (B) and 24 h blood glucose area under the curve (AUC) measured before (PRE) and 48–72 h after (POST) 6 week SIT in men and women using continuous glucose monitoring (CGM). Values are means ± SD (n = 7 per group for muscle data, n = 6 per group for CGM data). Representative Western blots for 2 men and 2 women are shown for GLUT4. *P<0.05, pre- vs. post-training; +p<0.05, men vs. women at same time point.

5.5±0.6 vs. 5.5±0.4 mmol/L, p>0.05). Similarly, 24 h glucose AUC was reduced in men only (Fig. 4C, interaction between training and sex, $p<0.05$). G_{max} was lower in men following training, but not in women (Table 2, interaction between training and sex, $p<0.01$)

Discussion

The main finding from the present study was that short-term interval training, using a protocol that involved only 1 min of very intense exercise within a total time commitment of 10 min, was a potent stimulus to induce physiological adaptations that are linked to improved health in overweight and obese adults. Our general design, which involved 3 sessions per week for 6 wk, was similar to recent studies by Metcalfe [10] and Ma [11], but clarified outstanding questions regarding the potential for very low-volume interval training to increase muscle oxidative capacity, resting blood pressure and aspects of glycemic control. Despite the small sample size, we also found evidence of potential sex-specific adaptations to this type of training that warrant further investigation.

Very low-volume interval training increases muscle oxidative capacity

A recent systematic review and meta-analysis [21] proposed a classification scheme for interval training in an effort to

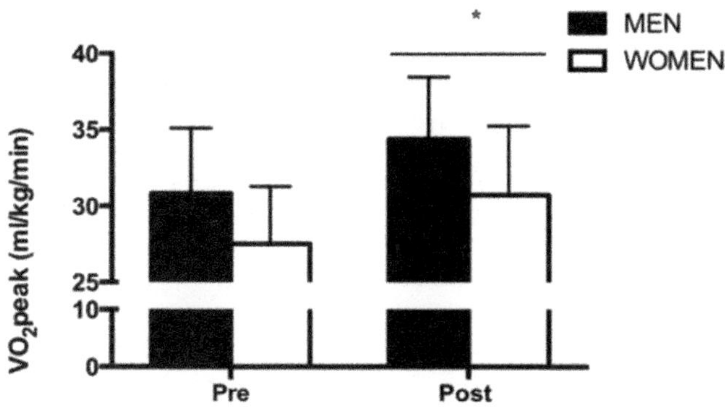

Figure 5. Very low-volume SIT increases VO_2 peak. Measured before (PRE) and 1 week following (POST) 6 wk SIT in men and women. Values are means ± SD (n = 7 per group). *$P<0.05$, pre- vs. post-training; line denotes a main effect.

standardize terminology employed in future studies. Using the descriptors proposed by Weston and colleagues, we have opted to classify the present protocol as "sprint interval training" (SIT) given the "all-out" efforts, as opposed to "high-intensity interval training" (HIIT), which the authors define as bouts performed at relatively intense but nonetheless submaximal workloads corresponding to 80–100% of maximal heart rate [21]. We report here for the first time that very low-volume SIT can increase the maximal activity of citrate synthase, which is reportedly one of the best indicators of mitochondrial content in human skeletal muscle, as it is highly correlated with gold-standard measures made by electron microscopy [22]. While skeletal muscle adaptations to SIT are well established, there are limited and equivocal data regarding the effect of very low-volume SIT on mitochondrial content. Skleryk et al. [23] reported that a protocol involving 8–12×10 s all-out cycle sprints against 5% body weight interspersed with 80 s rest, performed six times over 2 wk, did not improve mitochondrial capacity in overweight men as reflected by a lack of change in the protein content of COXII and COXIV. In contrast, Ma et al. [11] showed that a protocol consisting of 8, 20 s cycling efforts at an intensity of 170% of VO_2 peak and interspersed with 10 s of recovery, performed four times per week for 4 wk, increased the protein content of COXI and COXIV, however, the maximal activity of citrate synthase was unchanged. The results from the present study confirm that 6 wk of very low-volume SIT, involving a total of only 3 min of all out intermittent exercise within a 30 min time commitment per week, was a sufficient stimulus to elicit a robust increase in citrate synthase similar to what has been reported after protocols involving a larger volume of SIT or traditional moderate-intensity continuous training that involve a much greater total volume of exercise and training time commitment [24]. Clearly, there is some minimal total volume of SIT necessary to acutely stimulate mitochondrial biogenesis, which when performed repeatedly leads to measureable increases in enzyme protein content or maximal activity. The various short-term, very low-volume SIT protocols that have been employed to date are likely on the lower end of this threshold, which may in part explain the equivocal results to date. Additional studies, like the elegant work by Perry et al. [25], which characterized the early time course of adaptation to HIIT, will help to resolve this matter.

Effect of very low-volume interval training on markers of cardiometabolic health

Seminal work by Tabata and colleagues over two decades ago showed that 7–8 bouts of 20 s all out sprints, with 10 s rest in between, improved VO_2 peak in young men by 15%, when performed four times per week for 6 wk [26]. The beneficial effect of "Tabata style" training on VO_2 peak, which is a popular exercise strategy among many personal trainers, was recently confirmed by Ma et al. [11] who reported a 19% increase in young men after 4 wk. The present work, and recent studies by others [10–12,27], confirm that very brief bouts of all-out exercise, performed a few times per week, is a very time efficient strategy to improve VO_2 peak, which is a strong predictor of all-cause morbidity and mortality [28]. A novel, important finding from the present work was the significant reduction in MAP when measured 24 h after the final training bout, which is of similar magnitude to findings following traditional Wingate-based SIT in overweight/obese men and women [13], as well as 16 wk of high volume aerobic interval or continuous moderate intensity training in individuals with metabolic syndrome [29]. Based on findings from a recent systematic review and meta-analysis, the blood pressure reduction in the present study is of similar magnitude to those following intermittent isometric resistance training [30], which is emerging as a very effective exercise strategy for lowering resting blood pressure [30,31]. It is unclear if our findings represent an acute effect of the last training bout, however if one performs SIT every other day as in the present study, the beneficial effect on blood pressure would be maintained.

Potential sex-specific adaptations to low-volume interval training

SIT has been shown to improve insulin sensitivity, based on hyperinsulinemic euglycemic clamps performed on sedentary and recreationally active individuals [2] as well as oral glucose tolerance tests (OGTTs) performed on young healthy [4] and overweight/obese [13] men. Metcalfe et al. [10] recently reported that a 10 min low-intensity cycling protocol that included 2×20 s all-out sprints, performed 18 times over 6 wk, improved insulin sensitivity measured by OGTTs in men but not women [10]. Consistent with the observations of Metcalfe et al. [10], we found using CGM that 24 h average blood glucose concentration, glucose AUC and G_{max}, measured under standard dietary conditions from 48–72 h after the final training session, were improved in men but not women. Interestingly, the training-induced increase in total GLUT4 protein content was approximately 6-fold higher in men compared to women.

The lack of change in peripheral glucose control in women in the present study is consistent with recent reports by others [10,15], although this is not a universal finding [2]. It is possible that our low sample size (n = 6 for CGM data), or the fact that the women had higher 24 h blood glucose control at baseline, influenced our findings and resulted in a type 2 statistical error. Nonetheless, by way of a possible related mechanism, it has also been speculated that the rapid improvement in insulin sensitivity following SIT is attributed to high rates of glycogen breakdown and subsequent re-synthesis following each exercise bout [10], and women have been shown to break down 42% less muscle glycogen in type I fibers during a single Wingate sprint [32]. Future studies are needed to investigate if GLUT4 translocation following acute SIT is blunted in women, and definitively determine in larger cohorts of subjects if improvements in glucose control following SIT are sex-specific. HOMA-IR was improved in both men and women after training, owing to significant reductions in fasting plasma insulin, and consistent with previous studies [3,33].

We also found sex-specific differences in a marker of lipid oxidation capacity, based on changes in the maximal activity of β-HAD which were detected in men but not women. A similar period of Wingate-based SIT was reported to improve the maximal activity of β-HAD in both men and women, but that study did not involve a specific comparison between sexes [24]. Similar to the pre-training CGM data, it is possible that the higher baseline value for β-HAD in women in the present study reduced their potential to increase the capacity for lipid oxidation compared to men. Other recent studies however, have also highlighted sex-based differences in the skeletal muscle adaptive response to SIT in active young men and women [34]. Scalzo et al. [34] reported higher rates of muscle protein synthesis in men compared to women following a 3 wk SIT intervention, based on oral administration of deuterium oxide. Future research is needed, using designs which control for menstrual cycle phase and initial fitness level [35], to evaluate if sex-based differences exist in the skeletal muscle adaptive response low-volume SIT.

Conclusions

In summary, we report that 3 min of all-out exercise performed within a 30 min time commitment per week including warm-up and cool-down, improved skeletal muscle oxidative capacity and indices of cardiometabolic health including VO_2 peak and blood pressure, in overweight/obese adults. The protocol employed in the present study involved a training time commitment that was considerably lower than in previous Wingate-based SIT studies (i.e., 10 versus ~25 min per session) and provides further evidence of the potential for very brief, intense bursts of exercise to elicit physiological adaptations that are associated with improved health status in a time-efficient manner. Despite the small sample size, potential sex-specific adaptations were apparent that warrant further investigation.

Acknowledgments

We would like to thank Dr. Jonathan Little and Dr. Michael Riddell for their assistance in helping to facilitate the continuous glucose monitor measurements.

Author Contributions

Conceived and designed the experiments: JBG MJG. Performed the experiments: JBG MEP LES BJM RBT MAT MJG. Analyzed the data: JBG MEP LES BJM RBT. Contributed reagents/materials/analysis tools: MAT MJG. Wrote the paper: JBG MJG.

References

1. Gibala MJ, McGee SL (2008) Metabolic adaptations to short-term high-intensity interval training: a little pain for a lot of gain? Exerc Sport Sci Rev 36: 58–63. doi:10.1097/JES.0b013e318168ec1f.
2. Richards JC, Johnson TK, Kuzma JN, Lonac MC, Schweder MM, et al. (2010) Short-term sprint interval training increases insulin sensitivity in healthy adults but does not affect the thermogenic response to beta-adrenergic stimulation. J Physiol 588: 2961–2972. doi:10.1113/jphysiol.2010.189886.
3. Hood MS, Little JP, Tarnopolsky MA, Myslik F, Gibala MJ (2011) Low-Volume Interval Training Improves Muscle Oxidative Capacity in Sedentary Adults. Med Sci Sports Exerc 43: 1849–1856. doi:10.1249/MSS.0b013e3182199834.
4. Babraj JA, Vollaard NBJ, Keast C, Guppy FM, Cottrell G, et al. (2009) Extremely short duration high intensity interval training substantially improves insulin action in young healthy males. BMC Endocr Disord 9: 3. doi:10.1186/1472-6823-9-3.
5. Little JP, Gillen JB, Percival M, Safdar A, Tarnopolsky MA, et al. (2011) Low-volume high-intensity interval training reduces hyperglycemia and increases muscle mitochondrial capacity in patients with type 2 diabetes. J Appl Physiol 111: 1554–1560. doi:10.1152/japplphysiol.00921.2011.
6. Trost SG, Owen N, Bauman AE, Sallis JF, Brown W (2002) Correlates of adults' participation in physical activity: review and update. Med Sci Sports Exerc 34: 1996–2001. doi:10.1249/01.MSS.0000038974.76900.92.
7. Gillen JB, Gibala MJ (2014) Is high-intensity interval training a time-efficient exercise strategy to improve health and fitness? Appl Physiol Nutr Metab 39: 409–412. doi:10.1139/apnm-2013-0187.
8. Tremblay MS, Warburton DER, Janssen I, Paterson DH, Latimer AE, et al. (2011) New Canadian Physical Activity Guidelines. Appl Physiol Nutr Metab 36: 36–46. doi:10.1139/H11-009.
9. Garber CE, Blissmer B, Deschenes MR, Franklin BA, Lamonte MJ, et al. (2011) American College of Sports Medicine position stand. Quantity and quality of exercise for developing and maintaining cardiorespiratory, musculoskeletal, and neuromotor fitness in apparently healthy adults: guidance for prescribing exercise. Med Sci Sports Exerc 43: 1334–1359. doi:10.1249/MSS.0b013e318213fefb.
10. Metcalfe RS, Babraj JA, Fawkner SG, Vollaard NBJ (2011) Towards the minimal amount of exercise for improving metabolic health: beneficial effects of reduced-exertion high-intensity interval training. Eur J Appl Physiol 112: 2767–2775. doi:10.1007/s00421-011-2254-z.
11. Ma JK, Scribbans TD, Edgett BA, Boyd JC, Simpson CA, et al. (2013) Extremely low-volume, high-intensity interval training improves exercise capacity and increases mitochondrial protein content in human skeletal muscle. J Mol Integr Physiol 3: 202–210.
12. Hazell TJ, Macpherson REK, Gravelle BMR, Lemon PWR (2010) 10 or 30-S Sprint Interval Training Bouts Enhance Both Aerobic and Anaerobic Performance. Eur J Appl Physiol 110: 153–160. doi:10.1007/s00421-010-1474-y.
13. Whyte LJ, Gill JMR, Cathcart AJ (2010) Effect of 2 weeks of sprint interval training on health-related outcomes in sedentary overweight/obese men. Metabolism 59: 1421–1428. doi:10.1016/j.metabol.2010.01.002.
14. Little JP, Safdar A, Wilkin GP, Tarnopolsky MA, Gibala MJ (2010) A practical model of low-volume high-intensity interval training induces mitochondrial biogenesis in human skeletal muscle: potential mechanisms. J Physiol 588: 1011–1022. doi:10.1113/jphysiol.2009.181743.
15. Gillen JB, Percival ME, Ludzki A, Tarnopolsky MA, Gibala MJ (2013) Interval training in the fed or fasted state improves body composition and muscle oxidative capacity in overweight women. Obesity. doi:10.1002/oby.20379.
16. Frankenfield D, Roth-Yousey L, Compher C (2005) Comparison of predictive equations for resting metabolic rate in healthy nonobese and obese adults: a systematic review. J Am Diet Assoc 105: 775–789. doi:10.1016/j.jada.2005.02.005.
17. Tarnopolsky MA, Pearce E, Smith K, Lach B (2011) Suction-modified Bergström muscle biopsy technique: experience with 13,500 procedures. Muscle Nerve 43: 717–725. doi:10.1002/mus.21945.
18. Matsuda M, DeFronzo RA (1999) Insulin sensitivity indices obtained from oral glucose tolerance testing. Diabetes Care 22: 1462–1470.
19. Gibala MJ, Little JP, van Essen M, Wilkin GP, Burgomaster KA, et al. (2006) Short-term sprint interval versus traditional endurance training: similar initial adaptations in human skeletal muscle and exercise performance. J Physiol 575: 901–911. doi:10.1113/jphysiol.2006.112094.
20. Carter SL, Rennie CD, Hamilton SJ, Tarnopolsky MA (2001) Changes in skeletal muscle in males and females following endurance training. Can J Physiol Pharmacol 79: 386–392. doi:10.1139/cjpp-79-5-386.
21. Weston KS, Wisløff U, Coombes JS (2013) High-intensity interval training in patients with lifestyle-induced cardiometabolic disease: a systematic review and meta-analysis. Br J Sports Med. doi:10.1136/bjsports-2013-092576.
22. Larsen S, Nielsen J, Hansen CN, Nielsen LB, Wibrand F, et al. (2012) Biomarkers of mitochondrial content in skeletal muscle of healthy young human subjects. J Physiol 590: 3349–3360. doi:10.1113/jphysiol.2012.230185.
23. Skleryk JR, Karagounis LG, Hawley JA, Sharman MJ, Laursen PB, et al. (2013) Two weeks of reduced-volume sprint interval or traditional exercise training does not improve metabolic functioning in sedentary obese men. Diabetes Obes Metab 15: 1146–1153. doi:10.1111/dom.12150.
24. Burgomaster KA, Howarth KR, Phillips SM, Rakobowchuk M, Macdonald MJ, et al. (2008) Similar metabolic adaptations during exercise after low volume sprint interval and traditional endurance training in humans. J Physiol 586: 151–160. doi:10.1113/jphysiol.2007.142109.
25. Perry CGR, Lally J, Holloway GP, Heigenhauser GJF, Bonen A, et al. (2010) Repeated transient mRNA bursts precede increases in transcriptional and mitochondrial proteins during training in human skeletal muscle. J Physiol 588: 4795–4810. doi:10.1113/jphysiol.2010.199448.
26. Tabata I, Nishimura K, Kouzaki M, Hirai Y, Ogita F, et al. (1996) Effects of moderate-intensity endurance and high-intensity intermittent training on anaerobic capacity and VO2max. Med Sci Sports Exerc 28: 1327–1330.
27. Tjønna AE, Leinan IM, Bartnes AT, Jenssen BM, Gibala MJ, et al. (2013) Low- and high-volume of intensive endurance training significantly improves maximal oxygen uptake after 10-weeks of training in healthy men. PLoS One 8: e65382. doi:10.1371/journal.pone.0065382.

28. Blair SN, Brodney S (1999) Effects of physical inactivity and obesity on morbidity and mortality: current evidence and research issues. Med Sci Sports Exerc 31: S646–62.
29. Tjønna AE, Lee SJ, Rognmo Ø, Stølen TO, Bye A, et al. (2008) Aerobic interval training versus continuous moderate exercise as a treatment for the metabolic syndrome: a pilot study. Circulation 118: 346–354. doi:10.1161/CIRCULATIONAHA.108.772822.
30. Cornelissen VA, Smart NA (2013) Exercise training for blood pressure: a systematic review and meta-analysis. J Am Heart Assoc 2: e004473. doi:10.1161/JAHA.112.004473.
31. Brook RD, Appel LJ, Rubenfire M, Ogedegbe G, Bisognano JD, et al. (2013) Beyond medications and diet: alternative approaches to lowering blood pressure: a scientific statement from the american heart association. Hypertension 61: 1360–1383. doi:10.1161/HYP.0b013e318293645f.
32. Esbjörnsson-Liljedahl M, Sundberg CJ, Norman B, Jansson E (1999) Metabolic response in type I and type II muscle fibers during a 30-s cycle sprint in men and women. J Appl Physiol 87: 1326–1332.
33. Trapp E, Heydari M, Freund J, Boutcher SH (2008) The effects of high-intensity intermittent exercise training on fat loss and fasting insulin levels of young women. Int J Obes 32: 684–691. doi:10.1038/sj.ijo.0803781.
34. Scalzo RL, Peltonen GL, Binns SE, Shankaran M, Giordano GR, et al. (2014) Greater muscle protein synthesis and mitochondrial biogenesis in males compared with females during sprint interval training. FASEB J 28: 1–10. doi:10.1096/fj.13-246595.
35. Tarnopolsky MA (2008) Sex differences in exercise metabolism and the role of 17-beta estradiol. Med Sci Sports Exerc 40: 648–654. doi:10.1249/MSS.0b013e31816212ff.

14

Associations between Multiple Accelerometry-Assessed Physical Activity Parameters and Selected Health Outcomes in Elderly People – Results from the KORA-Age Study

Sandra Ortlieb[1,2], **Lukas Gorzelniak**[2], **Dennis Nowak**[3,4], **Ralf Strobl**[5,6], **Eva Grill**[5,6], **Barbara Thorand**[7], **Annette Peters**[7], **Klaus A. Kuhn**[2], **Stefan Karrasch**[1,8,9], **Alexander Horsch**[2,10,11¶], **Holger Schulz**[1*¶]

1 Institute of Epidemiology I, Helmholtz Zentrum München, German Research Center for Environmental Health, Neuherberg, Germany, **2** Institute of Medical Statistics and Epidemiology, Technische Universität München, Munich, Germany, **3** Institute and Outpatient Clinic for Occupational, Social and Environmental Medicine, Ludwig-Maximilians-Universität, Munich, Germany, **4** Comprehensive Pneumology Center Munich (CPC-M), Member of the German Center for Lung Research, Munich, Germany, **5** Institute for Medical Information Processing, Biometrics and Epidemiology, Ludwig-Maximilians-Universität München, Munich, Germany, **6** German Center for Vertigo and Balance Disorders, Ludwig-Maximilians-Universität München, Munich, Germany, **7** Institute of Epidemiology II, Helmholtz Zentrum München, German Research Center for Environmental Health, Neuherberg, Germany, **8** Institute and Outpatient Clinic for Occupational, Social and Environmental Medicine, Ludwig-Maximilians-Universität, Munich, Germany, **9** Institute of General Practice, University Hospital Klinikum rechts der Isar, Technische Universität München, Munich, Germany, **10** Department of Computer Science, University of Tromsø, Tromsø, Norway, **11** Department of Clinical Medicine, University of Tromsø, Tromsø, Norway

Abstract

Introduction: Accelerometry is an important method for extending our knowledge about intensity, duration, frequency and patterns of physical activity needed to promote health. This study has used accelerometry to detect associations between intensity levels and related activity patterns with multimorbidity and disability. Moreover, the proportion of people meeting the physical activity recommendations for older people was assessed.

Methods: Physical activity was measured in 168 subjects (78 males; 65–89 years of age), using triaxial GT3X accelerometers for ten consecutive days. The associations between physical activity parameters and multimorbidity or disability was examined using multiple logistic regression models, which were adjusted for gender, age, education, smoking, alcohol consumption, lung function, nutrition and multimorbidity or disability.

Results: 35.7% of the participants met the physical activity recommendations of at least 150 minutes of moderate to vigorous activity per week. Only 11.9% reached these 150 minutes, when only bouts of at least 10 minutes were counted. Differences in moderate to vigorous activity between people with and without multimorbidity or disability were more obvious when shorter bouts instead of only longer bouts were included. Univariate analyses showed an inverse relationship between physical activity and multimorbidity or disability for light and moderate to vigorous physical activity. A higher proportion of long activity bouts spent sedentarily was associated with higher risk for multimorbidity, whereas a high proportion of long bouts in light activity seemed to prevent disability. After adjustment for covariates, there were no significant associations, anymore.

Conclusions: The accumulated time in moderate to vigorous physical activity seems to have a stronger relationship with health and functioning when shorter activity bouts and not only longer bouts were counted. We could not detect an association of the intensity levels or activity patterns with multimorbidity or disability in elderly people after adjustment for covariates.

Editor: Nuria Garatachea, University of Zaragoza, Spain

Funding: The KORA research platform (KORA, Cooperative Health Research in the Region of Augsburg) was initiated and financed by the Helmholtz Zentrum München, German Research Center for Environmental Health (formerly GSF, National Research Center for Environment and Health), which is funded by the German Federal Ministry of Education and Research and by the State of Bavaria. KORA Age was financed by the German Federal Ministry of Education and Research (BMBF FKZ 01ET0713). Further support was provided by the BMBF funded Competence Network ASCONET, subnetwork COSYCONET (FKZ 01GI0882). The research was supported by the Graduate School of Information Science in Health (GSISH) and the Technische Universität München Graduate School. Lukas Gorzelniak received university grant monies as a PhD scholarship from 3/1/2009 to 6/30/2012. The funders had no role in study design, data collection and analysis, decision to publish, or preparation of the manuscript.

Competing Interests: The authors have declared that no competing interests exist.

* Email: schulz@helmholtz-muenchen.de

¶ These authors shared last authorship.

Introduction

Population aging will be a substantial societal phenomenon in the next half century. Due to the increase in life expectancy and the associated increase in the number of individuals at risk for chronic diseases and injuries, the aging of the population will produce crucial societal challenges [1]. Physical activity (PA) is a fundamental component targeted at preventing diseases and maintaining functional independence as well as in therapeutic intervention and rehabilitation programs for older adults.

Many studies have shown significant associations between PA and certain chronic diseases, including coexistence of selected diseases with high prevalence (e.g. cardiovascular diseases and diabetes) [2,3]. In contrast, studies about the associations of multimorbidity (the coexistence of multiple chronic diseases) and PA are rare. Only one article about this subject was included in the review by Marengoni et al. [4] in 2011, who examined occurrence, causes, and consequences of multimorbidity. Hudon et al. [5] did not identify an association between multimorbidity and PA. Recently, two further studies were published which showed an inverse association between PA and multimorbidity [6,7]. The relationship between PA and functional limitations or disability has been better investigated: two reviews dealt with this topic and reported consistent results demonstrating a positive influence of PA on the relationship of aging and disability [8,9]. However, all studies on the associations between disability or multimorbidity and PA used self-reports to assess PA.

Although moderate to vigorous physical activity (MVPA) has been shown to provide beneficial effects to the health and functioning of older people [10,11], little is known about the impact of light PA and the activity patterns needed to promote health in elderly people. The global recommendations on PA from the World Health Organization (WHO) [11] suggest that adults, including older adults, should perform a minimum of 150 min of at least moderate intensity PA per week for beneficial health effects. Moreover, the activity should be performed in bouts of at least 10 min duration. Moderate PA is defined as considerable increases in heart rate and breathing, such as brisk walking, and vigorous PA is even more exhausting [12]. The proportion of elderly people who meet the recommended PA guidelines diminishes from 47% −63%, found through questionnaires, to 6% −26%, when assessed by use of accelerometers [13].

Due to low costs and high feasibility, PA was usually measured by means of questionnaires in large epidemiological studies. The instrument requires a thorough and objective consideration of the questions addressed but it often comes along with recall bias, socially desirable responses, and the influence of mood, depression, anxiety, cognition, and disability on responses [14]. Accelerometers resolve some of the limitations of self-report instruments: they are not affected by random and systematic errors introduced by respondents and interviewers, and they provide valid and reliable estimates about basic characteristics (frequency, duration and intensity of PA) as well as of PA patterns [15,16]. Moreover, accelerometers have improved the ability to examine the relationship between PA and different health outcomes and thus present supportive statistics for public health planning and intervention [17].

Recently, sedentary PA, as characterized by activities involving mainly sitting, has been proposed as a risk factor for all-cause disease that is independent of MVPA [18]. The role of light PA (e.g. self-care, cooking, casual walking or shopping), measured by accelerometers, with regard to health effects has been less studied [19,20]. This might be of particular interest for older people who are limited in their exercise capacity due to age-related physical or mental restrictions [21]. In this respect, the patterns of PA have been proposed as a new group of PA outcomes that may offer additional information beyond reports of activity counts and activity type recognition [22].

In our study, we will examine the associations between the volume of PA (divided into sedentary PA: ≤100 counts per min (cpm), light PA: 101–1951 cpm, and MVPA: ≥1952 cpm) as well as PA patterns (with the so called GINI-Index [22,23] as quantification) measured by accelerometers and specific health outcomes (disability and multimorbidity). Each health outcome is a clinically distinct entity with different prognosis and health care implications [24] and should therefore be observed individually. In this context, we will answer the following research questions: 1) Is there an association between the volume of sedentary or light PA and the two health outcomes, independent of MVPA? 2) Is there an association between PA patterns and the two health outcomes? 3) Are there differences and similarities regarding the relationship of PA with disability and multimorbidity? The answers to these questions will allow us to present novel information about the associations between sedentary PA, light PA as well as PA patterns and different health outcomes. Furthermore, we will assess the proportion of people fulfilling the current global recommendations of PA for older people under different methodical conditions, i.e. assess the impact of different bout lengths varying between 1 and the WHO recommended 10 min in subjects with and without disability or multimorbidity, and translate our results into advice for the prevention of chronic diseases and disability in elderly people.

Methods

The KORA-Age study was approved by the Ethical Committee of the Bavarian medical association (Ethik-Kommission Nr. 08064), written informed consent has been obtained from the participants and all investigations have been conducted according to the principles expressed in the Declaration of Helsinki.

Study population

Data from the present study derived from the KORA (Cooperative Health Research in the Region of Augsburg)-Age cohort. The KORA-Age study investigates the determinants and consequences of health status changes of older adults in a representative population based sample over a period of 3 years. Details have been described previously [25]. Since lung function is an important predictor of morbidity and mortality [26], 200 eligible individuals with extreme lung function values within the normal range had been selected from the first and fourth quartiles of the study population and grouped into a 'better' and a 'worse' lung function group. Activity counts from the non-dominant side of the hip were measured in 191 subjects at a rate of 30 Hz and stored at an epoch length of 2 sec by means of a GT3X (ActiGraph, Pensacola, FL, USA) accelerometers during daily living. Data filtering was set to default ('normal') as recommended by ActiGraph. PA was recorded up to 10 days, starting from the day at the study center where the accelerometers were handed out, until the eleventh day, which was the day the subjects were instructed to return the devices. PA data from the first recorded day as well as any other day with a wear time of less than ten hours were excluded. To be included in the study, subjects had to have a minimum of four valid days. After exclusion of subjects with insufficient days of recordings (n = 19) or accelerometer malfunctions (n = 4), the final study sample comprised 78 men and 90 women. Participants had 8.1±1.5 (mean ± SD) days of valid accelerometer data. The mean wear time was 740±114 min per day.

Details about the study design, participants and other methodic procedures have been described previously [22].

Measures

Independent variables. The independent variables included: gender; age (65–69, 70–74, 75–79, >79); BMI (under-weight if <18.5 kg/m^2, normal weight if 18.5–24.9 kg/m^2, overweight if 25.0–29.9 kg/m^2 and obesity if ≥30.0 kg/m^2); education (≤10 years vs. >10 years); smoking habits (never, formerly smoked vs. currently smokes); alcohol consumption (teetotalism vs. no teetotalism); lung function ('better' vs. 'worse' lung function group) and risk of malnutrition measured by the Geriatric Nutritional Risk Index (GNRI) (major risk if <82, moderate risk if ≥82 and < 92), low risk if >92 and ≤98, and no risk if >98) [27]. No person was at major risk and only 4 people were on moderate risk. Therefore we merged moderate and low risk.

Physical activity: To represent the characteristics of PA, multiple variables were obtained from uniaxial accelerometer data. As an overall measure of PA average counts per minute (cpm) were calculated for each subject. Times in different intensity levels were calculated by the most commonly used PA cut points applied for adults: *sedentary PA* was defined as ≤100 cpm [14] and the cut points by Freedson et al. [28] were used for *light* (101−1951 cpm), *moderate* (1952−5724 cpm), and *vigorous PA* (5725−9498 cpm). *PA patterns:* In the present study, a *bout* is defined as consecutive min spent in a specific intensity level, i.e. sedentary PA, light PA or MVPA, without interruption. To determine the time participants spent in the MVPA level and the portion of people fulfilling the current PA recommendations of ≥ 150 min of MVPA per week [11], we applied different cut offs for the bout lengths, ranging from 1 min to 10 min: i.e. the recommended ≥150 min of MVPA per week had to be performed in bouts of at least 1 min up to at least 10 min. We averaged MVPA over all valid days of recordings and multiplied it by seven, in order to test if a person met the PA recommendations of ≥ 150 min per week.

Activity patterns are characterized by the distribution of frequency of bouts of different duration. This information is combined by the so-called *GINI-index (G)*, introduced by Chastin and colleagues [23]. The index expresses how the PA time in a specific intensity level is accumulated with respect to the bout lengths. The index value *G* ranges from 0 to 1 and has to be interpreted as follows: *High G values*: large difference between minimal and maximal bout lengths and relatively high proportion of few long bouts in relation to the overall time. *Low G values:* small difference between minimal and maximal bout length, i.e. the activity pattern is characterized by a lot of relatively short bouts of similar length. A G value of 0 would result if all the bouts were the same length. Note that this does not depend on the length of these bouts, but only on their relationship to each other.

Dependent variables. *Multimorbidity* was defined as the presence of ≥2 *chronic diseases* out of a list of 13 chronic diseases: hypertension, eye disease, heart disease, diabetes mellitus, joint disease, lung disease, gastrointestinal disease, mental disease, stroke, cancer, kidney disease, neurological disease, liver disease. Chronic health conditions were determined through a self-administered questionnaire and a standardized telephone interview adapted from the self-report-generated Charlson Comorbidity Index [29].

Disability was quantified using the Health Assessment Questionnaire Disability Index (HAQ-DI) [30] during a telephone interview. The instrument consists of 20 questions in eight domains (dressing and grooming, hygiene, arising, reach, eating, grip, walking, and common daily activities), which can be answered on a scale from 0 (no difficulty), 1 (some difficulty), 2 (much difficulty) to 3 (unable to perform). The HAQ-DI score is the mean of the eight domains. In line with the literature [31], disability was defined as HAQ-DI >0. The HAQ had shown high validity, a good test-retest reliability, and internal consistency, and can be applied very well to elderly people [31]. For more detailed information regarding disability within the KORA-Age framework see Strobl et al. [32].

Statistical analyses

Some of the metric variables were not normally distributed. Thus, the Wilcoxon two-sample test was used for metric variables to test for differences between people with and without a diagnosis of multimorbidity or disability, and Chi^2-test for categorical variables. For the multiple logistic regression models, we used the interquartile range (IQR) of each PA variable as scaling distance. The IQR is defined as the distance between the 25th and 75th percentiles and thus describes values of the predictor that are relatively well-represented in the sample [33]. The association between the six PA parameters (sedentary PA, light PA, MVPA, G for sedentary PA ($G_{sedentary}$), G for light PA (G_{light}) or G for MVPA (G_{MVPA})) and multimorbidity as well as disability was examined using multiple logistic regression models. Statistical models were adjusted for gender, age, BMI, education, smoking, alcohol consumption, lung function group, nutrition, and one of the health outcomes (multimorbidity, disability), as appropriate. Results are presented as odds ratios (OR) and 95% confidence intervals. Statistically significant differences were assumed at a significance level of $p<0.05$. Statistical analyses were conducted using SAS version 9.2 (SAS institute Cary, NC).

Results

Descriptive characteristics

Table 1 presents the characteristics of the study sample: 168 people (46.4% male, 53.6% female) were included in the study with a median (5%, 95%) age of 73 (65, 86) years and a median BMI of 27 (23, 35) kg/m^2. More than half of the study sample (51.8%) was multimorbid and 41.7% of the participants were disabled. 29.7% of all participants were both disabled and multimorbid (results not shown in the table). More detailed information about the subject characteristics and clinical parameters stratified by multimorbidity and disability are presented in table 1 (median values) and table S1 (mean values).

PA and bout length. Overall, most of the time in MVPA (55%) was performed in bouts of one min (Figure 1). 47.6% of the participants did not achieve at least one 10-min bout. 35.7% of the participants met the current PA recommendations [11] of performing ≥150 min of MVPA, regardless of bout length, and 11.9% reached this in bouts of at least 10 min (Figure 2A). Differences in terms of MVPA between people with and without a diagnosis of disability or multimorbidity were stronger under consideration of short bouts instead of only using longer bouts, and more obvious with regard to disablity compared to multimorbidity. Furthermore, there was little difference between disabled individuals and people which were both disabled and multimorbid (Figure 2A and 2B). In addition, mean values are presented in Figure S1.

Table 2 shows the PA variables stratified by presence of disability and presence of multimorbidity. The median (5%/95%) activity per day was 221 (67/487) cpm. Lower values were

Table 1. Characteristics of the participants, stratified by multimorbidity and disability. Median (5%, 95%).

	all	multimorbidity		disability	
	n = 168	no	yes	no	yes
		n = 81	n = 87	n = 98	n = 70
Age (years)	73 (65/86)	**69 (65/84)**	**77 (67/87)**	**71 (65/84)**	**76 (67/87)**
BMI (kg/m²)	27 (23/35)	27 (21/35)	27 (23/37)	**27 (21/34)**	**28 (23/38)**
Gender, m (n, (%))	78 (46.4)	40 (49.4)	38 (43.7)	**56 (57.1)**	**22 (31.4)**
Education ≤10 years (n (%))	110 (65.5)	56 (69.1)	54 (62.1)	59 (60.2)	51 (72.9)
Alcohol abstinence, yes (n (%))	23 (13.7)	8 (9.9)	15 (17.2)	**9 (9.2)**	**14 (20.0)**
Smoker or ex-smoker (n (%))	97 (57.7)	46 (56.8)	51 (58.6)	56 (57.1)	41 (58.6)
GNRI	109 (96/124)	108 (97/123)	109 (95/126)	108 (96/122)	110 (96/129)
Health outcomes					
Lung group, better (n (%))	92 (54.7)	47 (58.0)	45 (51.7)	58 (59.2)	34 (48.6)
Disability, yes (n (%))	70 (41.7)	**20 (24.7)**	**50 (57.5)**	–	–
Multimorbidity, yes (n (%))	87 (51.8)	–	–	**37 (37.8)**	**50 (71.4)**

Significant differences are written in bold, $p \leq 0.05$. Wilcoxon-test was used for metric variables and Chi²-test for categorical variables; GNRI = Geriatric Nutritional Risk Index.

observed in subjects with multimorbidity (181 (62/455) cpm) and disability (174 (57 439) cpm) while subjects without multimorbidity or disability showed significantly higher values. Overall, the participants passed a median time of 65% being sedentary, 32% in light activity and 2% in MVPA. Values of G tended to increase with decreasing intensity level: $G_{sedentary} = 0.63$, $G_{light} = 0.48$, and $G_{MVPA} = 0.43$ (see Table S2 for mean values). According to this, the accumulated PA time in the sedentary level was composed of a higher proportion of long bouts compared to the light or MVPA level. Multimorbid participants were generally less active. They spent 4% more of their time in the sedentary level ($p<0.01$), 2% less in the light level ($p = 0.02$) and 1% less in the MVPA level ($p< 0.01$) compared to people who were not multimorbid. Moreover, $G_{sedentary}$ was significantly higher in multimorbid people ($p<0.01$).

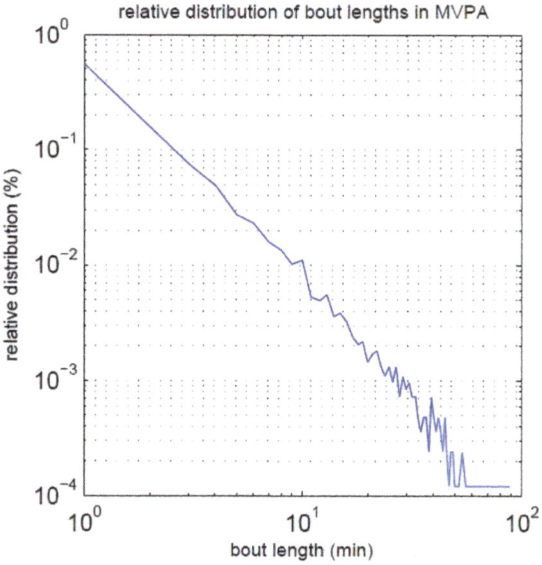

Figure 1. Distribution of PA bouts of moderate to vigorous physical activity.

The results for disability were similar with regard to the intensity levels, but not in terms of the PA patterns: G_{light} and G_{MVPA} were significantly lower in disabled people compared to people without diagnosis of disability ($p = 0.04$ and $p<0.01$).

Table 3 presents associations between the six PA variables and the prevalence of multimorbidity or disability, respectively. For the multiple regression models, each PA variable was scaled by its interquartile range (IQR). The resulting regression coefficient from IQR compares a person in the middle of the upper half of the predictor distribution to a person in the middle of the lower half of the distribution.

PA and multimorbidity. The risk of multimorbidity seemed to be 1.7 times higher for an elderly person with a typical 'high' (75th percentile) value on sedentary PA compared to a person with a typically 'low' (25th percentile) value (model 1). In contrast, high values of light PA and MVPA showed a protective effect ($OR = 0.88$, $p = 0.02$ and $OR = 0.99$, $p<0.01$). Since the participants spent little time in MVPA and the variance of MVPA was very low, even an OR of 0.99 emerged as a statistically significant risk. High $G_{sedentary}$ values appeared to increase the risk of multimorbidity by the factor 1.5 compared to low values. After adjustment for age and sex (model 2) all results tended into the same direction, however they were not significant, anymore. The same applied to model 3 (also adjusted for BMI, smoking, education, alcohol consumption, nutrition, lung function, and disability). Instead, higher age and presence of disability were significant predictors for multimorbidity, no matter which of the PA variables was included in the model.

PA and disability. The risk of disability appeared to be twice as high for participants with a typical 'high' value on sedentary PA compared to people with a typically 'low' value. In contrast, high values of light PA and MVPA showed a significant protective effect ($OR = 0.84$, $p<0.01$ and $OR = 0.99$, $p<0.01$). Due to the low variance of MVPA, even an OR of 0.99 emerged as a significant result. High G_{light} values reduced the risk of multimorbidity by 21% compared to low values. Significant associations between the three intensity levels and disability persisted, even after adjustment for age and sex (model 2). However, there were no significant relations, anymore, after controlling for further covariates (model

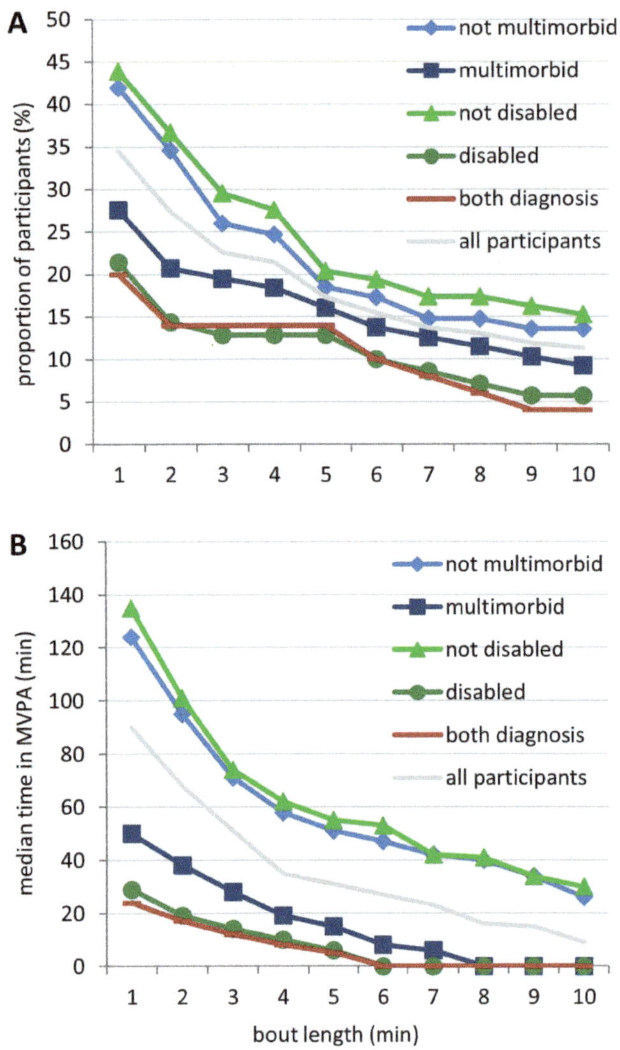

Figure 2. Moderate to vigorous physical activity (MVPA) in relation to different minimal bout lengths. A) Proportion of participants (%) fulfilling ≥150 min of MVPA/week vs. minimal bout length. B) Median time in MVPA per week (min). Each bout length refers to the minimal number of consecutive min in MVPA required for inclusion in the calculation of accumulated time in MVPA, i.e. if bout length is 3 then bouts of length 1 and 2 are excluded.

3). Instead, female gender and presence of multimorbidity emerged as significant risk factors for disability, no matter which of the PA variables was included in the model.

When comparing the models of the two health outcomes multimorbidity and disability, all results point in the same direction. According to model 2, the relationship between disability and PA seemed to be stronger than the relationship between multimorbidity and PA. The more variables were included in the model, the weaker became the associations between PA variables and health outcomes.

Discussion

To the best of our knowledge, this is the first study examining the association between PA patterns and multimorbidity or disability on a sample of elderly people using accelerometry. One striking finding was that shorter bouts (e.g. 1-min bouts) of MVPA seem to provide more distinct evidence about the positive effect of MVPA with multimorbidity and disability than longer bouts (e.g. 10-min bouts). An explanation for this may be the relatively short overall time that elderly people spend in this level and especially the low proportion of long bouts. This finding is in contrast to the current PA recommendations [11] which request that PA is performed in bouts of at least 10 min (in the following called '10-min bout rule') for beneficial health effects.

The majority of older adults (61.3%) failed to meet the PA recommendations [11] of 150 min of MVPA per week. When the 10-min bout rule was applied, only 11.9% fulfilled the recommendations. Differences in terms of MVPA between people with and without disability or multimorbidity were more obvious in connection with disability than with multimorbidity. Furthermore, disability seemed to be the limiting factor with regard to MVPA in people which were both disabled and multimorbid. Troiano et al. [34] reported that 7.6% of people ≥60 years met the recommendations of at least 150 min MVPA per week and according to MVPA performed in 10-min bouts only 2.4%. According to Tucker et al. [13] 8.5% of people aged 60–69 and 6.3% of people ≥70 years met the recommendations taking into account the 10-min bout rule. An explanation for the somewhat higher rates of people achieving the recommendations in our study might be that the participants had to attend the KORA study center and thus seemed to have better general health as compared to other studies: The prevalence of multimorbidity (defined as 2+ concurrent diseases) of older people widely varied (55−98%) across studies [4]. A large epidemiological study by van den Bussche et al. [35] determined a multimorbidity prevalence of 62% in Germany among people aged 65 or above and a comparable study about disability observed a prevalence of 63.6% [36] while we observed lower prevalence values, 52% of elderly people in our population were multimorbid and 42% were disabled.

There were differences between participants with and without a diagnosis of multimorbidity in terms of all intensity levels (sedentary PA, light PA, MVPA). The more time people spent actively, the lower was the risk of multimorbidity, regardless intensity of the movement. PA patterns of elderly people with and without multimorbidity only differed with regard to the PA level: people without a diagnosis seemed to get up more often. The associations were lost after adjusting for BMI, smoking, education, alcohol consumption, nutrition, lung function, and disability. Only higher age and disability showed significant associations with multimorbidity. Few large population-based health studies also investigated the relationship between PA and multimorbidity or the number of chronic diseases and reached inconsistent results: Hudon et al. [5] examined people aged 45–68 and found no relationship between multimorbidity and PA levels when age, education, income, employment, long-term limitations on activity, self-rated general health, and psychological distress were controlled for. In contrast, a study about Brazilian women aged 40 to 65 determined an increased likelihood of having two or more morbid conditions for inactive women after adjustment for sociodemographic, behavioral, clinical, and reproductive factors [6]. Likewise, two other studies reported an associations between multimorbidity and the frequency of PA (15 min, ≥12 times per month for positive effects) [37] or a mean PA score [7] in people aged ≥65 years of age after adjusting for predictor variables. However, comparisons between these studies and our results are limited because they used questionnaires to assess PA. Furthermore, the studies used different covariates, different definitions of PA (e.g. 'active' and 'inactive' vs. continuous), different definitions of multimorbidity (e.g. 'multimorbid' vs. 'not multimorbid' vs.

Table 2. PA variables by mulitmorbidity and disability. Median (5%/95%).

PA variables	all	n	not multimorbid	n	multimorbid	n
Average PA (cpm)	221 (67/487)	**168**	**250 (120/487)**	**81**	**181 (62/455)**	**87**
Sedentary PA time (%)	0.65 (0.48/0.82)	168	**0.63 (0.46/0.79)**	81	**0.67 (0.51/0.84)**	87
Light PA time (%)	0.32 (0.18/0.48)	168	**0.33 (0.20/0.51)**	81	**0.31 (0.16/0.48)**	87
MVPA time (%)	0.02 (0.00/0.08)	168	**0.02 (0.00/0.08)**	81	**0.01 (0.00/0.07)**	87
$G_{sedentary}$	0.63 (0.57/0.68)	168	**0.62 (0.57/0.68)**	81	**0.64 (0.58/0.68)**	87
G_{light}	0.48 (0.37/0.55)	168	0.48 (0.38/0.55)	81	0.47 (0.37/0.55)	87
G_{MVPA}	0.43 (0.00/0.66)	156	0.45 (0.00/0.67)	77	0.40 (0.00/0.65)	79
	all	**n**	**not disabled**	**n**	**disabled**	**n**
Average PA (cpm)	221 (67/487)	**168**	**269 (119/542)**	**98**	**174 (57/439)**	**70**
Sedentary PA time (%)	0.65 (0.48/0.82)	168	**0.64 (0.46/0.77)**	98	**0.68 (0.54/0.84)**	70
Light PA time (%)	0.32 (0.18/0.48)	168	**0.32 (0.21/0.51)**	98	**0.31 (0.16/0.45)**	70
MVPA time (%)	0.02 (0.00/0.08)	168	**0.02 (0.00/0.09)**	98	**0.01 (0.00/0.07)**	70
$G_{sedentary}$	0.63 (0.57/0.68)	168	0.63 (0.57/0.68)	98	0.63 (0.57/0.70)	70
G_{light}	0.48 (0.37/0.55)	168	**0.48 (0.40/0.55)**	98	**0.47 (0.35/0.55)**	70
G_{MVPA}	0.43 (0.00/0.66)	156	**0.46 (0.13/0.68)**	96	**0.37 (0.00/0.62)**	60

Results emerged from Wilcoxon-test. Significant differences are written in bold, $p \leq 0.05$; cpm = counts per minute; G = GINI-Index; high G = mainly few long bouts are responsible for the activity pattern; low G = mainly short bouts of similar length contribute to the activity pattern.

number of chronic conditions) and they partially included other age groups. Nonetheless, the present study supports the findings by Hudon et al. [5] that there is no association between multimorbidity and PA after controlling for covariates, based on objective assessment of PA.

According to the univariate results, PA was associated with disability. The risk for disability was twice as high in people with a high proportion of time spent sedentarily compared to people with less time in this level, whereas high levels of light PA and MVPA seemed protective (OR = 0.84 and OR = 0.99). Since the participants spent little time in MVPA and the variance of MVPA was very low, the OR of 0.99 emerged as significant risk. PA patterns of elderly people with and without disability only differed in terms of light PA. A high proportion of long bouts in light activity appeared protective against disability (OR = 0.8). After adjustment of the predictor variables, there were no significant associations,

Table 3. OR and 95% CI describing the associations between PA variables and prevalent diseases.

	Model 1[a]	p	Model 2[b]	p	Model 3[c]	p
Multimorbidity						
Sedentary PA, IQR	**1.66 (1.14, 2.40)**	**<.01**	1.32 (0.88, 2.00)	0.18	1.11 (0.70, 1.76)	0.67
Light PA, IQR	**0.88 (0.78, 0.98)**	**0.02**	0.93 (0.82, 1.06)	0.28	0.99 (0.86, 1.14)	0.86
MVPA, IQR	**0.99 (0.99, 1.00)**	**<.01**	1.00 (0.99, 1.00)	0.15	1.00 (0.99, 1.00)	0.30
$G_{sedentary}$, IQR	**1.48 (1.12, 1.97)**	**<.01**	1.33 (0.97, 1.82)	0.07	1.46 (1.03, 2.06)	0.03
G_{light}, IQR	0.90 (0.75, 1.08)	0.25	1.00 (0.81, 1.23)	0.98	1.13 (0.88, 1.46)	0.33
G_{MVPA}, IQR	1.02 (0.86, 1.21)	0.79	1.03 (0.86, 1.25)	0.73	1.07 (0.86, 1.33)	0.55
Disability						
Sedentary PA, IQR	**1.99 (1.33, 2.98)**	**<.01**	**1.74 (1.10, 2.75)**	**0.02**	1.52 (0.91, 2.53)	0.11
Light PA, IQR	**0.84 (0.75, 0.94)**	**<.01**	**0.86 (0.76, 0.99)**	**0.03**	0.89 (0.76, 1.03)	0.11
MVPA, IQR	**0.99 (0.98, 1.00)**	**<.01**	**0.99 (0.99, 1.00)**	**0.02**	1.00 (0.99, 1.00)	0.31
$G_{sedentary}$, IQR	1.19 (0.90, 1.58)	0.21	1.01 (0.74, 1.38)	0.94	0.89 (0.63, 1.25)	0.50
G_{light}, IQR	**0.79 (0.65, 0.95)**	**0.02**	0.85 (0.68, 1.06)	0.14	0.84 (0.65, 1.09)	0.18
G_{MVPA}, IQR	0.99 (0.83, 1.18)	0.88	0.96 (0.80, 1.16)	0.68	0.96 (0.79, 1.17)	0.70

Significant estimates are written in bold, $p \leq 0.05$. P-values result from multiple logistic regression models.
[a]unadjusted.
[b]adjusted for age and sex.
[c]also adjusted for BMI, smoking, education, alcohol consumption, nutrition, lung function, and multimorbidity or disability.
G = GINI-Index; high G = mainly few long bouts are responsible for the activity pattern; low G = mainly short bouts of similar length contribute to the activity pattern;

anymore. Even if PA parameters do not appear to be related to disability, it is related to other variables such as gender and multimorbidity. Strong evidence from questionnaire-based literature indicates that older adults who participate in regular PA have a reduced risk of functional limitations [32,38]. Significant results were shown for MVPA after controlling for potential predictors, whereas findings for light PA are inconsistent [39]. We found two other accelerometer-based studies which researched the relationship between PA and disability. They showed a significant association between daily PA and disability after controlling for other predictors [40,41]. However, they did not provide information about the exact intensity levels they applied.

Neither of the mentioned studies used a disability or multimorbidity index that accounted for the severity of the functional limitation or of any disease. A previous study showed that chronic diseases were only associated with another health outcome when the severity of the disease was considered [42].

To our knowledge, the present study is the first one that examined the association between accelerometry-assessed PA levels and multimorbidity in elderly people and the only one that presents information about the relationship of PA patterns with disability and multimorbidity. Due to the objective measurement, our results are not affected by recall biases associated with self-report in older people at risk for cognitive decline.

However, since our participants had to visit the study center, a selection bias is possible which may be responsible for somewhat lower rates of multimorbid and disabled people and slightly increased MVPA. As our study was cross-sectional, we cannot assure causality for any of the associations. For greater understanding of the associations, longitudinal or intervention studies are required. Another limitation of this study is the limited validity of the cut-points applied to classify activities into intensity levels [43] in elderly people [44]. We chose the algorithm by Freedson et al. [28] because it had the highest potential to provide comparable data [14,19,45]. More information on this issue can be found elsewhere [22]. Furthermore, the GT3X accelerometer used in this study is likely to underestimate activities due to its inability to measure water-related activities (e.g. swimming) and to detect the types of activities performed (e.g. cycling, gymnastics, or strength trainings) [16]. Other characteristics, such as self-rated health status or psychological distress level, may have been included in the model [5]. However, we wanted this study to be focused on the relationship of PA with multimorbidity and disability and decided not to include further covariates in the analysis.

Conclusion

In elderly people, MVPA seems to have a stronger relationship with multimorbidity and disability when shorter bouts and not only longer bouts were counted. In older people who are both disabled and multimorbid, disability seems to be the limiting factor for the performance of MVPA. From the univariate analysis presented, the following conclusions can be drawn: multimorbid people should interrupt their periods of inactivity more frequently, whereas disabled people should increase the proportion of long bouts in light activities. Again, associations between disability and PA were stronger than those between multimorbidity and PA. These conclusions should be treated with caution and are limited in their validity, since the findings were not significant after adjustment for covariates. According to multiple logistic regression analyses other variables emerged as significant predictors: higher age and disability were associated with higher risk of multimorbidity; female gender and multimorbidity were associated with higher risk of disability. Studies which take into account the severity of the disease of functional limitation could contribute to a greater understanding of the associations.

Supporting Information

Figure S1 Moderate to vigorous physical activity (MVPA) in relation to different minimal bout lengths. Mean (SD) time in MVPA per week (min). Each bout length refers to the minimal number of consecutive min in MVPA required for inclusion in the calculation of accumulated time in MVPA, i.e. if bout length is 3 then bouts of length 1 and 2 are excluded.

Table S1 Characteristics of the participants, stratified by multimorbidity and disability. Mean (SD). GNRI = Geriatric Nutritional Risk Index.

Table S2 PA variables by mulitmorbidity and disability. Mean (SD). cpm = counts per minute; G = GINI-Index; high G = mainly few long bouts are responsible for the activity pattern; low G = mainly short bouts of similar length contribute to the activity pattern.

Acknowledgments

Thanks to the subjects for their agreement to participate in the KORA-Age study and also to wear the accelerometers. Thanks to Claudia Flexeder (HMGU) for the statistical support.

Author Contributions

Conceived and designed the experiments: LG DN SK AP BT EG RS KAK HS AH. Performed the experiments: LG DN SK AP BT EG RS KAK HS AH. Analyzed the data: SO AH HS. Contributed reagents/materials/analysis tools: AH HS LG SK SO. Wrote the paper: SO. Manuscript revision and final approval of the version to be published: SO LG DN RS EG BT AP KAK SK AH HS.

References

1. Sidall C, Kjaeserud G, Dziworski W, Przywara B, Xavier A (2007) Healthy Ageing: Keystone for a Sustainable Europe. EU Health Policy in the Context of Demographic Change: Discussion Paper of the Services of DG SANCO, DG ECFIN.
2. Tanasescu M, Leitzmann M, Rimm E, Willett W, Stampfer M, et al. (2002) Exercise type and intensity in relation to coronary heart disease in men. JAMA 288: 1994–2000.
3. Knowler W, Barrett-Connor E, Fowler S, Hamman R, Lachin J, et al. (2002) Reduction in the incidence of type 2 diabetes with lifestyle intervention or metformin. NEnglJMed 346: 393–403.
4. Marengoni A, Angleman S, Melis R, Mangialasche F, Karp A, et al. (2011) Aging with multimorbidity: A systematic review of the literature. Ageing Research Reviews 10: 430–439.
5. Hudon C, Soubhi H, Fortin M (2008) Relationship between multimorbidity and physical activity: Secondary analysis from the Quebec health survey. BMC Public Health 8: 304.
6. de Souza Santos Machado V, Valadares A, da Costa-Paiva L, Moraes S, Pinto-Neto A (2012) Multimorbidity and associated factors in Brazilian women aged 40 to 65 years: a population-based study [Abstract]. Menopause 19: 569–575.
7. Autenrieth C, Kirchberger I, Heier M, Zimmermann A, Peters A, et al. (2013) Physical activity is inversely associated with multimorbidity in elderly men: Results from the KORA-Age Augsburg Study. Prev Med 57: 17–19.
8. Paterson D, Warburton D (2010) Physical activity and functional limitations in older adults: a systematic review related to Canada's Physical Activity Guidelines. Int J Behav Nutr Phys Act 7: 38.

9. Tak E, Kuiper R, Chorus A, Hopman-Rock M (2013) Prevention of onset and progression of basic ADL disability by physical activity in community dwelling older adults: A meta-analysis. Ageing Res Rev 12: 329–338.
10. Nelson ME, Rejeski WJ, Blair SN, Duncan PW, Judge JO, et al. (2007) Physical activity and public health in older adults: recommendation from the American College of Sports Medicine and the American Heart Association. Med Sci Sports Exerc 39: 1435–1445.
11. WHO (2010) Global Recommendations on Physical Activity for Health. Geneva: World Health Organization.
12. Haskell WL, Lee IM, Pate RR, Powell KE, Blair SN, et al. (2007) Physical activity and public health: updated recommendation for adults from the American College of Sports Medicine and the American Heart Association. Med Sci Sports Exerc 39: 1423–1434.
13. Tucker JM, Welk GJ, Beyler NK (2011) Physical activity in U.S.: adults compliance with the Physical Activity Guidelines for Americans. Am J Prev Med 40: 454–461.
14. Gorman E, Hanson H, Yang P, Khan K, Liu-Ambrose T, et al. (2014) Accelerometry analysis of physical activity and sedentary behavior in older adults: a systematic review and data analysis. Eur Rev Aging Phys Act 11: 35–49.
15. Troiano RP (2005) A Timely Meeting: Objective Measurement of Physical Activity. Med Sci Sports Exerc 37: S487–489.
16. Matthews CE, Hagströmer M, Pober DM, Bowles HR (2012) Best Practices for Using Physical Activity Monitors in Population Based Research - review. Med Sci Sports Exerc 44: 68–76.
17. Strath S, Pfeiffer K, Whitt-Glover M (2012) Accelerometer Use with Children, Older Adults, and Adults with Functional Limitations. Med Sci Sports Exerc 44: 77–85.
18. Bankoski A, Harris TB, McClain JJ, Brychta RJ, Caserotti P, et al. (2011) Sedentary Activity Associated With Metabolic Syndrome Independent of Physical Activity. Diabetes Care 34: 497–503.
19. Bento (2012) Use of accelerometry to measure physical activity in adults and the elderly. Rev Saúde Pública 46: 561–570.
20. Withall J, Stathi A, Davis M, Coulson J, Thompson J, et al. (2014) Objective indicators of physical activity and sedentary time and associations with subjective well-being in adults aged 70 and over. Int J Environ Res Public Health 11: 643–656.
21. Tudor-Locke C, Myers A (2001) Challenges and Opportunities for Measuring Physical Activity in Sedentary Adults. Sports Med 31: 91–100.
22. Ortlieb S, Dias A, Gorzelniak L, Nowak D, Karrasch S, et al. (2014) Exploring Patterns of Accelerometry-assessed Physical Activity in Elderly People. Int J Behav Nutr Phys Act 11: 28.
23. Chastin SFM, Granat MH (2010) Methods for objective measure, quantification and analysis of sedentary behaviour and inactivity. Gait & Posture 31: 82–86.
24. Fried L, Ferrucci L, Darer J, Williamson J, Anderson G (2004) Untangling the Concepts of Disability, Frailty, and Comorbidity: Implications for Improved Targeting and Care. Journal of Gerontology 59: 255–263.
25. Peters A, Döring A, Ladwig KH, Meisinger C, Linkohr B, et al. (2011) Multimorbidity and successful aging: the population-based KORA-Age study. Z Gerontol Geriatr 44: 41–54.
26. Mannino D, Buist A, Petty T, Enright P, Redd S (2003) Lung function and mortality in the United States: data from the First National Health and Nutrition Examination Survey follow up study. Thorax 58: 388–393.
27. Bouillanne O, Morineau G, Dupont C, Coulombel I, Vincent J-P, et al. (2005) Geriatric Nutritional Risk Index: a new index for evaluating at-risk elderly medical patients. Am J Clin Nutr 82: 777–783.
28. Freedson PS, Melanson E, Sirard J (1998) Calibration of the Computer Science and Applications, Inc. accelerometer. Med Sci Sports Exerc 30: 777–781.
29. Chaudhry S, Jin L, Meltzer D (2005) Use of a self-report-generated Charlson Comorbidity Index for predicting mortality. Med Care 43: 607–615.
30. Fries J, Spitz P, Young D (1982) The dimensions of health outcomes: the health assessment questionnaire, disability and pain scales. J Rheumatol 9: 789–793.
31. Krishnan E, Sokka T, Hakkinen A, Hubert H, Hannonen P (2004) Normative Values for the Health Assessment Questionnaire Disability Index. Arthritis Rheum 50: 953–960.
32. Strobl R, Müller M, Emeny R, Peters A, Grill E (2013) Distribution and determinants of functioning and disability in aged adults - results from the German KORA-Age study. BMC Public Health 13: 137.
33. Babyak M (2009) Statistical Tips from the Editors of Psychosomatic Medicine. Psychosom Med 24: 8.
34. Troiano RP, Berrigan D, Dodd KW, Masse LC, Tilert T, et al. (2008) Physical activity in the United States measured by accelerometer. Med Sci Sports Exerc 40: 181–188.
35. van den Bussche H, Schäfer I, Koller D, Hansen H, von Leitner E-C, et al. (2012) Multimorbidity in the German Elderly Population – Part 1: Prevalence in Ambulatory Medical Care. A Study Based on Statutory Health Insurance Data. Z Allg Med 88: 365–371.
36. Wilms H, Riedel-Heller S, Angermeyer M (2007) Limitations in activities of daily living and instrumental activities of daily living capacity in a representative sample: disentangling dementia- and mobility-related effects Compr Psychiatry 48: 95–101.
37. Kaplan M, Newsom J, McFarland B, Lu L (2001) Demographic and Psychosocial Correlates of Physical Activity in Late Life. Am J Prev Med 21: 306–312.
38. U.S. Department of Health and Human Services. Physical Activity Guidelines Advisory Committee Report, 2008. Available: http://www.health.gov/PAGuidelines/Report/. Accessed 2013 October 17.
39. He X, Baker D (2004) Body Mass Index, Physical Activity, and the Risk of Decline in Overall Health and Physical Functioning in Late Middle Age. Am J Public Health 94: 1567–1573.
40. Shah R, Buchman A, Leurgans S, Boyle P, Bennett D (2012) Association of total daily physical activity with disability in community-dwelling older persons: a prospective cohort study. BMC Geriatrics 12: 63.
41. Harris T, Owen C, Victor C, Adams R, Cook D (2009) What factors are associated with physical activity in older people, assessed objectively by accelerometry? Br J Sports Med 43: 442–450.
42. Fortin M, Bravo G, Hudon C, Lapointe L, Dubois M, et al. (2006) Psychological Distress and Multimorbidity in Primary Care. Ann Fam Med 4: 417–422.
43. Strath S, Bassett DJ, Swartz A (2003) Comparison of MTI accelerometer cut-points for predicting time spent in physical activity. Int J Sports Med 24: 298–303.
44. Santos-Lozano A, Santín-Medeiros F, Cardon G, Torres-Luque G, Bailón R, et al. (2013) Actigraph GT3X: Validation and Determination of Physical Activity Intensity Cut Points. Int J Sports Med 2013 34: 975–982.
45. Kaminsky L, Ozemek C (2012) A comparison of the Actigraph GT1M and GT3X accelerometers under standardized and free-living conditions. Physiol Meas 33: 1869–1876.

15

Longitudinal Associations between Self-Rated Health and Performance-Based Physical Function in a Population-Based Cohort of Older Adults

Willa D. Brenowitz[1]*, Rebecca A. Hubbard[2,3], Paul K. Crane[4], Shelly L. Gray[5], Oleg Zaslavsky[6], Eric B. Larson[2,4]

1 Department of Epidemiology, University of Washington School of Public Health, Seattle, Washington, United States of America, **2** Group Health Research Institute, Seattle, Washington, United States of America, **3** Department of Biostatistics, University of Washington School of Public Health, Seattle, Washington, United States of America, **4** Department of Medicine, Division of General Internal Medicine, University of Washington, Seattle, Washington, United States of America, **5** School of Pharmacy, University of Washington, Seattle, Washington, United States of America, **6** University of Haifa, Mount Carmel, Haifa, Israel

Abstract

Background: Although self-rated health (SRH) and performance-based physical function (PPF) are both strong predictors of mortality, little research has investigated the relationships between them. The objective of this study was to evaluate longitudinal, bi-directional associations between SRH and PPF.

Methods: We evaluated longitudinal associations between SRH and PPF in 3,610 adults aged 65–89 followed for an average of 4.8 (standard deviation [SD]: 4.4) years between 1994 and July 2011 in the Adult Changes in Thought study, a population-based cohort in the Seattle area. SRH was assessed with a single-item question in the ACT study. Participants were asked at each evaluation to rate their health as "excellent", "very good", "good", "fair", or "poor" in response to the question "In general, how would you rate your health at this time". PPF scores (ranging from 0–16, with higher indicating better performance) included walking speed, chair rises, grip strength, and balance.

Results: At the baseline visit, participants averaged 74.5 (SD: 5.8) years of age and 2,115 (58.6%) were female. In multivariable linear mixed models, PPF declined with age, with more rapid decreases associated with very good, good, and fair (vs. excellent) baseline SRH. Adjusted annual change in PPF was −0.17 points (95% confidence interval [CI]: −0.19, −0.15) for individuals with excellent baseline SRH and −0.21 points (95% CI: −0.22, −0.19) for participants with fair SRH. In multivariable generalized linear mixed models, lower baseline PPF quartiles were associated with lower odds of excellent/very good/good SRH at age 75, however, differences between baseline PPF quartiles diminished with age.

Conclusions: These results suggest that less than excellent SRH predicts decline in physical functioning, however, poor physical functioning may not predict change in SRH in a reciprocal fashion. SRH provides a simple assessment tool for identifying individuals at increased risk for decline in physical function.

Editor: Utpal Sen, University of Louisville, United States of America

Funding: This work was supported by National Institutes of Health (grant number U01-AG-06781). The funders had no role in study design, data collection and analysis, decision to publish, or preparation of the manuscript.

Competing Interests: EBL receives royalties from UpToDate. The remaining authors declare that no competing interests exist.

* Email: wbrenow@u.washington.edu

Introduction

Self-rated health (SRH) is a widely used measure of general health status that is typically assessed by asking an individual to rate their health [1]. Poor SRH is a consistent predictor of mortality [2–7] and morbidity [8–11] even after accounting for objective health indicators. The mechanisms underlying these associations are poorly understood. However, one possible mechanism is through decline in physical function [12,13].

Poor SRH is associated with faster decline in functional ability in older adults [8,10]. In turn, impairment in physical function is considered an early stage in the disablement process [14] and is linked to mortality [6,15,16]. Thus, it is hypothesized that decline in physical function may be an intermediary between SRH and mortality [12,13]. In this context, SRH may represent an individual's superior knowledge of their own health status and past health risks over objective health measures [1]. SRH is then perhaps statistically but not causally associated with decline in physical function and subsequently an increased risk of death [1]

(Figure 1). However, SRH is likely a dynamic evaluation of health [4]. Individuals may rate their health as poor due to their current health status or recent changes in health [17]. Thus, poor SRH may be both a predictor and an effect of worsening health (Figure 1). Research on the relationship between SRH and physical function may clarify the mechanisms by which each acts as a predictor of mortality.

Few studies have examined longitudinal relationships between SRH and physical function in older adults. Ratings of fair/poor SRH have been associated with future decline in gait speed [12,13]. Associations of SRH with decline in other measures of physical function have not been investigated. Summary measures of physical function, for instance, may be more robust than single items [18]. Furthermore, it remains unclear whether physical function predicts longitudinal change in SRH. Functional status has previously been associated with SRH but associations were found to be weaker for older adults [19–23]. Although SRH has been found to decline with worsening health [4,24], other studies have found that SRH improves with age [25,26]. Perceptions of health likely change with age [1]. Evaluating bi-directional associations between SRH and overall physical function may help elucidate factors influencing health perceptions and identify targets for early intervention.

The goal of this study was to evaluate bi-directional longitudinal relationships between SRH and performance-based physical function (PPF), a composite measure of tests that assess both upper and lower extremity function, among older adults [27]. PPF may capture functional limitations before difficulties are reported [28,29]. In particular, we sought to quantify relationships between PPF and the subjective component of SRH beyond its correlation with health status. We hypothesized that poorer baseline SRH would be associated with more rapid decline in PPF (Figure 1, pathway a), and that poorer baseline PPF would be associated with more rapid decline in SRH (Figure 1, pathway b), after adjusting for other health indicators.

Methods

Study Population

Participants were enrolled in the Adult Changes in Thought (ACT) study, a population based prospective cohort study of incident dementia and Alzheimer's disease, previously described [30]. Briefly, participants were cognitively intact older adults randomly sampled from Group Health Cooperative members

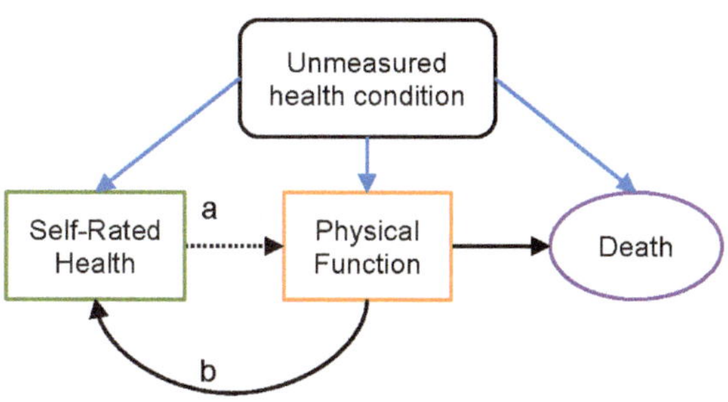

Figure 1. Hypothesized relationships between SRH and physical function. Poor SRH is likely a proxy for an individual's underlying health state that is not captured by other measures. SRH then is statically but perhaps not causally associated with decline in physical function and an increased risk of death (pathway a). Alternatively, poor physical function may lead people to rate their health as poor (pathway b).

aged 65 and older in the Seattle area. The original cohort of 2,581 participants was enrolled between 1994 and 1996. Between 2000 and 2002 an additional 811 participants were enrolled, and in 2004 continuous enrollment began to replace participants who dropped out, developed dementia, or died. Individuals with dementia at baseline were not enrolled in the ACT study. All participants were followed biennially until time of dementia diagnosis, death, or drop-out. At baseline and biennial follow-up evaluations, data collected included demographic characteristics, medical history, cognitive function, memory functioning, blood pressure, depression, and physical functioning. The research protocol for this study followed the Helsinki declaration and was reviewed and approved by the Group Health and University of Washington institutional review boards. Written informed consent was obtained from all participants.

The current analysis included ACT participants aged 65–89 years old who were followed between 1994 and July 2011. The sample was restricted to participants with complete data on SRH, PPF, and covariates at one or more visits. For this study, we defined the baseline visit as the first visit with non-missing SRH, PPF, and covariate information. Follow-up of participants ended at time of dementia diagnosis, death or drop-out; and did not include the visit at which a participant was diagnosed with dementia due to concern that dementia may influence SRH and PPF measures.

Measures

Self-Rated Health. SRH was assessed with a single-item question in the ACT study. This item is similar to SRH questions used in other questionnaires, particularly in the U.S. [1], such as the first question in the SF-36 health survey [31]. Participants were asked at each evaluation "In general, how would you rate your health at this time" with response options of excellent, very good, good, fair, and poor. The SRH question was asked before the physical function tests were performed. Although prior studies have used a variety of different wording and response options for SRH, they are considered to represent the same underlying variable [1], and concordance between different response options is good [32]. Prior studies have found dose-response relationships between original levels of SRH and adverse health outcomes, indicating the validity of SRH [7,9]. In analyses when SRH was the primary exposure, we used SRH at baseline retaining the original five categories. In analyses where SRH was the outcome, responses were dichotomized into excellent, very good, or good ("healthy") SRH vs. fair or poor ("unhealthy") [33,34].

Performance-Based Physical Function. The PPF score was created following methods developed by Wang and colleagues (2002) [28] for the ACT study population. The PPF score consisted of four performance measures that evaluate upper and lower extremity function: 10-foot timed walks (walking speed), five repeated chair stand time (chair rises), standing balance, and grip strength (in kilograms). These tests were chosen based on previously published research [35–37] and study logistics. Walking speed was tested by asking participants to walk a 10-foot distance at their usual speed, using assistive devices if needed. The average of two walks was recorded. Ability to rise from a chair was assessed by instructing participants to stand up from a straight-backed chair with their arms across their chest. Participants successful with one chair rise were then asked to stand up and sit down five times, as fast as possible. They were timed from the first sitting position to the final standing position. To test standing balance, participants were asked to stand close to a wall and were timed for how long they could stand with their feet side-by-side before touching the wall for support. Participants who were able to stand with their feet in the side-by-side position for 10 seconds were next asked to stand with their feet in a semi-tandem position for 10 seconds. Those able to maintain the semi-tandem position were then asked to stand with their feet in a full tandem position for 10 seconds. Grip strength was evaluated using a handheld dynamometer [JAMAR hydraulic hand dynamometer] and measured to the nearest 0.1 kg. Participants were asked to grip the handle as hard as possible using their dominant hand. The average of three attempts was recorded.

A score of 0 to 4 was determined for walking speed, chair rises, standing balance, and grip strength tests. For all tests a score of 0 was given if the participant could not complete the test. Scores of 1–4 for walking speed, chair rises, and grip strength tests were based on previously published sex-specific cutoffs, which corresponded to sex-specific quartiles in the ACT population [28]. Scores of 1–4 for standing balance were categorized based on ability to maintain standing in each position for at least 10 seconds. Score cutoffs are summarized in Table 1.

The sum of the four test scores determined an individual's PPF score (range: 0–16); higher scores corresponded to better performance. In analyses with PPF as the outcome, we used the total PPF score at each visit as a continuous variable. In analyses where PPF was the primary exposure, we categorized the baseline PPF score based on the study sample quartiles. We used baseline PPF quartiles because the relationship between baseline PPF and change in SRH may not be linear. In exploratory analyses, individual PPF components were dichotomized based on study sample quartiles into scores of 3–4 ("better" function), which generally corresponded to 75% of the participants vs. scores of 0–2; except balance, which had a highly skewed distribution, and "better" function was limited to a score of 4.

Covariates. At study baseline and follow-up visits, information was collected on demographics, health status, and chronic health conditions. Demographic factors measured included age, sex, self-reported race, and years of education. Health status-related covariates included cognitive functioning, functional status, depression, and body mass index, exercise (total number of occasions per week on which at least 15 minutes were performed for 8 activities), smoking (never, past, current), and alcohol use (never, past, current). Cognitive function was evaluated using the Cognitive Abilities Screening Instrument (CASI) [38], a 40-item test of global cognitive functioning, scaled such that the entire ACT cohort at baseline had a mean of 100 and standard deviation (SD) of 15. Self-reported functional status was measured using number of limitations in ADLs and instrumental activities of daily living (IADLs). Total number of ADL limitations was based on the participant's reported difficulty performing six ADLs (walking around inside the home, bathing/showering, dressing themselves, getting out of bed or a chair, feeding themselves, and using a toilet). Total number of IADL limitations was based on the

Table 1. Sex-specific Cutoffs for Scores (0 to 4) for Walking Speed, Chair Rises, Standing Balance, and Grip Strength Tests Based on Previously Published Scoring.

	Cutoff for Men	Cutoff for Women
Walking Speed		
0	Unable to complete	Unable to complete
1	>4.5 seconds	>5.0 seconds
2	4.5 - 4.0 seconds	5.0 - 4.0 seconds
3	4.0 - 3.0 seconds	4.0 - 3.0 seconds
4	≤3.0 seconds	≤3.0 seconds
Chair Rises		
0	Unable to complete	Unable to complete
1	>20 seconds	>21 seconds
2	17–20 seconds	18–21 seconds
3	11–17 seconds	12–18 seconds
4	≤11 seconds	≤12 seconds
Standing Balance		
0	Unable to balance side-by side	Unable to balance side-by side
1	Able to balance side-by-side, unable to balance semi-tandem	Able to balance side-by-side, unable to balance semi-tandem
2	Able to balance side-by-side and semi-tandem, unable to balance full tandem	Able to balance side-by-side and semi-tandem, unable to balance full tandem
3	Able to balance side-by-side, semi-tandem, and full tandem for 1–9 seconds	Able to balance side-by-side, semi-tandem, and full tandem for 1–9 seconds
4	Able to balance side-by-side, semi-tandem, and full tandem for 10 seconds	Able to balance side-by-side, semi-tandem, and full tandem for 10 seconds
Grip Strength		
0	Unable to complete	Unable to complete
1	<25.0 kg	<15.0 kg
2	25.0–30.0 kg	15.0–20.0 kg
3	30.0–40.0 kg	20.0–25.0 kg
4	≥40.0 kg	≥25.0 kg

participants reported difficulty in five IADLs (shopping, doing light housework, preparing meals, using a telephone, and managing money). Depressive symptoms were measured using the Center for Epidemiologic Studies Depression scale (CES-D) [39]. Scores were based on a standardized 10-question version [40]; each question contributed 0–3 points for possible range of 0 to 30 points. Height and weight were measured at each study visit. Body mass index was calculated from weight and height (kg/m^2) and categorized as underweight (<18.5), normal (18.5 to 24.9), overweight (25–29.9), and obese (30+). Participants were asked whether a doctor had ever told them they had cancer, cardiovascular disease, cerebrovascular disease, diabetes, hypertension, or rheumatoid or osteoarthritis. We did not obtain information on number of medications.

Statistical analysis

We used descriptive statistics to characterize the study population according to SRH. We described trends in PPF and SRH via their association with age. First, we estimated associations between baseline SRH and age-related change in PPF using linear mixed models with random intercepts to account for within-subject correlation. The primary exposures were age, baseline SRH, and their interactions. The outcome was the PPF score at each study visit. The interaction between age and baseline SRH allowed us to make inference on modifications to the relationship between age and PPF that were attributable to SRH. As sensitivity analyses, we re-ran models with missing PPF imputed first as the lowest PPF score and then as the highest PPF score. We also explored whether baseline SRH was associated with individual component measures of PPF.

Next, we estimated associations between baseline PPF and age-related change in SRH, repeating analyses but using a logistic link function in a generalized linear mixed model. Healthy SRH was the outcome and the primary exposures were age, quartiles of baseline PPF, and their interactions. Inference was based on the interaction between age and SRH, which described the extent to which the age-related differences in odds of healthy SRH were modified by baseline PPF. We also re-ran models with missing SRH values imputed as unhealthy SRH and then as healthy SRH.

We investigated three levels of time-varying covariate adjustment: Model 1 was adjusted for participant age at baseline; Model 2 was additionally adjusted for sex, race, education, cognitive functioning, limitations in ADLs and IADLS, depressive symptoms, body mass index, exercise, smoking status, and alcohol use; and Model 3 was additionally adjusted for chronic health conditions (cancer, cardiovascular disease, cerebrovascular disease, diabetes, hypertension, or arthritis). Potential confounders were selected a priori as factors previously found to be associated with SRH and PPF [21,28]. Values of SRH adjusted for other health indicators may reflect subjective and contextual evaluations and response styles [1]. We pre-specified Model 2 as the primary analysis.

To describe longitudinal trajectories across follow-up we report the estimated mean outcome for each level of the primary exposure at age 75 (corresponding to the average age at baseline for the sample) and the estimated annual change in the outcome for each level of the primary exposure from each model. In Models 2 and 3, we estimated the mean at age 75 based on regression model estimates using indirect standardization to account for possible confounding by other covariates included in the model. We used graphical analyses to illustrate estimated age-related trends in SRH and PPF. Model fit was assessed with residual plots. Analyses were conducted using R (version 2.12.1). All tests were two-sided with $\alpha = 0.05$.

Results

As of July 25, 2011, data were available on 4,513 participants without dementia who had ever been enrolled in the ACT study, of which 4,411 participants were aged 65–89. Age-eligible participants were excluded if they were missing SRH, PPF, or covariate data at all visits. The final study sample included 3,610 ACT participants (81.8% of 4,411 age-eligible participants) followed on average for 4.8 (SD: 4.4) years. Excluded age-eligible participants were primarily missing PPF (n = 326) and/or health conditions (n = 497); they tended to have higher education, more limitations in ADLs and IADLs, more health conditions, and shorter follow-up than included participants (Table S1). At the baseline visit in this analysis (the initial visit for>90%), participants averaged 74.5 (SD: 5.8) years of age and 14.3 (SD: 3.1) years of education; approximately 60% were female and 90% were white. There were 1,517 participants (41.7%) who died during follow-up. At baseline, 13% of participants had excellent SRH, 33% had very good SRH, 39% had good SRH, 14% had fair SRH, and 2% had poor SRH. The average PPF score was 12.5 (SD: 2.5). On average, participants with unhealthy SRH were older, had worse cognition and more depressive symptoms, and reported functional limitations and comorbidities; and they were more likely to have died during follow-up (Table 2).

Baseline SRH and Age-Related Changes in PPF

Among participants with at least one follow-up visit (n = 2,691), the average change in PPF score was −1.9 points over follow-up (SD: 2.7). Frequency and percentage of participants by trajectories of PPF are shown in Table 3. For a majority of participants (~70%), PPF declined by at least one point over follow-up (Table 3). However, many participants had fluctuations in PPF over time. In initial descriptive analyses, the relationship between PPF and age was approximately linear, on average.

In multivariable linear mixed models, poorer baseline SRH was associated with poorer mean PPF at age 75 (Table 4). On average, PPF declined with age even after adjustment for demographics and health status. There was a significant difference in rate of decline of PPF across levels of SRH ($P = 0.02$) (Table 4). Compared to participants with excellent baseline SRH, the average annual decline in PPF was slightly more rapid for participants with very good, good, and fair baseline SRH (Table 4, Figure 2). For participants with poor SRH, average annual decline was similar to participants with excellent SRH (Table 4). Results were similar across all models (Table S2). Very few participants with poor SRH at baseline (n = 21) had multiple visits; in examining PPF trajectories, we found that 9.5% had no change, 42.9% declined, 28.6% improved, and 19.0% fluctuated over follow-up. In exploratory analyses, annual change in odds of better function for individual PPF components was not consistently lower for poorer SRH (Table S3).

In sensitivity analyses, inference on variation in rates of decline in relation to baseline SRH was unchanged when all missing PPF values were imputed as the minimum, but when all missing PPF values were imputed as the maximum the mean rate of decline of PPF was slower for individuals with less than excellent baseline SRH (data not shown).

Baseline PPF and Age-Related Changes in SRH

Among 2,691 participants with at least one follow-up visit the vast majority (>80%) remained stable in SRH (healthy vs unhealthy) during follow-up (Table 3). In multivariable generalized linear mixed models, lower baseline PPF quartiles were associated with lower probability of healthy SRH at age 75

Table 2. Participant baseline characteristics by self-rated health (N = 3,610).

Participant Characteristics	Excellent/Very Good/Good SRH (n = 3,062)	Fair/Poor SRH (n = 548)
	Mean (SD)	Mean (SD)
Age	74.2 (5.8)	75.8 (5.9)
Cognitive Functioning		
CASI[a]	105.0 (10.5)	100.5 (10.3)
Depressive Symptoms		
CESD Score	3.4 (3.7)	6.6 (5.3)
Exercise		
Occasions per week of 15 minutes	5.6 (4.6)	4.1 (4.2)
	N (%)	N (%)
Female	1,796 (58.7)	319 (58.2)
Race		
White	2,819 (92.1)	467 (85.2)
Black	106 (3.5)	43 (7.8)
Asian	94 (3.1)	25 (4.6)
Other	43 (1.4)	13 (2.4)
Education		
<High school	295 (9.6)	109 (19.9)
Completed high school	689 (22.5)	177 (32.3)
At least some college	2078 (67.8)	262 (47.8)
ADL limitations (out of 6)		
0	2,582 (84.3)	318 (58.0)
1	382 (12.5)	125 (22.8)
≥2	98 (3.2)	105 (19.2)
IADL limitations (out of 5)		
0	2,770 (90.8)	374 (68.2)
1	234 (7.6)	96 (17.5)
≥2	49 (1.6)	78 (14.2)
Body Mass Index		
Underweight	27 (<1)	10 (1.8)
Normal	1,023 (33.4)	161 (29.4)
Overweight	1,264 (41.3)	210 (38.3)
Obese	748 (24.4)	167 (30.5)
Alcohol Use		
Never	565 (18.5)	145 (26.5)
Former	712 (23.3)	184 (33.6)
Current	1,785 (58.3)	219 (40.0)
Smoking		
Never	1,478 (48.2)	235 (42.9)
Former	1,425 (46.5)	270 (49.3)
Current	159 (5.2)	43 (7.8)
Health Conditions[b]		
None	723 (23.6)	54 (9.9)
One	1,141 (37.2)	137 (25.0)
Two or more	1,198 (39.1)	357 (65.1)
Death during follow-up	1,164 (38.0)	343 (62.6)

Abbreviations: SRH, self-rated health; CASI, Cognitive Abilities Screening Test; CESD, Center for Epidemiological Studies Depression Scale; ADL, Activities of Daily Living; IADL, Instrumental Activities of Daily Living.

[a]Scores are scaled such that at baseline the mean score for the entire ACT cohort was 100 and the standard deviation was 15.

[b]Health conditions included cancer, cerebrovascular disease, cardiovascular disease, diabetes, hypertension, and arthritis.

Table 3. Trajectories[a] in PPF and SRH level over follow-up for participants with two or more visits (N = 2,691).

	No change	Declined	Improved	Fluctuated, overall decline	Fluctuated, other
PPF score	184 (6.8)	944 (35.1)	265 (9.8)	900 (33.4)	398 (14.8)
SRH[b]	2052 (76.3)	259 (9.6)	137 (5.1)	32 (<1)	211 (7.1)

[a]No change, declined, and improved categories represent trajectories with one pattern; fluctuated categories represent trajectories with both decline and improvement (with either overall decline or another pattern).
[b]dichotomized (healthy vs. unhealthy).
Note: N(% of 2,691) shown for each category.

(Table 5). There was a significant difference in change of odds of healthy SRH across PPF quartiles ($P<0.001$) (Table 5). For those in the highest quartile of baseline PPF there was a 9% decrease in odds of healthy SRH per year (OR = 0.91). Participants in the upper middle and lower middle quartiles experienced a slower decrease in odds of healthy SRH (4 and 6% decrease per year, respectively) (Table 5). In adjusted models, odds of healthy SRH increased with age, for those in the lowest quartile (1% increase per year). This resulted in convergence of the estimated probability of healthy SRH across levels of baseline PPF for older compared to younger ages (Figure 3). Results were similar across all models (Table S4). Sensitivity analyses produced similar results when missing SRH values were imputed as excellent or as poor (data not shown).

Discussion

We investigated bi-directional longitudinal relationships between SRH and physical function among older adults without dementia, with adjustment for multiple health indicators. We found that lower baseline SRH was associated with lower PPF at age 75. Very good, good, or fair baseline SRH was associated with faster decline of PPF compared to excellent baseline SRH. Although we found that lower baseline PPF was associated with lower odds of healthy SRH at age 75, lower baseline PPF was associated with increasing odds of healthy SRH over time. This resulted in little difference in odds of healthy SRH at older ages.

Our results are consistent with previous studies that found fair/poor SRH to be associated with faster decline in timed gait [12,13]. We extend these findings to a measure of overall physical function. Furthermore, we found associations with even intermediate levels of SRH, which has shown graded associations with risk of mortality and self-reported functional limitations [7,9]. SRH

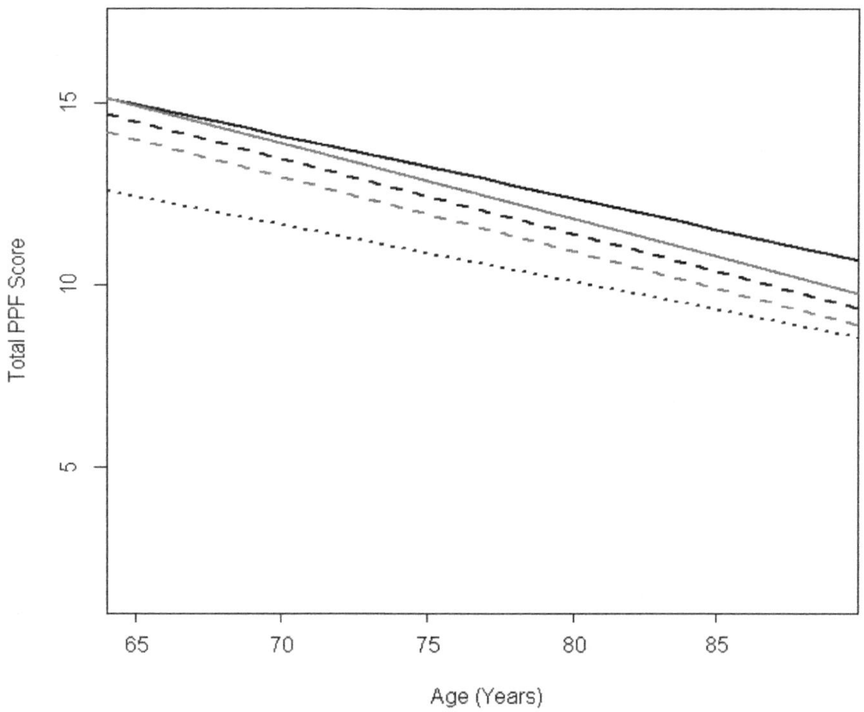

Figure 2. Population mean trajectories of performance-based physical functioning (PPF) score modified by self-rated health (SRH). Average trends in PPF for adults aged 65–89 were estimated from a linear mixed model adjusted for age at baseline, sex, race, education, cognitive functioning, depressive symptoms, functional limitations, body mass index, alcohol use, smoking status, and exercise. SRH levels are depicted as: excellent = black solid, very good = grey solid, good = black dashed, fair = grey dashed, poor = black dotted. PPF scores (y-axis) ranged from 0 to 16; higher scores corresponded to better performance.

Table 4. Linear mixed model results for the associations between baseline SRH and age-related changes PPF.[a]

Mean PPF at age 75 by SRH[b]			
	Mean	**95% CI**	***P*-value**[c]
Excellent	13.02	12.85, 13.19	<0.001
Very Good	12.63	12.53, 12.74	
Good	12.21	12.11, 12.31	
Fair	11.73	11.54, 11.91	
Poor	10.64	10.08, 11.21	
Annual rate of change in PPF by SRH level			
	β	**95% CI**	***P*-value**[c]
Excellent	−0.17	−0.19, −0.15	0.02
Very Good	−0.21	−0.22, −0.19	
Good	−0.21	−0.22, −0.19	
Fair	−0.21	−0.23, −0.18	
Poor	−0.16	−0.24, −0.07	

Abbreviations: PPF, performance-based physical function; SRH, self-rated health.
[a]Adjusted for age at baseline, sex, race, education, cognitive functioning, depressive symptoms, functional limitations, body mass index, alcohol use, smoking status, and exercise.
[b]Estimates are standardized to the distribution of all covariates included in the model via indirect standardization.
[c]P-values are for omnibus Wald test of any difference across categories of SRH.

may reflect a number of underlying constructs. SRH may represent an individual's superior knowledge of their own health over objective measures [2,9]. Alternatively, SRH may reflect psychosocial resources and health behaviors that influence changes in function [41,42]. Contrary to our expectations, poor baseline SRH did not predict more rapid decline in PPF compared to excellent SRH. This estimate may not be precise since very few participants with poor SRH had multiple visits. However, participants with poor SRH at baseline were more likely to have improved PPF scores in subsequent visits compared to those with higher levels of SRH. Perhaps for some participants poor SRH reflected acute or transient health effects that improved at later visits. On the other hand, participants with poor SRH at baseline were more likely to have died so there could also have been a bias toward follow-up of participants with poor SRH who had temporary health problems. Participants with poor SRH who had lasting impairments in functioning may have been more likely to die or be unable to return for additional study visits.

We provide new evidence describing the longitudinal change in healthy SRH according to baseline physical function. Our results complement prior findings that poor physical function did not predict decline in SRH [22], and that associations between

Table 5. Generalized linear mixed model results for the associations between baseline PPF and age-related changes in SRH.[a]

Probability of healthy SRH at age 75 by PPF quartile[b]			
	Prob	**95% CI**	***P*-value**[c]
Highest	0.95	0.95, 0.96	<0.001
Upper Middle	0.93	0.92, 0.94	
Lower Middle	0.93	0.92, 0.94	
Lowest	0.84	0.81, 0.87	
Annual multiplicative rate of change in odds of healthy SRH by PPF quartile			
	OR	**95% CI**	***P*-value**[c]
Highest	0.91	0.89, 0.93	<0.001
Upper Middle	0.94	0.91, 0.97	
Lower Middle	0.96	0.93, 0.99	
Lowest	1.01	0.97, 1.05	

Abbreviations: PPF, performance-based physical function; SRH, self-rated health.
[a]Adjusted for age at baseline, sex, race, education, cognitive functioning, depressive symptoms, functional limitations, body mass index, alcohol use, smoking status, and exercise.
[b]Estimates are standardized to the distribution of all covariates included in the model via indirect standardization.
[c]P-values are for omnibus Wald test of any difference across categories of SRH.

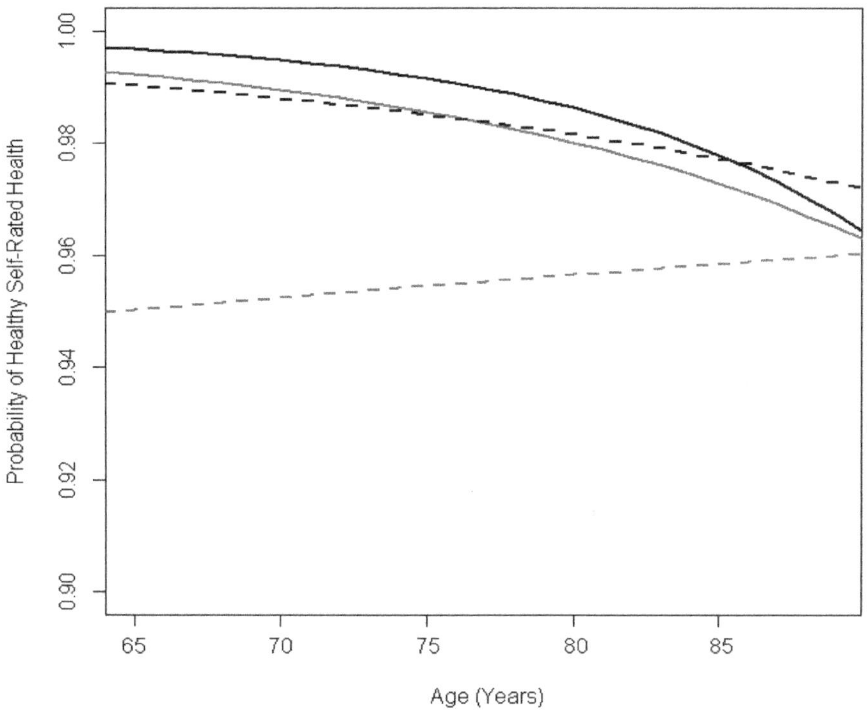

Figure 3. Population mean change in probability of excellent/very good/good (healthy) self-rated health (SRH) modified by quartiles of performance-based physical functioning (PPF). Average trends in PPF for adults aged 65–89 were estimated from a generalized linear mixed model adjusted for age at baseline, sex, race, education, cognitive functioning, depressive symptoms, functional limitations, body mass index, alcohol use, smoking status, and exercise. PPF Quartiles are depicted as: highest = black solid, upper-middle = grey solid, lower-middle = black dashed, lowest = grey dashed.

functional status and SRH weakened with age [20]. Current level of function may be a stronger determinant of SRH than prior level of function [20]. Alternatively, these results may be due to regression to the mean, the statistical phenomenon where extreme measurements tend to be closer to the mean on a second measurement [43]; other studies have found such trends in SRH [44,45]. Given that a large number of participants had fluctuating PPF trajectories, it is possible that non-uniform patterns of PPF over time explains the lack of predictive power of baseline PPF for subsequent changes in SRH. Another possible explanation is that with age, individuals may lower their expectations of good health after experiencing health declines [46]. This phenomenon, known as "response-shift", could differ across levels of physical functioning. Participants with worse baseline physical function may have lowered expectations for their health over time resulting in stable or higher SRH at subsequent visits compared to those with better function. On the other hand, participants with high levels of physical functioning may have had higher expectations for their health, and age-related decline in health may be more discordant to their expectations leading to more rapid declines in SRH.

Although our results suggest that SRH and physical function are interconnected, independent of demographics and health outcomes, worse baseline physical function did not predict decline in SRH in a reciprocal fashion as worse baseline SRH predicted decline in physical function. People with less than excellent SRH may be at an increased risk for future disability [11] and mortality [7,9] with decline in physical function as an intermediary [12,13]. Since overall decline in physical function was common and was associated with lower SRH, future research should determine whether decline in physical function could be prevented among individuals with lower SRH. Multi-component exercise interventions may effectively prevent disability in frail adults [51], and could be used to target individuals by their SRH level. Conversely, after adjustment for current health status, changes in SRH with age may be due to a more dynamic process that reflects changing self-assessment. Older adults consider a variety of factors when assessing their health including functional status, health behaviors and psychosocial factors; however the importance of each factor may differ according to an individual's demographics, psychological outlook, physical health status, and question framing [17,47,48]. In future research, it may be important to investigate whether the relationships between SRH and PPF differ by subgroups and response styles.

Our study has several limitations. Generalizability may be limited because participants were predominantly white and well educated. Participants in poor health may have been more likely to die, drop-out earlier, or skip visits, which may have attenuated associations between SRH and PPF. Due to our interest in the subjective processes behind SRH rather than global health status, our measure of SRH did not incorporate death, unlike an alternative coding of SRH [24]. Some ACT participants were excluded from this analysis due to missing data, especially in our PPF measures, which may not be assessed on participants with disabilities, poor health, or impaired cognition. This may have biased our results towards participants with better physical function and longer follow-up. However, there is excellent follow-up of ACT participants (completeness of follow-up index estimated to be 95.6% [49]) and sensitivity analyses in which missing PPF was imputed as poor gave similar results to the primary analyses.

This study also has several important strengths, including a large, representative sample of community-dwelling older adults with extensive follow-up with multiple measures of health indicators. We used a longitudinal analysis, which allowed us to average over fluctuations in individual measurements to help capture long-term trends in PPF and SRH. Since many participants had fluctuating PPF measures, longitudinal modelling of repeated PPF measures can help uncover trends that would otherwise be obscured. We recommend this approach for future studies of PPF and SRH. Additionally, we investigated the associations between SRH and an objective measure of overall physical function eliminating potential confounding arising in subjective measures of function [50]. Our composite measure of PPF is simple to assess and clinically relevant since interventions to improve overall function may be more effective at preventing disability than single components [51]. However, there are many tests of physical function [18]; future research should investigate optimal measures. We selected an analysis strategy that is robust to data missingness that can be predicted based on prior observations [52]. Furthermore, we conducted sensitivity analyses, which generally supported our results except in the unlikely situation when PPF measurements were more likely to be missing for those with good function. We tested specific hypotheses regarding the relationships between SRH and PPF; however, future studies could explore how multiple factors influence change in SRH and PPF as well as their relative impact.

In conclusion, we found longitudinal associations between SRH and PPF in a large prospective cohort study of older adults. However, there appears to be a complex relationship between SRH and PPF. Future research should also assess the mechanisms through which SRH may affect physical function as well as disentangle factors that influence longitudinal change in SRH. As a strong predictor of mortality and functional decline, SRH provides a simple tool that can be used to identify individuals at higher risk of future poor health outcomes. It is unclear whether future poor health outcomes can be prevented among individuals with lower SRH. However, interventions to maintain physical function may be especially beneficial for those with less than excellent SRH.

Supporting Information

Table S1 Baseline Characteristics of Included and Excluded ACT Participants Aged 65–89 (N = 4,411).

Table S2 Linear Mixed Model Results for the Association between Baseline SRH and Longitudinal PPF.

Table S3 Generalized Linear Mixed Effects Model Results for the Association between Baseline SRH and Odds of Better Function[a] for Individual Components of PPF. Estimates of individual PPF components at age 75 are standardized to the distribution of all covariates included in the model via indirect standardization.

Table S4 Generalized Linear Mixed Model Results for the Association between Baseline PPF Quartile and Odds of Excellent/Very Good/Good ("healthy") SRH.

Author Contributions

Conceived and designed the experiments: WDB RAH EBL PKC. Analyzed the data: WDB RAH PKC SLG OZ EBL. Wrote the paper: WDB RAH PKC SLG OZ EBL. Contributed to data aquisition: EBL PKC.

References

1. Jylhä M (2009) What is self-rated health and why does it predict mortality? Towards a unified conceptual model. Soc Sci Med 1982 69: 307–316. doi:10.1016/j.socscimed.2009.05.013.
2. Idler EL, Benyamini Y (1997) Self-Rated Health and Mortality: A Review of Twenty-Seven Community Studies. J Health Soc Behav 38: 21–37. doi:10.2307/2955359.
3. Benyamini Y, Idler EL (1999) Community Studies Reporting Association between Self-Rated Health and Mortality. Res Aging 21: 392–401. doi:10.1177/0164027599213002.
4. Ferraro KF, Kelley-Moore JA (2001) Self-Rated Health and Mortality Among Black and White Adults. J Gerontol B Psychol Sci Soc Sci 56: S195–S205. doi:10.1093/geronb/56.4.S195.
5. Wang C, Satariano WA (2007) Self-Rated Current and Future Health Independently Predict Subsequent Mortality in an Aging Population. J Gerontol A Biol Sci Med Sci 62: 1428–1434.
6. Cesari M, Onder G, Zamboni V, Manini T, Shorr RI, et al. (2008) Physical function and self-rated health status as predictors of mortality: results from longitudinal analysis in the ilSIRENTE study. BMC Geriatr 8: 34. doi:10.1186/1471-2318-8-34.
7. Bopp M, Braun J, Gutzwiller F, Faeh D (2012) Health risk or resource? Gradual and independent association between self-rated health and mortality persists over 30 years. PloS One 7: e30795. doi:10.1371/journal.pone.0030795.
8. Idler EL, Kasl SV (1995) Self-ratings of health: do they also predict change in functional ability? J Gerontol B Psychol Sci Soc Sci 50: S344–S353.
9. Idler EL, Russell LB, Davis D (2000) Survival, Functional Limitations, and Self-rated Health in the NHANES I Epidemiologic Follow-up Study, 1992. Am J Epidemiol 152: 874–883. doi:10.1093/aje/152.9.874.
10. Hubbard RA, Inoue LYT, Diehr P (2009) Joint modeling of self-rated health and changes in physical functioning. J Am Stat Assoc 104: 912. doi:10.1198/jasa.2009.ap08423.
11. Pietiläinen O, Laaksonen M, Rahkonen O, Lahelma E (2011) Self-rated health as a predictor of disability retirement–the contribution of ill-health and working conditions. PloS One 6: e25004. doi:10.1371/journal.pone.0025004.
12. Martinez DJ, Kasl SV, Gill TM, Barry LC (2010) Longitudinal association between self-rated health and timed gait among older persons. J Gerontol B P-sychol Sci Soc Sci 65: 715–719. doi:10.1093/geronb/gbp115.
13. Ashburner JM, Cauley JA, Cawthon P, Ensrud KE, Hochberg MC, et al. (2011) Self-ratings of health and change in walking speed over 2 years: results from the caregiver-study of osteoporotic fractures. Am J Epidemiol 173: 882–889. doi:10.1093/aje/kwq445.
14. Verbrugge LM, Jette AM (1994) The disablement process. Soc Sci Med 1982 38: 1–14.
15. Reuben DB, Rubenstein LV, Hirsch SH, Hays RD (1992) Value of functional status as a predictor of mortality: results of a prospective study. Am J Med 93: 663–669.
16. Guralnik JM, Simonsick EM, Ferrucci L, Glynn RJ, Berkman LF, et al. (1994) A short physical performance battery assessing lower extremity function: association with self-reported disability and prediction of mortality and nursing home admission. J Gerontol 49: M85–M94.
17. Benyamini Y, Leventhal EA, Leventhal H (2003) Elderly people's ratings of the importance of health-related factors to their self-assessments of health. Soc Sci Med 56: 1661–1667. doi:10.1016/S0277-9536(02)00175-2.
18. Freiberger E, Vreede P de, Schoene D, Rydwik E, Mueller V, et al. (2012) Performance-based physical function in older community-dwelling persons: a systematic review of instruments. Age Ageing 41: 712–721. doi:10.1093/ageing/afs099.
19. Hays JC, Schoenfeld DE, Blazer DG (1996) Determinants of poor self-rated health in late life. Am J Geriatr Psychiatry 4: 188–196.
20. Hoeymans N, Feskens EJM, Kromhout D, Van Den Bos GAM (1997) Ageing and the relationship between functional status and self-rated health in elderly men. Soc Sci Med 45: 1527–1536. doi:10.1016/S0277-9536(97)00089-0.
21. Jylhä M, Guralnik JM, Balfour J, Fried LP (2001) Walking difficulty, walking speed, and age as predictors of self-rated health: the women's health and aging study. J Gerontol A Biol Sci Med Sci 56: M609–M617.
22. Leinonen R, Heikkinen E, Jylhä M (2001) Predictors of decline in self-assessments of health among older people–a 5-year longitudinal study. Soc Sci Med 1982 52: 1329–1341.
23. Arnadottir SA, Gunnarsdottir ED, Stenlund H, Lundin-Olsson L (2011) Determinants of self-rated health in old age: a population-based, cross-sectional study using the International Classification of Functioning. BMC Public Health 11: 670. doi:10.1186/1471-2458-11-670.

24. Diehr P, Williamson J, Patrick DL, Bild DE, Burke GL, et al. (2001) Patterns of Self-Rated Health in Older Adults Before and After Sentinel Health Events. J Am Geriatr Soc 49: 36–44. doi:10.1046/j.1532-5415.2001.49007.x.
25. Ishizaki T, Yoshida H, Suzuki T, Shibata H (2009) The association between self-rated health status and increasing age among older Japanese living in a rural community over a 6-year period: a longitudinal data analysis. Gerontology 55: 344–352. doi:10.1159/000183749.
26. Dening TR, Chi LY, Brayne C, Huppert FA, Paykel ES, et al. (1998) Changes in self-rated health, disability and contact with services in a very elderly cohort: a 6-year follow-up study. Age Ageing 27: 23–33.
27. Reuben DB, Siu AL (1990) An objective measure of physical function of elderly outpatients. The Physical Performance Test. J Am Geriatr Soc 38: 1105–1112.
28. Wang L, van Belle G, Kukull WB, Larson EB (2002) Predictors of functional change: a longitudinal study of nondemented people aged 65 and older. J Am Geriatr Soc 50: 1525–1534.
29. Reuben DB, Siu AL, Kimpau S (1992) The Predictive Validity of Self-Report and Performance-based Measures of Function and Health. J Gerontol 47: M106–M110. doi:10.1093/geronj/47.4.M106.
30. Kukull WA, Higdon R, Bowen JD, McCormick WC, Teri L, et al. (2002) Dementia and Alzheimer disease incidence: a prospective cohort study. Arch Neurol 59: 1737–1746.
31. Ware JE, Gandek B (1998) Overview of the SF-36 Health Survey and the International Quality of Life Assessment (IQOLA) Project. J Clin Epidemiol 51: 903–912.
32. Jürges H, Avendano M, MacKenbach JP (2008) Are different measures of self-rated health comparable? An assessment in five European countries. Eur J Epidemiol 23: 773–781. doi:10.1007/s10654-008-9287-6.
33. Manor O, Matthews S, Power C (2000) Dichotomous or categorical response? Analysing self-rated health and lifetime social class. Int J Epidemiol 29: 149–157.
34. Ferraro KF, Wilmoth JM (2000) Measuring morbidity: disease counts, binary variables, and statistical power. J Gerontol B Psychol Sci Soc Sci 55: S173–S189.
35. Guralnik JM, Branch LG, Cummings SR, Curb JD (1989) Physical performance measures in aging research. J Gerontol 44: M141–M146.
36. Reuben DB, Valle LA, Hays RD, Siu AL (1995) Measuring physical function in community-dwelling older persons: a comparison of self-administered, interviewer-administered, and performance-based measures. J Am Geriatr Soc 43: 17–23.
37. Cress ME, Schechtman KB, Mulrow CD, Fiatarone MA, Gerety MB, et al. (1995) Relationship between physical performance and self-perceived physical function. J Am Geriatr Soc 43: 93–101.
38. Teng EL, Hasegawa K, Homma A, Imai Y, Larson E, et al. (1994) The Cognitive Abilities Screening Instrument (CASI): A Practical Test for Cross-Cultural Epidemiological Studies of Dementia. Int Psychogeriatr 6: 45–58. doi:10.1017/S1041610294001602.
39. Radloff LS (1977) The CES-D Scale A Self-Report Depression Scale for Research in the General Population. Appl Psychol Meas 1: 385–401. doi:10.1177/014662167700100306.
40. Andresen EM, Malmgren JA, Carter WB, Patrick DL (1994) Screening for depression in well older adults: evaluation of a short form of the CES-D (Center for Epidemiologic Studies Depression Scale). Am J Prev Med 10: 77–84.
41. Xu J, Roberts RE (2010) The power of positive emotions: it's a matter of life or death–subjective well-being and longevity over 28 years in a general population. Health Psychol Off J Div Health Psychol Am Psychol Assoc 29: 9–19. doi:10.1037/a0016767.
42. Halford C, Ekselius L, Anderzen I, Arnetz B, Svärdsudd K (2010) Self-rated health, life-style, and psychoendocrine measures of stress in healthy adult women. Ups J Med Sci 115: 266–274. doi:10.3109/03009734.2010.496910.
43. Barnett AG, Pols JC van der, Dobson AJ (2005) Regression to the mean: what it is and how to deal with it. Int J Epidemiol 34: 215–220. doi:10.1093/ije/dyh299.
44. Miller TR, Wolinsky FD (2007) Self-Rated Health Trajectories and Mortality Among Older Adults. J Gerontol B Psychol Sci Soc Sci 62: S22–S27.
45. Zajacova A, Dowd JB (2011) Reliability of self-rated health in US adults. Am J Epidemiol 174: 977–983. doi:10.1093/aje/kwr204.
46. Galenkamp H, Huisman M, Braam AW, Deeg DJH (2012) Estimates of prospective change in self-rated health in older people were biased owing to potential recalibration response shift. J Clin Epidemiol 65: 978–988. doi:10.1016/j.jclinepi.2012.03.010.
47. Schüz B, Wurm S, Schöllgen I, Tesch-Römer C (2011) What do people include when they self-rate their health? Differential associations according to health status in community-dwelling older adults. Qual Life Res Int J Qual Life Asp Treat Care Rehabil 20: 1573–1580. doi:10.1007/s11136-011-9909-4.
48. Sargent-Cox KA, Anstey KJ, Luszcz MA (2010) Patterns of longitudinal change in older adults' self-rated health: the effect of the point of reference. Health Psychol Off J Div Health Psychol Am Psychol Assoc 29: 143–152. doi:10.1037/a0017652.
49. Siskind V (2002) Quantification of completeness of follow-up. The Lancet 360: 724. doi:10.1016/S0140-6736(02)09861-6.
50. Leibson CL, Garrard J, Nitz N, Waller L, Indritz M, et al. (1999) The role of depression in the association between self-rated physical health and clinically defined illness. The Gerontologist 39: 291–298.
51. Daniels R, van Rossum E, de Witte L, Kempen GIJM, van den Heuvel W (2008) Interventions to prevent disability in frail community-dwelling elderly: a systematic review. BMC Health Serv Res 8: 278. doi:10.1186/1472-6963-8-278.
52. Little RJA, Rubin DB (1987) Statistical analysis with missing data. New York: Wiley.

16

Physiological Comparison of Concentric and Eccentric Arm Cycling in Males and Females

C. Martyn Beaven[1]*, Sarah J. Willis[1], Christian J. Cook[2], Hans-Christer Holmberg[1]

1 Swedish Winter Sports Research Centre, Department of Health Sciences, Mid Sweden University, Östersund, Sweden, **2** School of Sport, Health and Exercise Sciences, Bangor University, Bangor, United Kingdom

Abstract

Lower body eccentric exercise is well known to elicit high levels of muscular force with relatively low cardiovascular and metabolic strain. As a result, eccentric exercise has been successfully utilised as an adaptive stressor to improve lower body muscle function in populations ranging from the frail and debilitated, to highly-trained individuals. Here we investigate the metabolic, cardiorespiratory, and energy costs of upper body eccentric exercise in a healthy population. Seven men and seven women performed 4-min efforts of eccentric (ECC) or concentric (CON) arm cycling on a novel arm ergometer at workloads corresponding to 40, 60, and 80% of their peak workload as assessed in an incremental concentric trial. The heart rate, ventilation, cardiac output, respiratory exchange ratio, and blood lactate concentrations were all clearly greater in CON condition at all of the relative workloads (all $p<0.003$). Effect size calculations demonstrated that the magnitude of the differences in VO_2 and work economy between the ECC and CON exercise ranged from very large to extremely large; however, in no case did mechanical efficiency (η_{MECH}) differ between the conditions (all $p>0.05$). In contrast, delta efficiency (η_{Δ}), as previously defined by Coyle and colleagues in 1992, demonstrated a sex difference (men>women; $p<0.05$). Sex differences were also apparent in arteriovenous oxygen difference and heart rate during CON. Here, we reinforce the high-force, low cost attributes of eccentric exercise which can be generalised to the muscles of the upper body. Upper body eccentric exercise is likely to form a useful adjunct in debilitative, rehabilitative, and adaptive clinical exercise programs; however, reports of a shift towards an oxidative phenotype should be taken into consideration by power athletes. We suggest delta efficiency as a sensitive measure of efficiency that allowed the identification of sex differences.

Editor: Alejandro Lucia, Universidad Europea de Madrid, Spain

Funding: The authors have no support or funding to report.

Competing Interests: The authors have declared that no competing interests exist.

* Email: Martyn.Beaven@miun.se

Introduction

In 1892 Adolf Fick clearly demonstrated in thermometric studies on isolated muscle that more heat is produced when the muscle is actively stretched than during active shortening [1]. While in 1896, Chauveau reported that in human subjects the cost of descending stairs backwards (negative work or travail négatif) was substantially less than ascending them forwards (positive work or travail positif) [2]. Since this time, it has become abundantly clear that excentric (eccentric) exercise can be performed with a lower metabolic, ventilatory, and haemodynamic cost when compared to concentric exercise [3–10].

Consequently, lower limb eccentric training has been applied to populations for whom high-intensity training is contraindicated such as the elderly [11–13] and COPD patients [14]. Further, eccentric training generates extensive mechanical muscle tension [15] which is associated with activation of mitogen-activated protein kinases [16]. This property has led to the utilization of lower limb eccentric training in athletic populations to induce muscular overload and enhance maximal strength, muscular stiffness, and muscle accretion [15,17,18].

Unsurprisingly, using a novel arm ergometer fabricated in-house, our laboratory has previously confirmed that the low metabolic cost and high force generating capacities of eccentric contractions are not constrained to the muscles of the lower limbs. Specifically, we found that arm ergometry at three absolute power outputs (40, 80, and 120 W) performed at 60 revolutionsmin^{-1} were demonstrably and significantly less metabolically demanding (as assessed by oxygen uptake VO_2) when performed eccentrically as compared to concentrically [19]. An acknowledged limitation of our previous study design is that the absolute workloads imposed may have taxed the participants differentially and influenced the observed responses to concentric and eccentric arm cycling. Herein, we address this shortcoming by prescribing relative workloads.

We were also interested in the effect of sex on the observed responses as our earlier study included only men. It is apparent that there exists an innate disparity in the relative strength and muscular endurance characteristics of men and women that are specific to the muscles of the upper body [20]. There are also known differences between upper and lower body oxygen kinetics [21,22]. A relationship between cardiac output (Q_C) and metabolic demand has been described in the lower limbs indicating that exercise-induced circulatory responses are mainly under metabolic control [9]; however, no such information is currently available for upper-body exercise.

In the present study, we tested the hypothesis that our previous observations of a significantly decreased metabolic cost of exercise at absolute work rates would be confirmed with relative work rates.

Further, we hypothesized that sex differences in upper body muscle efficiency would be apparent. Lastly we sought to investigate the relationship between Q_C and metabolic demand in the muscles of the upper limbs.

Methods

Ethics Statement

The investigation was conducted according to the principles expressed in the Declaration of Helsinki. All participants provided informed written consent prior to participation and pre-approval was obtained from the Umeå Regional Ethical Review Board (# 2012-114-31M).

Participants

Seven men and seven women (physical characteristics described in Table 1) volunteered to participate in this study. Participants were physically active in a variety of sports a minimum of three times per week. The protocol and procedures were explained verbally and all participants provided written informed consent prior to testing.

Experimental Protocol

The week before the experimental data collection, participants performed three sessions of eccentric (ECC) and concentric (CON) arm cycling in order to become familiar with the arm cycle ergometers and testing protocol. In addition, these practice trials enabled participants to acquire the specific coordination patterns required for eccentric arm cycling. It is important to point out that eccentric exercise to which an individual is unaccustomed is commonly associated with direct and indirect measures of reversible muscle damage as well as subjective increases in pain [23,24]. To minimize the occurrence of such muscle soreness, the duration and intensity of the eccentric arm cycling trials were progressively increased over the three practice sessions (e.g. from 4 to 10 min and from 60 to 120 W). After this familiarization period, participants entered the experimental protocol only if they reported no residual muscle soreness as assessed using the perceived recovery status scale [25]. Following the three practice sessions, and at least 48 h prior to entering the experimental week, individual W_{PEAK} was determined from an incremental concentric arm cycling test that started at 60 W and increased by 15 W every 60 seconds.

During the experimental week, participants reported to the laboratory on two separate occasions to perform either eccentric or concentric arm cycling trials that were assigned in a random fashion. On each day, participants performed a concentric arm cycling warm-up for 5 min at 60 W. Subsequently, participants performed either eccentric or concentric arm cycling trials with 4-min efforts at 40, 60, and 80% of their individual W_{PEAK}. Physiological responses were constantly measured as described below. A recovery period of 3.5 min was provided between each 4 min effort. All experimental visits were separated by at least 48 h and completed at the same time of day.

The eccentric and concentric arm cycle ergometers used in this investigation have been described in detail in a recent paper from our Swedish laboratory [19]. Briefly, an isokinetic eccentric arm cycle ergometer was constructed using a Monark 891E cycle ergometer frame, stand, and flywheel (Monark Exercise AB, Vansbro, Sweden). A 2.2 kW electric motor (BEVI 2SIE1004A, BEVI AB, Blomstermåla, Sweden) was connected to the flywheel via a pulley and a belt. Motor speed and pedaling rate were controlled by a variable frequency drive (Invertek Optidrive-E i55, Invertek Drives Ltd., Welshpool, UK). Cycling power was quantified using a power meter (Schoberer Rad Meßtechnik [SRM], Jülich, Germany), a system that has previously been shown to accurately quantify power output [26].

For the eccentric arm cycling trials, participants were instructed to resist the motor-driven handles of the ergometer at their individually specified target powers (i.e. 40, 60, or 80% of W_{PEAK}). Pedaling rate was set at 60 revolutionsmin^{-1} and the SRM power meter (sampling at 1 Hz) displayed the power that the participant was absorbing. An illustration of the eccentric arm ergometer can be seen in Figure 1 of our previous article [19]. During each trial, participants were given at least 10 s to stabilize at this target power, which was then maintained for 4 min during which physiological responses were monitored and recorded.

The concentric arm cycling ergometer was fabricated by adapting a mechanically braked Monark 839E cycle ergometer.

Table 1. Participant characteristics.

Variable	Group (n = 14)	Men (n = 7)	Women (n = 7)
Age (yr)	25.3±5.4	26.6±6.8	24.0±3.7
Height (cm)	174±9	179±9	169±6*
Body Mass (kg)#	74.2±9.6	82.0±7.5	67.5±5.0**
Lean Body Mass (kg)#	54.6±11.6	65.4±6.6	45.4±4.0**
Body Fat Mass (kg)#	16.3±4.3	12.9±2.3	19.2±3.4**
Body Fat Mass (%)#	23.5±7.6	16.5±2.9	29.5±4.0**
Arm Lean Mass (kg)#	6.8±2.2	8.9±0.9	5.0±0.7**
Arm Fat Mass (kg)#	1.9±0.5	1.5±0.2	2.2±0.3**
Arm Fat Mass (%)#	22.8±9.0	14.2±2.1	30.1±4.5**
VO_{2PEAK} (L·min^{-1})	2.7±0.6	3.0±0.6	2.3±0.4*
VO_{2PEAK} (mL·kg^{-1}·min^{-1})	35.8±5.7	38.0±6.2	34.0±5.0
HR_{PEAK} (beats·min^{-1})	182±9	180±9	185±9
W_{PEAK} (W)	138±29	157±22	119±23**

All values are reported as mean ± standard deviation. VO_{2PEAK} Peak oxygen consumption, HR_{PEAK} Peak heart rate, W_{PEAK} Peak power production. All peak values refer to those obtained in an incremental concentric arm cycling test (60+15 W·60 s). # As assessed by dual-energy X-ray absorptiometry (GE, Lunar iDXA). *$p<0.05$, **$p<0.01$.

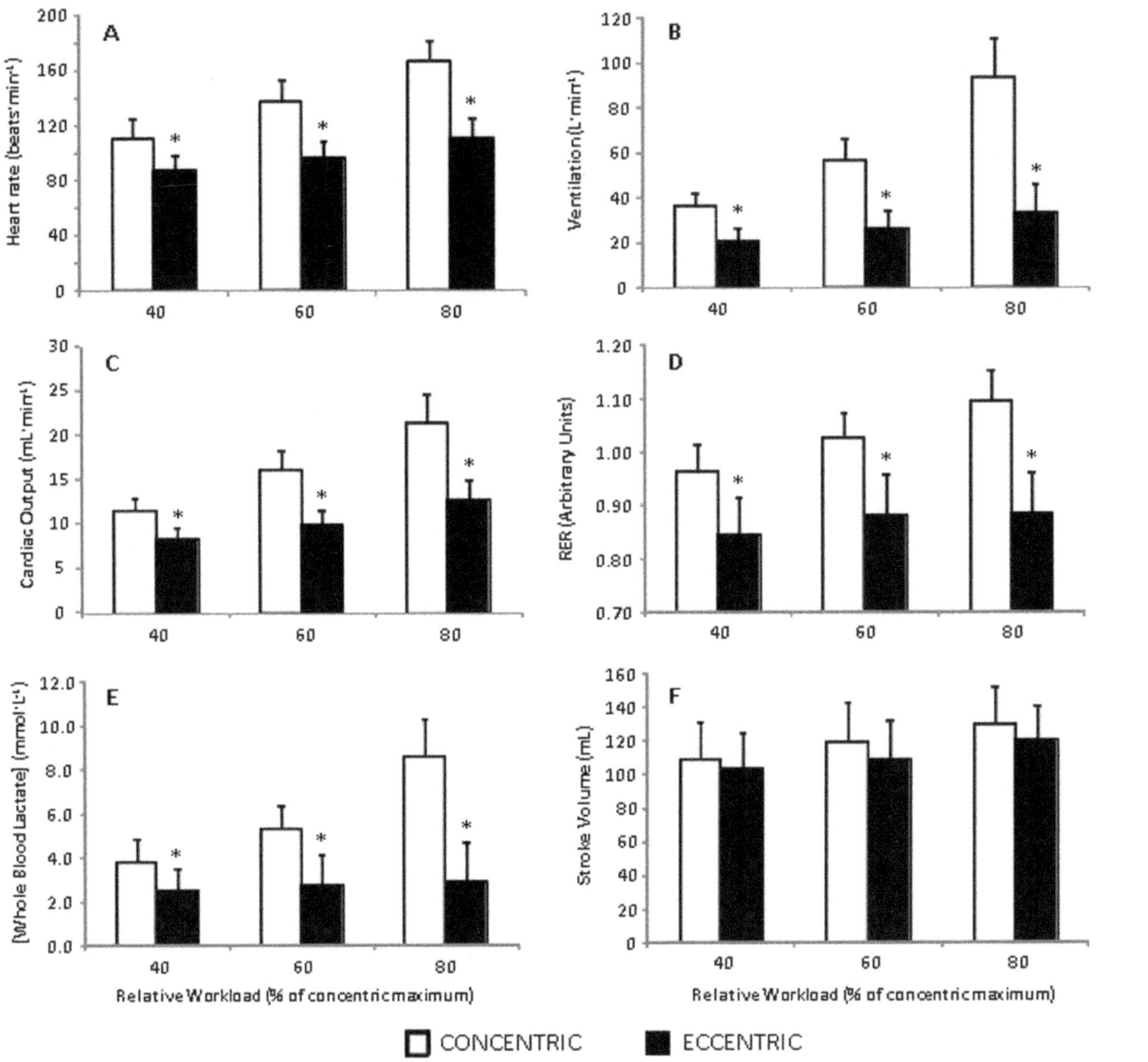

Figure 1. Metabolic and cardiorespiratory responses to eccentric and concentric arm cycling. Values are reported as mean ± standard deviation. *$p<0.05$ vs concentric exercise modality.

For the concentric arm cycling trials, participants were instructed to cycle at 60 revolutionsmin^{-1} whilst the ergometer (in constant power mode) maintained the prescribed power (i.e. 40, 60, or 80% of W_{PEAK}). The SRM power meter (sampling at 1 Hz) displayed pedalling rate and the power produced by the participant.

Although the cycle ergometers differed for the eccentric and concentric arm cycling trials (i.e. constant pedalling rate vs. constant power) SRM crank power was measured at the same location in both cases. Both SRM power meters were calibrated using the same static procedures with the average calibration factor (Hz·N·m^{-1}) entered into the SRM power control unit from four different positions [19,27]. Finally, individual ergometer and seat positions were carefully adjusted and standardized such that the crank axle was located just below the level of the heart and the elbow positioned at a comfortable angle (~20° between the ulnar notch and humoral head when the cranks were horizontal), since posture is known to influence force production capacity [28]. Both arm cycle ergometers were set up in an asynchronous configuration, with the pedal arms of the flywheel oriented at 180° relative to one another.

Physiological Measures

Gas exchange values were measured with a mixed expired procedure using an ergospirometry system (AMIS 2001 model C; Innovision A/S, Odense, Denmark), equipped with an inspiratory flowmeter. The gas analyzers were calibrated with a high-precision mixture of 16.0% O_2 and 4.5% CO_2 (Air Liquide, Kungsängen, Sweden), and calibration of the flowmeter was performed at low, medium, and high flow rates with a 3-L air syringe (Hans Rudolph, Kansas City, MO). Ambient conditions were monitored with an external apparatus (Vaisala PTU 200; Vaisala Oy, Helsinki, Finland). Oxygen consumption (VO_2; Lmin^{-1}), ventilation (V_E; Lmin^{-1}) and the respiratory exchange ratio (RER) were monitored continuously, and values were averaged over the final

30 s of each trial. Heart rate was recorded using a Polar monitor (Polar S610, Polar Electro Oy, Kempele, Finland). Overall rating of perceived exertion (RPE_{BODY}) as well as arm-specific RPE (RPE_{ARMS}) were assessed during the final 30 s of each trial using a Borg 6–20 scale [29]. Whole blood lactate (20 μL, Biosen 5140, EKF-diagnostic GmbH, Magdeburg, Germany) was collected from the fingertip within 1 min after each trial.

Stroke volume (SV; ml), cardiac output (Q_C; $mLmin^{-1}$), arterial pressure (mmHg), and systemic vascular resistance (SVR; $dyn \cdot s \cdot cm^{-5}$) were determined employing thoracic electrical bioimpedance utilizing Signal-Morphology Impedance Cardiology (SM-ICG) and High Definition Impedance (HD-Z) technologies (Physio Flow, Manatec type PF05L1, Paris, France) during the final 30 s of each trial. The PhysioFlow device emits high-frequency (75 kHz) and low-amperage (3.8 mA peak-to-peak) alternating electrical current via skin electrodes and calculates SV independently of baseline impedance signal (Z0) relying on changes in the impedance signal (ΔZ) that is independent of hydration status, the inter-electrode distance, and the resistivity of the blood [30]. A cardiac index ($Lmin^{-1}m^{-2}$) was calculated from the Q_C/BSA, where BSA is the body surface area (m^{-2}) calculated using the Haycock method: $BSA = 0.024265 \times Height^{0.3964} \times Weight^{0.5378}$.

Before each test, the bioimpedance device was calibrated according to the manufacturer's instructions. The participant's skin was shaved and then abraded with a specialized skin preparation gel (Nuprep, Weaver and Co., Aurora, CO, USA), and cleaned with a 70% ethanol solution prior to the application of 6 self-adhesive AgCl electrodes (PhysioFlow, PF-50, Leonhard Lang GmbH, Innsbruck, Austria). The clinical acceptability of this bioimpedance device has previously been established against the direct Fick method over a wide range of Q_C values (3.55 to 26.75 $Lmin^{-1}$) during repeated incremental exercise separated by three days in healthy subjects [31,32]. Bioimpedance cardiography has also been demonstrated to exhibit superior reproducibility (as estimated from the variability between repeated measures) compared to other non-invasive methods of cardiac output estimation [33]. Mean arterial pressure was calculated as [(2 × diastolic arterial pressure)+systolic arterial pressure]/3 [9]. The arteriovenous oxygen difference $[(A\text{-}V)O_2]$ was was assessed indirectly via the Fick Principle: $VO_2 = Q_C \times (C_aO_2 - C_vO_2)$, where C_aO_2 is the arterial oxygen content and C_vO_2 is the venous oxygen content.

Work economy ($WL^{-1}min^{-1}$) as well as both gross mechanical efficiency (η_{MECH}) and delta efficiency (η_Δ) were calculated. η_Δ was assessed as it eliminates the influence of metabolic processes that do not contribute to the work performed and thus has been suggested as a more valid indicator of muscular efficiency [34,35]. Specifically, work economy was calculated as the mechanical work performed per litre of oxygen consumed in one minute. η_{MECH} (%) during sub-maximal steady-state was calculated by dividing the internally liberated metabolic power by the external power output as described by Hopman and colleagues [36]: $\eta_{MECH} = W/(VO_2 \times 340)$, where W represents the internally liberated mechanical power and 340 represents the power equivalent of 1 L of O_2min^{-1}. Finally, the η_Δ (%) was calculated from the reciprocal of the slope of the linear regression line that described the relationship between energy expenditure and work rate [34].

Data Analysis

Requisite transformations of the efficiency (arcsineroot transformation) and physiological (log transformation) data was performed prior to statistical analysis to reduce bias arising from non-uniformity of error (Hopkins et al. 2009). Separate analyses of variance procedures were performed to assess differences in physiological responses between the CON and ECC conditions. Subsequent paired student's t-tests were performed on relevant comparisons. The magnitude of between-condition differences in the means were expressed as an effect size (ES), which were calculated using the pooled standard deviations [37]. Threshold values for ES statistics were >0.2 (small), >0.6 (moderate), >1.2 (large), >2.0 (very large) and >4.0 (extremely large). Confidence intervals (90%) for the (true) mean changes or between-group differences were estimated (Hopkins et al. 2009). Quantitative chances of the likelihood of between condition differences were assessed qualitatively as follows: ≤1% almost certainly not, >1–5% very unlikely, >5–25% unlikely, >25–75% possible, >75–95% likely, >95–99 very likely, >99% almost certain. The effect was deemed 'clear' if its confidence interval did not overlap the thresholds for small positive and negative effects [38]. Bi-variate relationships between variables of interest were examined via multiple regression to control for between subject variation (r). Magnitudes of correlations were interpreted using thresholds of 0.1, 0.3, 0.5, 0.7 and 0.9 for small-, moderate-, large-, very large- and nearly perfect correlations respectively. Significance was set at an alpha level of $p \leq 0.05$.

Results

The incremental concentric arm cycling test established work loads of 55±11, 84±18 and 111±23 W corresponding to 40, 60 and 80% of W_{PEAK}. The actual work performed in the three CON and ECC trials was 40.5±1.5, 60.6±1.0, and 80.2±1.0 and 40.6±1.2, 60.3±1.4, and 78.8±1.3% of W_{MAX}, respectively, demonstrating excellent agreement with the prescribed workloads. Notably, the 120-W absolute workload imposed in our prior work corresponded to a relative workload that ranged from 65 to 99% of W_{PEAK} in the current male cohort; thus reinforcing the importance of prescribing relative work when assessing physiological load in this type of experiment. Also note that for clarity and ease of comparison, all power values measured during eccentric cycling are expressed as absolute values herein. The average pre-trial rating on the perceived recovery status scale was 7.9±1.6 corresponding to nominal values associated with an expectation of similar performance [25].

When compared with the ECC condition, the HR responses (all $p<0.0001$), V_E (all $p<0.0001$), Q_C (all $p<0.0001$), RER (all $p<0.0001$) and blood lactate concentration (all $p<0.003$) were all almost certainly higher in the CON condition at all three workloads (Figure 1A to 1E). RPE_{BODY} (all $p<0.016$) and RPE_{ARMS} (all $p<0.002$) were also clearly elevated in the CON compared to the ECC condition. There was no clear difference in SV between the conditions (Figure 1F). We also noted a near perfect correlation between the HR obtained from the PhysioFlow and Polar monitors (r = 0.99).

Extremely large or very large differences in VO_2 were observed between the CON and ECC conditions at 40 (ES: 3.62±0.63; $p<0.0001$), 60 (ES: 4.16±0.63; $p<0.0001$), and 80% of W_{PEAK} (ES: 4.08±0.63; $p<0.0001$; Figure 2A). VO_2 consistently increased as workload increased in both conditions (all $p<0.004$). The qualitative magnitudes of the differences in economy (all ES > 3.83), and η_{MECH} (all ES >3.83) between the CON and ECC conditions were either very large or extremely large (Figure 2B & 2C). In no case did η_{MECH} differ at the different workloads (all $p>0.05$; Figure 2C). It was noteworthy that a clear sex difference of 1.7±1.7% (ES: 0.95) in concentric η_Δ was observed (men> women), that was not apparent in the η_{MECH} metrics (Figure 3).

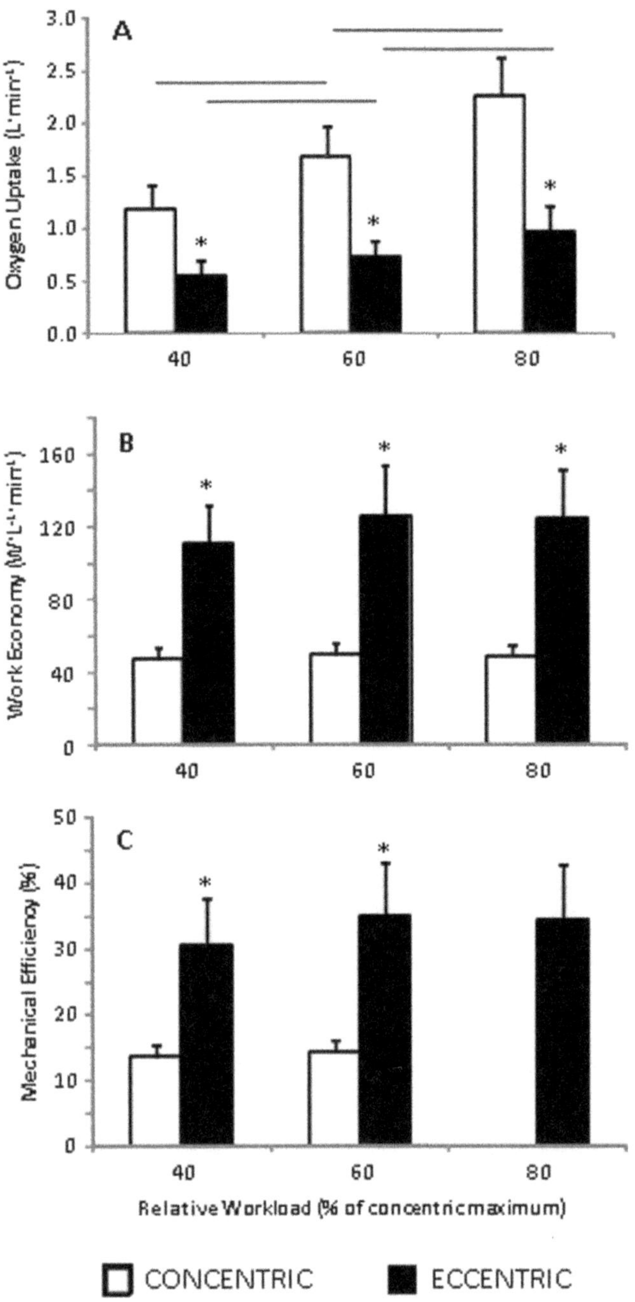

Figure 2. Energy cost of eccentric and concentric arm cycling. Values are reported as mean ± standard deviation. *$p<0.05$ vs concentric exercise modality. Horizontal bars represent significant differences between the indicated workloads $p<0.05$.

While no sex differences were apparent in Q_C (all p>0.5), the HR was consistently and substantially higher in females by 10 to 16 bpm during concentric exercise (ES 0.71 to 1.23) which corresponded to a 4.2 to 6.4% higher percentage of the maximum heart rate observed in the incremental concentric arm cycling test (Figure 4A). The cardiac index was also higher in women at all concentric workloads by 0.85 to 1.62 $Lmin^{-1}m^{-2}$ (ES 0.84 to 1.12; Figure 4B). Interestingly, despite the relative loads prescribed, VO_2 during concentric exercise was lower in women at all workloads by 0.30 to 0.43 $Lmin^{-1}$ ($p \leq 0.0172$; ES: 1.40 to 1.83; Figure 4C) and thus the internally liberated metabolic power of concentric arm cycling was also lower in women (all $p \leq 0.0182$; ES: 1.49 to 1.95). A corollary of the fact that VO_2 was lower in women, despite no difference between the sexes for Q_C, was that the (A-V)O_2 was of lesser magnitude in women (all $p \leq 0.0340$; Figure 4D). Overall, the (A-V)O_2 was greater during concentric than eccentric exercise at 40% (ES: 1.98±0.65), 60% (ES: 1.62±0.65), and 80% (ES: 1.45±0.65) of W_{PEAK} (all $p \leq 0.001$). In both exercise conditions, the (A-V)O_2 tended to increase with workload (CON: 102 to 106 ml $O_2 \cdot L^{-1}$, 4.2±4.1%, p = 0.0831; ECC: 66 to 78 ml $O_2 \cdot L^{-1}$, 15.4±8.3%, p = 0.0028).

Using multiple regression to control for between subject variation, VO_2 was significantly related to Q_C ($R^2 = 0.84$; $p<0.0001$) and HR ($R^2 = 0.87$; $p<0.0001$), but not SV ($R^2 = 0.31$; $p = 0.24$). Plotting VO_2 against absolute work output resulted in distinct slopes for the CON (0.0173) and ECC (0.007) conditions (Figure 5). These linear relationships revealed that the oxygen requirement was 206% greater in the CON compared to ECC condition at the wattage corresponding to the lowest VO_2 observed (26.8 W; 0.36 $Lmin^{-1}$), a value that increased to 235% at the highest VO_2 observed (152.2 W; 2.91 $Lmin^{-1}$). When individual plots of VO_2 against absolute work output were plotted the slopes for the CON (0.0198; range: 0.0158 to 0.0245) and ECC conditions (0.008; range 0.004 to 0.0160) were similar to the grouped data (Figure 5). Finally, it was apparent that, despite higher systolic arterial pressure in the CON trials (all $p<0.0015$; Figure 6A), the mean arterial pressure was not different between the conditions (all $p>0.4$; Figure 6B). This observation was explained by greater systemic vascular resistance in the ECC condition compared to the CON condition at all workloads (all ES >2.50; all $p<0.0001$; Figure 6C) with a decrease in vascular resistance as workload (VO_2) increased (Figure 6 inset).

Discussion

Our data clearly demonstrate the magnitude of the differences in metabolic and cardiovascular responses, and efficiency between eccentric and concentric arm cycling, extending previous observations in the lower-limbs. Thus, our hypothesis that eccentric arm cycling at the same *relative* workload is substantially less physiologically taxing than concentric arm cycling was confirmed. Further, we demonstrate that delta efficiency was sensitive enough to allow the detection of sex differences and thus suggest a greater relevance of delta efficiency, as compared to gross mechanical efficiency, as a measure of muscular efficiency. Together, these results emphasize the high-force, low-cost nature of multi-joint eccentric muscle actions and indicate that eccentric arm cycling may serve as a unique modality for training muscles in the upper body across a range of populations.

Our results document physiological responses to eccentric arm cycling that are in general agreement with those previously reported during eccentric leg cycling, even with considerable differences in muscle mass. Three key similarities can be identified that highlight the consistent nature of submaximal multi-joint eccentric muscle actions. First, VO_2 during eccentric arm cycling was only a fraction of that during concentric arm cycling performed at an equivalent relative workload (Figure 2A) with the eccentric cycling being relatively more metabolically efficient at higher loads as suggested previously [8]. These extremely large differences in VO_2 are consistent with the early work of Abbott and colleagues [39] and others [8–10] who have demonstrated that VO_2 during eccentric leg cycling is ~1/7 to 1/2 of that during concentric leg cycling. The reduced oxygen demand during eccentric exercise has been attributed to lower muscle activation or

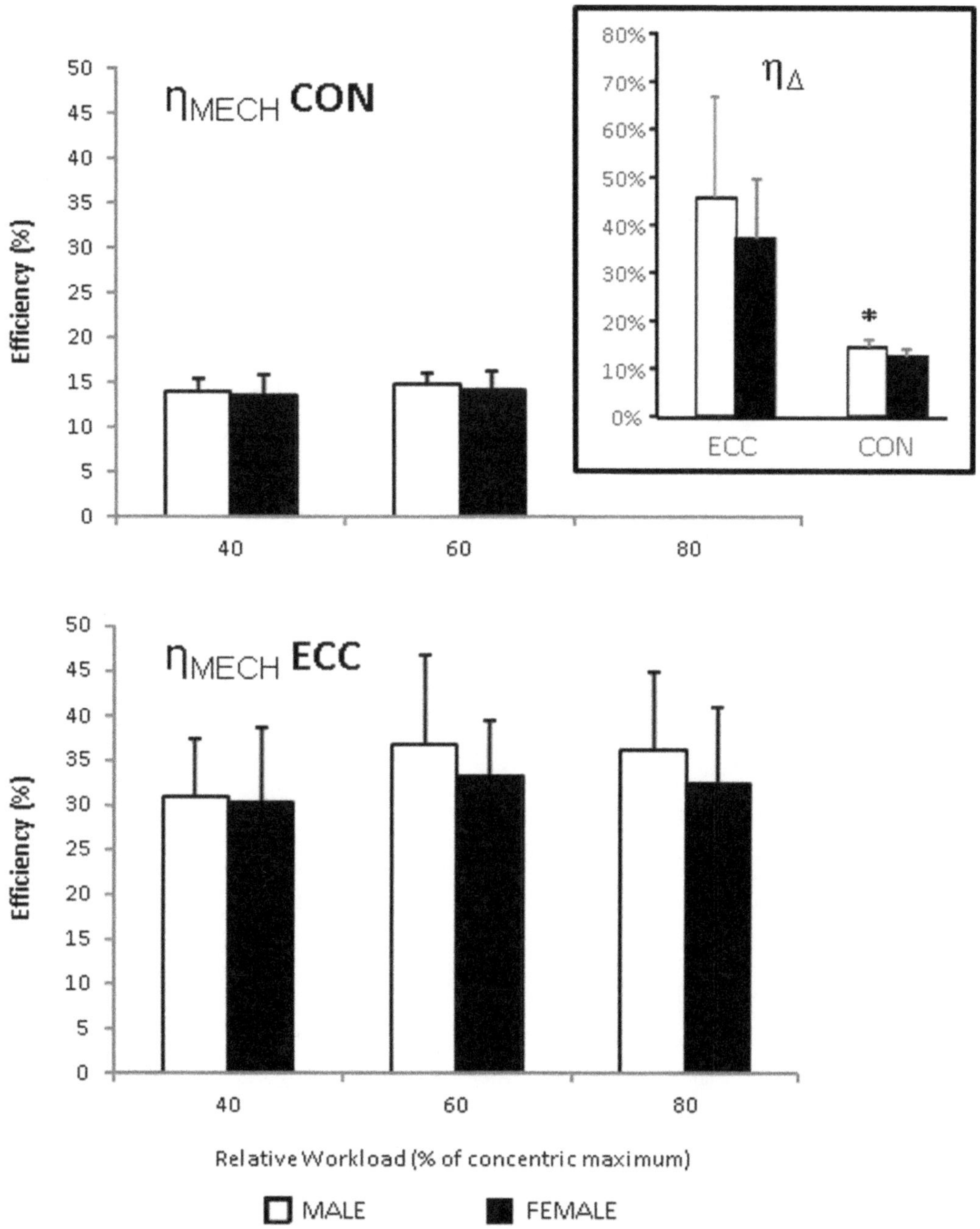

Figure 3. Sex differences in efficiency measures of eccentric and concentric arm cycling. Values are reported as mean ± standard deviation. *clear difference vs male participants.

may result from the active muscle fibers consuming less oxygen [3,9,10].

Secondly, at a similar metabolic demand, the power produced during eccentric arm cycling was 2 to 3 fold greater than during concentric trials (Figure 4). These values are in agreement with previous reports that power absorption during eccentric leg cycling can be as much as five times greater than power production during concentric leg cycling [9,10]. Thus, both lower- and upper-body eccentric cycling can facilitate mechanical overloading of muscle groups to a greater extent than concentric cycling, which has important ramifications for increasing muscle mass and strength [16,40].

Thirdly, the exercise intensity during eccentric arm cycling was well below the blood lactate threshold of 4 $mmol \cdot L^{-1}$ (2.5 to 2.9 $mmol \cdot L^{-1}$) and whole-body and arm-specific perceived exertion ratings was low (6 to 12 on the Borg scale). Consequently, the novel aspect of eccentric arm cycling is that only low to moderate levels of perceived exertion are required to generate relatively high work rates, which lends this exercise modality to use for counteracting sarcopenia and maintaining muscle mass in populations that would otherwise be contraindicated (e.g. the elderly or COPD patients). These features have been well documented in eccentric leg cycling, demonstrating that the distinct physiological responses to submaximal multi-joint eccen-

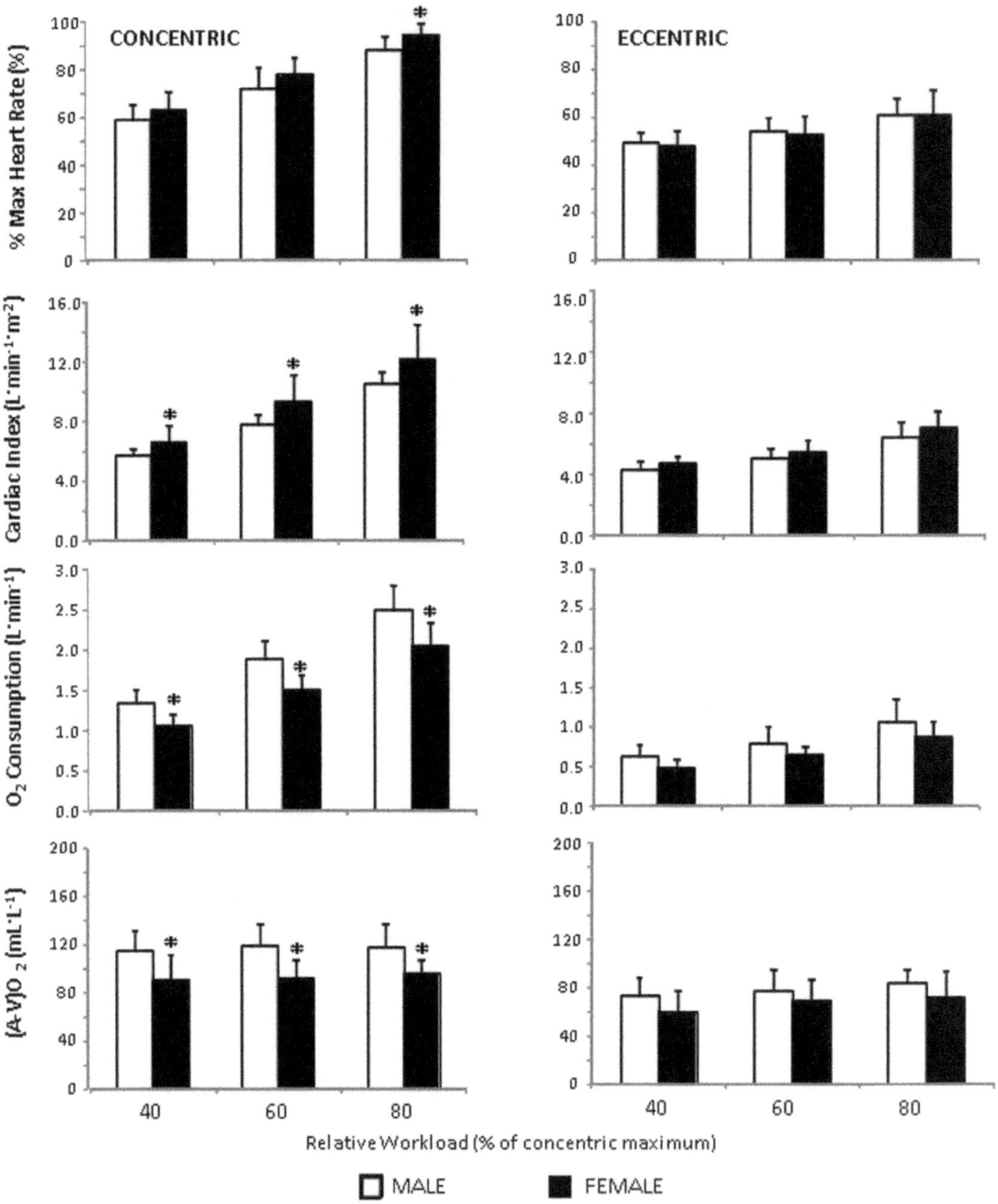

Figure 4. Sex differences in cardiovascular measures of eccentric and concentric cycling. Values are reported as mean ± standard deviation. *clear difference vs male participants. $(A\text{-}V)O_2$, arteriovenous difference.

tric muscle actions are rather consistent for different muscle groups.

The distinct economy, η_{MECH} and η_{Δ} parameters of the eccentric contractions in the current study agree with the body of literature describing the superior efficiency of eccentric versus concentric contractions [6,41–45]. η_{Δ} has been suggested to possess "conceptual advantages" over η_{MECH} in that the former is independent of metabolic processes that do not contribute to the work accomplished and therefore may provide a more valid measure of muscular efficiency [34,35,46]. We report a clear sex difference in η_{Δ} during CON contractions that was not apparent in η_{MECH}. While, greater muscular endurance in the elbow flexors of women has previously been reported, which is suggestive of greater muscular efficiency [20], only one previous study has investigated η_{Δ} in arm cycling efficiency and found no difference between men and women [47]. However, these authors did not use a magnitude-based approach to identify differences and Figure 2b from their 2008 paper is suggestive of a difference in the mean in the order of one standard deviation when assessing work rates between 70 and 85% of individually prescribed ventilatory threshold putatively similar to that observed herein.

Other sex differences of note include the elevated heart rate and decreased $(A\text{-}V)O_2$ apparent in the women during concentric exercise. In a study designed to investigate the difference between

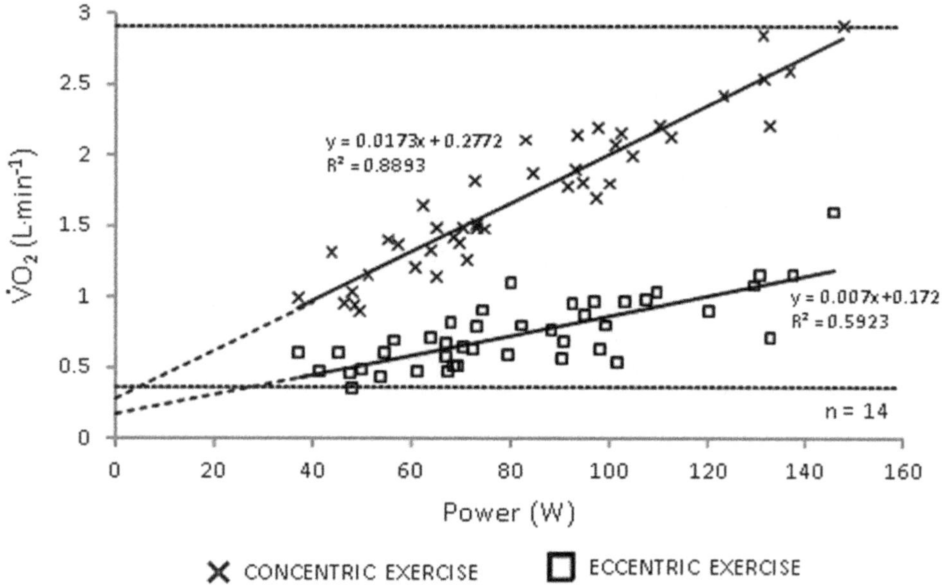

Figure 5. Absolute power output and oxygen consumption for eccentric and concentric arm cycling. Data represents all 14 individuals assessed across three relative workloads.

upper and lower body oxygen extraction, Calbet and colleagues [21] demonstrated that arm oxygen extraction was less efficient than in the muscles of the lower limbs. Similarly, Jensen-Urstad and Ahlborg [22] reported average (A-V)O_2 between leg exercise (170 ml $O_2 \cdot L^{-1}$) and arm exercise (143 ml $O_2 \cdot L^{-1}$) preformed at 80% of VO_{2MAX}, suggestive of the validity of the current measures (range 85 to 138 ml $O_2 \cdot L^{-1}$ at 80% of W_{PEAK}). This prior research posited that lesser arm oxygen extraction capacity could be attributed to: a lower mass-normalized arm capillary muscle oxygen conductance; a lower diffusional area combined with a greater diffusional distance and; an inferior ability to counteract the exercise-induced vasodilatory response. Sex differences in these three physiological aspects could potentially explain the decreased efficiency observed in the current study. The markedly elevated absolute and relative heart rate and lower oxygen extraction during concentric exercise by the women in the current study provide evidence of a greater cardiovascular strain when maintaining a given workload and this was further evidenced by the disparity in cardiac output relative to body surface area (CI).

In an elegant assessment of the metabolic and mechanical factors that contribute to circulatory control, Dufour and colleagues [9] found that Q_C was primarily under metabolic control, demonstrating significant relationships between VO_2 and Q_C ($R^2 = 0.75$), HR ($R^2 = 0.84$) and SV ($R^2 = 0.50$) in the lower body. Here, we report similar relationships in the upper body between VO_2 and Q_C ($R^2 = 0.84$) and HR ($R^2 = 0.87$) but not SV ($R^2 = 0.31$). It is known that vascular reactivity differs between the arms and the legs, with greater changes in blood flow in response to physiological vasodilatory stimuli in the arms [48]. Indeed, the lower capacity of the arms to extract O_2 from the blood implies that a greater cardiovascular effort is required to maintain a given metabolic rate in the upper limbs [21]. The relatively high systemic vascular resistance observed during our ECC condition may reflect an enhanced sympathetic drive, with decoupling of functional sympatholysis from the low metabolic demand [49]. "Differential circulatory adjustments" to muscle contraction type have been suggested to be related to muscle mechanoreceptor activation [50], and/or may simply reflect the lower demand for oxygen. Clinicians should be cognizant of the elevated vascular resistance when applying eccentric workloads in populations where raised arterial pressure would be contraindicated.

While there is little dispute as to the benefit of eccentric loading on muscle hypertrophy and strength measures [18,51,52], it is worth considering the possible implications of upper-body ergometry in athletic populations. Specifically, gains associated with eccentric training are highly specific to the velocity of movement and this may "compromise the transferability of strength gains to more functional movements" [40]. Such an assertion is supported by Cook et al. [18] who demonstrated "relatively negative" running sprint speed adaptations in well trained athletes exposed to an eccentric training program. Indeed, eccentrically biased contractions have been associated with specific adaptations which reflect a more oxidative muscle phenotype [12,53,54]. Interestingly, fast contractions ($180°s^{-1}$) have been shown to activate proteolytic pathways, whereas slow contractions ($30°s^{-1}$) lead to an upregulation of protein synthesis [55]. Indeed, Chapman and colleagues [56] demonstrated that, with equal time-under-tension, fast eccentric contractions ($210°s^{-1}$) elicit more pronounced muscle damage than slow contractions ($30°s^{-1}$). Collectively, these data suggest that the inclusion of high velocity eccentric contractions during training to more closely mimic dynamic actions common in sports should be carefully considered based on the desired outcomes.

In summary, the participants in this investigation performed repetitive multi-joint, eccentric upper-body exercise at substantially lower levels of metabolic, cardiovascular and ventilatory demand and perceived exertion than was associated with traditional concentric arm cycling. These data reinforce the distinct physiological responses to eccentric exercise and extend the application of lower body eccentric cycling to the muscles of the upper body. It is noted that delta efficiency (η_Δ) allowed the identification of sex differences with men demonstrating a greater muscular efficiency. These findings suggest clear applications for upper body eccentric exercise in both debilitative and rehabilitative environments. Upper body eccentric exercise is also likely to form a useful adjunct for athlete training programs although the

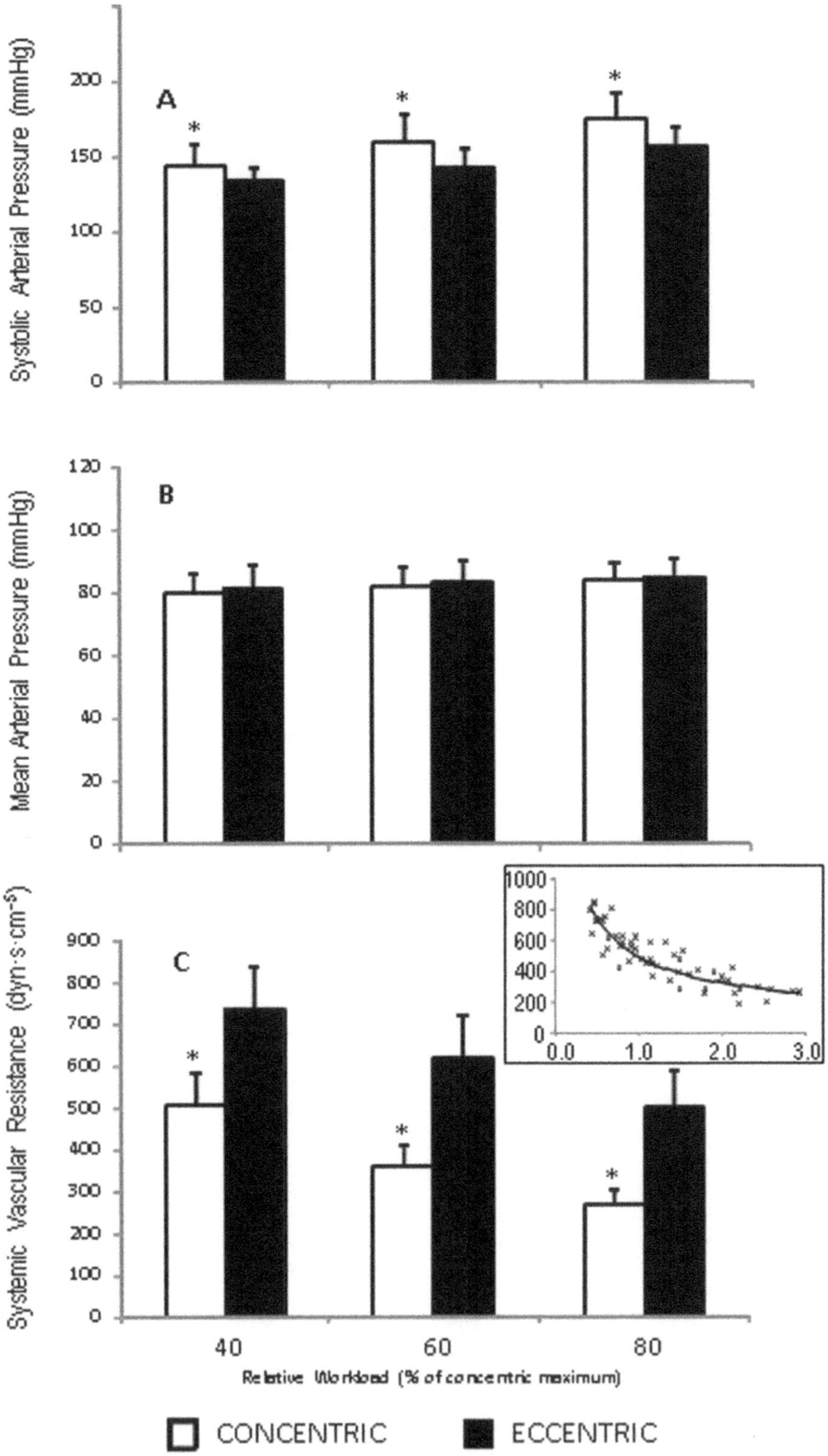

Figure 6. Arterial pressure and systemic vascular resistance plots responses to eccentric and concentric arm cycling. Values are reported as mean ± standard deviation. $*p<0.05$ vs concentric exercise modality. A: Systolic Arterial Pressure; B: Mean Arterial Pressure; C: Systemic Vascular Resistance; Inset: relationship between VO2 (x-axis: $Lmin^{-1}$) and Systemic Vascular Resistance (y-axis: $dyn \cdot s \cdot cm^{-5}$).

possible impact on dynamic actions highlighted by a shift to a more oxidative phenotype should be taken into consideration in the case of power athletes.

Acknowledgments

We sincerely thank Andreas Kårström and Malin Jonsson for their assistance with the data collection. We also extend our appreciation to

Mikael Therell, for his technical assistance with all aspects of the arm ergometer construction and maintenance.

Author Contributions

Conceived and designed the experiments: CMB SW HCH. Performed the experiments: CMB SW. Analyzed the data: CMB SW. Contributed reagents/materials/analysis tools: CMB SW. Wrote the paper: CMB SW CJC HCH.

References

1. Fick A (1892) Neue beiträge zur kenntniss von der wärme-entwicklung im muskel. Pflügers Archiv 51: 541–569.
2. Chauveau MA (1896) La dépense énergétique respectivement engagée dans le travail positif et le travail négatif des muscles, d'après les échanges respiratoires. Applications à la vérification expérimentale de la loi de l'equivalence dans les transformations de la force chez les êires organisés Exposition des principes de la méthode qui a servi à cette vérification. Comptes rendus hebdomadaires des séances de l'Académie des sciences 122: 58–64.
3. Bigland-Ritchie B, Woods JJ (1976) Integrated electromyogram and oxygen uptake during positive and negative work. J Physiol 260: 267–277.
4. Hill AV (1938) The heat of shortening and the dynamic constants of muscle. Proceedings of the Royal Society of London Series B, Biological Sciences 126: 136–195.
5. Henriksson J, Knuttgen HG, Bonde-Petersen F (1972) Perceived exertion during exercise with concentric and eccentric muscle contractions. Ergonomics 15: 537–544.
6. Aura O, Komi PV (1986) The mechanical efficiency of locomotion in men and women with special emphasis on stretch-shortening cycle exercises. European Journal of Applied Physiology and Occupational Physiology 55: 37–43.
7. Asmussen E (1953) Positive and negative muscular work. Acta Physiologica Scandinavica 28: 364–382.
8. Peñailillo L, Blazevich A, Numazawa H, Nosaka K (2013) Metabolic and muscle damage profiles of concentric versus repeated eccentric cycling. Med Sci Sports Exerc.
9. Dufour SP, Doutreleau S, Lonsdorfer-Wolf E, Lampert E, Hirth C, et al. (2007) Deciphering the metabolic and mechanical contributions to the exercise-induced circulatory response: insights from eccentric cycling. American Journal of Physiology - Regulatory, Integrative and Comparative Physiology 292: R1641–R1648.
10. Perrey S, Betik A, Candau R, Rouillon JD, Hughson RL (2001) Comparison of oxygen uptake kinetics during concentric and eccentric cycle exercise. Journal of Applied Physiology 91: 2135–2142.
11. LaStayo PC, Ewy GA, Pierotti DD, Johns RK, Lindstedt S (2003) The positive effects of of negative work: Increased muscle strength and decreased fall risk in a frail elderly population. The Journals of Gerontology Series A, Biological Sciences and Medical Sciences 58: M419–M424.
12. Mueller M, Breil F, Vogt M, Steiner R, Lippuner K, et al. (2009) Different response to eccentric and concentric training in older men and women. Eur J Appl Physiol 107: 145–153.
13. Vallejo AF, Schroeder ET, Zheng L, Jensky NE and Sattler FR (2006) Cardiopulmonary responses to eccentric and concentric resistance exercise in older adults. Age and Ageing 35: 291–297.
14. Rocha Vieira DS, Baril J, Richard R, Perrault H, Bourbeau J, et al. (2011) Eccentric cycle exercise in severe COPD: feasibility of application. COPD 8: 270–274.
15. Lindstedt SL, LaStayo PC, Reich TE (2001) When active muscles lengthen: Properties and consequences of eccentric contractions. News in Physiological Science 16: 256–261.
16. Martineau LC, Gardiner PF (2001) Insight into skeletal muscle mechanotransduction: MAPK activation is quantitatively related to tension Journal of Applied Physiology 91: 693–702.
17. Gross M, Lüthy F, Kroell J, Müller E, Hoppeler H, et al. (2010) Effects of eccentric cycle ergometry in alpine skiers. Int J Sports Med 31: 572–576.
18. Cook CJ, Kilduff LP, Beaven CM (2013) Three weeks of eccentric training combined with over-speed exercises enhances power and running speed performance gains in trained athletes. The Journal of Strength & Conditioning Research 27: 1280–1286.
19. Elmer SJ, Danvind J, Holmberg HC (2013) Development of a novel eccentric arm cycle ergometer for training the upper body. Med Sci Sports Exerc 45: 206–211.
20. Miller AE, MacDougall JD, Tarnopolsky MA, Sale DG (1993) Gender differences in strength and muscle fiber characteristics. European Journal of Applied Physiology and Occupational Physiology 66: 254–262.
21. Calbet JAL, Holmberg HC, Rosdahl H, van Hall G, Jensen-Urstad M, et al. (2005) Why do arms extract less oxygen than legs during exercise? American Journal of Physiology - Regulatory, Integrative and Comparative Physiology 289: R1448–R1458.
22. Jensen-Urstad M, Ahlborg G (1992) Is the high lactate release during arm exercise due to a low training status? Clinical Physiology 12: 487–496.
23. Isner-Horobeti ME, Dufour SP, Vautravers P, Geny B, Coudeyre E, et al. (2013) Eccentric exercise training: modalities, applications and perspectives. Sports Medicine (Auckland, NZ) 43: 483–512.
24. Chen Y, Hubal MJ, Hoffman EP, Thompson PD, Clarkson PM (2003) Molecular responses of human muscle to eccentric exercise. Journal of Applied Physiology 95: 2485–2494.
25. Laurent CM, Green JM, Bishop PA, Sjökvist J, Schumacker RE, et al. (2011) A practical approach to monitoring recovery: development of a perceived recovery status scale. Journal of Strength and Conditioning Research 25: 620–628.
26. Abbiss CR, Quod MJ, Levin G, Martin DT, Laursen PB (2009) Accuracy of the Velotron ergometer and SRM power meter. Int J Sports Med 30: 107–112.
27. Wooles AL, Robinson AJ, Keen PS (2005) A static method for obtaining a calibration factor for SRM bicycle power cranks. Sports Engineering 8: 137–144.
28. Jacquier-Bret J, Faupin A, Rezzoug N, Gorce P (2013) A new postural force production index to assess propulsion effectiveness during handcycling. Journal of Applied Biomechanics [Epub ahead of print].
29. Borg G (1970) Perceived exertion as an indicator of somatic stress. Scand J Rehabil Med 2: 92–98.
30. Billat VL, Petot H, Landrain M, Meilland R, Koralsztein JP, et al. (2012) Cardiac output and performance during a marathon race in middle-aged recreational runners. Scientific World Journal 810859.
31. Richard R, Lonsdorfer-Wolf E, Charloux A, Doutreleau S, Buchheit M, et al. (2001) Non-invasive cardiac output evaluation during a maximal progressive exercise test, using a new impedance cardiograph device. Eur J Appl Physiol 85: 202–207.
32. Richard R, Lonsdorfer-Wolf E, Dufour S, Doutreleau S, Oswald-Mammosser M, et al. (2004) Cardiac output and oxygen release during very high-intensity exercise performed until exhaustion. Eur J Appl Physiol 93: 9–18.
33. Christensen TB, Jensen BV, Hjerpe J, Kanstrup IL (2000) Cardiac output measured by electric bioimpedance compared with the CO_2 rebreathing technique at different exercise levels. Clinical Physiology 20: 101–105.
34. Coyle EF, Sidossis LS, Horowitz JF, Beltz JD (1992) Cycling efficiency is related to the percentage of Type I muscle fibers. Med Sci Sports Exerc 24: 782–788.
35. Coyle EF (2008) Reply to Gore, Ashenden, Sharpe, and Martin. Journal of Applied Physiology 105: 1021.
36. Hopman MTE, Teeffelen WM, Brouwer J, Houtman S, Binkhorst RA (1995) Physiological responses to asynchronous and synchronous arm-cranking exercise. European Journal of Applied Physiology and Occupational Physiology 72: 111–114.
37. Cohen J (1988) Statistical Power Analysis for the Behavioural Sciences. Hillside, NJ.
38. Hopkins WG, Marshall SW, Batterham AM, Hanin J (2009) Progressive statistics for studies in sports medicine and exercise science. Med Sci Sports Exerc 41: 3–12.
39. Abbott BC, Bigland B, Ritchie JM (1952) The physiological cost of negative work. Journal of Physiology 117: 380–390.
40. Roig M, O'Brien K, Kirk G, Murray R, McKinnon P, et al. (2009) The effects of eccentric versus concentric resistance training on muscle strength and mass in healthy adults: a systematic review with meta-analysis. Br J Sports Med 43: 556–568.
41. Aura O, Komi PV (1986) Mechanical efficiency of pure positive and pure negative work with special reference to the work intensity. Int J Sports Med 7: 44–49.
42. Pimental NA, Shapiro Y, Pandolf KB (1982) Comparison of uphill and downhill walking and concentric and eccentric cycling. Ergonomics 25: 373–380.
43. Menard MR, Penn AM, Lee JW, Dusik LA, Hall LD (1991) Relative metabolic efficiency of concentric and eccentric exercise determined by 31P magnetic resonance spectroscopy. Archives of Physical Medicine and Rehabilitation 72: 976–983.
44. Komi PV, Kaneko M, Aura O (1987) EMG activity of the leg extensor muscles with special reference to mechanical efficiency in concentric and eccentric exercise. Int J Sports Med 8 22–29.
45. Ryschon TW, Fowler MD, Wysong RE, Anthony, Balaban RS (1997) Efficiency of human skeletal muscle in vivo: comparison of isometric, concentric, and eccentric muscle action. Journal of Applied Physiology 83: 867–874.
46. Hansen EA, Sjøgaard G (2007) Relationship between efficiency and pedal rate in cycling: significance of internal power and muscle fiber type composition. Scandinavian Journal of Medicine and Science in Sports 17: 408–414.
47. Yasuda N, Gaskill SE, Ruby BC (2008) No gender-specific differences in mechanical efficiency during arm or leg exercise relative to ventilatory threshold. Scandinavian Journal of Medicine & Science in Sports 18: 205–212.
48. Richardson RS, Secher NH, Tschakovsky ME, Proctor DN, Wray DW (2006) Metabolic and vascular limb differences affected by exercise, gender, age, and disease. Med Sci Sports Exerc 38: 1792–1796.
49. Calbet JA, Gonzalez-Alonso J, Helge JW, Sondergaard H, Munch-Andersen T, et al. (2007) Cardiac output and leg and arm blood flow during incremental

exercise to exhaustion on the cycle ergometer. Journal of Applied Physiology 103: 969–978.
50. Dufour SP, Lampert E, Doutreleau S, Lonsdorfer-Wolf E, Billat VL, et al. (2004) Eccentric cycle exercise: training application of specific circulatory adjustments. Med Sci Sports Exerc 36: 1900–1906.
51. LaStayo PC, Pierotti DJ, Pifer J, Hoppeler H, Lindstedt SL (2000) Eccentric ergometry: increases in locomotor muscle size and strength at low training intensities. American Journal of Physiology - Regulatory, Integrative and Comparative Physiology 278: R1282–R1288.
52. Farthing JP, Chillibeck PD (2003) The effects of eccentric and concentric training at different velocities on muscle hypertrophy. Eur J Appl Physiol 89: 578–586.
53. Hody S, Lacrosse Z, Leprince P, Collodoro M, Croisier JL, et al. (2013) Effects of eccentrically and concentrically biased training on mouse muscle phenotype. Med Sci Sports Exerc 45: 1460–1468.
54. Hody S, Leprince P, Sergeant K, Renaut J, Croisier JL, et al. (2011) Human muscle proteome modifications after acute or repeated eccentric exercises. Med Sci Sports Exerc 43: 2281–2296.
55. Ochi E, Hirose T, Hiranuma K, Min SK, Ishii N, et al. (2010) Elevation of myostatin and FOXOs in prolonged muscular impairment induced by eccentric contractions in rat medial gastrocnemius muscle. Journal of Applied Physiology 108: 306–313.
56. Chapman D, Newton M, Sacco P, Nosaka K (2006) Greater muscle damage induced by fast versus slow velocity eccentric exercise. Int J Sports Med 27: 591–598.

Yoga for Multiple Sclerosis: A Systematic Review and Meta-Analysis

Holger Cramer[1]*, Romy Lauche[1], Hoda Azizi[2], Gustav Dobos[1], Jost Langhorst[1]

1 Department of Internal and Integrative Medicine, Kliniken Essen-Mitte, Faculty of Medicine, University of Duisburg-Essen, Essen, Germany, 2 Department of Complementary Medicine, Mashhad University of Medical Sciences, Mashhad, Iran

Abstract

While yoga seems to be effective in a number of neuropsychiatric disorders, the evidence of efficacy in multiple sclerosis remains unclear. The aim of this review was to systematically assess and meta-analyze the available data on efficacy and safety of yoga in patients with multiple sclerosis. Medline/PubMed, Scopus, the Cochrane Central Register of Controlled Trials, PsycINFO, CAM-Quest, CAMbase, and IndMED were searched through March 2014. Randomized controlled trials (RCTs) of yoga for patients with multiple sclerosis were included if they assessed health-related quality of life, fatigue, and/or mobility. Mood, cognitive function, and safety were defined as secondary outcome measures. Risk of bias was assessed using the Cochrane tool. Seven RCTs with a total of 670 patients were included. Evidence for short-term effects of yoga compared to usual care were found for fatigue (standardized mean difference [SMD] = −0.52; 95% confidence intervals (CI) = −1.02 to −0.02; p = 0.04; heterogeneity: $I^2 = 60\%$; $Chi^2 = 7.43$; p = 0.06) and mood (SMD = −0.55; 95%CI = −0.96 to −0.13; p = 0.01; heterogeneity: $I^2 = 0\%$; $Chi^2 = 1.25$; p = 0.53), but not for health-related quality of life, muscle function, or cognitive function. The effects on fatigue and mood were not robust against bias. No short-term or longer term effects of yoga compared to exercise were found. Yoga was not associated with serious adverse events. In conclusion, since no methodological sound evidence was found, no recommendation can be made regarding yoga as a routine intervention for patients with multiple sclerosis. Yoga might be considered a treatment option for patients who are not adherent to recommended exercise regimens.

Editor: Lamberto Manzoli, University of Chieti, Italy

Funding: This review was supported by a grant from the Rut- and Klaus-Bahlsen-Foundation. The funding source had no influence on the design or conduct of the review; the collection, management, analysis, or interpretation of the data; or in the preparation, review, or approval of the manuscript.

Competing Interests: The authors have declared that no competing interests exist.

* Email: h.cramer@kliniken-essen-mitte.de

Introduction

Multiple sclerosis is the most common chronic autoimmune inflammatory disease of the central nervous system and the leading cause of disability in young adults [1,2]. Multiple sclerosis is mainly characterized by impaired health-related quality of life, fatigue, and reduced mobility [1–3]. Other common symptoms include cognitive impairment, depression, and emotional lability [1,2].

Yoga is rooted in Indian philosophy and has been a part of traditional Indian spiritual practice for millennia [4]. Yoga traditionally is a complex intervention that comprises not only physical activity but also advice for ethical lifestyle, spiritual practice, breathing exercises, and meditation. While the ultimate goal of traditional yoga has been described as uniting mind, body, and spirit, yoga has become a popular means to promote physical and mental well-being [4,5]. In North America and Europe, yoga is most often associated with physical postures (asanas), breathing techniques (pranayama), and meditation (dhyana); and different yoga forms have emerged that put varying focus on physical and mental practices [4]. In North America and Europe, yoga is gaining increased popularity as a therapeutic method. About 14 million adult Americans (more than 6% of the population) reported that yoga had been recommended to them by a physician or therapist [6]. Indeed, about half of American yoga practitioners (more than 13 million people) reported that they had started practice explicitly to improve their health [7,8].

While systematic reviews and meta-analyses have evaluated the efficacy and safety of yoga for a number neuropsychiatric disorders [9–11], the evidence of efficacy of yoga in multiple sclerosis has not yet been systematically assessed. Thus, the aim of this review was to systematically evaluate and meta-analyze the available data on efficacy and safety of yoga in improving health-related quality of life, fatigue, mobility, mood, and cognitive function in patients with multiple sclerosis.

Methods

This review was planned and conducted in accordance with the Preferred Reporting Items for Systematic Reviews and Meta-Analyses (PRISMA) guidelines [12] (Checklist S1) and recommendations of the Cochrane Collaboration [13]. The review protocol was developed a priori and not modified during the conduct of the review.

Eligibility criteria

Types of studies. Randomized controlled trials (RCTs), randomized cross-over studies, and cluster-randomized trials were eligible. No language restrictions were applied.

Types of participants. Studies on adult patients (≥18 years) with a diagnosis of multiple sclerosis were eligible.

Types of interventions. *Experimental:* Studies on yoga interventions including at least one of the following: physical activity, breath control, meditation, and/or lifestyle advice (based on yoga theory and/or traditional yoga practices) were eligible. No restrictions were made regarding yoga tradition, length, frequency or duration of the program. Studies on multimodal interventions that include yoga amongst others were excluded. Studies allowing individual co-interventions were eligible.

Control: Studies comparing yoga to usual care, exercise, or other active non-pharmacological control interventions were eligible.

Types of outcome measures. To be eligible for inclusion, studies had to assess at least one primary outcome as recommended by an international, multi-disciplinary consensus meeting [14]:

1. Health-related quality of life, assessed using validated disease-specific instruments such as the Multiple Sclerosis Impact Scale or the Multiple Sclerosis Quality of Life Scale; or generic instruments. Where available, disease-specific instruments were preferred.
2. Fatigue, assessed using validated instruments such as the Fatigue Severity Scale or the Modified Fatigue Impact Scale.
3. Mobility/muscle function, assessed using objective physician-rated tests such as the 6 minute walk test.

Secondary outcomes included:

1. Mood, assessed using validated instruments for depression or anxiety.
2. Cognitive function, assessed using validated neuropsychological tests.
3. Safety of the intervention, assessed as number of patients with adverse events (AEs).

Search methods

The search strategy comprised seven electronic databases from their inception through March 01, 2014: Medline/PubMed, Scopus, the Cochrane Central Register of Controlled Trials, PsycINFO, CAM-Quest, CAMbase, and IndMED. The literature search was constructed around search terms for 1. "yoga" and 2. "multiple sclerosis" and adapted for each database as necessary. The complete search strategy for Medline was as follows: ("Multiple Sclerosis"[Mesh] OR "Multiple Sclerosis"[Title/Abstract] OR "MS"[Title/Abstract] OR "Disseminated Sclerosis" [Title/Abstract]) AND ("Yoga"[Mesh] OR "Yoga"[Title/Abstract] OR "Yogic"[Title/Abstract] OR "Asana"[Title/Abstract] OR "Pranayama"[Title/Abstract] OR "Dhyana"[Title/Abstract]). Additionally, reference lists of identified original articles or reviews; and the tables of contents of the International Journal of Yoga Therapy and the Journal of Yoga & Physical Therapy were searched manually.

Two reviewers independently screening and selected abstracts; potentially eligible articles were read in full by two reviewers. Disagreements were settled through a discussion with a third reviewer until consensus was reached. If necessary, additional information was obtained from the authors of the primary study.

Data extraction and management

Two reviewers independently extracted data on patients (e.g. age, gender, ethnicity), methods (e.g. randomization, allocation concealment), interventions (e.g. yoga type, frequency, and duration), control interventions (e.g. type, frequency, duration), outcomes (e.g. outcome measures, assessment time points), and results using an a priori developed data extraction form. Discrepancies were discussed with a third reviewer until consensus was reached.

Assessment of risk of bias in individual studies

Two reviewers independently assessed risk of bias using the Cochrane risk of bias tool [13]. This tool assesses risk of bias on seven domains: random sequence generation, allocation concealment, blinding of participants and personnel, blinding of outcome assessment, incomplete outcome data, selective reporting, and other sources of bias. For each domain, risk of bias was assessed as low; unclear; or high risk of bias. Discrepancies were discussed with a third reviewer until consensus was achieved.

Data analysis

Assessment of overall effect size. Separate meta-analyses were conducted for comparisons of yoga to different control interventions. Meta-analyses were conducted using Review Manager 5 software (Version 5.1, The Nordic Cochrane Centre, Copenhagen) by random effects models if at least two studies assessing this specific outcome were available. For continuous outcomes, standardized mean differences (SMD) with 95% confidence intervals (CI) were calculated as the difference in means between groups divided by the pooled standard deviation using Hedges's correction for small study samples [13]. Where no standard deviations were available, they were calculated from standard errors, confidence intervals or t-values [13], or attempts were made to obtain the missing data from the trial authors by email.

A positive SMD (i.e. higher values in the yoga group) was defined to indicate beneficial effects of yoga compared to the control intervention for quality of life, mobility, and cognitive function while a negative SMD (i.e. lower values in the yoga group) was defined to indicate beneficial effects for fatigue and mood. If necessary, values were inverted [13].

Cohen's categories were used to evaluate the magnitude of the overall effect size with SMD = 0.2–0.5: small; SMD = 0.5–0.8: medium; and SMD>0.8: large effect sizes [15].

Assessment of heterogeneity

Statistical heterogeneity between studies was analyzed using the I^2 statistics, a measure of how much variance between studies can be attributed to differences between studies rather than chance. The magnitude of heterogeneity was categorized as (1) $I^2 = 0$–24%: low heterogeneity; $I^2 = 25$–49%: moderate; $I^2 = 50$–74%: substantial; and $I^2 = 75$–100%: considerable [13,16]. The Chi^2 test was used to assess whether differences in results are compatible with chance alone. Given the low power of this test when only few studies or studies with low sample size are included in a meta-analysis, a P-value≤0.10 was regarded to indicate significant heterogeneity [13].

Subgroup and sensitivity analyses

Subgroup analyses were planned for the type of yoga intervention (yoga interventions including physical postures vs. yoga interventions without physical postures). As all included

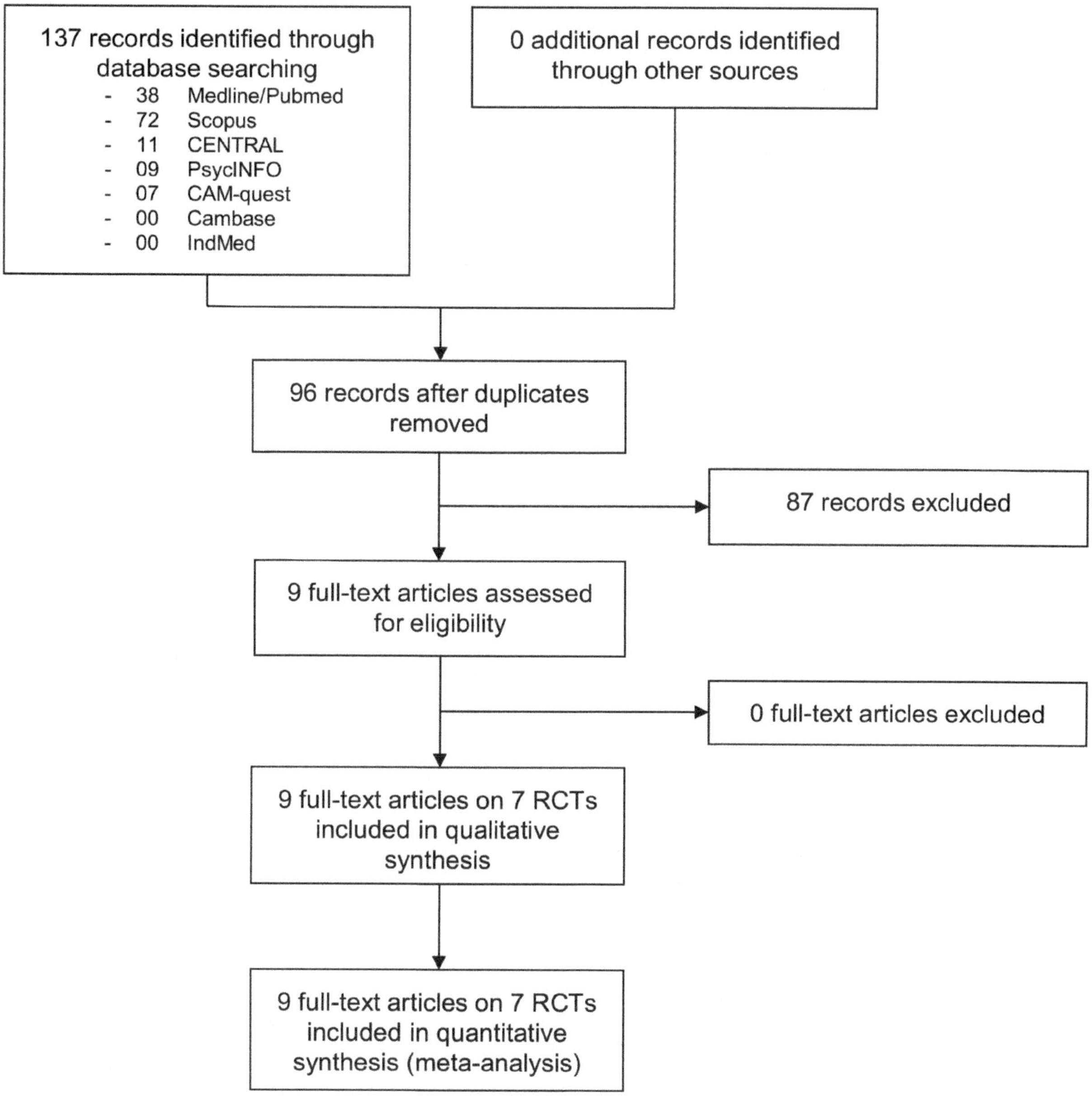

Figure 1. Flowchart of the results of the literature search.

studies comprised yoga postures, subgroup analyses could not be performed.

To test the robustness of significant results, sensitivity analyses were conducted for studies with high versus low risk of bias at the following domains: selection bias (random sequence generation and allocation concealment), detection bias (blinding of outcome assessment), and attrition bias (incomplete outcome data).

If present in the respective meta-analysis, subgroup and sensitivity analyses were also used to explore possible reasons for statistical heterogeneity.

Risk of bias across studies

If at least 10 studies were included in a meta-analysis, assessment of publication bias was originally planned by using funnel plots generated using Review Manager software [13,17]. As less than 10 studies were included in each meta-analysis, funnel plots could not be analyzed.

Results

Literature search

The literature search retrieved 96 non-duplicate records of which 87 were excluded on the basis of title and abstract because they did not meet all pre-defined inclusion criteria (Table S1). Nine full-text articles were assessed for eligibility [18–26]. All nine full-text articles reporting on seven RCTs involving a total of 670 patients met the inclusion criteria and were included in the qualitative analysis and meta-analysis (Figure 1). One full-text article was published in Persian [25], the others in English.

Table 1. Characteristics of the included studies.

Reference	Origin	Sample	Intervention	Control group	Outcome assessment time point	Outcome measures:	Results post-intervention (between group differences, if not otherwise stated)
	Country; Recruited from	Sample size; diagnosis; current treatment; mean age; ethnicity	Intervention; program length; frequency; duration	Intervention; program length; frequency; duration	Post-intervention; longest follow-up	1. Quality of life; 2. Fatigue; 3. Muscle function/mobility (walking distance); 4. Mood; 5. Cognitive function; 6. Safety	1. Quality of life; 2. Fatigue; 3. Muscle function/mobility (walking distance); 4. Mood; 5. Cognitive function; 6. Safety
Ahmadi, 2010, 2013 [18,19]	Iran; physiotherapy clinic	31 women; MS diagnosed by physician; disease modifying drugs were allowed; 35.2±9.0 years; ethnicity NR	Hatha Yoga; 8 weeks; 3x/weeks; 60–70 min each (postures, breathing techniques, meditation)	Control group 1) Exercise (treadmill training) 8 weeks; 3x/weeks; 30 min each; Control group 2) Usual care	8 weeks	1. MSQOL54: physical health composite, mental health composite; 2. FSS; 3. 10-m timed walk test, 2-min walk test; 4. BDI, BAI; 5. NA; 6. Exacerbation	1. Sign. improvements in Yoga, but not in Usual care; 2. Sign. improvements in Yoga and Exercise, but not in Usual care; 3. Sign. improvements in Yoga and Exercise, but not in Usual care; 4. BDI, BAI: sign. Improvements in Yoga and Exercise, but not in Usual care; 5. NA; 6. No exacerbations
Doulatabad 2013 [20]	Iran; university hospital	60 women; MS not in acute phase; current treatment NR; 31.6±8.0 years; ethnicity NR	Hatha Yoga; 12 weeks; 2x/week; 60–90 min. each (postures, breathing techniques, meditation)	Usual care	12 weeks	1. MSQOL54; 2.-6. NA	1. Sign. improvements in Yoga, but not in Usual care; 2.-6. NA
Garret 2013 [21,22]	Ireland; Multiple Sclerosis Society of Ireland	314; MS diagnosed by physician or neurologist; no steroid treatment; 48.8±11.0 years; ethnicity NR	Yoga, not predefined; 10 weeks; 1x/week; 1 hour each (postures, breathing techniques, relaxation)	Control group 1) Physiotherapist led exercise (aerobic, resistance); 10 weeks; 1x/week; 1 hour each; Control group 2) Fitness instructor led exercise (aerobic, resistance); 10 weeks; 1x/week; 1 hour each; Control group 3) Usual care	12 weeks; 24 weeks	1. MSIS-29v2: physical health composite, mental health composite; 2. MFIS; 3. 6-min walk test; 4.-5. NA; 6. Drop outs due to medical reasons	1. Sign. improvements in Yoga and Exercise groups, but not in Usual care; sign. larger improvement in Yoga compared to Usual care for mental health composite only; 2. Sign. improvements in Yoga and Exercise groups, but not in Usual care; sign. larger improvement in Yoga compared to Usual care; 3. NS; 4.-5. NA; 6. N = 3/77 in Yoga, N = 4/80 in Physiotherapist led exercise; N = 5/86 in Fitness instructor led exercise, N = 8/71 in Usual care
Hogan 2014 [23]	Ireland; Multiple Sclerosis Society of Ireland	146; MS diagnosed by physician or neurologist; no steroid treatment; 54.4 years; ethnicity NR	Yoga, not predefined; 10 weeks; 1x/week; 1 hour each (postures, breathing techniques, relaxation)	Control group 1) Individual physiotherapy (aerobic, resistance exercise); 10 weeks; 1x/week; 1 hour each; Control group 2) Group led physiotherapy (aerobic, resistance exercise); 10 weeks; 1x/week; 1 hour each; Control group 3) Usual care	12 weeks	1. MSIS-29v2: physical health composite, mental health composite; 2. MFIS; 3. 6-min walk test; 4.-5. NA; 6. Drop outs due to medical reasons	1. Sign. improvements in Group Physiotherapy, but not Yoga or Usual Care; Sign. improvements in individual physiotherapy for physical health composite only; 2. Sign. improvements in exercise groups, but not Yoga or Usual Care; 3. Sign. improvements in group physiotherapy, but not Yoga or Usual Care; 4.-5. NA; 6. N = 0/16 in Yoga, N = 2/66 in Group Physiotherapy; N = 2/45 in Individual Physiotherapy, N = 1/19 in Usual care

Table 1. Cont.

Reference	Origin	Sample	Intervention	Control group	Outcome assessment time point	Outcome measures:	Results post-intervention (between group differences, if not otherwise stated)
Oken 2004 [24]	North America; adverts and newsletters of MS societies	69 patients with MS; medical records; no change in CNS-active medications; 49.0 years; ethnicity NR	Iyengar yoga; 6 months; 1x/week; 90 min each; daily home practice (postures, breathing techniques, relaxation)	Control group 1) Aerobic exercise; 6 months; 1x/week; 90 min each; daily home practice; Control group 2) Usual care	6 months	1. SF-36: physical health composite, mental health composite; 2. MFI; 3. 25-foot timed walk test; 4. POMS; CES-D; STAI; 5. Attention (Stroop Color and Word Test, modified Useful Field of View task, adapted attentional shift task, PASAT, Wechsler Memory Scales III Logical Memory, Wechsler Adult Intelligence Scale III Similarities); alertness (EEG, SSS); 5. NA; 6. Adverse events	1.-4. NS; 5. NA; 6. 3 surgeries; 1 exacerbation in Yoga and Exercise each
Rahnama 2011 [25]	Iran; Multiple Sclerosis Foundation	30 women with MS; under medication therapy; 33.4 years, ethnicity NR	Yoga; 8 weeks; 2x/week; 60–75 min each; 1x/week home practice (postures, relaxation)	Usual care	8 weeks	1.-3. NA; 4. BDI; 5.-6. NA	1.-3. NA; 4. Sign. improvement in Yoga, but not in Usual care; 5.-6. NA
Velikonja 2010 [26]	Slovenia; recruitment NR	20 patients with MS; primary or secondary progressive MS; current treatment NR; age between 26 and 50 years; ethnicity NR	Hatha Yoga; 10 weeks; 1x/week (postures, breathing techniques)	Exercise (Sports climbing)	10 weeks	1. NA; 2. MFIS; 3. NA; 4. CES-D 5. Executive functions (NAB, TOL), attention (d2CP); 6. NA	1. NA; 2. Sign. improvement in Exercise, but not in Yoga; 3. NA; 4. NS; 5. Sign. improvement in Yoga, but not in Exercise; 6. NA

Abbreviations: BAI – Beck Anxiety Inventory; BDI – Beck Depression Inventory; CES-D - Center for Epidemiological Studies Depression Scale; d2CP – Brickenkamp d2 test concentration performance; FSS – Fatigue Severity Scale; MAS – Modified Ashworth Scale; MFI – Multidimensional Fatigue Inventory; MFIS – Modified Fatigue Impact Scale; MS – multiple sclerosis; MSIS-29v2– Multiple Sclerosis Impact Scale-29, version2; MSQOL54 - Multiple Sclerosis Quality of Life 54; NA – Not assessed; NAB – Neuropsychological Assessment Battery; NR – not reported; NS – not significant; PASAT – Paced Auditory Serial Addition Test; POMS – Profile of Mood States; SF-36 - Short Form-36 Health Survey; SSS – Stanford Sleepiness Scale; STAI – State Trait Anxiety Inventory; TOL – Tower of London Test.

Table 2. Sensitivity analysis: effect sizes when only trials with low risk of detection bias were included.

Comparison/Outcome	No. of studies	No. of patients (yoga)	No. of patients (control)	Standardized mean difference (95% confidence interval)	P (overall effect)	Heterogeneity I^2; Chi^2; P
Yoga versus usual care						
Quality of life	3	98	84	−0.00 (−0.30; 0.29)	0.98	0%; 0.17; 0.92
Fatigue	3	98	84	−0.32 (−0.72; 0.08)	0.12	36%; 3.14; 0.21
Mobility	1	22	20	−0.20 (−0.80; 0.41)	0.52	-
Mood	1	22	20	−0.63 (−1.25; −0.01)	0.05	-
Yoga versus exercise						
Quality of life	3	98	230	0.09 (−0.15; 0.34)	0.46	0%; 0.16; 0.92
Fatigue	3	98	230	0.05(−0.21; 0.31)	0.70	5%; 2.11; 0.35
Mobility	1	22	16	−0.20 (−0.85; 0.44)	0.54	-
Mood	1	22	16	0.31 (−0.34; 0.96)	0.35	-
Cognitive function	1	22	16	0.26 (−0.39; 0.91)	0.43	-

Study characteristics

Characteristics of the sample, interventions, outcome assessment, and results are shown in Table 1.

Study and participant characteristics. Of the seven studies that were included, three originated from Iran [18–20,25]; two from Ireland [21–23]; and one each from the USA [24]; and Slovenia [26]. Patients were recruited from hospitals [18–20], multiple sclerosis societies [21–24] or multiple sclerosis foundations [25]. Only three studies reported on the type of multiple sclerosis, all three studies included patients with all types of multiple sclerosis [21–23,26]. The sample size ranged from 20 to 314 with a median of 60. Participant's mean age ranged from 31.6 to 54.4 years with a median of 42 years. Between 75.2% and 100.0% of participants were female (median 96.5%). Ethnicity was not reported in any study.

Intervention characteristics. Three studies used Hatha Yoga [18–20,26]; one used Iyengar Yoga [24]; two did not predefine the yoga intervention but let the yoga teachers decide on content of the intervention [21–23]; and one did not report the yoga style used [25]. All seven studies used yoga postures and meditation or relaxation; six also used yogic breathing techniques [18–24,26]. The duration of yoga programs ranged from eight weeks to six months with a median of 10 weeks; frequency of yoga interventions ranged from one to three (median: 1) weekly yoga sessions of 60 to 90 (median: 66.25) minutes length. Six studies compared yoga to usual care or no specific treatment [18–25]. Five studies compared yoga to exercise including treadmill training [18,19]; aerobic exercise [24]; mixed aerobic and resistance exercise [21–23]; or sports climbing [26]. Except for one study where the yoga sessions were longer in duration than the exercise session [18,19], the yoga and exercise interventions were exactly matched for program length, and frequency and duration of the sessions.

Outcome measures. All seven studies assessed outcomes immediately after the end of the intervention; one study also assessed longer-term effects 12 weeks after the end of the intervention [21,22]. Health-related quality of life was assessed in five studies using the Multiple Sclerosis Quality of Life 54 [18–20], the Multiple Sclerosis Impact Scale-29 [21–23], or the Short Form-36 Health Survey [24]. Five studies assessed fatigue with the Fatigue Severity Scale [18,19], the Modified Fatigue Impact Scale [21–23,26], or the Multidimensional Fatigue Inventory [24]. Mobility was assessed using the 10-m timed walk test [18,19], the 25-foot timed walk test [24], the 2-minute walk test [18,19], or the 6-minute walk test [21–23]. Mood was assessed in three studies using the Beck Depression Inventory [18,19,25], the Beck Anxiety Inventory [18,19], the Profile of Mood States [24], the Center for Epidemiological Studies Depression Scale [24,26], and/or the State Trait Anxiety Inventory [24]. Two studies assessed cognitive function using standardized neuropsychological test batteries [24,26] (table 2). Four studies reported safety-related data [18,19, 21,22,23,24].

Risk of bias in individual studies

Risk of bias in individual studies is shown in figure 2. One study each had reported adequate random sequence generation [24] or allocation concealment [21,22]; and three studies each reported adequate blinding of outcome assessement [21–24] or were free of suspected selective reported [21,22,26].

Analysis of overall effect

Primary outcomes. Meta-analyses revealed evidence for short-term effects of yoga compared to usual care on fatigue (SMD = −0.52; 95% CI = −1.02 to −0.02; p = 0.04) but not on health-related quality of life (SMD = 0.06; 95% CI = −0.19 to 0.30; p = 0.64) or mobility (SMD = −0.20; 95% CI = −0.69 to 0.30; p = 0.42). No evidence for effects of yoga compared to exercise was found for fatigue (SMD = 0.03; 95% CI = −0.24 to 0.30; p = 0.83), health-related quality of life (SMD = 0.09; 95% CI = −0.15 to 0.34; p = 0.46), or mobility (SMD = −0.11; 95% CI = −0.63 to 0.41; p = 0.68) was found (figure 3). while no meta-analysis was possible, based on single RCTs no evidence for longer-term effects of yoga compared to exercise on health-related quality of life, fatigue, or mobility was found [21,22].

Secondary outcomes. Evidence for short-term effects of yoga compared to usual care was found for mood (SMD = −0.55; 95% CI−0.96, −0.12; p = 0.01) (figure 4). No evidence for short-term effects of yoga compared to exercise on mood (SMD = 0.16; 95% CI−0.40 to 0.72; p = 0.58) or cognitive function (SMD = 0.41; 95% CI−0.11 to 0.94; p = 0.12) was found (figure 4, table 2).

Safety. Four studies reported safety-related data. One of those reported adverse events: one exacerbation in each group occurred, and four further adverse events were reported that were not related to the study interventions [24]. In another study, no

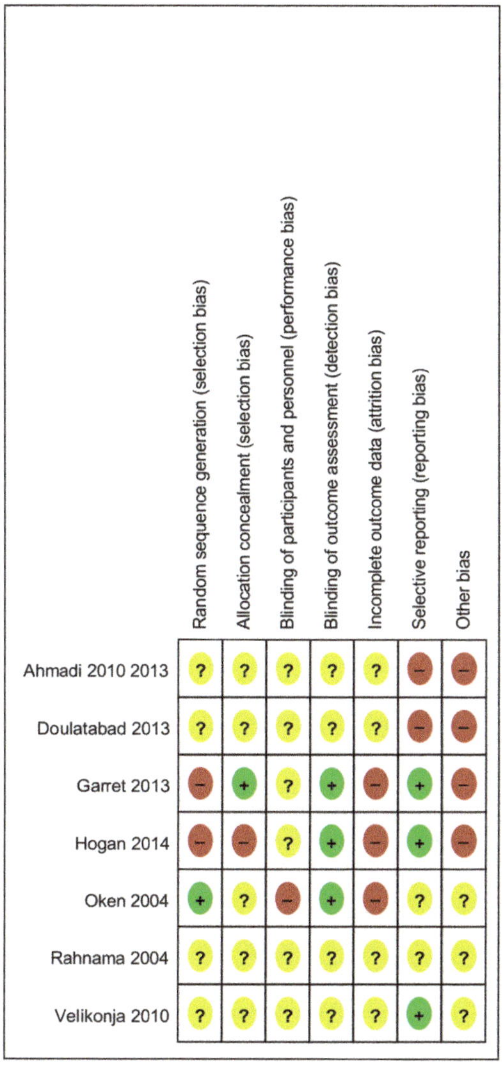

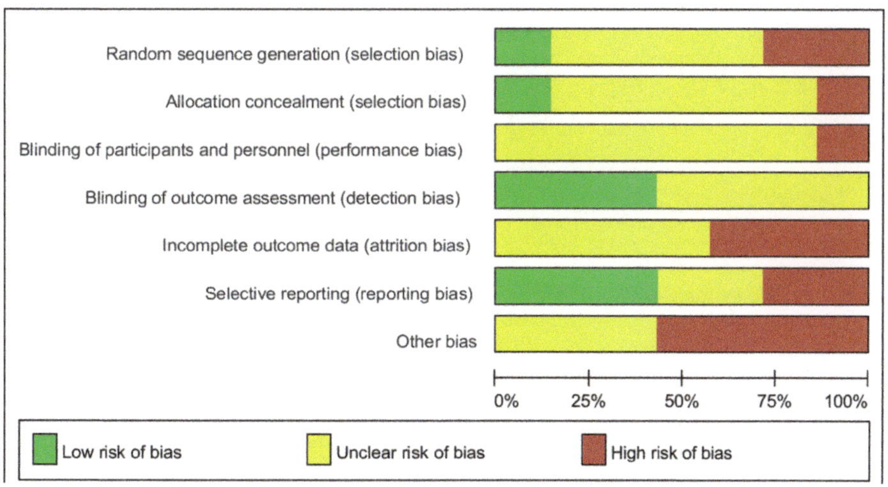

Figure 2. Risk of bias for each criterion for each included study (top) and risk of bias for each criterion presented as percentages across all included studies (bottom).

Health-related Quality of Life

Study or Subgroup	Yoga Mean	Yoga SD	Yoga Total	Control Mean	Control SD	Control Total	Weight	Std. Mean Difference IV, Random, 95% CI
Yoga vs. usual care								
Ahmadi 2010 2013	65.7	11.5	11	66.64	12.3	10	8.0%	-0.08 [-0.93, 0.78]
Doulatabad 2013	7.4	2.16	30	6.8	1.9	30	22.8%	0.29 [-0.22, 0.80]
Garret 2013	29.4	19.4	63	29.9	20.7	49	42.4%	-0.02 [-0.40, 0.35]
Hogan 2014	49.6	11.6	13	50.5	11.3	15	10.7%	-0.08 [-0.82, 0.67]
Oken 2004	61	31.6	22	58.1	23.3	20	16.1%	0.10 [-0.50, 0.71]
Subtotal (95% CI)			**139**			**124**	**100.0%**	**0.06 [-0.19, 0.30]**
Heterogeneity: Chi² = 1.23, df = 4 (P = 0.87); I² = 0%								
Test for overall effect: Z = 0.47 (P = 0.64)								
Yoga vs. exercise								
Garret 2013	29.4	19.4	63	27.9	18.59	130	67.4%	0.08 [-0.22, 0.38]
Hogan 2014	49.6	11.6	13	47.4	11.14	84	17.9%	0.19 [-0.39, 0.78]
Oken 2004	61	31.6	22	60	27.9	16	14.7%	0.03 [-0.61, 0.68]
Subtotal (95% CI)			**98**			**230**	**100.0%**	**0.09 [-0.15, 0.34]**
Heterogeneity: Chi² = 0.16, df = 2 (P = 0.92); I² = 0%								
Test for overall effect: Z = 0.74 (P = 0.46)								

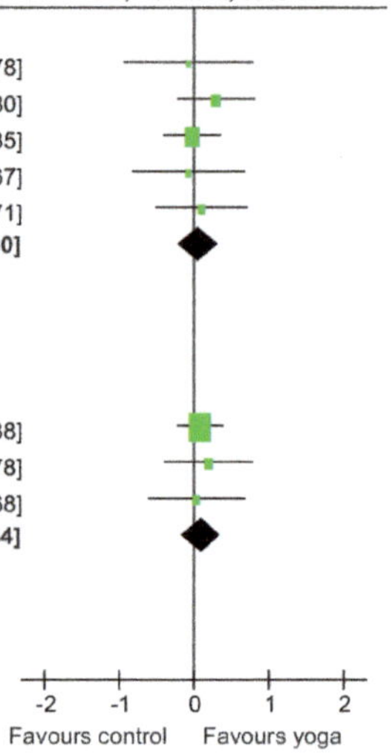

Fatigue

Comparison/Study	Yoga Mean	Yoga SD	Yoga Total	Control Mean	Control SD	Control Total	Weight	Std. Mean Difference IV, Random, 95% CI
Yoga vs. usual care								
Ahmadi 2010 2013	2.44	1.5	11	4.23	1.04	10	16.8%	-1.32 [-2.28, -0.36]
Garret 2013	34.2	17.9	63	35.1	20.1	49	35.1%	-0.05 [-0.42, 0.33]
Hogan 2014	32.5	19.5	13	42.6	17.1	15	21.9%	-0.54 [-1.30, 0.22]
Oken 2004	13	2.9	22	14.9	3	20	26.2%	-0.63 [-1.25, -0.01]
Subtotal (95% CI)			**109**			**94**	**100.0%**	**-0.52 [-1.02, -0.02]**
Heterogeneity: Chi² = 7.43, df = 3 (P = 0.06); I² = 60%								
Test for overall effect: Z = 2.03 (P = 0.04)								
Yoga vs. exercise								
Ahmadi 2010 2013	2.44	1.5	11	1.9	0.73	10	8.8%	0.43 [-0.44, 1.30]
Garret 2013*	34.2	17.9	63	32.57	17.27	130	49.9%	0.09 [-0.21, 0.39]
Hogan 2014*	32.5	19.5	13	37.27	14.79	84	18.0%	-0.31 [-0.89, 0.28]
Oken 2004	13	2.9	22	12.1	2.8	16	15.0%	0.31 [-0.34, 0.96]
Velikonja 2010**	26.6	9.12	10	34	15.59	10	8.3%	-0.55 [-1.45, 0.34]
Subtotal (95% CI)			**119**			**250**	**100.0%**	**0.03 [-0.24, 0.30]**
Heterogeneity: Chi² = 4.59, df = 4 (P = 0.33); I² = 13%								
Test for overall effect: Z = 0.22 (P = 0.83)								

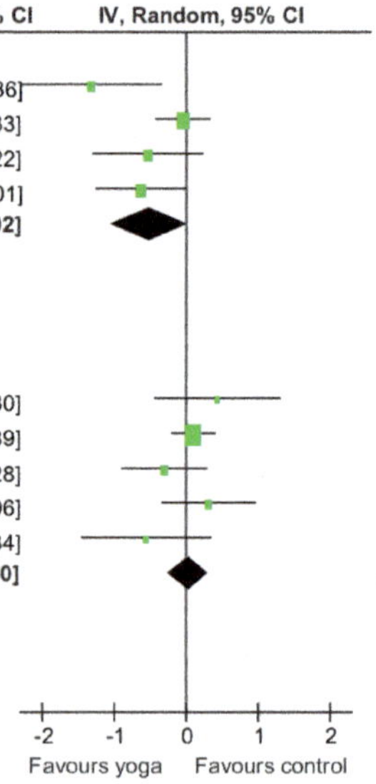

Mobility

Comparison/Study	Favours yoga Mean	Favours yoga SD	Favours yoga Total	Control Mean	Control SD	Control Total	Weight	Std. Mean Difference IV, Random, 95% CI
Yoga vs. usual care								
Ahmadi 2010 2013	8.78	1.79	11	9.16	1.88	10	33.3%	-0.20 [-1.06, 0.66]
Oken 2004	7.2	3.7	22	8.1	5.2	20	66.7%	-0.20 [-0.80, 0.41]
Subtotal (95% CI)			**33**			**30**	**100.0%**	**-0.20 [-0.69, 0.30]**
Heterogeneity: Chi² = 0.00, df = 1 (P = 1.00); I² = 0%								
Test for overall effect: Z = 0.78 (P = 0.43)								
Yoga vs. exercise								
Ahmadi 2010 2013	8.78	1.79	11	8.68	1.93	10	36.2%	0.05 [-0.80, 0.91]
Oken 2004	7.2	3.7	22	8.3	7	16	63.8%	-0.20 [-0.85, 0.44]
Subtotal (95% CI)			**33**			**26**	**100.0%**	**-0.11 [-0.63, 0.41]**
Heterogeneity: Chi² = 0.21, df = 1 (P = 0.64); I² = 0%								
Test for overall effect: Z = 0.42 (P = 0.68)								

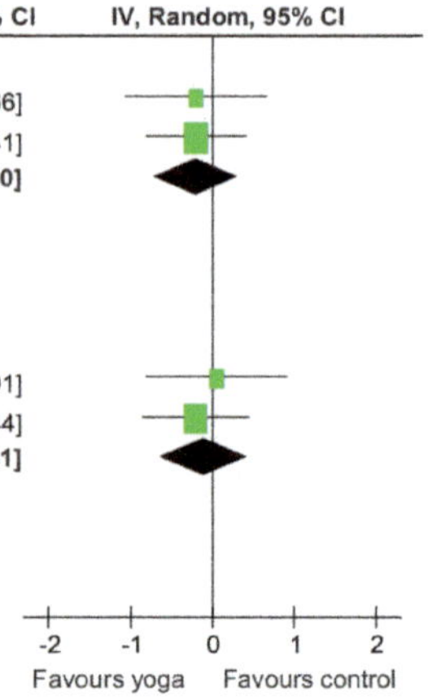

Figure 3. Effect sizes for the primary outcomes quality of life, fatigue, and mobility. *both exercise groups combined; **means and standard deviations provided upon request.

exacerbation occurred in any of the three groups [18,19]. In another study, three patients in the yoga group were lost to follow-up after the intervention due to medical reasons (including exacerbations) compared to four, five, and eight patients in the physiotherapist-led exercise, fitness instructor-led exercise, and usual care group, respectively [21,22]. In the fourth study, zero, two, three, and one patients were lost to follow-up after the intervention due to medical reasons in the yoga, group physiotherapy, individual physiotherapy, and control group, respectively [23].

Sensitivity analyses

Since no study had low risk of selection or attrition bias, no effect remained significant in sensitivity analyses for low risk of selection or attrition bias. In studies with low risk of detection bias, the effect of yoga compared to usual care on mood did not change substantially (SMD = −0.63; 95% CI−1.25, −0.01; p = 0.05). No other effects remained significant (table 2).

Discussion

Summary of evidence

In this systematic review of seven randomized trials on yoga for multiple sclerosis, evidence for positive short-term effects of yoga on fatigue and mood, but not on more objective physician-rated outcomes such as mobility or cognitive function were found. No effect was robust against potential methodological bias. Although the overall high risk of bias hinders definite conclusions, yoga seems to be equally effective as exercise interventions in improving both patient-reported and physician-rated outcomes.

Safety of the intervention was insufficiently reported. Specifically, only one study explicitly assessed adverse events. However, exacerbations of multiple sclerosis were fewer or equal in number in the groups compared to the usual care or exercise groups. This is in line with previous cross-sectional studies [27,28] and systematic reviews of yoga interventions in other patient populations that found no evidence for serious yoga-associated adverse events [29–33]. It should however be considered that yoga has occasionally been associated with serious adverse events in case studies [34].

Agreements with prior systematic reviews

No systematic review specifically on yoga for multiple sclerosis was available. However, a recent review on studies on mind-body medicine for multiple sclerosis published until March 2012 [35] included one RCT on yoga [24]. This review concluded that while yoga improved multiple sclerosis-related fatigue with fewer side

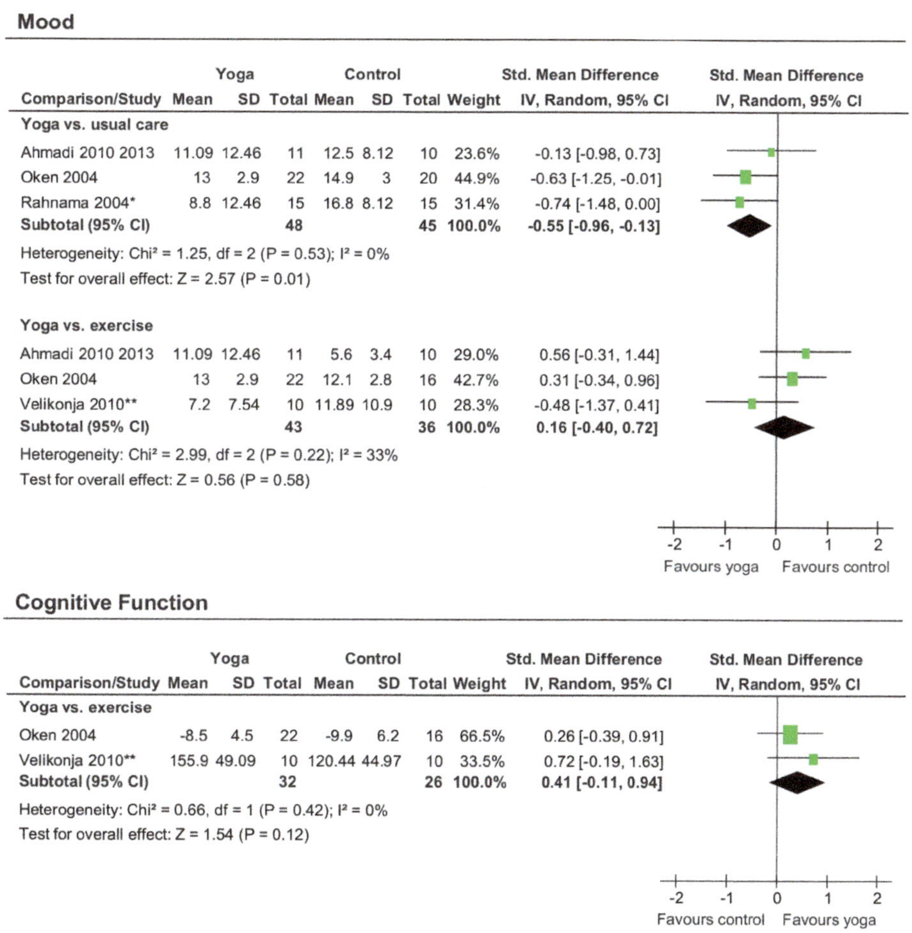

Figure 4. Effect sizes for the secondary outcomes mood and cognitive function. *standard deviation imputed from other studies; **means and standard deviations provided upon request.

effects than conventional treatment, more research was needed to draw definite conclusions. A recent systematic review on exercise for multiple sclerosis concluded that exercise therapy including yoga [24] may have beneficial effects on patients with multiple sclerosis without adverse events and might thus be recommended for the rehabilitation of multiple sclerosis patients [36]. A systematic review on yoga for fatigue that also conducted a meta-analysis included two trials on multiple sclerosis [24,26] amongst trials other conditions. This meta-analysis found moderate evidence for effects of yoga on fatigue with larger effect sizes in non-cancer populations [37]. The recent guideline on complementary and alternative medicine in multiple sclerosis by the American Academy of Neurology included a systematic review on studies of yoga for multiple sclerosis [38,39]. This review included four studies [19,21,24,26] and concluded that, mainly due the low power of the available trials, the data were inadequate to assess the effect of yoga on disability, spasticity, fatigue, cognition, mood, balance, or walking speed in patients with multiple sclerosis [38,39].

External and internal validity

Mainly patients from the Middle East and Europe were included. Given that ethnical and geographical factors influence the incidence and severity of multiple sclerosis [1,2], the applicability of these findings in other geographical regions is limited. Moreover, since mainly female patients were included, the results might not be fully applicable to male patients. Four studies did not report on the eligible types of multiple sclerosis [18–20,24,25]. This further limits the applicability of the results.

Overall, risk of bias of the included studies was unclear or high. Most importantly, only one study each reported adequate random sequence generation [24] or allocation concealment [21,22]. As inadequate allocation concealment has been empirically demonstrated to be the most important source of bias in RCTs [40], this strongly limits the interpretability of results. In sensitivity analyses, no effect was robust against all potential sources of bias. The internal validity of the results is thus limited.

Strengths and weaknesses

To the best of our knowledge, this is the first systematic review and/or meta-analysis available on yoga for patients with multiple sclerosis. Strengths of this review include the comprehensive literature search without language restrictions and the assessment of applicability of the results [41]. The primary limitation of this review is the paucity of eligible studies, rendering subgroup analyses impossible and resulting in a relatively limited overall sample size. Another major limitation is the insufficient reporting and/or low methodological quality of the included studies, limiting the interpretability of the results. Moreover, the reliability of the Cochrane risk of bias tool in systematic reviews on clinical trials of behavioral interventions has been questioned. It has been demonstrated that there is poor inter-rater reliability for several of the domains, specifically for the domain 'blinding of participants and personnel' [42]. Since it is generally regarded impossible to blind patients and therapists in trials of behavioral interventions such as yoga, different research groups tend to rate this domains differently if no information on blinding is provided. Accordingly, this domain was not used in sensitivity analyses. The applicability of the findings was limited. As only one study reported longer-term effects [21,22], the results of this review are only applicable to the short-term. No unpublished studies or studies published in 'grey literature' were included. The usefulness of including unpublished trials is still under debate [13]. Meant to address publication bias, only few unpublished trials can normally be located for systematic reviews and the located studies may be an unrepresentative sample of all unpublished studies [13,43]. Investigators are often unwilling to provide unfavorable results; thus publication bias may still remain an issue [13]. Moreover, unpublished studies tend to be of lower methodological quality than published studies [44] and normally lack peer-review [13].

Implications for further research

Given that the main drawback of this review was the insufficient reporting of trial methodology, authors of prospect research should improve the reporting of yoga trials and follow commonly accepted reporting guidelines (e.g. CONSORT) [45]. Future studies should ensure rigorous methodology, mainly adequate randomization, allocation concealment, intention-to-treat analysis, and blinding of at least outcome assessors [45].

Implications for clinical practice

While this review found evidence for effects of yoga on fatigue and mood in patients with multiple sclerosis, due to the insufficient reporting of the included trials and the limited external validity, this evidence should be applied in clinical practice with care. Thus, no recommendation can be made regarding yoga as a routine intervention for patients with multiple sclerosis at this point. Given that yoga was not associated with severe adverse events, its practice needs not be discouraged in this patient population. Given its evident effectiveness [36], exercise is strongly encouraged by international guideline for the treatment of multiple sclerosis-associated symptoms, especially for improving fatigue [46,47,48]. Since fatigue seems to be equally improved by yoga and exercise, yoga might be considered a treatment option for patients who are not adherent to recommended exercise regimens.

Acknowledgments

The authors would like to express their appreciation to Dr. Ana Ožura, Ljubljana, Slovenia for providing additional data for Ref [26].

Author Contributions

Conceived and designed the experiments: HC RL JL. Performed the experiments: HC RL HA. Analyzed the data: HC. Contributed to the writing of the manuscript: HC RL GD JL.

References

1. Compston A, Coles A (2008) Multiple sclerosis. Lancet 372: 1502–1517.
2. Noseworthy JH, Lucchinetti C, Rodriguez M, Weinshenker BG (2000) Multiple sclerosis. N Engl J Med 343: 938–952.
3. Riazi A, Hobart JC, Lamping DL, Fitzpatrick R, Freeman JA, et al. (2003) Using the SF-36 measure to compare the health impact of multiple sclerosis and Parkinson's disease with normal population health profiles. J Neurol Neurosurg Psychiatry 74: 710–714.
4. Feuerstein G (1998) The yoga tradition. Prescott: Hohm Press.
5. Iyengar BKS (1966) Light on yoga. New York: Schocken Books.

6. Macy D (2008) Yoga journal releases 2008 "Yoga in America" market study. Yoga Journal. Available: http://www.yogajournal.com/advertise/press_releases/10. Accessed 7 March 2014.
7. Barnes PM, Bloom B, Nahin RL (2008) Complementary and alternative medicine use among adults and children: United States, 2007. Natl Health Stat Report (12): 1–23.
8. Barnes PM, Powell-Griner E, McFann K, Nahin RL (2004) Complementary and alternative medicine use among adults: United States, 2002. Advance data (343): 1–19.
9. Vancampfort D, Vansteelandt K, Scheewe T, Probst M, Knapen J, et al. (2012) Yoga in schizophrenia: a systematic review of randomised controlled trials. Acta Psychiatr Scand 126: 12–20.
10. Cramer H, Lauche R, Klose P, Langhorst J, Dobos G (2013) Yoga for schizophrenia: a systematic review and meta-analysis. BMC Psychiatry 13: 32.
11. Cramer H, Lauche R, Langhorst J, Dobos G (2013) Yoga for depression: a systematic review and meta-analysis. Depress Anxiety 20: 1068–83.
12. Moher D, Liberati A, Tetzlaff J, Altman DG (2009) Preferred reporting items for systematic reviews and meta-analyses: the PRISMA statement. BMJ 339: b2535.
13. Higgins JPT, Green S (2008) Cochrane handbook for systematic reviews of interventions. West Sussex: John Wiley & Sons Ltd.
14. Paul L, Crosbie J, Coote S, Dixon D, Hale L, et al. (2013) Outcome measures for studies of exercise in multiple sclerosis: recommendations from an international, multi-disciplinary consensus meeting. 29th Congress on the European Committee for Treatment and Research in Multiple Sclerosis. Available: http://registrationakmch/einsichtphp?XNABSTRACT_ID=179215&XNSPRACHE_ID=2&XNKONGRESS_ID=195&XNMASKEN_ID=900. Accessed 7 March, 2014.
15. Cohen J (1988) Statistical Power Analysis for the Behavioral Sciences. Hillsdale: Lawrence Erlbaum Associates.
16. Higgins JP, Thompson SG, Deeks JJ, Altman DG (2003) Measuring inconsistency in meta-analyses. BMJ 327: 557–560.
17. Egger M, Davey Smith G, Schneider M, Minder C (1997) Bias in meta-analysis detected by a simple, graphical test. BMJ 315: 629–634.
18. Ahmadi A, Arastoo AA, Nikbakht M, Zahednejad S, Rajabpour M (2013) Comparison of the Effect of 8 weeks Aerobic and Yoga Training on Ambulatory Function, Fatigue and Mood Status in MS Patients. Iran Red Crescent Med J 15: 449–454.
19. Ahmadi A, Nikbakh M, Arastoo A, Habibi AH (2010) The Effects of a yoga intervention on balance, speed and endurance of walking, fatigue and quality of life in people with multiple sclerosis. J Hum Kinet 23: 71–78.
20. Doulatabad SN, Nooreyan K, Doulatabad AN, Noubandegani ZM (2012) The effects of pranayama, hatha and raja yoga on physical pain and the quality of life of women with multiple sclerosis. Afr J Tradit Complement Altern Med 10: 49–52.
21. Garrett M, Hogan N, Larkin A, Saunders J, Jakeman P, et al. (2013) Exercise in the community for people with minimal gait impairment due to MS: an assessor-blind randomized controlled trial. Mult Scler 19: 782–789.
22. Garrett M, Hogan N, Larkin A, Saunders J, Jakeman P, et al. (2013) Exercise in the community for people with multiple sclerosis - A follow-up of people with minimal gait impairment. Mult Scler 19: 790–798.
23. Hogan N, Kehoe M, Larkin A, Coote S (2014) The Effect of Community Exercise Interventions for People with MS Who Use Bilateral Support for Gait. Mult Scler Int 2014: 109142.
24. Oken BS, Kishiyama S, Zajdel D, Bourdette D, Carlsen J, et al. (2004) Randomized controlled trial of yoga and exercise in multiple sclerosis. Neurology 62: 2058–2064.
25. Rahnama N, Namazizadeh M, Etemadifar M, Bambaeichi E, Arbabzadeh S, et al. (2011) Effects of yoga on depression in women with multiple sclerosis. Journal of Isfahan Medical School 29: 483–490.
26. Velikonja O, Curic K, Ozura A, Jazbec SS (2010) Influence of sports climbing and yoga on spasticity, cognitive function, mood and fatigue in patients with multiple sclerosis. Clin Neurol Neurosurg 112: 597–601.
27. Cramer H, Lauche R, Langhorst J, Dobos G, Paul A (2013) Quality of life and mental health in patients with chronic diseases who regularly practice yoga and those who do not: a case-control study. Evid Based Complement Alternat Med: 2013: 702914.
28. Cramer H, Lauche R, Langhorst J, Paul A, Michalsen A, et al. (2013) Predictors of yoga use among internal medicine patients BMC Complement Altern Med 13: 172.
29. Cramer H, Lange S, Klose P, Paul A, Dobos G (2012) Yoga for breast cancer patients and survivors: a systematic review and meta-analysis. BMC cancer 12: 412.
30. Cramer H, Lauche R, Haller H, Dobos G (2013) A systematic review and meta-analysis of yoga for low back pain. Clin J Pain 29: 450–460.
31. Cramer H, Lauche R, Haller H, Dobos G, Michalsen A (2014) A systematic review of yoga for heart disease. Eur J Prev Cardiol. doi:10.1177/2047487314523132.
32. Cramer H, Lauche R, Haller H, Steckhan N, Michalsen A, et al. (2014) Effects of yoga on cardiovascular disease risk factors: a systematic review and meta-analysis. Int J Cardiol 173: 170–183.
33. Cramer H, Lauche R, Langhorst J, Dobos G (2012) Effectiveness of yoga for menopausal symptoms: a systematic review and meta-analysis of randomized controlled trials. Evid Based Complement Alternat Med 2012: 863905.
34. Cramer H, Krucoff C, Dobos G (2013) Adverse Events Associated with Yoga: A Systematic Review of Published Case Reports and Case Series. PLoS ONE 8: e75515.
35. Senders A, Wahbeh H, Spain R, Shinto L (2012) Mind-body medicine for multiple sclerosis: a systematic review. Autoimmune Dis 2012: 567324.
36. Sá MJ (2013) Exercise therapy and multiple sclerosis: a systematic review. J Neurol. doi:10.1007/s00415-013-7183-9.
37. Boehm K, Ostermann T, Milazzo S, Bussing A (2012) Effects of yoga interventions on fatigue: a meta-analysis. Evid Based Complement Alternat Med 2012: 124703.
38. Yadav V, Bever C Jr, Bowen J, Bowling A, Weinstock-Guttman B, et al. (2014) Summary of evidence-based guideline: complementary and alternative medicine in multiple sclerosis: report of the guideline development subcommittee of the American Academy of Neurology. Neurology 82: 1083–1092.
39. Yadav V, Bever C Jr, Bowen J, Bowling A, Weinstock-Guttman B, et al. (2014) Summary of evidence-based guideline: complementary and alternative medicine in multiple sclerosis: report of the guideline development subcommittee of the American Academy of Neurology. Available: https://www.aan.com/Guidelines/Home/GetGuidelineContent/643. Accessed 5 June, 2014.
40. Schulz KF, Chalmers I, Hayes RJ, Altman DG (1995) Empirical evidence of bias. Dimensions of methodological quality associated with estimates of treatment effects in controlled trials. JAMA 273: 408–412.
41. Gartlehner G (2008) Assessment of adverse effects and applicability–two areas not (yet) covered adequately in Cochrane reports. Z Evid Fortbild Qual Gesundhwes 102: 497–502.
42. Armijo-Olivo S, Ospina M, da Costa BR, Egger M, Saltaji H, et al. (2014) Poor reliability between Cochrane reviewers and blinded external reviewers when applying the Cochrane risk of bias tool in physical therapy trials. PLOS One 9: e96920.
43. Hetherington J, Dickersin K, Chalmers I, Meinert CL (1989) Retrospective and prospective identification of unpublished controlled trials: lessons from a survey of obstetricians and pediatricians. Pediatrics 84: 374–380.
44. Egger M, Jüni P, Bartlett C, Holenstein F, Sterne J (2003) How important are comprehensive literature searches and the assessment of trial quality in systematic reviews? Empirical study. Health Technology Assessment 7: 1.
45. Schulz KF, Altman DG, Moher D (2010) CONSORT 2010 statement: updated guidelines for reporting parallel group randomized trials. Ann Intern Med 152: 726–732.
46. National Multiple Sclerosis Society (2008) Management of MS-related fatigue. New York: National Multiple Sclerosis Society.
47. Latimer-Cheung AE, Martin Ginis KA, Hicks AL, Motl RW, Pilutti LA, et al. (2013) Development of evidence-informed physical activity guidelines for adults with multiple sclerosis. Arch Phys Med Rehabil: 94: 1829–1836.
48. National Collaborating Centre for Chronic Conditions (2004) Multiple Sclerosis: National clinical guideline for diagnosis and management in primary and secondary care. London: Royal College of Physicians (UK).

18

Influence of Aerobic Training on the Reduced Vasoconstriction to Angiotensin II in Rats Exposed to Intrauterine Growth Restriction: Possible Role of Oxidative Stress and AT_2 Receptor of Angiotensin II

Vanessa Oliveira[1], Eliana Hiromi Akamine[2], Maria Helena C. Carvalho[2], Lisete Compagno Michelini[3], Zuleica Bruno Fortes[2], Tatiana Sousa Cunha[4], Maria do Carmo Franco[1,5]*

1 Nephrology Division, School of Medicine, Federal University of São Paulo, São Paulo, Brazil, **2** Pharmacology Department, University of São Paulo, São Paulo, Brazil, **3** Physiology Department, University of São Paulo, São Paulo, Brazil, **4** Science and Technology Institute, Federal University of São Paulo, São Paulo, Brazil, **5** Physiology Department, School of Medicine, Federal University of São Paulo, São Paulo, Brazil

Abstract

Intrauterine growth restriction (IUGR) is associated with impaired vascular function, which contributes to the increased incidence of chronic disease. The aim of this study was to investigate whether aerobic training improves AngII-induced vasoconstriction in IUGR rats. Moreover, we assess the role of superoxide dismutase (SOD) isoforms and NADPH oxidase-derived superoxide anions in this improvement. Female Wistar rats were randomly divided into two groups on day 1 of pregnancy. A control group was fed standard chow *ad libitum*, and a restricted group was fed 50% of the *ad libitum* intake throughout gestation. At 8 weeks of age, male offspring from both groups were randomly assigned to 4 experimental groups: sedentary control (SC), trained control (TC), sedentary restricted (SRT), and trained restricted (TRT). The training protocol was performed on a treadmill and consisted of a continuous 60-min session 5 days/week for 10 weeks. Following aerobic training, concentration–response curves to AngII were obtained in endothelium-intact aortic rings. Protein expression of SOD isoforms, AngII receptors and the NADPH oxidase component $p47^{phox}$ was assessed by Western blot analysis. The dihydroethidium was used to evaluate the *in situ* superoxide levels under basal conditions or in the presence of apocynin, losartan or PD 123,319. Our results indicate that aerobic training can prevent IUGR-associated increases in AngII-dependent vasoconstriction and can restore basal superoxide levels in the aortic rings of TRT rats. Moreover, we observed that aerobic training normalized the increased $p47^{phox}$ protein expression and increased MnSOD and AT_2 receptor protein expression in thoracic aortas of SRT rats. In summary, aerobic training can result in an upregulation of antioxidant defense by improved of MnSOD expression and attenuation of NADPH oxidase component $p47^{phox}$. These effects are accompanied by increased expression of AT_2 receptor, which provide positive effects against Ang II–induced superoxide generation, resulting in attenuation of AngII-induced vasoconstriction.

Editor: Michael Bader, Max-Delbrück Center for Molecular Medicine (MDC), Germany

Funding: This study was supported by project grants from Fundação de Amparo a Pesquisa do Estado de São Paulo (FAPESP) (2007/58044-2 and 2010/51904-9). The funders had no role in study design, data collection and analysis, decision to publish, or preparation of the manuscript.

Competing Interests: The authors have declared that no competing interests exist.

* Email: maria.franco@unifesp.br

Introduction

Several approaches that reverse endothelial dysfunction have important applications in a variety of cardiovascular diseases (CVDs). Various pharmacological and nonpharmacological interventions can improve endothelial function [1–4]. For example, an epidemiological study suggests that aerobic exercise training is associated with lower morbidity and mortality due to CVDs [5]. Although the mechanisms involved in the reduction of cardiovascular morbidity by aerobic exercise training remain unclear, the reduction of blood pressure levels, modulation of the renin-angiotensin system (RAS), improvement of vascular function, and maintenance of redox balance appear to contribute to decreasing cardiovascular risk [6–10].

In recent decades, some metabolic and cardiovascular comorbidities have been associated with an unfavorable intrauterine environment. Several insults (e.g., diet manipulation, hormonal treatments, or surgical procedures) during fetal life can contribute to the development of CVDs in adulthood [11–15]. The occurrence of these insults during a critical period of development can result in intrauterine growth restriction (IUGR) and lead to fetal programming [11–15]. IUGR significantly correlates with high blood pressure levels, abnormalities in RAS components, and endothelial dysfunction [16–18]. In this regard, these comorbidities perpetuate a vicious positive-feedback cycle that can lead to subsequent CVD development.

There is a growing recognition of the need to reduce the negative effects of IUGR. Although clear beneficial roles exist for aerobic exercise in the development and progression of cardiometabolic disease, this influence has been poorly investigated in an experimental model of IUGR. Exercise training has been previously reported to improve insulin sensitivity and restores deficits in pancreatic β-cell mass associated with IUGR in adult rats [19–20]. However, the mechanisms underlying the beneficial effects of aerobic exercise training on blood pressure and vascular function in IUGR rats remain unclear.

Thus, we evaluated whether aerobic training improves AngII-induced vasoconstriction in IUGR rats. Moreover, we assess the role of superoxide dismutase (SOD) isoforms and NADPH oxidase-derived superoxide anions in this improvement.

Materials and Methods

Animal Care and Protocol

All experimental procedures were approved by the Ethical Committee for Animal Research (Approval Number: 0092/10) at the Federal University of São Paulo and conformed to the guidelines for ethical conduct in the care and use of animals established by the Brazilian Society of Laboratory Animal Science (SBCAL/COBEA). During all of the procedures, the rats were housed in a constant room temperature environment; with a 12:12 h light–dark cycle and free access to standard rat chow and tap water. The female rats were mated overnight with male breeders (age range of 12–14 weeks) that were obtained from colonies maintained at the Institute of Biomedical Sciences of the University of São Paulo, and the day on which spermatozoa were found in the vaginal smear was designated as the day of conception (day 0). Pregnant rats were transferred to individual standard cages and randomly allocated into one of two groups: the control group (C, n = 10) was fed with a standard chow laboratory animal diet (Nuvilab CR1 - based on the recommendation of the National Research Council and National Institutes of Health, USA) *ad libitum*, and the restricted group (RT, n = 16) was fed with 50% of the typical daily food intake determined by the amount of food consumed by the C group through the gestation period. The amount of food provided daily was weighed, and food intake was monitored. At least four females from the RT group were unable to complete the gestation period due to miscarriages during pregnancy and/or occurrence of fetal resorption, and were excluded from the present study. To prevent any variation in neonatal growth due to the availability of milk intake during suckling, the litter size was standardized to eight pups, and the gender ratio was kept as close to 1:1 as possible. The offspring was nursed by their mothers until weaning at day 21, after that was fed with a standard chow laboratory animal diet. Beginning at 8 weeks of age, male offspring from each experimental group (C = 40; RT = 40) were randomly assigned to 4 experimental groups: sedentary control (SC, n = 20 from 10 litters), trained control (TC, n = 20 from 10 litters), sedentary restricted (SRT, n = 20 from 12 litters), and trained restricted (TRT, n = 20 from 12 litters).

Aerobic Training Protocol

Rats were initially adapted to walking/running on a motor treadmill (8 to 10 sessions at 0.4 up to 0.6 km/h; 0% grade; 10 minutes). Subsequently, rats were subjected to a maximal exercise test (graded exercise with increments of 0.3 km/h every 3 minutes, beginning at 0.3 km/h up to the maximal intensity attained for each animal), which was necessary to establish the

Table 1. Birth Weight, Hemodynamic Measurements, and Maximal Response to Angiotensin II in the experimental groups.

	SC (n)	TC (n)	SRT (n)	TRT (n)	*P* (Two-Way ANOVA)		
					IUGR Effect	Trained Effect	Interaction IUGR×Trained
Blood Pressure (mmHg)	111±2 (20)	109±3 (20)	122±3 (20)#	110±2 (20)			0.001
Heart Rate (bpm)	321±4 (20)	299±3 (20)‡	325±8 (20)	300±5 (20)‡‡		<0.001	
R_{Max} Ang II (grams of tension)	0.37±0.66 (7)	0.40±0.03 (7)	0.66±0.03 (7)#	0.38±0.02 (7)	0.002	0.005	0.001

Data are mean ±SEM. (n) number of rats.
#$P<0.05$ *vs.* SC; TC and TRT after a Tukey's *post hoc* test.
‡$P<0.05$ *vs.* SC and ‡‡ *vs.* SRT after a *Tukey post hoc* test.

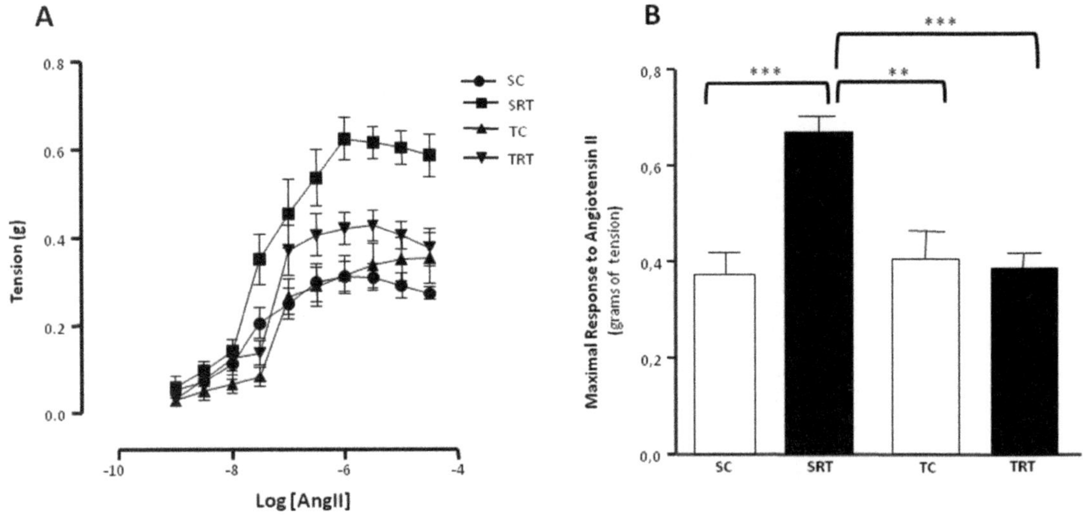

Figure 1. Effect of the IUGR and aerobic training on the vascular reactivity to Angiotensin II. (**A**) Dose-dependent contractions (**B**) Maximal response to angiotensin II in aortic rings isolated from the sedentary control (SC), sedentary restricted (SRT), trained control (TC), and trained restricted (TRT) groups. Values are expressed as the mean ± SEM from seven animals per group. Two-way ANOVA analysis was performed to assess the effects of IUGR, aerobic training and of their interaction (IUGR X Trained) on the aortic contractile responses. ***P = 0.001* and ****P<0.001* in Tukey's post Hoc test.

intensity of the aerobic training. The aerobic training protocol was performed over 10 weeks, 5 day/week, with intensity between 50–60% (low-intensity training) of the maximal capacity test. The duration was progressively increased until 1 hour/day. At 5 weeks, the maximal capacity test was repeated to readjust the running speed. The untrained animals were handled every day and subjected once per week to a period of aerobic exercise (0.4 up to 0.6 km/h; 0% grade; 10 minutes). This approach has been used in order of submitting untrained animals to the same handled stress that the trained rats, however, it is unable to promote the aerobic training adaptations.

Measurement of Blood Pressure (BP) and Heart Rate (HR)

Resting BP and HR were noninvasively determined using a computerized tail-cuff system (PowerLab 4/S ADInstruments Pty Ltd, Castle Hill, Australia) prior to and following the aerobic training protocol. Rats were acclimatized to the apparatus during daily sessions over 5 days, 1 week prior to the commencement of the experimental period.

Vascular Reactivity Study

Forty-eight hours after the last training session, the rats were decapitated and vascular function was evaluated. Segments of the thoracic aorta (4 mm in length), which were free of connective tissue, were mounted in an isolated tissue chamber containing Krebs–Henseleit solution, which consisted of 118 mM NaCl, 4.7 mM KCl, 25 mM $NaHCO_3$, 2.5 mM $CaCl_2{\cdot}2H_2O$, 1.2 mM KH_2PO_4, 1.2 mM $MgSO_4{\cdot}7H_2O$, 11 mM glucose, and 0.01 mM EDTA. The solution was gassed with 95% O_2–5% CO_2 and was maintained at a resting tension of 1.5 g at 37°C and pH 7.4. Isometric tension was recorded using an isometric force transducer (Letica TRI 210, Barcelona, Spain) connected to an acquisition system (PowerLab 8/30, ADInstruments Pty Ltd, Castle Hill, Australia). After 60 min of equilibration, concentration–response curves to angiotensin II (AngII, 10^{-9} to 3×10^{-5} M) were obtained in endothelium-intact aortic rings. Vascular responses to AngII are expressed as grams of tension. At the end of the experiment, the presence of functional endothelium was verified in all aortic rings by observing whether relaxation occurred upon exposure to acetylcholine (ACh, 10^{-5} M). The endothelium was considered intact if the aortic ring relaxed more than 80% upon ACh treatment. The maximal response (R_{max}) and the log agonist concentration resulting in 50% of the R_{max} (log EC_{50}) were calculated for each concentration-response curve using nonlinear regression analysis (GraphPad Prism Software, USA).

Detection of Superoxide Anions in the Aorta

The oxidation-sensitive fluorescent dye dihydroethidium (DHE) was used to evaluate the *in situ* concentration of superoxide, as previously described [21]. Thoracic aortas were carefully dissected and cleaned of connective tissue. Aortas were then divided into cylindrical segments of 4 mm in length and were first immersed in an embedding medium (tissue freezing medium) and then frozen and stored at −80°C until the determination of superoxide anion levels. Transverse aortic sections (7 μm) were obtained in a cryostat from the previously frozen aortas, collected on glass slides, and allowed to reach equilibrium for 30 min at 37°C in phosphate-buffered saline (PBS). Fresh PBS containing DHE (5 μmol L^{-1}) was topically applied to each tissue section and incubated in a light-protected, humidified chamber at 37°C for 30 min. Control sections received an identical volume of PBS. Some assays were performed in the presence of AngII (10^{-4} M), apocynin (an inhibitor of NADPH oxidase, 10^{-4} M), losartan (an AT_1 receptor antagonist, 10^{-4} M), or PD 123,319 (an AT_2 receptor antagonist, 10^{-4} M). Images were obtained using a Nikon E1000 microscope equipped for epifluorescence (excitation at 488 nm; emission at 610 nm). Fluorescence was detected using a 585-nm long-pass filter. The fluorescence intensity was quantified using ImageJ software (Wayne Rasband, National Institutes of Health, USA) and is expressed in arbitrary units. The fluorescence ratio was evaluated in at least three locations in each image.

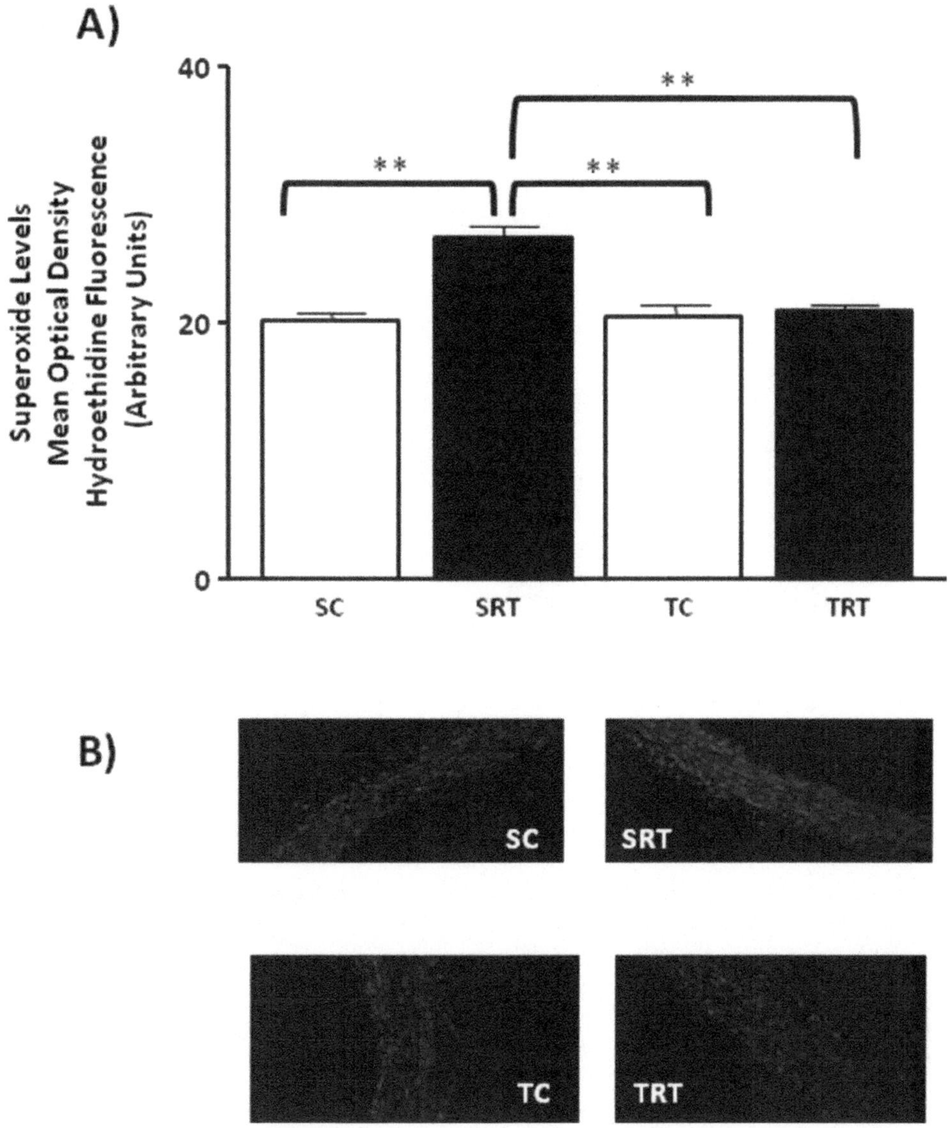

Figure 2. Effect of the IUGR and aerobic training on the vascular superoxide concentration. (**A**) Histogram and (**B**) digital images illustrate the presence of superoxide in dihydroethidium (DHE)-treated sections of aortic rings from SC, SRT, TC, and TRT rats. Values are expressed as the means ± SEM from six animals per group. Two-way ANOVA analysis was performed to assess the effects of IUGR, aerobic training and of their interaction (IUGR X Trained). $^{**}P = 0.001$ in Tukey's post Hoc test.

Tissue Preparation for Western Blot Analysis

Forty-eight hours after the last training session, the rats were decapitated, and the thoracic aorta samples were harvested, weighed, frozen, stored at −80°C, and used for Western blot analysis. For the analysis of CuZnSOD, MnSOD, and p47^{phox}, the total tissue lysates were prepared using lysis buffer [100 mM Tris-HCl at pH 7.4, 100 mM sodium pyrophosphate, 10 mM sodium orthovanadate, 100 mM NaF, 10 mM EDTA, 2 mM phenylmethylsulfonyl fluoride (PMSF), 0.01 mg/mL aprotinin, and 1% Triton X-100]. For the analysis of the AT_1 and AT_2 receptors, the aortas were homogenized in a buffer containing 50 mM Tris-HCl at pH 7.4, 1 mM EDTA, 10% sucrose, 2 mM PMSF, 0.01 mg/mL leupeptin, and 0.01 mg/mL aprotinin. Homogenates were centrifuged (15,000 *g*, 30 min, 4°C), and the supernatant was collected. The protein content of the lysates was determined using the BCA (bicinchoninic acid) Protein Assay Kit (Pierce Biotechnology, Rockford, IL, USA). Proteins from homogenized aortas (70 µg of protein extracts) were treated with Laemmli buffer containing 200 mmol/L dithiothreitol (DTT) and then subjected to SDS-PAGE in 10% polyacrylamide gels. Following electrophoresis, proteins were electrotransferred onto PVDF membranes (BioRad, Hercules, USA).

Western Blot Analysis

The protein expression of CuZnSOD, MnSOD, p47^{phox}, and the AT_1 and AT_2 receptors was analyzed using Western blot analysis. After blocking nonspecific sites with T-TBS buffer containing 5% nonfat dry milk and 3% bovine serum albumin (BSA) at room temperature for 1 hour, the membranes were incubated overnight at 4°C with the following primary antibodies:

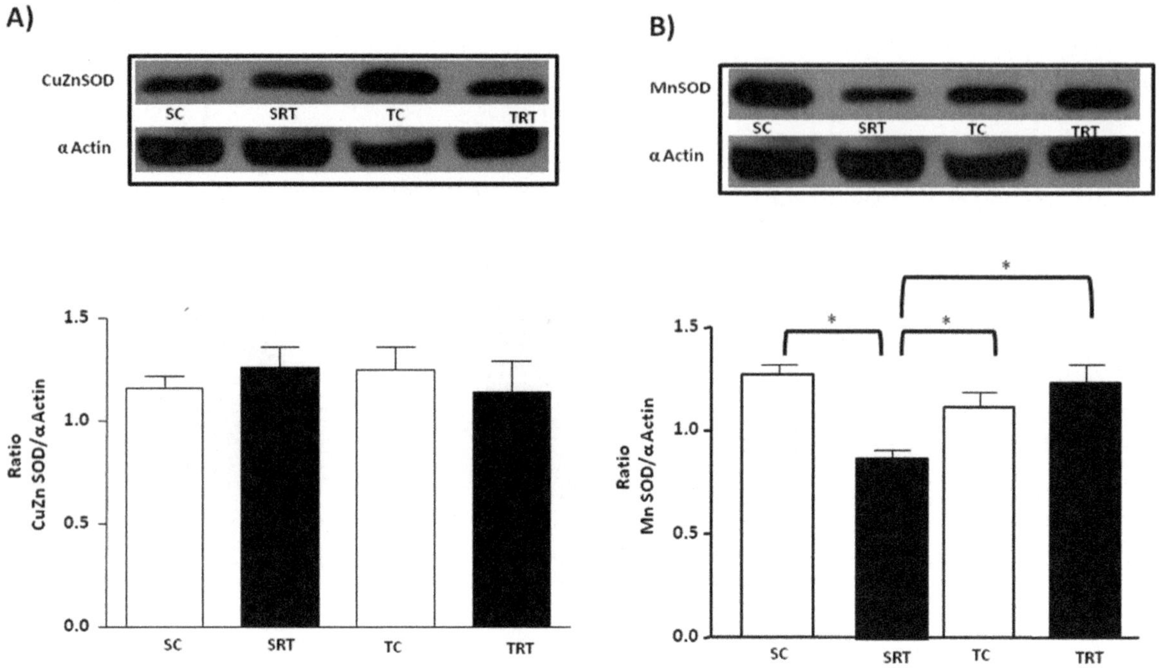

Figure 3. Expression profile of aortic SOD isoforms. Western blot analyses of CuZnSOD (**A**) and MnSOD (**B**) protein expression in thoracic aortas from SC, SRT, TC, and TRT rats. Representative immunoblots and the corresponding optical density normalized to the optical density of α-actin. Values are expressed as the mean ± SEM from five animals per group. Two-way ANOVA analysis was performed to assess the effects of IUGR, aerobic training and of their interaction (IUGR X Trained). **P<0.05* in Tukey's post Hoc test.

anti-CuZnSOD (1:1000, Upstate Biotechnology, USA); anti-MnSOD (1:2000, Upstate Biotechnology, USA); anti-p47^{phox} (1:1500, Upstate Biotechnology, USA); anti-AT_1 (1:1000, Proteimax Inc., Brazil); and anti-AT_2 (1:1000, Proteimax Inc., Brazil). The primary antibody was detected using peroxidase-conjugated secondary anti-rabbit IgG antibodies (MnSOD and p47^{phox}, 1:4000; CuZnSOD, 1:2000; AT_1 and AT_2, 1:15,000). Identical membranes were used to determine α-actin protein expression using a mouse monoclonal antibody (1:1500, Sigma-Aldrich). The immune complexes were detected using an enhanced luminol chemiluminescence system (ECL Plus, GE Healthcare, UK), which was subsequently exposed to a photographic film. The film was developed, and the bands were analyzed using ImageJ software (Wayne Rasband, National Institutes of Health, USA). The total expression of the analyzed proteins was normalized to α-actin protein expression levels and is expressed as the ratio between the optical density of the specific protein and the optical density of α-actin.

Statistical Analysis

Statistical analysis was carried out using the SPSS (v17, SPSS Inc., Chicago, IL, USA). Concentration–response curves were constructed using Prism (v.6; GraphPad Software, San Diego, CA, USA) and sigmoidal curves fitted to the data using the least squares method. The results are expressed as the means ± S.E.M. The normality of distribution of each variable was tested and transformed data were used when necessary. Where appropriate, data were analyzed using a Student's unpaired *t* test, two-way ANOVA to determine IUGR/aerobic training interaction or three-way ANOVA to determine IUGR/aerobic training/treatment interaction effects for dependent variables. A subsequent Tukey's *post-hoc* test was used to examine data for specific intergroup differences. A level of 5% probability was considered significant.

Results

Maternal nutrient restriction during pregnancy resulted in IUGR, as indicated by a marked reduction in the birth weight (C: 6.8±0.2; RT: 4.1±0.1, n = 40, P<0.001). Higher BP was observed in SRT rats, however, after 10 weeks of aerobic training the BP levels was reduced in these rats (Table 1). Two-way ANOVA revealed significant interaction between IUGR and aerobic training on BP (F (1,34) = 9.491, P = 0.001), indicating that these factors acted dependently. However, the HR significantly decreased after 10 weeks of aerobic training for both TRT and TC rats in comparison to the sedentary groups (Table 1). Two-way ANOVA indicated no significant interaction between IUGR and aerobic training on HR (P = 0.736), but very significant main effects for trained (F (1,26) = 23.99, P<0.01).

In comparison to the aortic rings from SC rats, the aortic rings from SRT rats were more responsive to AngII. Aerobic exercise training decreased the hyperreactivity to AngII of aortic rings isolated from TRT rats to levels that are similar to those observed in SC rats, but aerobic exercise training did not alter the corresponding responses in aortic rings from TC rats (Table 1, Figure 1). A significant interactive effect of IUGR and aerobic training on maximal contractile responses to AngII was confirmed by two-way ANOVA (F (1, 25) = 14.4, P = 0.001). Moreover, main effects for IUGR (P = 0.002) and aerobic training (P = 0.005) were also significant.

As shown in Figure 2, in DHE fluorescence intensity the two-ANOVA revealed significant IUGR-dependent differences (F (1, 14) = 23.584, P<0.001, main effect of IUGR) with highest values

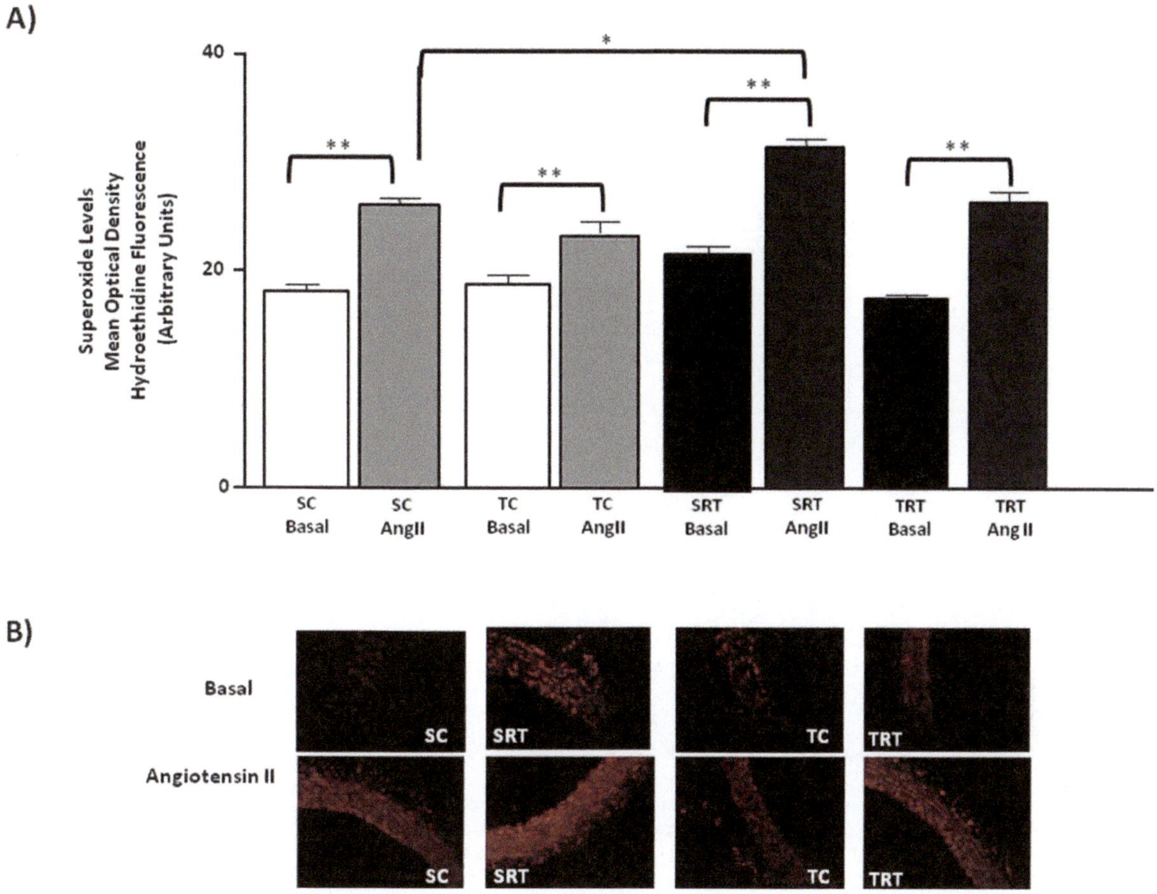

Figure 4. Role of the angiotensin II stimulation on the vascular superoxide production. (**A**) Histogram and (**B**) digital images illustrate the presence of superoxide in dihydroethidium (DHE)-treated sections of aortic rings from SC, SRT, TC, and TRT rats under basal conditions and following stimulation with angiotensin II (Ang II: 10^{-4} M). Three-way ANOVA analysis was performed to assess the effects of IUGR, aerobic training, Ang II treatment and of their interactions. Values are expressed as the mean ± SEM from six animals per group. ***P = 0.001* and **P<0.05* in Tukey's post Hoc test.

found in SRT rats than in SC rats, suggesting increased superoxide production in IUGR rats. Aerobic exercise training for 10 weeks significantly reduced superoxide levels in the aortas of TRT rats. Superoxide production remained unaltered in the aortas of TC rats (Figure 2). Moreover, we found significant interaction between IUGR and aerobic training in superoxide production (F (1, 14) = 17.554, $P = 0.001$).

As shown in Figure 3, we did not observe any significant differences in the protein expression of CuZnSOD among all groups. However, MnSOD protein expression was significantly decreased in SRT rats compared with SC rats, whereas this alteration was normalized by aerobic exercise training (Figure 3B). In contrast, MnSOD protein expression was significantly decreased in SRT rats compared with SC rats, whereas this alteration was normalized by aerobic exercise training (Figure 3B). A significant interaction between IUGR and aerobic training was observed for the MnSOD protein expression (F (1, 16) = 4.290, $P = 0.05$) and main effects for IUGR ($P = 0.022$) and aerobic training status ($P = 0.034$). In all experimental groups, we observed that treatment of the aorta segments with AngII promoted an increase in superoxide levels, although this effect was greater in aortic rings isolated from SRT rats (Figure 4). This was confirmed by three-way ANOVA that indicated significant main effect of IUGR (F (1, 29) = 27.350, $P<0.001$) and treatment (F (1, 29) = 28.671, $P<0.001$) on superoxide production. As shown in Figure 5, treatment of the aorta segments with losartan significantly reduced basal superoxide levels in the aortas of SRT rats. Three-way ANOVA revealed significant IUGR-dependent differences in superoxide concentration (F (1,30) = 9.797, $P = 0.004$, main effect of IUGR) with IUGR/treatment interactions (F (1,30) = 15.087, $P = 0.001$). Furthermore, IUGR or aerobic exercise training did not alter the protein expression of the AT_1 receptor in the isolated thoracic aortas (Figure 5C).

To determine whether NADPH oxidase was involved in the production of superoxide, we evaluated the effect of the inhibitor apocynin. Indeed, treatment with apocynin reduced basal superoxide production in only SRT rats, suggesting that vascular NADPH oxidases may participate in this production of superoxide (Figure 6). This was confirmed by three-way ANOVA between groups analysis that showed a significant main effect for IUGR (F (1,30) = 25.809, $P<0.001$) with IUGR/treatment interaction (F (1,30) = 19.280, $P<0.001$). Apocynin inhibits the release of superoxide anions by NADPH oxidase by preventing the translocation of the $p47^{phox}$ subunit to the membrane. The aortas from SRT rats exhibited increased $p47^{phox}$ protein expression (Figure 6C). However, aerobic exercise training reduced $p47^{phox}$ protein expression in the aortas of TRT rats but did not alter $p47^{phox}$ protein expression in TC rats (Figure 6). In this case two-

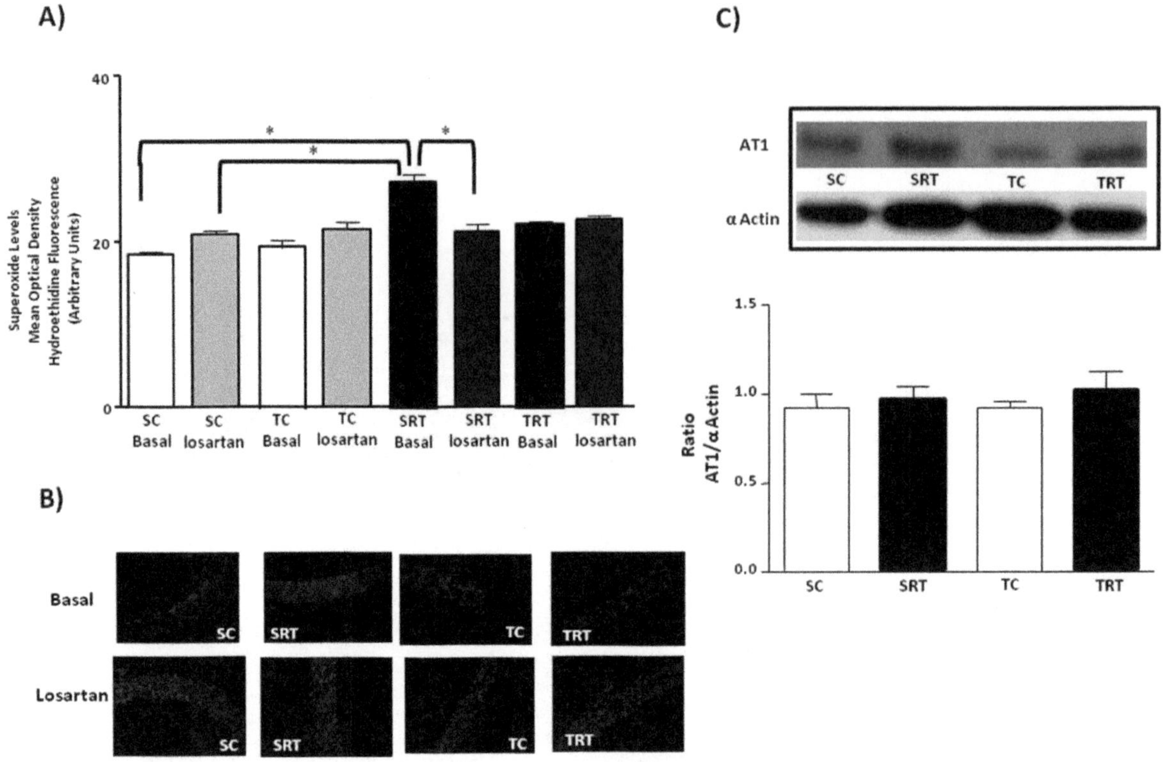

Figure 5. Effect of the AT_1 receptor antagonist on the vascular superoxide production and expression profile of aortic AT_1 receptor. (**A**) Histogram and (**B**) digital images illustrate the presence of superoxide in dihydroethidium (DHE)-treated sections of aortic rings from SC, SRT, TC, and TRT rats under basal conditions and in the presence of losartan (Los: 10^{-4} M). Three-way ANOVA analysis was performed to assess the effects of IUGR, aerobic training, losartan treatment and of their interactions. (**C**) Representative immunoblots and the corresponding optical density of AT_1 receptors normalized to the optical density of α-actin. Two-way ANOVA analysis was performed to assess the effects of IUGR, aerobic training and of their interaction. Values are expressed as the mean ± SEM from six animals per group. *$*P<0.05$* in Tukey's post Hoc test.

way ANOVA revealed a significant interaction between IUGR and aerobic training on $p47^{phox}$ protein expression (F (1,16) = 7.807, $P = 0.013$).

Given that AT_2 receptors exert a beneficial vascular effect, we further examined superoxide levels following antagonism with the AT_2 receptor antagonist PD 123,319. Interestingly, we observed increased superoxide levels following PD 123,319 treatment in only SRT and TRT rats, whereas PD 123,319 treatment did not demonstrate an effect in SC or TC rats (Figure 7). Three-way ANOVA did not reveal a significant interaction between IUGR/aerobic training/treatment on superoxide concentration. Instead, main effects were confirmed for IUGR (F (1,32) = 23.095, $P<0.001$) and PD 123,319 treatment (F (1,32) = 14.004, $P = 0.001$), indicating that these factors acted independently. To gain additional insight into this response, we investigated the protein expression of AT_2 receptors. We observed that AT_2 protein levels were reduced in the aortas of SRT rats and were restored following aerobic exercise training, whereas AT_2 protein expression in TC rats was unaltered (Figure 7C). A significant interaction between IUGR and aerobic training affected the AT2 protein expression in aorta (F (1,15) = 4.540, $P = 0.050$). Additionally, the AT_1/AT_2 ratio was significantly increased in SRT rats compared with SC rats (Figure 8), whereas aerobic exercise training resulted in the normalization of AT_1/AT_2 levels in TRT rats. No changes were observed in the AT_1/AT_2 ratio in TC rats. Consistent with these results, the two-way ANOVA also reveal significant interaction between IUGR and aerobic exercise training on ratio (F (1,15) = 4.955, $P = 0.042$).

Discussion

It is well recognized that IUGR can lead to several pathologies including hypertension, type 2 diabetes mellitus, and cardiovascular disorders [11–18]. In contrast, aerobic exercise training promotes several beneficial cardiovascular adaptations [6–10]. This study highlights five important findings. First, aerobic exercise training can prevent the IUGR-associated increase in AngII-dependent vasoconstriction in the aortic rings of TRT rats. Second, exercise training reversed the increase in basal levels of superoxide in TRT rats. Third, exercise training reversed the downregulation of MnSOD protein expression in TRT rats. Fourth, aerobic exercise training significantly upregulated AT_2 receptor protein expression in TRT rats. Fifth, exercise training significantly attenuated $p47^{phox}$ protein expression, which is a subunit of NADPH oxidase.

In this study, we found that the thoracic aorta vasoconstriction to AngII were higher in SRT rats. The modulation of AngII-induced vasoconstriction exhibited a biphasic response, in which the most potent vasoconstriction occurs at lower concentrations of AngII. Additionally, we found that aerobic exercise training for 10 weeks attenuates AngII-induced vasoconstriction in aortic rings from TRT rats. Although the possible beneficial effect of aerobic exercise training on the endothelial dysfunction induced by IUGR

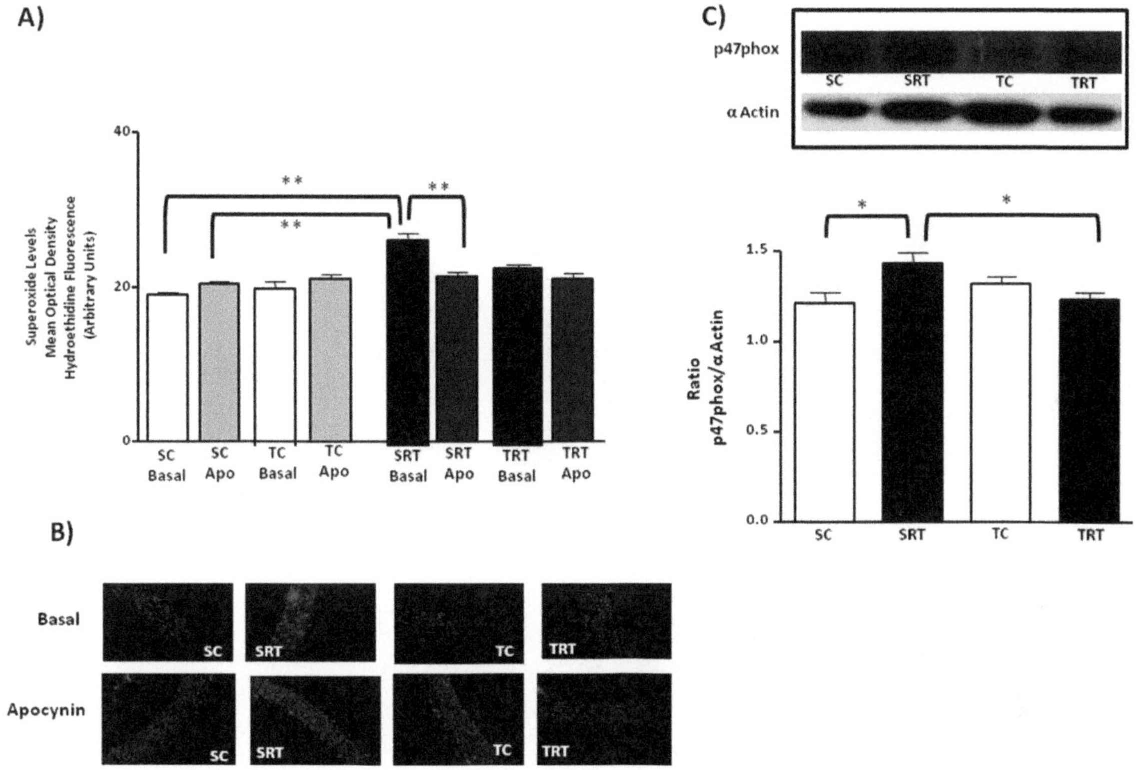

Figure 6. Effect of the NADPH-oxidase inhibitor on the vascular superoxide production and protein expression of aortic NADPH subunit. (**A**) Histogram and (**B**) digital images illustrate the presence of superoxide in dihydroethidium (DHE)-treated sections of aortic rings from SC, SRT, TC, and TRT rats under basal conditions and in the presence of apocynin (Apo: 10^{-4} M). Three-way ANOVA analysis was performed to assess the effects of IUGR, aerobic training, apocynin treatment and of their interactions. (**C**) Representative immunoblots and the corresponding optical density of the $p47^{phox}$ subunit normalized to the optical density of α-actin. Two-way ANOVA analysis was performed to assess the effects of IUGR, aerobic training, apocynin treatment and of their interaction. Values are expressed as the mean ± SEM from six animals per group. ***P = 0.001* and **P<0.05* in Tukey's post Hoc test.

was not investigated in this study, the notion that exercise training primarily affects the modulatory function of endothelial cells is supported by findings in animal models of hypertension [22], diabetes [23], aging [24], and acute myocardial infarction [25]. However, the mechanisms involved in this beneficial effect on IUGR-induced vascular dysfunction remain unclear.

Increasing studies suggest that superoxide anions are not only implicated but also play an important role in the endothelial dysfunction induced by IUGR [26–28]. Scavengers of superoxide anions and treatment with other antioxidants have been shown to improve IUGR-related endothelial dysfunction by restoring NO bioavailability [26,28]. In this study, aerobic exercise training for 10 weeks significantly reduced superoxide generation, but only in TRT rats. Several studies have demonstrated that an antioxidant effect is induced by exercise training *via* the enhancement of the activity of radical scavenger enzymes [29–33]. Aerobic training decreases oxidative stress by increasing the efficiency of the antioxidant system in isolated arteries from SHR [32] and diabetic [33] rats. Consistent with these findings, our results indicated that MnSOD protein expression levels were decreased in SRT rats in comparison to SC rats, and aerobic exercise reversed this downregulation. Numerous studies indicate that MnSOD is abundantly expressed in endothelial cells compared with other cell types, suggesting that MnSOD protects against endothelial dysfunction [34–37]. Our results support the hypothesis that the positive effect of aerobic exercise observed in the TRT rats is, in part, due to an enhanced capacity of MnSOD to scavenge superoxide.

The ability of AngII to stimulate the vascular production of superoxide by mediating NADPH oxidase activation has been widely recognized [38–40]. Our results support this finding by a marked increase in superoxide production following AngII treatment, which is inhibited by the addition of both losartan and apocynin in SRT rats. Additionally, we observed that AT_1 receptor protein expression was unaltered by IUGR or by aerobic exercise training. Conversely, we found that the protein expression of the NADPH oxidase subunit $p47^{phox}$ was higher in SRT rats, whereas aerobic exercise training was effective in normalizing $p47^{phox}$ expression. Physical training performed prior to lung ischemia/reperfusion has been reported to be effective in normalizing $p47^{phox}$ protein expression in mesenteric arteries [41]. $p47^{phox}$ plays an important role in superoxide production in response to AngII [42]. Recently, it has been shown the effects of IUGR on AngII-mediated activation of the NADPH oxidase complex [29]. Results presented here suggest that Ang II-mediated generation of superoxide in a p47phox-dependent manner in SRT rats, whereas 10 weeks of aerobic exercise training was effective in downregulation of p47phox subunit protein expression.

The activation of AT_1 receptors is known to promote vasoconstriction through increased smooth muscle intracellular Ca^{2+} availability, whereas AngII binding to AT_2 receptors on the endothelium causes vasodilation through the activation of the NO-

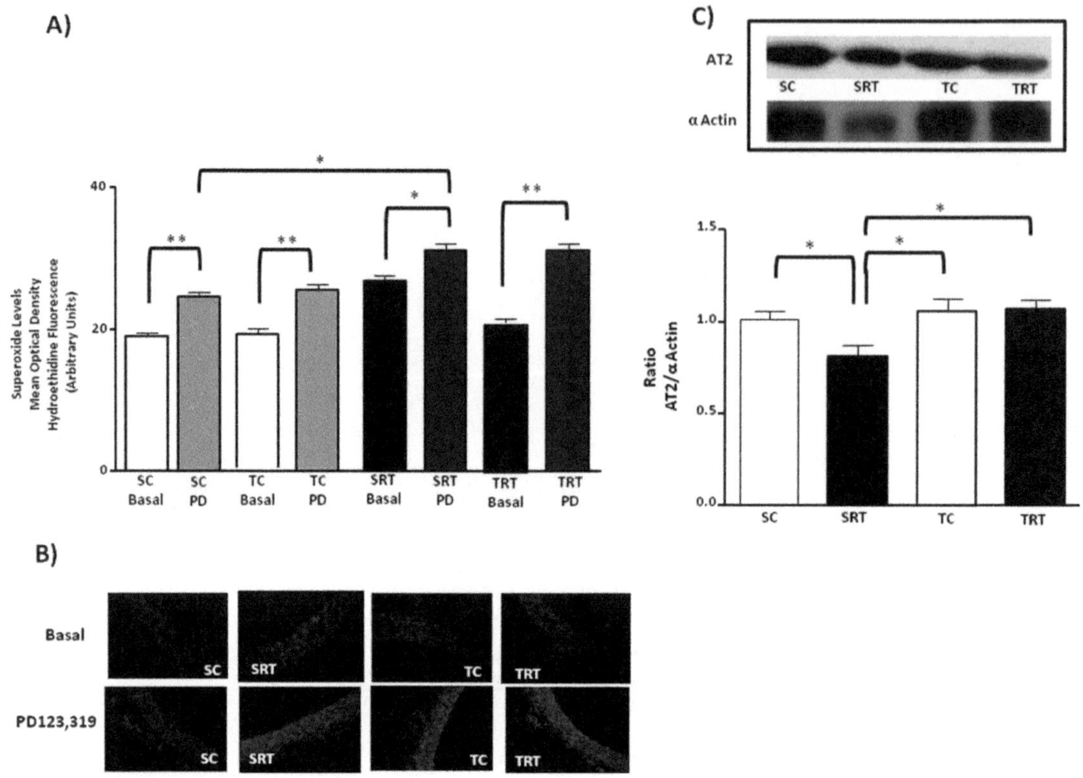

Figure 7. Effect of the AT_2 receptor antagonist on the vascular superoxide production and expression profile of aortic AT_2 receptor. (**A**) Histogram and (**B**) digital images illustrate the presence of superoxide in dihydroethidium (DHE)-treated sections of aortic rings from SC, SRT, TC, and TRT rats under basal conditions and in the presence of PD 123,319 (PD: 10^{-4} M). Three-way ANOVA analysis was performed to assess the effects of IUGR, aerobic training, PD 123,319 treatment and of their interactions. (**C**) Representative immunoblots and the corresponding optical density of AT_2 receptors normalized to the optical density of α-actin. Two-way ANOVA analysis was performed to assess the effects of IUGR, aerobic training and of their interaction. Values are expressed as the mean ± SEM from six animals per group. *$^{**}P = 0.001$* and *$^{*}P < 0.05$* in Tukey's post Hoc test.

cGMP axis [43,44]. Our results indicate that an increased response to AngII stimulation occurred with a decrease in AT_2 receptor protein expression in isolated aortas of SRT rats. Moreover, a higher ratio of AT_1/AT_2 receptors was also found in these rats. The role of AT_2 receptor stimulation in cardiovascular cells is not entirely understood. The AT_2 receptor is a counter-regulatory component of the RAS, and AngII stimulation of this receptor opposes the effects mediated by the AT_1 receptor on cell growth, vascular function, and fluid balance [44]. Studies have reported that AT_2 activation increased NO production, which significantly, but not entirely, contributes to the beneficial effects observed following AT_1 receptor antagonism [45,46]. Furthermore, some metabolites of AngII degradation (e.g., Ang (1–7) and Ang III) are known to exert their biological actions, at least partially, by binding to the AT_2 receptor [47]. This versatility of the AT_2 receptor appears to be highly cell-type and tissue specific in determining the complex cross-talk between angiotensin receptors and certain metabolites.

A correlation exists between the AT_2 receptor and aerobic exercise. Some reports indicate an upregulation of AT_2 receptor protein levels in heart, ventricular tissue, and vessels in several animal models [48]. In this study, we found that aerobic exercise training for 10 weeks restores AT_2 receptor protein expression in aortic rings from TRT rats. The AT_1/AT_2 ratio in the aorta was also normalized by exercise training, thereby locally modifying the actions of AngII. Moreover, we observed that AT_2 antagonism with PD 123,319 increased superoxide formation, but only in SRT and TRT rats, supporting the inhibitory role of AT_2 receptors on superoxide production in restricted rats. Knowledge of how AT_2 mediates superoxide anion generation is limited, and little is known regarding the likely beneficial effects of aerobic exercise on the modulation of this receptor. Studies suggest that AngII receptors differentially modulate endothelial superoxide generation [49]. Sohn *et al.* [49] reported that AT_1 activates superoxide formation and that AT_2 receptors appear to attenuate this AT_1-induced effect, most likely *via* a pathway that involves tyrosine phosphatases. A study by Sabuhi *et al.* [50] suggests that the activation of AT_2 receptors lowers oxidative stress by increasing SOD activity and decreasing the expression of the NADPH oxidase component $gp91^{phox}$. Our study suggests the possibility of an association between AT_2 modulation and exercise training. However, the exact mechanisms of these effects remain to be elucidated.

In summary, the results of this study provide evidence that aerobic training demonstrates a beneficial effect on antioxidant capacity *via* the upregulation of MnSOD protein expression. The vascular protective effects of exercise training may partially be due to the downregulation of $p47^{phox}$ and, subsequently, the reduced activation of NADPH oxidase. Finally, the increase in AT_2 receptor protein levels may also provide beneficial effects against superoxide generation. Nevertheless, we did not directly evaluate the role of nitric oxide (NO) regarding the beneficial effects of

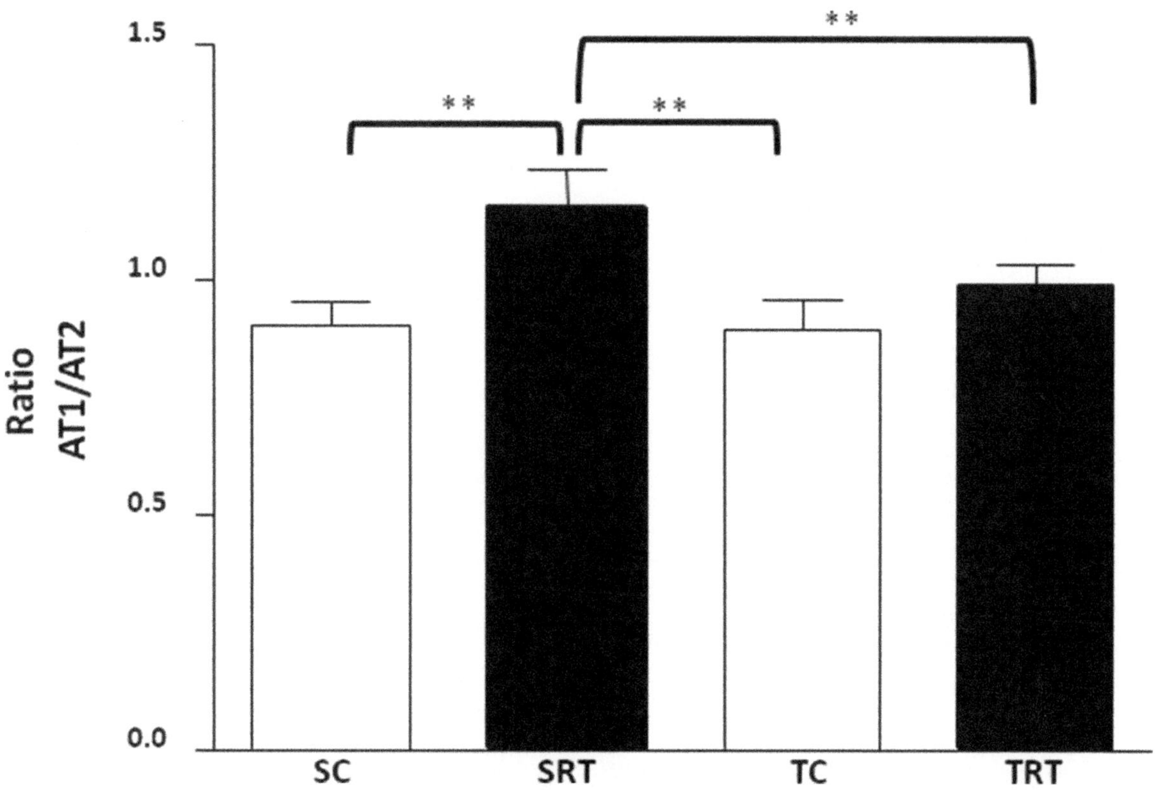

Figure 8. Representative histogram of the AT_1/AT_2 ratio in thoracic aortas of SC, SRT, TC, and TRT rats. Values are expressed as the mean ± SEM from six animals per group. Two-way ANOVA analysis was performed to assess the effects of IUGR, aerobic training and of their interaction (IUGR X Trained). $^{**}P = 0.001$ in Tukey's post Hoc test.

exercise training; assessment of this pathway would add considerable clarity to the mechanisms that regulate vascular function and NO–redox–based signaling in IUGR rats submitted to aerobic training.

Author Contributions

Conceived and designed the experiments: MF TSC EHA LCM ZBF VO. Performed the experiments: VO. Analyzed the data: MF VO EHA LCM TSC. Contributed reagents/materials/analysis tools: MF MHCC ZBF EHA. Contributed to the writing of the manuscript: MF VO EHA.

References

1. Green DJ, Maiorana A, O'Driscoll G, Taylor R (2004) Effect of exercise training on endothelium-derived nitric oxide function in humans. J Physiol 561: 1–25.
2. Maiorana AJ, Naylor LH, Exterkate A, Swart A, Thijssen DH, et al. (2011) The impact of exercise training on conduit artery wall thickness and remodeling in chronic heart failure patients. Hypertension 57: 56–62.
3. McAllister RM, Newcomer SC, Laughlin MH (2008) Vascular nitric oxide: effects of exercise training in animals. Appl Physiol Nutr Metab 33: 173–178.
4. Pal S, Radavelli-Bagatini S, Ho S (2013) Potential benefits of exercise on blood pressure and vascular function. J Am Soc Hypertens 7: 494–506.
5. Bacon SL, Sherwood A, Hinderliter A, Blumenthal JA (2004) Effects of exercise, diet and weight loss on high blood pressure. Sports Medicine 34: 307–316.
6. Hagberg JM, Park J-J, Brown MD (2000) The role of exercise training in the treatment of hypertension: an update. Sports Medicine 30: 193–206.
7. Whelton SP, Chin A, Xin X, He J (2002) Effect of aerobic exercise on blood pressure. Annals of Internal Medicine 136: 493–503.
8. da Rocha RF, de Oliveira MR, Pasquali MA, Andrades ME, Oliveira MW, et al. (2010) Vascular redox imbalance in rats submitted to chronic exercise. Cell Biochem Funct 28: 190–196.
9. Tinken TM, Thijssen DHJ, Hopkins N (2010) Shear Stress Mediates Endothelial Adaptations to Exercise Training in Humans. Hypertension 55: 312–318.
10. Ciampone S, Borges R, de Lima IP, Mesquita FF (2011) Long-term exercise attenuates blood pressure responsiveness and modulates kidney angiotensin II signalling and urinary sodium excretion in SHR. J Renin Angiotensin Aldosterone Syst 12: 394–403.
11. Barker DJP, Oosmond C, Bull AR, Simonds (1999) Fetal and placental size and risk of hypertension in adult life. B M J 301: 259–262.
12. Barker DJP, Osmond C, Simmonds SJ, Wield GA (1993) The relation of small head circuference and thinness at birth to death from cardiovascular disease in adult life. British Med J 306: 422–426.
13. Gluckman PD, Hanson MA (2004) Living with the past: evolution, development, and patterns of disease. Science 305: 1733–1736.
14. Gluckman PD, Hanson MA, Pinal C (2005) The developmental origins of adult disease. Maternal and Child Nutrition 1: 130–141.
15. Brawley L, Itoh S, Torrens C, Barker A, Bertram C, et al. (2003) Dietary protein restriction in pregnancy induces hypertension and vascular defects in rat male offspring. Pediatric Research 54: 83–90.
16. Langley-Evans SC, Sherman RC, Welham SJ, Nwagwu MO, Gardner DS, et al. (1999) Intrauterine programming of hypertension: the role of the renin-angiotensin system. Biochem Soc Trans 27: 88–93.
17. Torrens C, Hanson MA, Gluckman PD, Vickers MH (2009) Maternal undernutrition leads to endothelial dysfunction in adult male rat offspring independent of postnatal diet. Br J Nutr 101: 27–33.
18. Ceravolo GS, Franco MC, Carneiro-Ramos MS, Barreto-Chaves ML, Tostes RC, et al. (2007) Enalapril and losartan restored blood pressure and vascular reactivity in intrauterine undernourished rats. Life Sci 80: 782–787.
19. Cambri LT, Dalia RA, Ribeiro C, Rostom de Mello MA (2010) Aerobic capacity of rats recovered from fetal malnutrition with a fructose-rich diet. Appl Physiol Nutr Metab 35(4): 490–497.
20. Cambri LT, de Araujo GG, Ghezzi AC, Botezelli JD, Mello MA (2011) Metabolic responses to acute physical exercise in young rats recovered from fetal protein malnutrition with a fructose-rich diet. Lipids Health Dis 10: 164.
21. Miller FJ Jr, Gutterman DD, Rios CD, Heistad DD, Davidson BL (1988) Superoxide production in vascular smooth muscle contributes to oxidative stress and impaired relaxation in atherosclerosis. Circ Res 82: 1298–1305.
22. Roque FR, Briones AM, García-Redondo AB, Galán M, Martínez-Revelles S, et al. (2013) Aerobic exercise reduces oxidative stress and improves vascular changes of small mesenteric and coronary arteries in hypertension. Br J Pharmacol 168: 686–703

23. Chakraphan D, Sridulyakul P, Thipakorn B, Bunnag S, Huxley VH, et al. (2005) Attenuation of endothelial dysfunction by exercise training in STZ-induced diabetic rats. Clin Hemorheol Microcirc. 32: 217–226.
24. Trotti DW, Gunduz F, Laughlin MH (2009) Exercise training reverses age-related decrements in endothelium-dependent dilation in skeletal muscle feed arteries. J Appl Physiol 106: 1925–1934.
25. Kemi OJ, Haram PM, Høydal MA, Wisløff U, Ellingsen Ø (2013) Exercise training and losartan improve endothelial function in heart failure rats by different mechanisms. Scand Cardiovasc J. 47: 160–167.
26. Franco Mdo C, Dantas AP, Akamine EH, Kawamoto EM, Fortes ZB, et al. (2002) Enhanced oxidative stress as a potential mechanism underlying the programming of hypertension in utero. J Cardiovasc Pharmacol 40: 501–509
27. Franco M, Akamine EH, Dimarco GS, Casarinil DE, Fortes ZB, et al. (2003) NADPH Oxidase and Enhanced Superoxide Generation in the Intrauterine Undernourished Rats: Involvement of the Renin-Angiotensin System Cardiovasc Res 59: 767–775.
28. Franco Mdo C, Akamine EH, Aparecida de Oliveira M, Fortes ZB, Tostes RC, et al. (2003) Vitamins C and E improve endothelial dysfunction in intrauterine-undernourished rats by decreasing vascular superoxide anion concentration. J Cardiovasc Pharmacol 42: 211–217.
29. Alessio HM, Goldfarb AH (1988) Lipid peroxidation and scavenger enzymes during exercise: adaptive response to training. J Appl Physiol 64:1333–1336.
30. Fukai T, Siegfried MR, Ushio-Fukai M, Cheng Y, Kojda G, et al. (2000) Regulation of the vascular extracellular superoxide dismutase by nitric oxide and exercise training. J Clin Invest 105: 1631–1639.
31. Lawler JM, Kwak HB, Kim JH, Suk MH (2009) Exercise training inducibility of MnSOD protein expression and activity is retained while reducing prooxidant signaling in the heart of senescent rats. Am J Physiol Regul Integr Comp Physiol 296: R1496–R1502.
32. Kimura H, Kon N, Furukawa S, Mukaida M, Yamakura F, et al. (2010) Effect of endurance exercise training on oxidative stress in spontaneously hypertensive rats (SHR) after emergence of hypertension. Clin Exp Hypertens 32: 407–415.
33. Rosety-Rodriguez M, Rosety I, Fornieles-Gonzalez G, Diaz-Ordonez AJ, Camacho A, et al. (2012) A 6-week training program increased muscle antioxidant system in elderly diabetic fatty rats. Med Sci Monit 18: BR346–BR350.
34. Fukai T, Folz RJ, Landmesser U, Harrison DG (2002) Extracellular superoxide dismutase and cardiovascular disease. Cardiovasc Res 55: 239–249.
35. Faraci FM, Didion SP (2004) Vascular protection: superoxide dismutase isoforms in the vessel wall. Arterioscler Thromb Vasc Biol 24: 1367–1373.
36. Andresen JJ, Faraci FM, Heistad DD (2004) Vascular responses in Mn-SOD deficient mice. Am J Physiol Heart Circ Physiol 287: H1141–H1148.
37. Chrissobolis S, Faraci FM (2010) Sex differences in protection against angiotensin II-induced endothelial dysfunction by manganese superoxide dismutase in the cerebral circulation. Hypertension 55: 905–910.
38. Warnholtz A, Nickenig G, Schulz E, Macharzina R, Bräsen JH, et al. (1999) Increased NADH-oxidase-mediated superoxide production in the early stages of atherosclerosis: evidence for involvement of the renin-angiotensin system.-Circulation 20: 2027–2033.
39. Doughan AK, Harrison DG, Dikalov SI (2008) Molecular mechanisms of angiotensin II-mediated mitochondrial dysfunction: linking mitochondrial oxidative damage and vascular endothelial dysfunction. Circ Res 29: 488–496.
40. Selemidis S, Sobey CG, Wingler K, Schmidt HH, Drummond GR (2008) NADPH oxidases in the vasculature: molecular features, roles in disease and pharmacological inhibition. Pharmacology & Therapeutics 120: 254–291.
41. Delbin MA, Davel AP, Rossoni LV, Antunes E, Zanesco A (2011) Beneficial effects of physical training on the cardio-inflammatory disorder induced by lung ischemia/reperfusion in rats. Inflammation 34: 319–325.
42. Li JM, Shah AM (2003) Mechanism of endothelial cell NADPH oxidase activation by angiotensin II. Role of the p47phox subunit. J Biol Chem 278: 12094–12100.
43. Wagenaar LJ, Voors AA, Buikema H, Van Gilst WH (2002) Angiotensin receptors in the cardiovascular system. Can J Cardiol 18: 1331–1339.
44. Li Y, Li XH, Yuan H (2012) Angiotensin II type-2 receptor-specific effects on the cardiovascular system Cardiovasc Diagn Ther 2: 56–62.
45. Wollert KC, Drexler H (1999) The renin-angiotensin system and experimental heart failure. Cardiovasc Res 43: 838–849.
46. Toda N, Ayajiki K, Okamura T (2007) Interaction of endothelial nitric oxide and angiotensin in the circulation. Pharmacol Rev 59: 54–87.
47. Gaspari TA, Vinh A, Jones ES, Widdop RE (2012) Ganging up on angiotensin II type 1 receptors in vascular remodeling. Hypertension 60: 17–19.
48. Li Y, Li XH, Yuan H (2012) Angiotensin II type-2 receptor-specific effects on the cardiovascular system. Cardiovasc Diagn Ther 2: 56–62.
49. Sohn HY, Raff U, Hoffmann A, Gloe T, Heermeier K, et al. (2000) Differential role of angiotensin II receptor subtypes on endothelial superoxide formation. Br J Pharmacol 131: 667–672.
50. Sabuhi R, Ali Q, Asghar M, Al-Zamily NR, Hussain T (2011) Role of the angiotensin II AT2 receptor in inflammation and oxidative stress: opposing effects in lean and obese Zucker rats. Am J Physiol Renal Physiol 300: F700–F706.

19

The Road to Gold: Training and Peaking Characteristics in the Year Prior to a Gold Medal Endurance Performance

Espen Tønnessen[1]*, Øystein Sylta[2], Thomas A. Haugen[1], Erlend Hem[1], Ida S. Svendsen[3], Stephen Seiler[2]

1 The Norwegian Olympic Federation, Oslo, Norway, **2** Faculty of Health and Sport Sciences, University of Agder, Kristiansand, Norway, **3** School of Sport, Exercise and Health Sciences, Loughborough University, Leicestershire, United Kingdom

Abstract

Purpose: To describe training variations across the annual cycle in Olympic and World Champion endurance athletes, and determine whether these athletes used tapering strategies in line with recommendations in the literature.

Methods: Eleven elite XC skiers and biathletes (4 male; 28±1 yr, 85±5 mL. min^{-1}. kg^{-1} $\dot{V}O_{2max}$, 7 female, 25±4 yr, 73±3 mL. min^{-1}. kg^{-1} $\dot{V}O_{2max}$) reported one year of day-to-day training leading up to the most successful competition of their career. Training data were divided into periodization and peaking phases and distributed into training forms, intensity zones and endurance activity forms.

Results: Athletes trained ~800 h/500 sessions.year^{-1}, including ~500 h. year^{-1} of sport-specific training. Ninety-four percent of all training was executed as aerobic endurance training. Of this, ~90% was low intensity training (LIT, below the first lactate threshold) and 10% high intensity training (HIT, above the first lactate threshold) by time. Categorically, 23% of training sessions were characterized as HIT with primary portions executed at or above the first lactate turn point. Training volume and specificity distribution conformed to a traditional periodization model, but absolute volume of HIT remained stable across phases. However, HIT training patterns tended to become more polarized in the competition phase. Training volume, frequency and intensity remained unchanged from pre-peaking to peaking period, but there was a 32±15% ($P < .01$) volume reduction from the preparation period to peaking phase.

Conclusions: The annual training data for these Olympic and World champion XC skiers and biathletes conforms to previously reported training patterns of elite endurance athletes. During the competition phase, training became more sport-specific, with 92% performed as XC skiing. However, they did not follow suggested tapering practice derived from short-term experimental studies. Only three out of 11 athletes took a rest day during the final 5 days prior to their most successful competition.

Editor: Matjaz Perc, University of Maribor, Slovenia

Funding: The authors received no specific funding for this work.

Competing Interests: The authors have declared that no competing interests exist.

* Email: espen.tonnessen@olympiatoppen.no

Introduction

Winning a gold medal in a major international championship requires not only outstanding athletic ability and long-term training progression, but also that the athlete achieves peak performance at the right time. In recent years, increased attention has been given to quantifying the training characteristics of elite endurance athletes [1–3] and this information has provided a fruitful foundation for hypothesis testing regarding training load and physiological adaptation. At the same time, a strong knowledge base has developed regarding best practice for the tapering and peaking process, based largely on experimental interventions [4–6]. However, studies linking the characteristics of the long-term training process to those of the short term pre-peaking and peaking process are lacking.

Recently, a number of descriptive studies, both retrospective and prospective, have been published on the training characteristics of athletes from endurance sports such as running [7–12], cycling [13–14], XC skiing [15–17], swimming [18–19], rowing [20–21], triathlon [22–23], speed skating [24–25] and kayaking [26]. Training load variables such as volume, frequency and intensity distribution appear to play an interactive role in maximizing physical capacity and performance [27]. Depending on the specific muscular loading characteristics of the sport, athletes typically train 500 h (distance running) [7,8,11,12,28,29] to well in excess of 1000 h per year (rowing, swimming, cycling, triathlon) [13–14,18–23] performed during 400–800 annual training sessions [11–12,15–17,23], in order to reach an internationally elite level. When examining the intensity distribution of this large training volume, a number of studies across a broad range of sports converge on the finding that 75–90% of all endurance training time is performed as low intensity training (LIT, below the first lactate turn point) for athletes training >

500 h per year. The remaining 10–25% is comprised of high intensity training (HIT) performed above the first lactate turn point [7–8,14–15,22–23]. This approximate "80–20" distribution between low and high intensity training among high-level performers is a robust finding [3], even if mechanistic explanations for its ubiquity remain speculative. Furthermore, the "best practice" magnitude and distribution of HIT remains unclear. In addition, the training-dose response relationship has a significant individual variation component, which further complicates the generalizability of the picture. While the influx of descriptive data on the training of elite endurance athletes has informed training practice, and stimulated new experimental studies, methodological compromises are inherent to the challenge of measuring behavior reliably and precisely in highly selected groups. Available descriptive studies typically only present data over a shorter time frame [7–8,12], at a sub-elite level [9,14–15,17,21–22] or as single case studies [11,23,28–29]. Accuracy in training monitoring is also unclear, due to weaknesses in methods such as questionnaires [10] or compilation and analysis of data that are in part or completely based on training plans instead of strict quantification of actual training performed [7–8,20]. Limited data currently exist on the long-term training of highly trained and elite athletes, based on accurate training monitoring [30].

Short-term training manipulations to achieve peaking for optimal sports performance have been investigated for more than 20 years. A synthesis of studies on well-trained athletes from a variety of different sports has shown a performance improvement of up to 3%, providing the final 4–28 days of training are executed correctly [5–6,31–33]. All other things being equal, a well-executed peaking phase can therefore dramatically increase the odds of winning a gold medal at a championship event for an individual athlete with finalist potential. In the research literature, the peaking process is typically divided into two phases: a pre-tapering phase, and the final taper period culminating with the intended competition. The aim of the pre-tapering phase is to stimulate a controlled "over-reaching" state and elicit a super-compensatory adaptive response in the following taper. Experimentally, the optimal duration of the actual taper depends on the training executed in the pre-taper [6,33–34]. The taper is initiated approximately 14 days prior to the desired peak performance, and the aim of this phase is to facilitate regeneration and reduce fatigue, while maintaining or increasing fitness and technical/psychological readiness in order to mobilize maximal performance in competition [4–6,35]. The optimal training volume, frequency and intensity in each phase is debated [4–6,31,35], but a reduction in training load of between 41–60% from pre-taper to taper has been recommended. This reduction appears to be best achieved via reduced training duration per session, while maintaining session frequency [5]. Maintaining training intensity is considered to be a key factor in a successful peaking regime, and it is therefore recommended that the frequency of HIT sessions be maintained during the taper [36–39]. Despite 20 years of research on tapering and peaking for athletic performance, we are unaware of any study that has successfully quantified the "real life" peaking strategies of athletes achieving ultimate success in Olympic Games or World Championship events. It is therefore unclear how the models developed from controlled experimental studies are translated to the actual peaking practices of elite endurance athletes. Furthermore, few studies havelinked peaking strategies to annual training characteristics and the competitive season of elite athletes [30].

The current study therefore aimed to: 1) present highly accurate day-to-day annual training data from a cohort of endurance athletes that all won Olympic or World Championship gold medals and, 2) quantify and examine relationships between annual training and peaking characteristics in these athletes.

Methods

Subjects

Four male and seven female former and current Norwegian elite XC skiers and biathletes were included in the study (Table 1). All athletes had won a least one individual Olympic or World Championship senior gold medal during their career. In total, included males had won 41 (5–26) and females 25 (1–9) gold medals (includes both individual and relays from 1985 through 2011). In addition, included athletes had systematically and accurately recorded their day-to-day training in detail from junior through to senior level. In the current study, we have analyzed and reported the year specifically leading up to their most successful competition at senior level. The regional ethics committee of Southern Norway reviewed the study and concluded that, due to the nature of the investigation, it did not require their approval. The study was therefore submitted to and approved by the Norwegian Social Science Data Services (NSD), and all athletes gave their oral and written informed consent prior to study participation.

Physiological testing

All athletes underwent regular physiological testing during their career. The test values presented in Table 1 represent the highest result achieved during the analyzed year. There were no physiological tests performed during the competition period, and the presented results therefore represent tests from October or November, while Olympic or World Championship events were typically held in February-March. All physiological testing was conducted at the Norwegian Olympic training center. $\dot{V}O_{2max}$ testing was performed as running at 10.5% inclination on a motorized treadmill (Woodway Gmbh, Weil am Rhein, Germany) calibrated for speed and incline. The procedure started with an extensive warm-up sequence, followed by a stepwise increase in running velocity every minute thereafter until volitional exhaustion, normally occurring after 4–6 minutes. Starting velocity for all athletes corresponded to 85–90% of $\dot{V}O_{2max}$. The increase was 1 $km.h^{-1}.min^{-1}$, and the last velocity step was held for at least 1 min. The test was terminated before voluntary exhaustion if the $\dot{V}O_2$values leveled off or decreased despite increasing workload and ventilation, in addition to respiratory exchange ratio (RER) > 1.10. $\dot{V}O_{2max}$ was defined as the highest average of two consecutive 30 s measurements. Oxygen uptake was measured using EOS Sprint (Jaeger-Toennis, Wurtzburg, Germany) until 2002, after which an Oxycon Pro (Jaeger-Toennis, Wurtzburg, Germany) metabolic test system was used. An internal comparison between the two analyzers was conducted during the transition in 2002 and showed identical regression lines for the treadmill running velocity $-\dot{V}O_2$ relationship with both systems. Primarily two exercise physiologists supervised all testing during the entire period.

Training monitoring

Athletes included in the study recorded their day-to-day training during their most successful year in paper diaries designed by the Norwegian Ski Association [40–41], the Norwegian Biathlon Association [42] or, since ~2005, in the digital version developed by the Norwegian Olympic Federation (OLT). The training recorded for each session included total training time distributed across training form (strength, endurance, sprint), activity form

Table 1. General characteristics of athletes included in the study.

Subject	Gender	Age	Height	Weight	$\dot{V}O_{2max}$ (ml·kg^{-1}.min^{-1})	$\dot{V}O_{2max}$ (l.min^{-1})
1	M	28	180	77	92.5	7.13
2	M	26	190	82	81.9	6.73
3	M	29	189	83	84.8	7.07
4	M	28	179	66	81.2	5.25
5	F	23	172	55	72.9	3.90
6	F	23	176	63	73.6	4.64
7	F	29	173	63	76.6	4.81
8	F	20	175	69	70.4	4.83
9	F	28	166	61	69.1	4.24
10	F	22	162	51	76.0	3.93
11	F	30	169	64	71.4	4.60
Mean ± SD, Male		28±1	185±6	77±8	85.1±5.2	6.5±0.9
Mean ± SD, Female		25±4	170±5	61±6	72.9±2.8	4.4±0.4

Values are reported from the analyzed year in the current study.

(skiing, roller-skiing, running, cycling etc.), and intensity zone, as well as specific comments regarding session details. All paper training diaries were transferred session by session to digital format by persons from the current research group. Total training time and frequency of sessions was distributed in line with the structure in Figure 1. Digitized diary data was rigorously cross-checked for internal consistency among different training distribution breakdowns at the individual level. Internal consistency of digitized training records from all included athletes was ≥99%.

All the athletes included in the study used a 5 intensity zone model, where zones 1–2 are classified as LIT and zones 3–5 as HIT. The intensity scale presented in Table 2 represents average self-reported zone-cut offs from 29 elite XC-skiers from a previous study [43]. In the results section we have presented the data either in a binary model (LIT/HIT) or a 5-zone model were zones 1–2 are below the first lactate threshold (LT^1), zone 3 between LT^1 and LT^2, and zones 4–5 above LT^2 [3,44]. The intensity distribution is classified both according to a time in training zone approach and a frequency based session goal approach (SG). These methods and the intensity zones cut-offs have been described in detail recently [43].

Annual periodization phases and peaking model

General training data from the entire year are either presented as annual training characteristics or divided into different periodization phases as presented in Table 3. Peaking characteristics were quantified based on the final 6 weeks of training prior to the gold medal winning performance, as delineated in Table 3.

Statistical analyses

All data in text, tables or figures are presented as mean ± standard deviation (SD) and/or range. Statistical comparisons between different periodization phases are focused on the general preparation period (GP), specific preparation period (SP) and competition period (CP) in addition to comparing the actual peaking phase with pre-peaking phase, GP and SP. Data were not normally distributed. Therefore each variable from the GP, SP and CP (overall, pre-peaking and peaking phase) was tested with a non-parametric Friedman test, followed by a post-hoc test (Wilcoxon Signed Rank) to locate statistical differences. Male and female athlete data are merged, as a Mann-Whitney U Test revealed no significant differences in any relevant variables across gender (data not shown). All figures and statistical analyses were performed using Microsoft Excel or SPSS 18.0 (SPSS Inc, Chicago, IL, USA) and statistical significance was accepted at the $P<.05$ level or Bonferroni adjusted alpha level.

Results

Annual training characteristics

Total training volume was 770±99 h (622–942) distributed across 470±68 sessions (375–585) throughout the gold medal year. Endurance training accounted for 94±3% of all training time with the remaining 5±2% composed of strength training and 1±1% ski sprint training. Time in training zone based intensity distribution showed that 91±1% of all endurance training time was executed as LIT (zone 1–2) and 9±1% as HIT (zone 3–5).

Monthly training distribution of specific and non-specific activity forms during each training phase are presented in Figure 2. Endurance and sprint training was executed with sport-specific movement patterns (ski or roller ski) for 64±3% (465±56 h/min-max: 376–569 h) of total training time, with the remaining 36±3% (265±47 h/min-max: 196–337 h), composed of non-specific activity forms (running, cycling etc.) throughout the year. The proportion of sport-specific training increased significantly from GP (48±6%) to SP (87±8%) and CP (92±4%) ($P<.01$).

The distribution across all five intensity zones was: zone 1: 86.0±3.4%, zone 2: 5.3±3.0%, zone 3: 3.3±0.9%, zone 4: 3.3±1% and zone 5: 2.1±1.0%. When all endurance sessions were nominally categorized using the SG approach, the distribution was 77±2% LIT and 23±2% HIT (Figure 3, A). Weekly training patterns during each training phase are presented in Table 4.

Total annual HIT duration (including competitions) was 63±14 h (46–85 h) distributed across 106±20 sessions (85–147) throughout the year. The relative distribution of HIT duration in intensity zones 3, 4 and 5 was 39±10%, 37±13% and 24±13% respectively, and 32±6%, 38±14% and 30±13% according to a SG distribution. Monthly frequency of HIT sessions increased

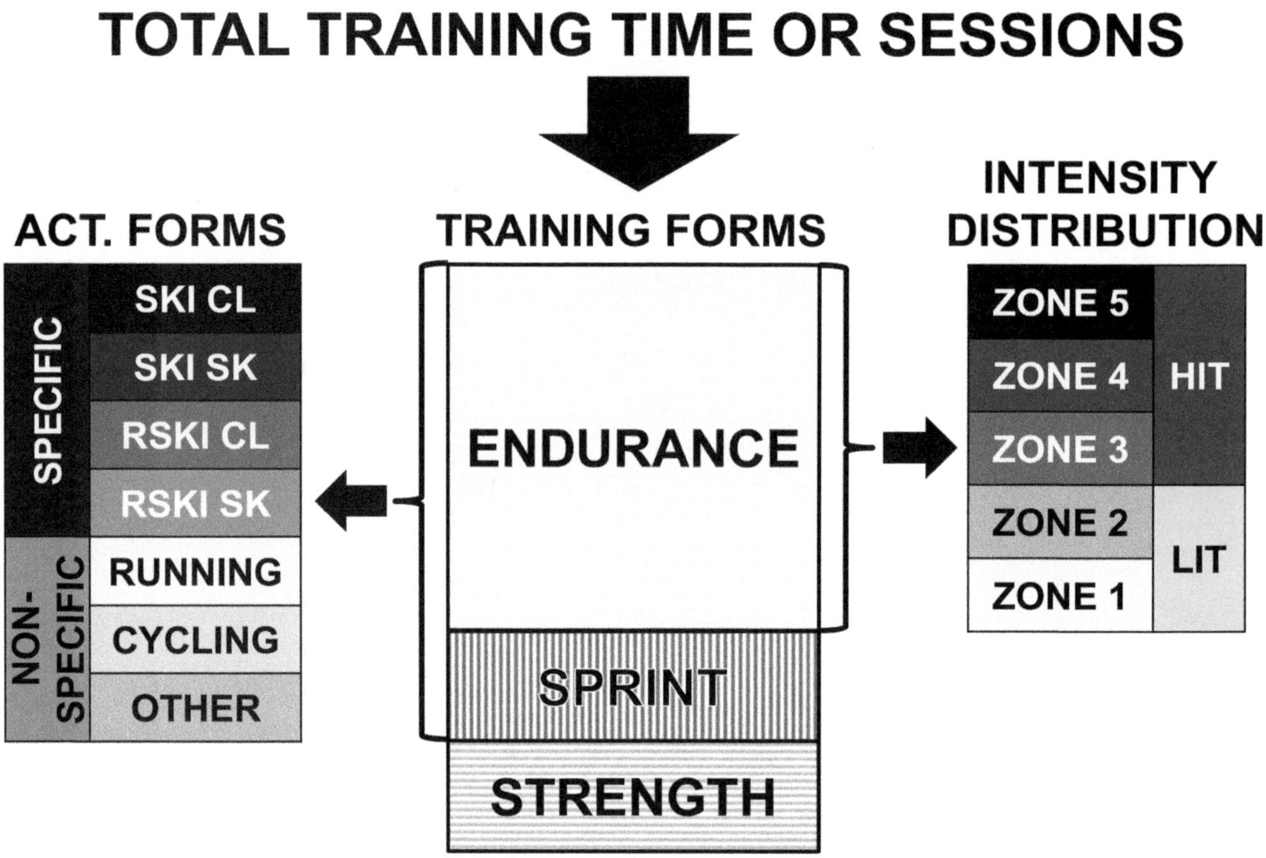

Figure 1. Training distribution methods. Total training time was divided into training forms (endurance, sprint and strength). Endurance time and frequency were further distributed into 5 intensity zones in line with table 2. Zones 1–2 are LIT and zones 3–5 are HIT. Endurance and sprint time together were divided into activity forms. Ski and roller ski were classified as specific, and running, cycling or other as non-specific activity forms.

from GP to SP (P<.01). In addition, the monthly frequency of intensity zone 5 sessions increased from GP to SP and then remained unchanged in the CP (P<.01) (Figure 3, B). Weekly HIT patterns during each training phase are presented in Table 4.

Peaking characteristics

Total training time ($h.wk^{-1}$) decreased by 9±14% from the pre-peaking to peaking phase, but this did not reach statistical significance. However, the reduction from GP, when training volume was highest, to the peaking phase, was 32±15% (P<.01). This decrease in total training volume was entirely due to a reduction in non-sport-specific training. Individual data for each of the 11 athletes are presented in Figure 4. The decrease in training volume from GP and pre-peaking phase to the peaking phase was achieved via a reduction in both endurance and strength training, while sprint training time remained stable, although there was a tendency for sprint training time to increase slightly from the pre-peaking phase to the peaking phase. There were no significant changes in total session frequency per week between the peaking phase and any of the other phases (Figure 5 A and Table 4).

There was non-significant decrease of 9±15% in LIT endurance training ($h.wk^{-1}$) from the pre-peaking phase to the peaking phase. However, LIT training volume decreased by 31±17% (P<.01) from GP to the peaking phase. In contrast, HIT time ($h.wk^{-1}$) remained stable from both pre-peaking phase to the

Table 2. The 5-zone, 3-zone, and binary intensity scales used in the current study.

Intensity Zone	Typical Blood lactate[A] (mmol. L^{-1})	Typical Heart Rate (% max)	Three zone model	Binary model
5	>5.8	>94	>LT^2	
4	3.7–5.7	89–93		HIT
3	2.1–3.6	84–88	LT^1–LT^2	
2	1.3–2.0	74–83		LIT
1	<1.2	54–73	<LT^1	

[A]Measured with Lactate Pro LT-1710. Reference values presented are derived from the average self-reported zone-cut offs of 29 elite XC-skiers [43], and individual adjustments are required.

Table 3. Training phases in annual cycle, including peaking phases.

Period in annual training cycle	Duration
Preparation period (PP)	May-December
Transition period	*May*
General preparation period (GP)	*June-October*
Specific preparation period (SP)	*November-December*
Competition Period (CP)	January-March
Pre-peaking phase	*6–3 weeks before championship event*
Peaking phase	*Last 14 days before championship event*
Regeneration period	April

peaking phase and from GP to the peaking phase (Figure 5 A and Table 4).

LIT endurance session frequency decreased from GP to the peaking phase by 21±24% (P=.016) but remained stable from pre-peaking phase to the peaking phase. Weekly HIT session frequency increased by 40±27% (P<.01) from GP to the peaking phase, but remained stable from pre-peaking phase to the peaking phase (Figure 5 B). Training volume and frequency distribution among zones 3, 4 and 5 through the different phases are presented in Figure 5 B and Table 4.

Discussion

To the authors' knowledge, this is the first study to connect accurate annual day-to-day training data to a specific peaking period in a group of athletes achieving ultimate international success in an endurance sport. The main findings of the present study are: 1) The annual training data for these Olympic and World champion XC skiers and biathletes conforms to previously reported training patterns amongst elite endurance athletes. 2) In contrast, peaking characteristics for these gold medalists did not conform to suggested best practice for tapering strategies in elite endurance athletes, as derived from partly experimental studies.

Annual training characteristics

Training volume. High training volume has emerged as a key commonality in successful endurance training [20,1–3,25]. Athletes in the current study trained ~800 h.year^{-1}across ~500 annual training sessions although there were individual differences. This finding is in line with previous studies reporting training volume in elite XC skiers [1,16–17]. Muscular loading differences and stress associated with different activities probably explain why there is large variation in reported annual training volume across sports. For example, top international runners are reported to train "only" 500–600 h.year^{-1} [7–8] while a case study of an international level triathlete reports >1000 h.year^{-1} [23]. The current data show a tendency for developments in training

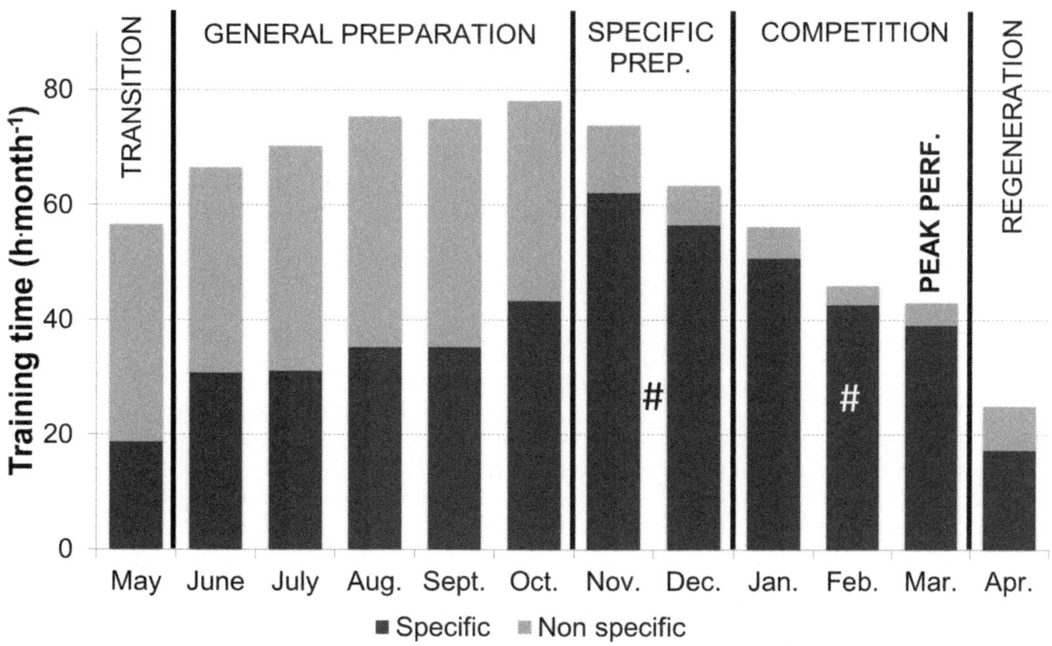

Figure 2. Annual organization of specific and non-specific activity forms. Endurance and sprint training time (h) distributed into specific (ski and roller ski) and non-specific (running, cycling and other) activity forms during each month and divided in phases. # Difference in specific training time vs. GP (P<.01).

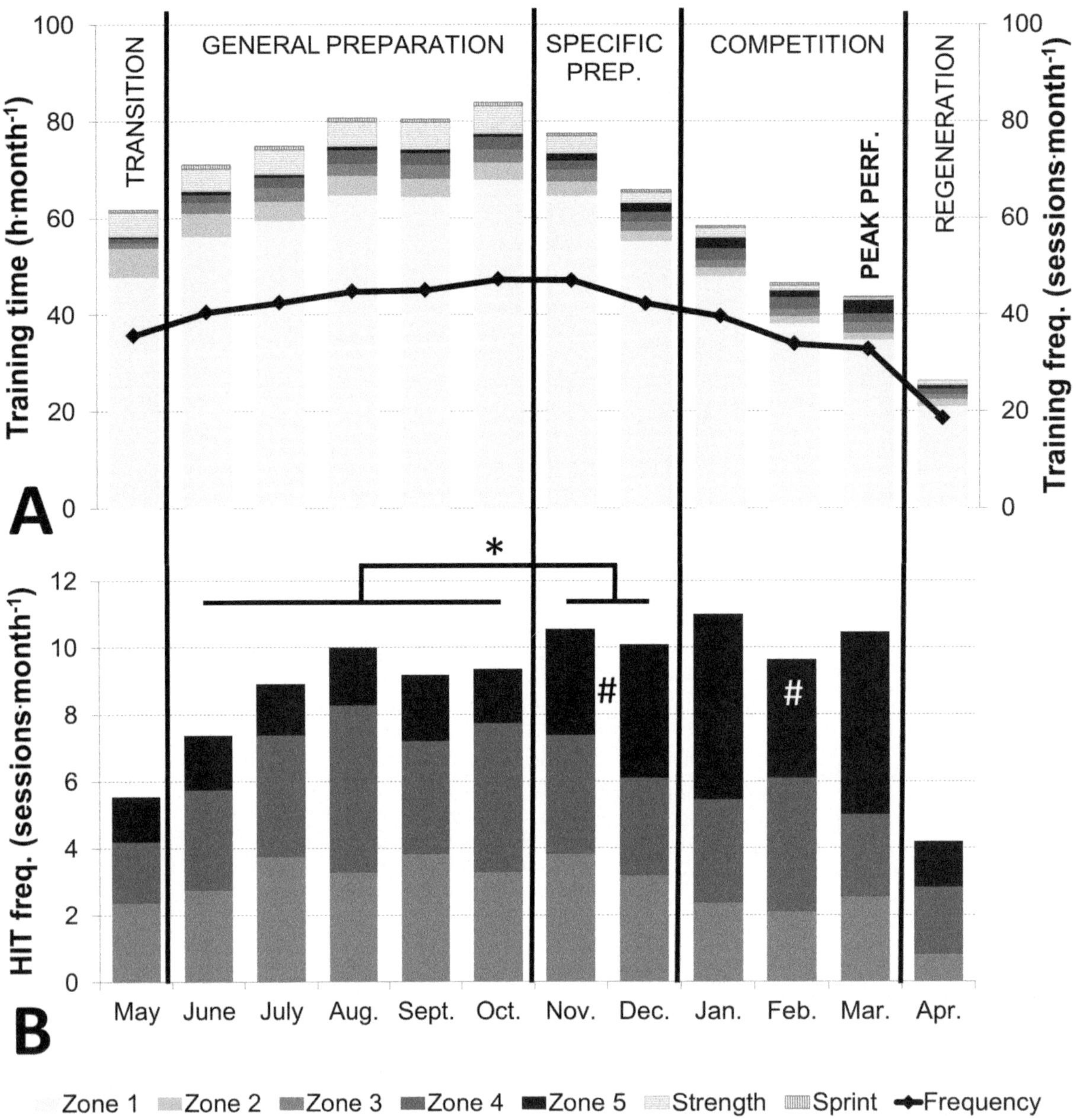

Figure 3. Annual training characteristics. A: Total training time (h) distributed into endurance training (zones 1–5), strength and sprint (bars, y-axis), and total training frequency (sessions) (line, z-axis) during each month and divided into phases. B: HIT frequency (sessions) distributed into zones 3, 4 and 5 (bars, y-axis) during each month and divided in phases. There was a statistically significant difference ($P<.05$) in total HIT sessions and zones 3, 4 and 5 respectively across the GP, SP and CP. Pairwise post-hoc tests showed: * Difference in total HIT sessions across phases ($P<.01$). # Difference between zone 5 sessions vs. GP ($P<.01$).

patterns during the time period from 1985 to 2011, with a positive relationship between total training volume and year of championship title ($r = .59$, $P = .055$). Increased training volume appears to be mainly due to increased frequency of training sessions from 1985 to 2011, while average duration per training session has remained relatively stable at 1.7 ± 0.2 h.

During the entire training year, 94% of all training *time* was executed as endurance training. However, strength and sprint training appear to play an important role in the training of XC skiers [45]. Strength training was carried out as general, specific or maximal, while sprints included both specific ski sprint-related exercises and jumps. Interestingly, ~90% of all strength and sprint training was executed during the preparation period (PP). In practice, this means two to three strength and sprints sessions.-week^{-1} in PP compared to one weekly session during CP, typically conducted at the end of endurance training sessions. The main underlying philosophy for these athletes was to build up a prescribed strength level during PP and then maintain this level during CP. Unfortunately, systematic strength testing documentation was not available for these athletes. We are therefore not able to verify whether strength characteristics of these athletes were stable during CP. However, previous research suggests that one bout of strength training per week is sufficient to maintain strength levels over shorter time frames [46].

Table 4. Weekly training patterns during different phases throughout the season.

				Competition phase			
Weekly training patterns	**Transition phase**	**General preparation phase**	**Specific preparation phase**	**Overall**	**Pre-peaking**	**Peaking**	**Regeneration phase**
Total training:							
Training time (h.wk^{-1})	13.9±5.3	17.9±2.5	16.5±2.4	11.6±2.2 $^{\#\beta}$	13.5±3.1 $^{\#\beta}$	12.1±2.4 $^{\#\beta}$	6.1±3.7
Tr. sessions·wk^{-1}	8.1±2.8	10.1±1.0	10.3±1.7	8.3±2.1 $^{\#\beta}$	8.9±1.9 $^{\#\beta}$	9.2±2.3	4.3±2.3
Training forms:							
Endurance (h·wk^{-1})	12.7±4.9	16.5±2.6	15.7±2.2	11.2±2.0 $^{\#\beta}$	12.9±2.8 $^{\beta}$	11.7±2.3 $^{\#\beta}$	5.9±3.6
Strength (h·wk^{-1})	1.1±1.0	1.2±0.5	0.7±0.4 *	0.3±0.2 $^{\#\beta}$	0.5±0.4 $^{\#}$	0.2±0.2 $^{\#\beta}$	0.2±0.3
Sprint (h·wk^{-1})	0.1±0.1	0.2±0.2	0.1±0.1	0.1±0.1	0.1±0.1	0.2±0.2	0.0±0.0
Intensity distribution:							
Zone 1 (h·wk^{-1})	10.8±4.7	14.3±2.6	13.8±2.1	9.4±2.3 $^{\#\beta}$	11.2±2.8 $^{\beta}$	9.7±2.0 $^{\#\beta}$	4.9±2.9
Zone 2 (h·wk^{-1})	1.3±0.9	0.9±0.6	0.6±0.5 *	0.4±0.3 $^{\#}$	0.4±0.5 $^{\#}$	0.6±0.8	0.3±0.5
Zone 3 (h·wk^{-1})	0.3±0.2	0.6±0.2	0.5±0.2	0.4±0.3	0.4±0.2 $^{\#}$	0.4±0.4	0.2±0.3
Zone 4 (h·wk^{-1})	0.2±0.2	0.5±0.2	0.4±0.3	0.5±0.3	0.5±0.4	0.7±0.4 $^{\beta}$	0.3±0.3
Zone 5 (h·wk^{-1})	0.1±0.1	0.2±0.1	0.4±0.2 *	0.5±0.3	0.4±0.3	0.2±0.3	0.2±0.2
Activity forms:							
Specific (h·wk^{-1})	4.3±3.3	8.1±1.7	13.7±2.3 *	10.3±1.5 $^{\#\beta}$	12.2±2.6 $^{\#}$	10.8±1.8 $^{\#}$	4.1±3.2
Non-Specific (h·wk^{-1})	8.5±4.6	8.6±1.5	2.1±1.2 *	1.0±0.6 $^{\#\beta}$	0.8±0.6 $^{\#\beta}$	1.0±1.0 $^{\#\beta}$	1.8±1.5

Values are mean ± SD and represent training hours per week in different phases. A non-parametric Friedman test indicated that there was a statistically significant difference in all variables across the GP, SP and CP (P<.05 level). A pairwise post-hoc test (Wilcoxon Signed Rank) was used to determine whether there was a statistically significant difference between the GP, SP or CP, as well as pre-peaking and peaking phases (P<.01 level).
*P<.01, GP vs. SP;
$^{\#}$P<.01, GP vs. CP, pre-peaking or peaking;
$^{\beta}$P<.01, SP vs. CP, pre-peaking or peaking;
†P<.01, pre-peaking vs. peaking.

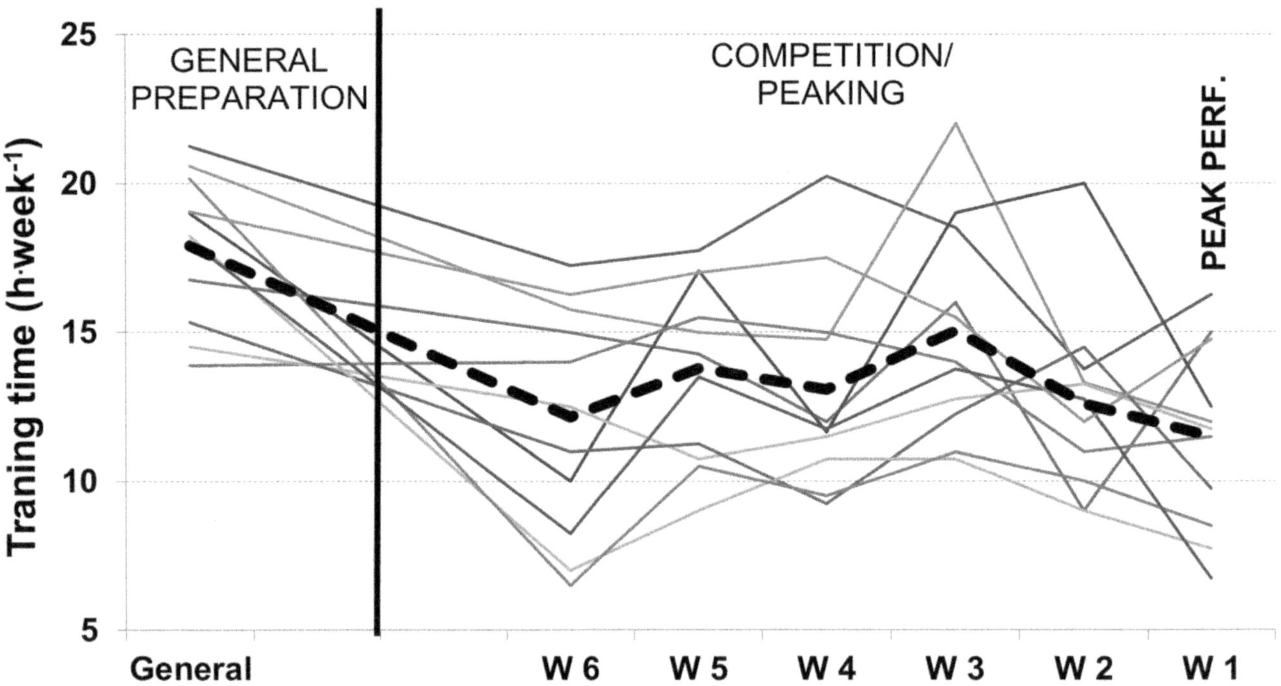

Figure 4. Individual peaking characteristics. Individual (lines) and average (dotted bold line) total weekly training volume during GP, and the last 6 weeks prior to championship title.

Activity forms. During the entire training year, 64% (~500 h) of all training was executed with sport-specific movement patterns (skiing/roller-skiing). However, over the course of the training year the amount of specific training increased from ~50 to 90%. That is, in line with the early periodization models [48], when training load was highest in PP only ~50% of all training was executed as ski or roller-ski. Otherwise, when training load was lowest in CP, >90% was performed as sport-specific training.

Sport-specific training is outlined as a key to improving $\dot{V}O_{2\max}$ [51–52]. Hence, a high portion of sport-specific training during the CP for these athletes appears to be essential in order to reach an international performance level. However, we maintain that a large volume of non-specific activity forms during PP serve an important purpose in increasing trainability and improving general aerobic capacity [53–54].

Intensity distribution. Recently there has been some debate regarding findings suggesting that HIT induces superior physiological and performance adaptations compared with LIT [47]. The trend among endurance athletes is to adopt a polarized intensity distribution model integrating both intensity domains [7,9,16,20,25]. The present data consistently demonstrate that these 11 gold medalists executed a large proportion of their total training as LIT throughout the annual cycle. Total LIT time was progressively increased during PP, in line with some key features from the early periodization models of Matwejew [48], before being reduced dramatically during CP. However, it is important to emphasize that the marked intensity shift to more HIT described in Matwejew's models was not observed in this group of elite athletes.

The current study contributes unique knowledge to our understanding of the self-selected duration and distribution of HIT in elite endurance sports. Depending on the quantification methods used [43], results from several other studies suggest that an approximate 80/20% LIT/HIT distribution is optimal, although the percentage of HIT varies from ~10–30% [7–9,14–16,44,49–50] using a time in training zone method [43]. However, in the current study only 9% of annual endurance training time, or ~60 h/~100 sessions were reported to be above LT[1]. This is in contrast to other top Olympic athletes reported to perform a greater amount of HIT in addition to high total training volume [23,28–29]. The total volume of HIT training was evenly distributed throughout the year with an average of 5±2 h or 9±3 sessions·month^{-1}. Interestingly, it was also found that HIT training sessions were distributed virtually equally among zones 3, 4 & 5, with average durations of 0.8/0.6/0.5 h in zones 3/4/5 respectively. However, from the PP to CP, both duration and frequency in zones 3 and 4 were maintained, while the frequency of zone 5 training sessions increased. That is, as the main performance peak came closer, LIT time decreased dramatically while HIT patterns shifted towards a more polarized model, despite virtually constant HIT training time.

Peaking practice

Training volume and specificity. Optimizing the reduction in training load during the peaking phase is believed to be a key to optimal championship performance [6,30]. Training load is described as a combination of training volume, intensity and frequency [27]. A meta-analysis conducted by Bosquet et al [5] concluded that athletes could maximize taper-associated benefits by reducing training volume by ~50%, without reducing training frequency or training intensity.

In line with current best practice [4–6], we defined the peaking phase as the last 14 days prior to the athletes' most successful competition (Olympic/World Championship gold medal), and compared training patterns in this final training phase to the penultimate phase beginning 4 weeks prior to the peaking phase (pre-peaking phase). With regards to training volume, we found

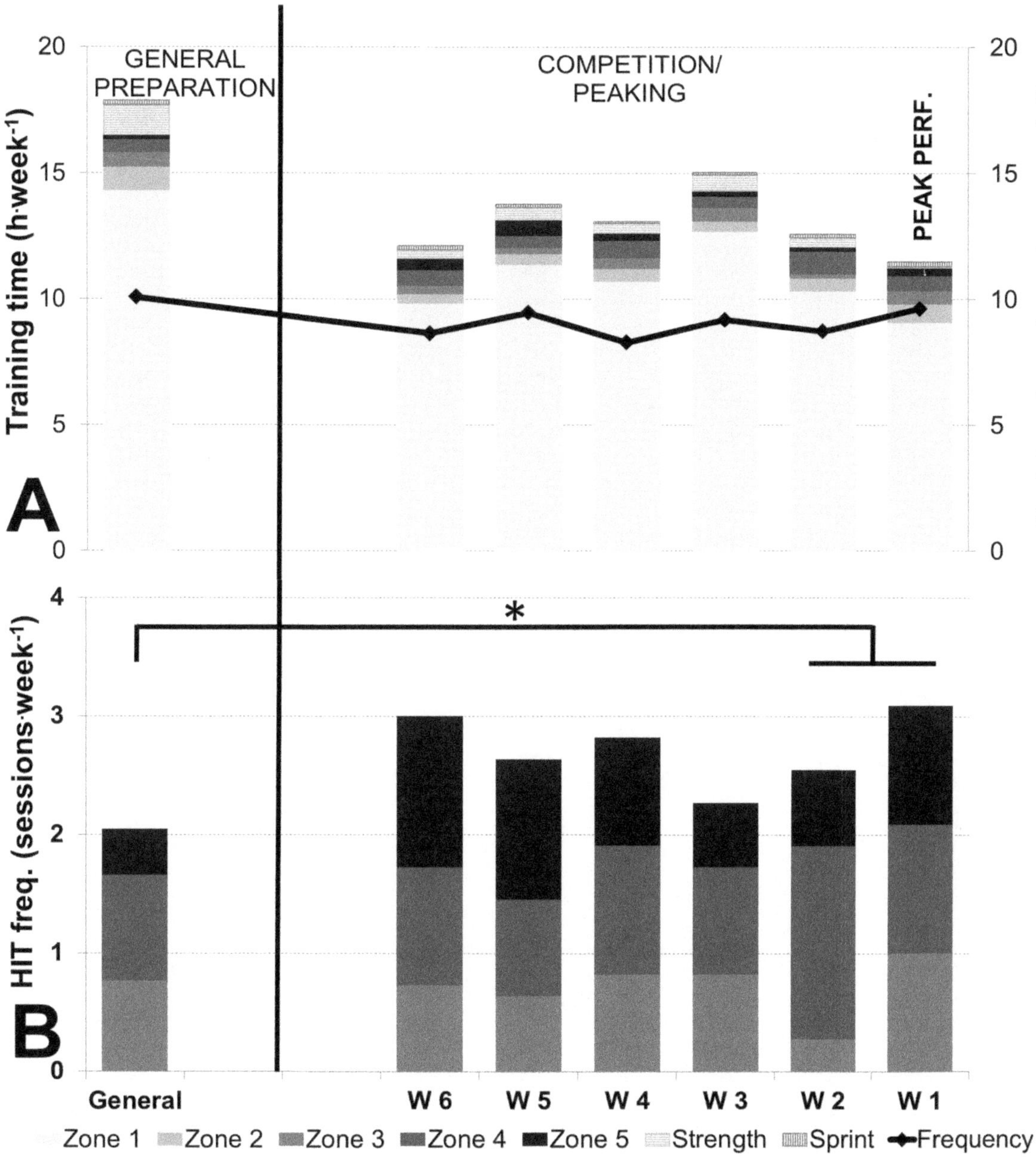

Figure 5. Peaking characteristics. A: Weekly training time (h) distributed into endurance training (zones 1–5), strength and sprints (bars, y-axis), and total training frequency (sessions) (line, z-axis) during GP, and during the last 6 weeks prior championship title. B: HIT frequency (sessions) distributed into zones 3, 4 and 5 (bars, y-axis) during GP, and during the last 6 weeks prior to championship title. There was a statistically significant difference ($P<.05$) in total HIT sessions and zones 3 and 5 respectively across GP, pre-peaking phase and peaking phase. Pairwise post-hoc tests showed: * Difference in total HIT sessions across phases ($P<.01$). There were no statistically significant differences in zones 3, 4 or 5 across phases.

only a 4 and 15% (NS) decrease in training volume during days -14 to -8 and days -7 to-1 respectively, compared to the pre-peaking phase. This is substantially less than the current taper recommendations of a ~50% reduction (Figure 6). It is possible to speculate as to why these champion athletes chose a strategy very different from experimentally derived optimum. Bosquet et al [5] reported no effect on performance if the reduction in training volume was 20% or less. However, there was large individual variation in peaking behavior in the current study, and no clear patterns emerged. In fact, 4 of the 11 athletes increased their training volume during the last seven days. However, existing research has limitations in terms of narrow focus on one single competition [32]. In contrast, our results demonstrate that competitions are frequently integrated into the peaking process in elite sports. The competition schedule, designed by the International Ski Federation, is crucial in planning a taper and must be integrated into the peaking regime. The WC season in these sports typically consists of two competition days per week over up to 14 weeks with a maximum of two to four competition free weeks. Such a schedule may interfere with an optimal tapering process. Rather than incorporating a single tapering phase, such a schedule may rather require the athlete to perform repeated "mini-tapers" prior to each competition.

Since there was minimal decrease (NS) in overall training volume during the four-week pre-peaking period, we chose to compare training performed during the peaking phase to GP, where weekly training volume was highest. Once the athletes started their WC season, in either XC or biathlon, their total training volume was consistently lower than that reported during GP. Relative to GP, training volume was, respectively, 29 and 35% lower during the penultimate and final weeks before each athlete's gold medal race. High competition stress load and frequent travel may dictate the reduced training volume during this phase, rather than a predetermined periodization model. These data indicate that peak training volume for these athletes was markedly dissociated in time from peak performance by up to 4 months, even accepting individual variations. It is unclear whether high training volume executed during PP 4–9 months prior still influences physical capacity during the peaking phase, following an extended period of reduced training volume where competitions themselves become a key source of HIT.

Several decades ago, Hickson et al [55] reported that trained athletes retain most of their physiological and endurance performance adaptations during 15 subsequent weeks of reduced training. However, for an Olympic athlete, even a small performance decrement associated with reduced training could be the difference between a medal and fourth place. Unfortunately, similar to strength performance, we do not have data for endurance tests throughout the year. Our objective testing data for these athletes terminates 3–4 months prior to their gold medal performances. In elite practice, laboratory testing typically ends when the competitive season begins. However, in a similar group of athletes with virtually identical training patterns as in the current study, Losnegaard et al [17] found that aerobic physiological adaptations were maintained, and performance and anaerobic adaptations were even enhanced, several months after peak training volume.

To our knowledge, no data are available providing mechanistic links that span such an extended time period. It is possible to speculate that a prolonged period of high training volume during PP could favorably alter genomic sensitivity to training during the season through epigenetic mechanisms [51]. Such cellular level adaptations to high training volume could be a mechanistic bridge linking PP training characteristics to training effects several months later, when high training volumes are precluded by the competition and travel stress load.

During both the pre-peaking phase and the peaking phase, virtually all (92%) training was conducted as XC skiing. This shift towards more specific movement patterns when competition approaches may explain why peak performance is possible even after several months with reduced training volume [51–52].

Training frequency. The athletes in the current study trained, on average, 8–10 sessions·week^{-1}, with no significant differences in training frequency between the peaking phase and other phases (Table 2). This finding is in line with current taper recommendations [4–6]. Nor were there any significant differences in the number of LIT or HIT sessions from the pre-peaking

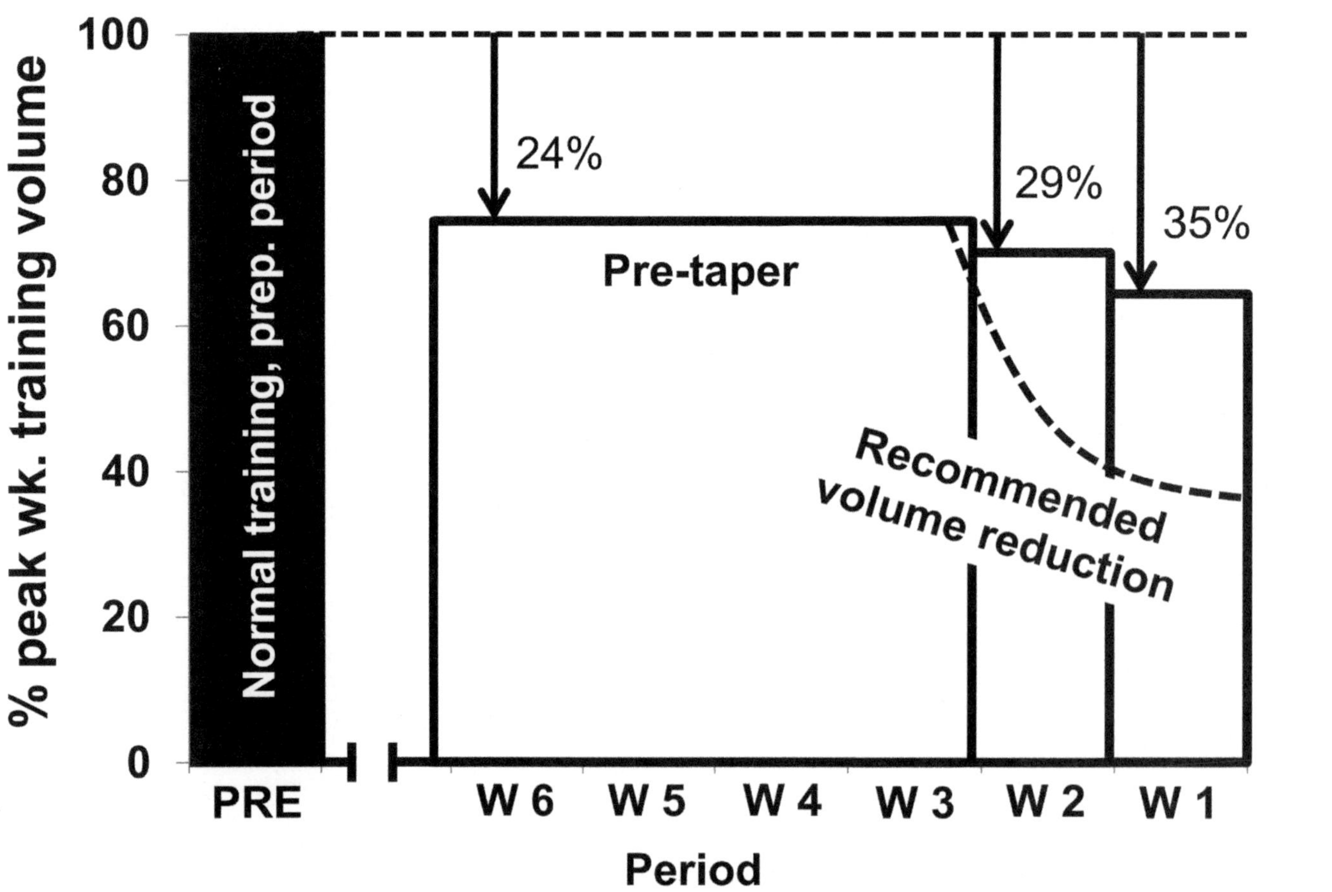

Figure 6. Taper comparison. Schematic representation of the actual taper observed in current study compared to recommended volume reduction. Adapted from Mujika & Padilla [4].

phase to the peaking phase. However, LIT frequency decreased from GP (8 sessions·week^{-1}) to the peaking phase (6 sessions·week^{-1}), indicating that the observed reduction in total LIT time was a result of both reduced session frequency and session duration.

Intensity distribution and rest days. Adaptive stimuli from HIT sessions appear to be a key component in maintaining and enhancing physiological and performance adaptations q during a taper period [36–37,39]. McNeely & Sandler [31] reported that frequent short HIT bouts >90% $\dot{V}O_{2max}$ are more effective than LIT to enhance endurance performance, and that, during a taper, steady-state workouts should be replaced by HIT intervals and short sprints in order to improve performance. Interestingly, we found that HIT duration did not change (1.3 h·week^{-1}) during any of the phases. However, HIT frequency increased from 2 sessions·week^{-1} in GP to 3 sessions·week^{-1} in the peaking phase ($P<.01$). In addition, there was a tendency towards increased sprint training duration from the pre-peaking phase to the peaking phase. Hence, HIT sessions during the peaking phase were typically executed more frequently but with shorter duration than during GP, alongside more frequent bouts of sport-specific "anaerobic sprint training". Examining distribution of training among intensity zones 3, 4 and 5, we observed a tendency toward a decrease in zones 3 and 4 and an increase in zone 5 in both duration and frequency from GP to CP. This suggests that total HIT duration did not change throughout the year, but that the actual executed intensity shifted towards a more polarized model as the major competition approached.

To our knowledge, details regarding best practice models of HIT patterns and recovery strategies during the final days prior to peak performance are lacking in the literature. However, the current data show that short bouts of HIT were performed evenly throughout the final 14 days (~5 sessions in total per athlete) (Figure 7). Interestingly, 10 out of 11 athletes performed a HIT session within 48 h of competition. The exact intensity during these HIT sessions is somewhat inconsistent, but was typically above LT^2. Competitions performed during the final days but not seen as "primary events" were also integrated into the peaking strategy. Whether these contribute to a beneficial peaking regime, or interfere with the optimal strategy is not clear. Eight of 11 athletes in the present study competed in at least one championship final prior to the event in which they won a gold medal. With regard to recovery strategies, rest days were typically concentrated in days 12 to 6. Among all 11 athletes, only 3 athletes took a rest day during the last 5 days, compared with 14 athlete rest days taken in the middle period of the peaking phase. That is, rest days were 3 times more likely to be taken during the middle portion of the peaking phase (days 12–6) compared with the final 5 days. However, it is not clear whether this organization of HIT and rest days during the final 14 days was the result of strategic planning to optimize performance, or merely coincidental. It has been previously reported that runners taking a rest every third day during a six day taper performed worse than those athletes who trained every day [56], and this topic may be a fruitful area for future research.

Altitude training. Altitude training is incorporated into the training of most world-class XC skiers, and is a consistent feature of Norwegian endurance training. For athletes in the current study, precise records are not available regarding all days spent at altitude or the specific altitude at which each training session was performed. For the last 2–3 decades, 4–6 annual training camps of 14–21 d duration living at 1800–2000 m above sea level and training at 1200 to 2800 m above sea level, have been integrated throughout the annual cycle. The aim of these altitude training camps is to stimulate increased hemoglobin mass, and specifically acclimate to competition venues located above 1400 m. The athletes in the current study typically spent 60 to 100 days training at altitude during the season quantified, although this was likely somewhat lower for those athletes winning gold prior to 1992. In addition, where championship events were held at moderate altitude (e.g. in Salt Lake City, 2002) altitude camps were also an important feature of the final weeks of training. Based on a previous study of 29 XC skiers training at altitude [43], objective data suggest that intensity distribution during altitude camps shifts towards lower intensity. Training at the highest aerobic intensities during such camps is essentially absent, unless it is performed at reduced altitudes. The likely impact of this emphasis on altitude training was to somewhat reduce the amount of HIT performed during PP.

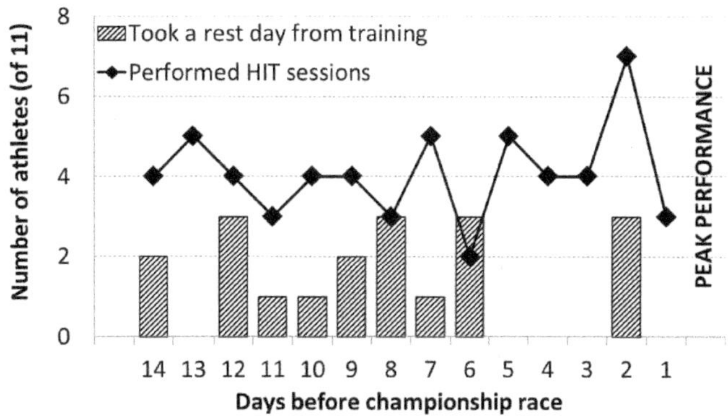

Figure 7. Peaking phase. Number of athletes (of 11) who performed HIT sessions (line) and number of athletes who took a rest day from training (bars) during the final 14 days prior to peak performance.

Winning an international title in endurance sports clearly requires outstanding physiological capacity and performance level. Controlled laboratory trials of world-class elite athletes are challenging, and training literature based on less well-trained individuals may be misleading when linking findings to elite athletes. Our current data outlines unique and accurate day-to-day training data throughout a season that concluded with each athlete winning an Olympic or World championship title. Experimental approaches may in many ways be artificial, while descriptive training studies allow investigation of elite endurance athletes in a real-life situation. This may therefore provide a fruitful foundation from which to generate novel experimental research questions.

We did not find evidence of athletes following the current tapering recommendations regarding training volume reduction. However, when comparing training patterns during the peaking phase to training executed during PP several months earlier, we found a picture more analogous to that derived from experimental studies, although the magnitude of training time reduction was still lower. It is possible to speculate as to whether the medal-winning performances of these athletes was truly representative of their best possible performance, or if they could have skied even faster had they followed recommended tapering strategies specifically for that one event. On the other hand, the more progressive reduction in training time from GP to CP observed in the current study, continued to a lesser degree throughout the CP up until the major competition, may be the ideal strategy in sports where the competition schedule is organized as it is in XC skiing and biathlon. A three month competition phase during which athletes are typically required to compete once or twice every week, precludes the application of the recommended tapering strategy presented in the research literature. Regardless, the performance of these athletes was sufficient to beat the rest of the field on the day, and take home the gold medal.

A central concern in a descriptive study such as this, where training self-report is the key data source, is whether the data are accurate and valid. We have recently demonstrated that elite endurance athletes report their training accurately, although we found some small discrepancies related to intensity distribution [57]. We believe the current data represent the same validity as shown in Sylta et al [57], since both athlete groups used similar monitoring routines, and some of the athletes are, in fact, represented in both papers. In addition, athletes recorded their training on a daily basis, which likely reduced reporting error.

Conclusions

These data show that winning an international title in XC skiing or biathlon requires a training load of ~800 h/500 sessions·year^{-1}, of which ~500 h is executed as sport-specific movement patterns. Endurance training time for these athletes was distributed as approximately 90% LIT and 10% HIT, equal to a ~80/20% SG distribution. Training volume was highest during GP and decreased progressively during SP and CP. Concurrently, the proportion of sport-specific training increased markedly. Total amount of HIT remained stable across all phases, although HIT training patterns tended to become more polarized in CP.

These athletes did not appear to incorporate a taper in the final weeks leading up to competition, with training volume, frequency and intensity remaining unchanged from the pre-peaking phase to the peaking phase. Hence, we did not observe the recommended ~50% training volume reduction that has been proposed as the optimal tapering strategy based on previous experimental studies. However, there was a clear reduction in training volume from GP to the peaking phase. This reduction was almost entirely due to a reduction in non-sport-specific LIT with virtually all training during the pre-peaking phase and the peaking phase composed of ski training. Only three out of 11 athletes incorporated a rest day in the final five days leading up to the best athletic performance of their career, A very large training load during the GP appears to be an important precondition for exceptional athletic performance several months later, although exactly how training loads in June-October are mechanistically connected to performance several months later remains unclear.

Author Contributions

Conceived and designed the experiments: ET SS. Performed the experiments: EH IS ET ØS. Analyzed the data: ET ØS SS IS TH. Contributed reagents/materials/analysis tools: ET EH. Contributed to the writing of the manuscript: ET EH ØS SS IS TH.

References

1. Tønnessen E (2009) Hvorfor ble de beste best? En casestudie av kvinnelige verdensenere i orientering, langrenn og langdistanseløp. Oslo: Norges Idrettshøgskole. 299 p.
2. Seiler S, Tønnessen E (2009) Intervals, Thresholds, and Long Slow Distance: the Role of Intensity and Duration in Endurance Training. Sportscience 13: 1–27.
3. Seiler S (2010) What is Best Practice for Training Intensity and Duration Distribution in Endurance Athletes? Int J Sports Physiol Perform 5: 276–291.
4. Mujika I, Padilla S (2003) Scientific bases for precompetition tapering strategies. Med Sci Sports Exerc 35: 1182–7.
5. Bosquet L, Montpetit J, Arvisais D, Mujika I (2007) Effects of tapering on performance: a meta-analysis. Med Sci Sports Exerc 39: 1358–65.
6. Le Meur Y, Hausswirth C, Mujika I (2012) Tapering for competition: A review. Science & Sports 27: 77–87.
7. Billat V, Demarle A, Slawinski J, Paiva M, Koralsztein JP (2001) Physical and training characteristics of top-class marathon runners. Med Sci Sports Exerc 33: 2089–2097.
8. Billat V, Lepretre PM, Heugas AM, Laurence MH, Salim D, et al. (2003) Training and bioenergetic characteristics in elite male and female Kenyan runners. Med Sci Sports Exerc 35: 297–304.
9. Esteve-Lanao J, San Juan AF, Earnest CP, Foster C, Lucia A (2005) How Do Endurance Runners Actually Train? Relationship with Competition Performance. Med Sci Sports Exerc 37: 496–504.
10. Karp J R (2008) Training characteristics of US Olympic Marathon Trials qualifiers. New Studies in Athletics 23: 31–37.
11. Ingham SA, Fudge BW, Pringle JS (2012) Training Distribution, Physiological Profile, and Performance for a Male International 1500-m Runner. Int J Sports Physiol Perform 7: 193–195.
12. Stellingwerff T (2012) Case study: Nutrition and training periodization in three elite marathon runners. Int J Sport Nutr Exerc Metab 22: 392–400.
13. Schumacher OY, Mueller P (2002) The 4000-m team pursuit cycling world record: Theoretical and practical aspects. Med Sci Sports Exerc 34: 1029–1036.
14. Zapico AG, Calderón FJ, Benito PJ, González CB, Parisi A, et al. (2007) Evolution of physiological and haematological parameters with training load in elite male road cyclists: A longitudinal study. J Sports Med Phys Fitness 47: 191–196.
15. Seiler KS, Kjerland GØ (2006) Quantifying training intensity distribution in elite endurance athletes: is there evidence for an "optimal" distribution? Scand J Med Sci Sports 16: 49–56.
16. Sandbakk O, Holmberg HC, Leirdal S, Ettema G (2011) The physiology of world-class sprint skiers. Scand J Med Sci Sports 21: 9–16.
17. Losnegard T, Myklebust H, Spencer M, Hallén J (2013) Seasonal variations in VO2max, O2-cost, O2-deficit and performance in elite cross-country skiers. J Strength Cond Res 27: 1780–1790.
18. Gao J (2008) A Study on Pre-Game Training Characteristics of Chinese Elite Swimmers. J Beijing Sport Univ 31: 832–834.
19. Siewierski M (2010) Volume and structure of training loads of top swimmers in direct starting preparation phase for main competition. Pol J Sport Tourism 17: 227–232.
20. Fiskerstrand Â, Seiler KS (2004) Training and performance characteristics among Norwegian International Rowers 1970–2001. Scand J Med Sci Sports 14: 303–310.
21. Guellich A, Seiler S, Emrich E (2009) Training Methods and Intensity Distribution of Young World-Class Rowers. Int J Sports Physiol Perform 4: 448–460.
22. Neal CM, Hunter AM, Galloway SD (2011) A 6-month analysis of training-intensity distribution and physiological adaptation in Ironman triathletes. J Sports Sci 29: 1515–23.
23. Mujika I (2013) Olympic Preparation of a World-Class Female Triathlete. Int J Sports Physiol Perform: In press.
24. Hongjun Y, Chen X, Zhu W, Cao C (2012) A Quasi-Experimental Study of Chinese Top-Level Speed Skaters' Training Load: Threshold Versus Polarized Model. Int J Sports Physiol Perform 7: 103–112.
25. Orie J, Hofman N, de Koning JJ, Foster C (2014) Thirty-eight years of training distribution in olympic speed skaters. Int J Sports Physiol Perform 9: 93–9.
26. Garcia-Pallares J, García-Fernández M, Sánchez-Medina L, Izquierdo M (2010) Performance changes in world-class kayakers following two different training periodization models. Eur J Appl Physiol 110: 99–107.
27. Wenger HA, Bell GJ (1986) The Interactions of Intensity, Frequency and Duration of Exercise Training in Altering Cardiorespiratory Fitness. Sports Med 3: 346–356.
28. Tjelta LI (2013) A Longitudinal Case Study of the Training of the 2012 European 1500 m Track Champion. Int J Appl Sports Sci 25: 11–18.
29. Tjelta LI, Tønnessen E, Enoksen E (2014) A case study of the training of nine times New York Marathon winner Grete Waitz. Int J Sports Sci Coach 9: 139–159.
30. Mujika I, Chatard JC, Busso T, Geyssant A, Barale F, et al. (1995) Effects of training on performance in competitive swimming. Can J Appl Physiol 20: 395–406.
31. Mujika I, Padilla S, Pyne D (2002) Swimming performance changes during the final 3 weeks of training leading to the Sydney 2000 Olympic Games. Int J Sports Med 23: 582–7.
32. McNeely E, Sandler D (2007) Tapering for endurance athletes. Strength Cond J 29: 18–24.
33. Pyne D B, Mujika I, Reilly T (2009) Peaking for optimal performance: Research limitations and future directions. J Sports Sci 27: 195–202.
34. Thomas L, Busso T (2005) A theoretical study of taper characteristics to optimize performance. Med Sci Sports Exerc 37: 1615–1621.
35. Mujika I (1998) The influence of training characteristics and tapering on the adaptation in highly trained individuals: a review. Int J Sports Med 19: 439–46.
36. Hickson RC, Foster C, Pollock ML, Galassi TM, Rich S (1985) Reduced Training Intensities and Loss of Aerobic Power, Endurance, and Cardiac Growth. J Appl Physiol 58: 492–499.

37. Shepley B, MacDougall JD, Cipriano N, Sutton JR, Tarnopolsky MA, et al. (1992) Physiological-Effects of Tapering in Highly Trained Athletes. J Appl Physiol 72: 706–711.
38. Houmard JA, Scott BK, Justice CL, Chenier TC (1994) The Effects of Taper on Performance in Distance Runners. Med Sci Sports Exerc 26: 624–631.
39. Mujika I (2010) Intense training: the key to optimal performance before and during the taper. Scand J Med Sci Sports 20: 24–31.
40. NSF (1992) Treningsdagbok – Langrenn. Oslo: Norges Skiforbund.
41. NSF (1985) Treningsdagbok - Langrenn. Oslo: Norges Skiforbund.
42. NSSF (1991) Treningsdagbok - Skiskyting. Oslo: Norges Skiskytterforbund.
43. Sylta O, Tonnessen E, Seiler S (2014) From heart-rate data to training quantification: a comparison of 3 methods of training-intensity analysis. Int J Sports Physiol Perform 9: 100–7.
44. Lucia A, Hoyos J, Carvajal A, Chicharro JL (1999) Heart rate response to professional road cycling: the Tour de France. Int J Sports Med 20: 167–172.
45. Sandbakk O, Holmberg HC (2014) A reappraisal of success factors for olympic cross-country skiing. Int J Sports Physiol Perform 9: 117–121.
46. Rønnestad B, Hansen E, Raastad T (2010) In-season strength maintenance training increases well-trained cyclists' performance. Eur J Appl Physiol 110: 1269–1282.
47. Laursen PB (2010) Training for intense exercise performance: high-intensity or high-volume training? Scand J Med Sci Sports 20: 1–10.
48. Matwejew L (1975) Periodisierung des sportlichen trainings, 2nd ed. Berlin: Bartels & Wernitz.
49. Lucia A, Hoyos J, Santalla A, Earnest C, Chicharro JL (2003) Tour de France versus Vuelta a Espana: which is harder? Med Sci Sports Exerc 35: 872–878.
50. Esteve-Lanao J, Foster C, Seiler S, Lucia A (2007) Impact of training intensity distribution on performance in endurance athletes. J Strength Cond Res 21: 943–949.
51. Tanaka H (1994) Effects of cross-training – transfer of training effects on VO_{2max} between cycling, running and swimming. Sports Med 18: 330–339.
52. Foster C, Hector LL, Welsh R, Schrager M, Green MA, et al. (1995) Effects of specific versus cross-training on running performance. Eur J Appl Physiol 70: 367–372.
53. Steinacker JM, Lormes W, Lehmann M, Altenburg D (1998) Training of rowers before world championships. Med Sci Sports Exerc 30: 1158–1163.
54. Bompa T (1999) Periodization: Theory and methodology of training (4th ed.). Champaign, IL: Human Kinetics.
55. Hickson RC, Kanakis C Jr, Davis JR, Moore AM, Rich S (1982) Reduced Training Duration Effects on Aerobic Power, Endurance, and Cardiac Growth. J Appl Physiol 53: 225–229.
56. Mujika I, Goya A, Ruiz E, Grijalba A, Santisteban J, Padilla S (2002) Physiological and performance responses to a 6-day taper in middle-distance runners: influence of training frequency. Int J Sports Med 23: 367–373.
57. Sylta O, Tonnessen E, Seiler S (2014) Do elite endurance athletes report their training accurately? Int J Sports Physiol Perform 9: 85–92.

Influence of Exercise on Bone Remodeling-Related Hormones and Cytokines in Ovariectomized Rats: A Model of Postmenopausal Osteoporosis

Lihui Li[1¶], Xi Chen[1,4¶], Shuang Lv[1], Miaomiao Dong[1], Li Zhang[1], Jiaheng Tu[1], Jie Yang[1], Lingli Zhang[1], Yinan Song[1], Leiting Xu[1,3]*, Jun Zou[2]*

1 School of Kinesiology, Shanghai University of Sport, Shanghai, China, **2** Scientific Research Department, Shanghai University of Sport, Shanghai, China, **3** Medical School of Ningbo University, Ningbo, China, **4** School of Sports Science, Wenzhou Medical University, Wenzhou, China

Abstract

This study aims to explore the effects of exercise on postmenopausal osteoporosis and the mechanisms by which exercise affects bone remodeling. Sixty-three Wistar female rats were randomly divided into five groups: (1) control group, (2) sham-operated group, (3) OVX (Ovariectomy) group, (4) DES-OVX (Diethylstilbestrol-OVX) group, and (5) Ex-OVX (Exercise-OVX) group. The rat osteoporosis model was established through ovariectomy. The Ex-OVX rats were made to run 251.2 meters every day, 6 d/wk for 3 months in a running wheel. Trabecular bone volume (TBV%), total resorption surface (TRS%), trabecular formation surface (TFS%), mineralization rate (MAR), bone cortex mineralization rate (mAR), and osteoid seam width (OSW) were determined by bone histomorphometry. The mRNA and protein levels of interleukin-1β (IL-1β_2), interleukin-6 (IL-6), and cyclooxygenase-2 (Cox-2) were determined by *in situ* hybridization and immunohistochemistry, respectively. Serum levels of estrogen estradiol (E_2), calcitonin (CT), osteocalcin (BGP), and parathyroid hormone (PTH) were determined by ELISA assays. The investigation revealed that compared to the control and the sham-operated groups, the OVX group showed significantly lower levels of TBV%, E_2, and CT, but much higher levels of TRS%, TFS%, MAR, OSW, BGP, and PTH. The Ex-OVX group showed increased TBV% and serum levels of E_2 and CT compared to the OVX group. Ovariectomy also led to a significant increase in IL-1β mRNA and protein levels in the bone marrow and IL-6 and Cox-2 protein levels in tibias. In addition, the Ex-OVX group showed lower levels of IL-1 mRNA and protein, IL-6 mRNA, and Cox-2 mRNA and protein than those in the OVX group. The upshot of the study suggests that exercise can significantly increase bone mass in postmenopausal osteoporosis rat models by inhibiting bone resorption and increasing bone formation, especially in trabecular bones.

Editor: Luc Malaval, Université de Lyon - Université Jean Monnet, France

Funding: This work was supported by Shanghai Key Lab of Human Sport Competence Development and Maintenance (Shanghai University of sport) (NO. 11DZ2261100), The National Natural Science Foundation of China (Grant No. 81170323). The funders had no role in study design, data collection and analysis, decision to publish, or preparation of the manuscript.

Competing Interests: The authors have declared that no competing interests exist.

* Email: zoujun777@126.com (JZ); xuleiting@nbu.edu.cn (LX)

¶ These authors are co-first authors on this work.

Background

Osteoporosis is a major health problem among the elderly and is characterized by low bone mineral density (T score for bone mineral density below 2.5) and microarchitectural deterioration of bone, leading to increased fracture risks [1]. Osteoporosis is prevalent among women, in particular postmenopausal women. Estrogen shortage/deficiency results in an increase in bone turnover, wherein the rate of osteoclastic resorption exceeds the rate of osteoblastic osteogenesis, leading to a net loss of bone mass. Many studies have indicated that hormone replacement therapies (HRT) can be used to prevent and/or treat postmenopausal osteoporosis. However, long-term estrogen supplementation poses several risks, e.g., endometrial cancer, breast cancer, ovarian cancer, and cardiovascular diseases, and is no longer recommended [2,3].

Previous studies suggest that estrogen may inhibit osteoclast activity through regulating the levels of serum CT and PTH [4]. Estrogen stimulates the synthesis of CT, which directly inhibits osteoclast differentiation and activity, and thus reduces the number of osteoclasts and serum concentration of Ca^{2+} [5]. PTH is one of the most important peptide hormones that regulate calcium and phosphorus homeostasis and bone remodeling [6]. Estrogen can decrease the expression of PTH and lead to a decrease in serum levels of PTH [7]. Estrogen also inhibits PTH-stimulated adenylate cyclase activity and thus PTH-stimulated bone resorption [8]. In addition, estrogen shortage has been found to increase serum levels of BGP (Bone Gla Protein) in postmenopausal women. BGP, also known as γ-carboxyglutamic acid protein, is a hormone-like peptide synthesized and secreted by osteoblasts [9]. BGP is not only an indicator of *in vivo* bone formation rate but also a positive regulator of bone mineralization.

In addition to these hormones, estrogen inhibits bone resorption by suppressing secretion of key osteolytic cytokines such as IL-1 and IL-6 by bone marrow stromal cells and osteoblasts. These cytokines are positive regulators of osteoclast activity and bone resorption [10,11]. Besides, these cytokines may crosstalk with each other to synergistically promote osteoclastogenesis and bone resorption. For example, IL-1, including both IL-1α and IL-1β subunits, can induce osteoblasts to secrete IL-6 to further promote bone resorption [11]. Estrogen, IL-1β, and IL-6 also regulate PGE production, which promotes proliferation and differentiation of osteoclast precursors. Previous studies have reported that PGE_2 could also stimulate bone resorption by increasing IL-6 transcription [12,13]. Furthermore, IL-1 was found to increase COX-2 expression at the mRNA and protein levels, leading to an increase in prostaglandin production. The stabilization of COX-2 mRNA is the most important basis of continued increase in COX-2 protein [14].

Previous studies have shown that increased physical activity is effective in maintaining or even increasing bone and muscle mass in postmenopausal women [15]. Appropriate long-term exercise helps to prevent the development of postmenopausal osteoporosis [16]. Exercise is also effective in maintaining BMD in early postmenopausal women. Kemmler et al. reported that exercises that can improve muscle function might improve overall fitness, maintain bone health, and reduce fall risk [17]. Thus, exercise has been proposed as a preventative measure for osteoporosis. However, the exact mechanisms by which exercise regulates bone remodeling and improves bone quality remain unclear. In animal studies, exercise is generally considered to increase the peak bone mass. Joo et al. showed that treadmill running improves trabecular bone microarchitecture, bone density, and cortical geometry in young growing female rats [18]. Tromp et al. showed that mechanical loading has beneficial effects on bone mineral content (BMC) and bone mineral density of ovariectomized rats [19]. Sakakura et al. showed that exercise has a beneficial effect on tibia and the neck of the condyloid process in ovariectomized rats, probably by increasing serum levels of progesterone [20]. However, how exercise exerts its beneficial effects on bone is not well understood.

We hypothesize that exercise executes its positive influence on bone mass and quality by regulating the synthesis of hormones and cytokines that are involved in bone remodeling. We found that exercise escalates the levels of estrogen in OVX rats, which may suppress the expression of bone resorption stimulators such as CT, IL-1, and IL-6, to inhibit bone resorption. Moreover, we found that exercise also increases bone formation in ovariectomized rats although the mechanisms need further investigation. The results demonstrate that exercise assists in preventing bone loss in rat model of postmenopausal osteoporosis.

Materials and Methods

Animals

This study was carried out in strict accordance with the recommendations from the Ethical Committee of Shanghai University of Sports on the Care and Use of Animal Subjects in Research (Permit Number: [2008](2)), following the protocols approved by the committee. All animals were housed in a temperature- and humidity-controlled environment with a 12 h light/12 h dark cycle with free access to food (standard laboratory chow) and water *ad libitum*. All surgery was performed under sodium pentobarbital anesthesia, and all possible efforts were made to minimize suffering.

Surgical Procedures

A total of 63 female Wistar rats (200 g to 220 g) were obtained from the Laboratory Animal Center of the Academy of Military

Table 1. The mRNA sequence of IL-1β target genes.

Group	The mRNA sequence of IL-1β target genes							
No.1	5′	ACAAA	ATACC	TGTGG	CCTTG	GGCCT	CAAGG	3′
No.2	5′	GAAGA	AGATG	GAAAA	GCGAT	TTGTC	TTCAA	3′
No.3	5′	CAACT	GGTAC	ATCAG	CACCT	CTCAA	GCAGA	3′

Table 2. The mRNA sequence of IL-6 target genes.

Group	The mRNA sequence of IL-6 target genes							
No.1	5′	CTCCG	CAAGA	GACTT	CCAGC	CAGCT	GCCTT	3′
No.2	5′	CTTCC	AAACT	GGATA	TAACC	AGGAA	ATTTG	3′
No.3	5′	ATTTC	TAAAG	GTCAC	TATGA	GGTCT	ACTCG	3′

Table 3. The mRNA sequence of COX-2 target genes.

Group	The mRNA sequence of COX-2 target genes							
No.1	5′	ATGTA	TGAGT	GTGGG	ATTTG	ACCAG	TATAA	3′
No.2	5′	GAACG	TTGTG	AATAA	CATTC	CCTTC	CTTCG	3′
No.3	5′	TGCCT	CAATT	CAGTC	TCTCA	TCTGC	AATAA	3′

Medical Sciences, PCLA (License No. SCXK-(military) 2002-001) and maintained in the Laboratory Animal Rooms (License No. SYK11-00-0039) of the Institute of Basic Theory, Chinese Academy of Chinese Medical Sciences. The rats were randomly divided into five groups: control group (n = 13), sham-operated group (n = 13), OVX group (n = 13), DES-OVX group (n = 13), and Ex-OVX group (n = 11). Rats in the OVX group, the DES-OVX group, and the Ex-OVX group were ovariectomized. To remove the ovaries, rats were anesthetized using an intraperitoneal injection of pentobarbital sodium (48 mg/kg) while in prone position. They were shaved along the midaxillary line, 0.5 cm away from the lateral border of the spine below the last rib, exposing the surgical field. An incision on the skin was made on one side through the musculature and peritoneum, and the ovary was subsequently retracted and removed. Tubal ligation was performed, and then the wound was closed. The same procedure was repeated on the other side. The procedure was also performed on rats belonging to the sham-operated group, except that the ovaries of these rats were retracted and put back into their abdomen and some adipose tissues around their ovaries were removed.

Physical exercise protocol for animals

Two and a half months after surgery, a two-week acclimation period of wheel running training was conducted. Rats in the Ex-OVX group were given access to a running wheel (40 cm diameter, homemade) for 10 min on d 1, with an increase of 10 min/d thereafter until 1 h/d was reached. Wheel revolutions and running distance were counted and automatically recorded using a counter. Three months after surgery, rats in the Ex-OVX group were made to run 200 revolutions (251.2 meters) in the running wheel every day, 6 d/wk for 3 months. Rats belonging to the DES-OVX group were intragastrically administered with Diethylstilbestrol (0.045 mg/kg; concentration, 0.0045 mg/ml; Beijing Yimin Pharmaceutical Co., Ltd., Batch No. H11020899). The control, OVX, and sham-operated groups were given distilled water every day, 6 d/wk for 3 months.

Animal tissue preparation

Rats in all groups were given two intraperitoneal injections of tetracycline hydrochloride (30 mg/kg; Aozehui Technology and Trade Company, US22105) 3 and 16 d before exercising. Five and a half months after surgery, all rats were anesthetized using an intraperitoneal injection of pentobarbital sodium (45 mg/kg; Beijing Tongxian Yucai Fine Chemical Works, Batch No. 950427). When rats appeared to clamping as judged by independent animal care personnel with no knowledge of the protocol design, they were euthanized by Carbon monoxide in a box. Then rats' blood samples were collected from the femoral arteries. The tibias were harvested, with the right tibias being used for undecalcified bone sections to determine bone morphometric indices and the left ones being used for decalcified bone frozen sections for in situ hybridization to detect IL-1β, IL-6, and COX-2 mRNA levels. The blood obtained from the femoral arteries was centrifuged (2000 r/min) and the supernatant was collected. The serum was transferred to an Eppendorf tube and preserved at −20°C for future detection of E2, calcitonin, osteocalcin, and parathyroid hormone.

Bone histomorphometry

The proximal one-third of the right tibias of the rats were obtained and the soft tissues, along with some cortex at both ends, were removed. The samples were dehydrated in increasing concentrations of ethanol (twice at each concentration, each time for 24 h), and xylene was used as a transparency agent (50% ethanol + 50% xylene 30 min, and xylene 30 min twice). The next step was resination of the samples by immersing them in the solutions described below: Solution I: 75 ml methyl methacrylate (Beijing Yili Fine Chemical Co. Ltd., Batch No. 960523), 25 ml dibutyl phthalate (DBP; Beijing Chemical Reagent Company, Batch No. 970628); Solution II: 1 g benzoyl peroxide (Beijing Jinlong Chemical Reagent Co. Ltd., Batch No. 20000420) added to Solution I; Solution III: 2.5 g benzoyl peroxide added to Solution I. Each of these solutions was mixed using a magnetic stirrer. The specimens were sequentially immersed in Solutions I, II, and III, for 36 hrs each. Afterwards, 5 ml of Solution III was injected into a small bottle containing penicillin. The specimens were placed in the bottle. The closed bottle was then placed in an incubator. Polymerization was performed at 40°C for 3 d to 4 d. A hard, colorless, transparent block with embedded samples was formed. The block was taken out and shaped using a file. The resulting undecalcified bone sections were cut at a thickness of 5 or 10 μm on a microtome (Autocut 2040, Reichert-Jung, Heidelberg, Germany) with a tungsten steel blade. The 5 μm-thick undecalcified bone sections were placed in methyl methacrylate for 2 h and then twice in xylene, each time for 1 h. After deresination, the sections were again dehydrated with increasing concentrations of ethanol and stained with toluidine blue. The 10 μm-thick undecalcified bone sections were directly subjected to fluorescence observation.

Leica QWin image analysis software was used to determine the morphometric indices of the undecalcified bone sections using the method reported by Liu [21]. The morphometric indices of trabecular bone, including trabecular bone volume (TBV%), total

Table 4. TBV, TRS, and TFS percentages in the five groups.

Group	TBV%	TRS%	TFS%
control group	31.75±6.23	3.65±1.32	4.07±1.21
sham-operated group	31.05±5.88	3.76±1.37	3.91±1.29
OVX group	13.21±3.91$^{□□**}$	9.48±2.63$^{□□**}$	7.92±1.76$^{□□**}$
DES-OVX group	25.81±4.79$^{□*△△}$	5.09±1.79$^{□*△△}$	5.31±1.37$^{□*△△}$
Ex-OVX group	16.90±4.52$^{□□**△▲▲}$	8.59±1.65$^{□□**▲▲}$	9.58±1.56$^{□□**△▲▲}$

compared with the control group: $^{□}p<0.05$, $^{□□}p<0.01$;
compared with the sham-operated: $^{*}p<0.05$, $^{**}p<0.01$;
compared with the OVX group: $^{△}p<0.05$, $^{△△}p<0.01$;
compared with the DES-OVX group: $^{▲▲}p<0.01$.

Table 5. The levels of MAR, mAR, and OSW in the five groups.

Group	MAR (μm/d)	mAR (μm/d)	OSW (μm)
control group	1.31±0.25	1.98±0.38	10.17±1.90
sham-operated group	1.49±0.27	2.11±0.32	9.77±1.90
OVX group	2.52±0.40□□**	3.31±0.56□□**	16.79±3.85□□**
DES-OVX group	1.73±0.33△△	2.06±0.31△△	10.32±2.63△△
Ex-OVX group	2.22±0.33□□**▲▲	2.62±0.36□□**△△▲▲	14.85±2.25□□**▲▲

compared with the control group: □□$p<0.01$;
compared with the sham-operated: **$p<0.01$;
compared with the OVX group: △△$p<0.01$;
compared with the DES-OVX group: ▲▲$p<0.01$.

resorption surface (TRS%), trabecular formation surface (TFS%), and mineralization rate (MAR), as well as those of the inner surface of the cortex bone, including osteoid seam width (OSW) and bone cortex mineralization rate (mAR), were calculated.

Quantitation of IL-1β, IL-6, and COX-2

The proximal one-third of the left tibias of the rats was harvested with the soft tissues removed. The tibias were then fixed in 4% paraformaldehyde for 24 h, fully rinsed using PBS, and decalcified for 3 wk at 4°C using 10% EDTA/PBS. The decalcification solution was changed every other day. The decalcified bones were rinsed with PBS and then dehydrated in 15% sucrose solution/PBS for 24 h. Frozen sections were later cut at 10 μm on a refrigerated microtome (BRIGHT–5030, UK).

Immunohistochemical staining was used to detect IL-1β, IL-6, and COX-2 protein levels. IL-1β, IL-6, and COX-2 mRNA levels in the rat tibias were determined using in situ hybridization kits (Wuhan Boster Biological Technology, Ltd.). Oligonucleotide probes for IL-1β, IL-6, and COX-2 were labeled with digoxin. The mRNA sequences transcribed from the human IL-1β genes are shown in **Table 1**. The only difference among the sequences of rat, mouse, and human lies on 1 bp/90 bp. The mRNA sequences transcribed from the rat and mouse IL-6 genes are shown in **Table 2**. The mRNA sequences transcribed from the human COX-2 target genes are shown in **Table 3**. The only difference among the sequences of rat, mouse, and human lies on 5 bp/90 bp. In the morphometric analysis that used the Leica Q Win image analysis software, a positive reaction was indicated by brown coloration of the cytoplasm. More than five high-power fields (×400) below the epiphyseal plate within the medullary cavity were randomly picked and analyzed. The mRNA and protein level of IL-6 and COX-2 in osteoblasts was determined by the ratio of positive cells area per trabecular area in high-power field, and the mRNA and protein level of IL-1β in bone marrow was determined by the ratio of positive cells area per high-power field (without trabecular area), the mean was calculated and recorded as the percentage of positively reacting cells (%).

Measurement of serum CT, BGP, PTH, and E_2

ELISA assays were adapted to determine the levels of serum CT, BGP, PTH, and E_2. ELISA kits for rat BGP, CT, and PTH were purchased from Market Company (Batch Nos. RE030, IR108, and IR067) and the E_2 kit was purchased from Tianjing Jiuding Biomedical Engineering Ltd. (Batch No. ESBL4287).

Statistical analysis

Data are presented as mean ± standard deviation. Statistical evaluation was performed using one-way ANOVA. Data were compared between groups, and a Q-test was performed.

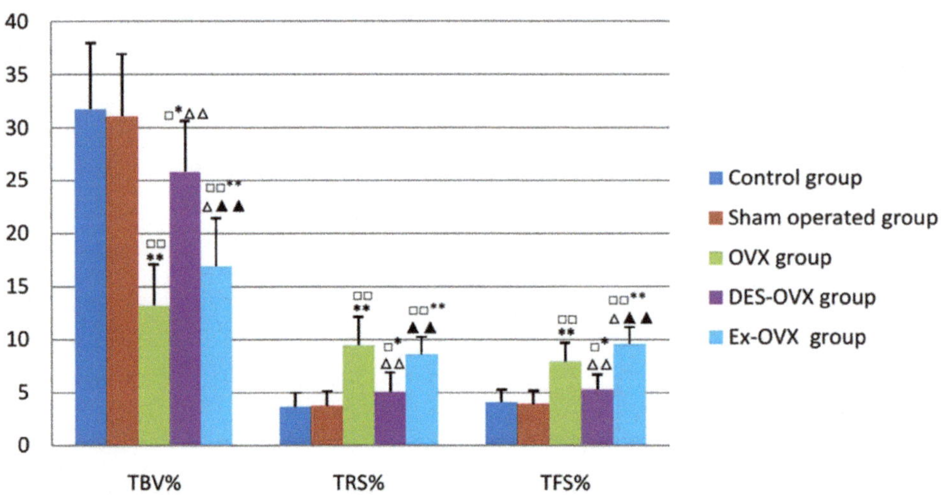

Figure 1. TBV, TRS, and TFS percentages in the five groups. compared with the control group: □$p<0.05$, □□$p<0.01$; compared with the sham-operated: *$p<0.05$, **$p<0.01$; compared with the OVX group: △$p<0.05$, △△$p<0.01$; compared with the DES-OVX group: ▲▲$p<0.01$.

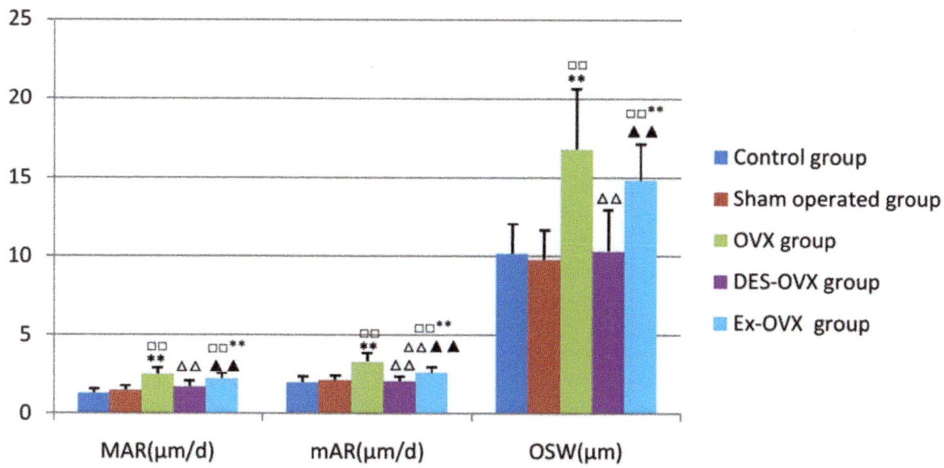

Figure 2. MAR, mAR, and OSW in the five groups. compared with the control group: $^{\square\square}p<0.01$; compared with the sham-operated: $^{**}p<0.01$; compared with the OVX group: $^{\triangle\triangle}p<0.01$; compared with the DES-OVX group: $^{\blacktriangle\blacktriangle}p<0.01$.

Significant differences were considered at $p<0.05$ and highly significant differences at $p<0.01$.

Results

In this study, we studied the effects of exercise on bone remodeling parameters of ovariectomized rats by histomorphometry and explored whether bone remodeling-related hormones and cytokines are involved.

Effect of exercise on bone histomorphometric parameters

As shown in **Table 4 and Figure 1**, the TBV% of the OVX group was significantly lower than the control and the sham-operated groups, which was accompanied by increased TRS, confirming that ovariectomy led to increased bone resorption and bone loss in rats. Moreover, the OVX group rats also showed higher levels of TFS%, MAR, mAR, and OSW than the control and sham-operated group rats (**Table 5 and Figure 2**), suggesting that these rats also displayed increased bone formation, which is likely caused by the coupling between bone resorption and formation. Thus, ovariectomized rats showed high bone turnover rate, with the increase in bone resorption being greater than that in bone formation. These findings are in accordance with previous studies and suggest that the surgery was successful in this study. To confirm these findings, we also treated ovariectomized rats with DES and found that DES almost completely reversed the bone loss and restored the bone parameters. In addition, none of the parameters was significantly different between the sham-operated group and the normal control group, which excludes the impact of surgical factors.

More importantly, exercise significantly increased the bone mass in the Ex-OVX group rats, which could be attributable to a decrease in bone resorption and an increase in bone formation, as TRS% was decreased whereas TFS% was increased compared to the OVX group. These bone histomorphometric parameters were measured in trabecular bones. On the other hand, the cortical bone parameters including MAR, mAR, and OSW were slightly decreased in the EX-OVX rats compared to OVX rats. These results suggest exercise can inhibit bone resorption and increase trabecular bone formation, which helps to prevent further bone loss in ovariectomized rats.

Effect of exercise on serum levels of CT, BGP, PTH, and E_2

We then analyzed some of the hormones that are involved in bone remodeling, especially the hormones whose levels are altered in post-menopausal osteoporotic patients and animal models. As shown in **Table 6 and Figure 3**, rats in the OVX group had much lower E_2 whereas DES-OVX rats showed E2 levels that were comparable to the control rats. Interestingly, exercise significantly increased serum levels of E2, which might be

Table 6. The levels of CT, BGP, PTH, and E_2 in the five groups.

Group	CT (pg/ml)	BGP (ng/ml)	PTH (pg/ml)	E2 (pg/ml)
control group	9.98 ± 1.33	4.76 ± 0.90	41.72 ± 9.14	40.36 ± 15.91
sham-operated group	10.13 ± 1.24	4.94 ± 1.03	42.30 ± 12.52	40.87 ± 19.61
OVX group	$5.88\pm1.02^{\square\square**}$	$10.14\pm1.06^{\square\square**}$	$54.03\pm10.27^{\square\square*}$	$5.09\pm1.07^{\square\square**}$
DES-OVX group	$8.78\pm1.09^{\square**\triangle\triangle}$	$3.09\pm1.06^{\square\square**\triangle\triangle}$	$44.13\pm6.60^{\triangle\triangle}$	$37.38\pm12.78^{\triangle\triangle}$
Ex-OVX group	$7.30\pm1.61^{\square\square**\triangle\blacktriangle}$	$8.85\pm1.81^{\square\square**\triangle\blacktriangle\blacktriangle}$	$51.65\pm11.83^{\square}$	$6.98\pm1.46^{\square\square**\triangle\triangle\blacktriangle\blacktriangle}$

compared with the control group: $^{\square}p<0.05$, $^{\square\square}p<0.01$;
compared with the sham-operated: $^{*}p<0.05$, $^{**}p<0.01$;
compared with the OVX group: $^{\triangle}p<0.05$, $^{\triangle\triangle}p<0.01$;
compared with the DES-OVX group: $^{\blacktriangle}p<0.05$, $^{\blacktriangle\blacktriangle}p<0.01$.

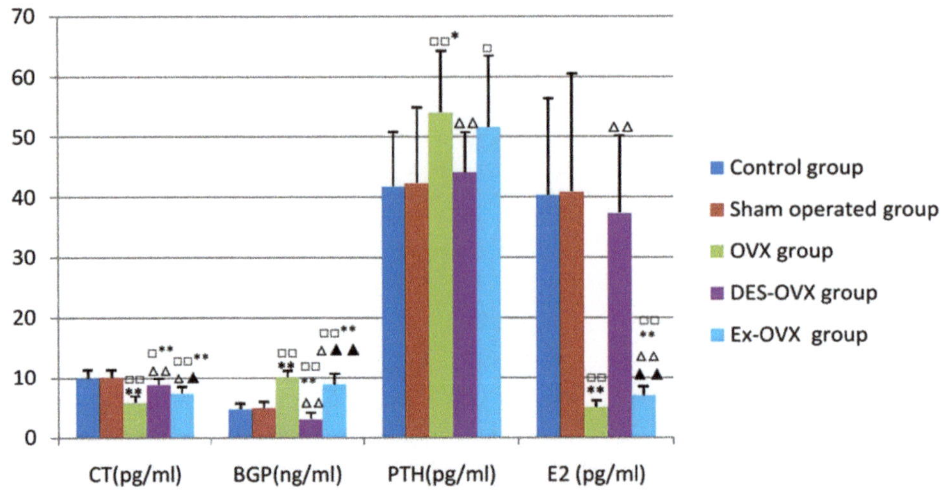

Figure 3. CT, BGP, PTH, and E_2 in the five groups. compared with the control group: □$p<0.05$, □□$p<0.01$; compared with the sham-operated: *$p<0.05$, **$p<0.01$; compared with the OVX group: △$p<0.05$, △△$p<0.01$; compared with the DES-OVX group: ▲$p<0.05$, ▲▲$p<0.01$.

synthesized and secreted by organs other than the ovary [22]. The increase in E2 levels was expected to inhibit bone resorption.

Moreover, the levels of CT, a negative regulator of osteoclast differentiation and activity, were decreased in OVX rats. On the other hand, the levels of PTH, a positive regulator of bone resorption, were increased in the OVX group compared to the control and the sham-operated groups. Additionally, the change in these two hormones was restored to close to normal levels in the DES-OVX group. These results suggest that estrogen deficiency led to a decrease in CT but an increase in PTH in ovariectomized rat. Furthermore, the levels of BGP, an osteoblast-produced hormone that promotes bone mineralization and acts as an indicator of in vivo bone formation rate, was also increased in ovariectomized rats. These results are consistent with our finding that estrogen deficiency leads to enhanced bone formation, in which BGP might play a positive role.

We also found that rats in the Ex-OVX group showed higher levels of CT and lower levels of BGP than the OVX rats, without significantly changing the levels of PTH. Note that the Ex-OVX group still showed lower levels of CT and E2, as well as higher levels of BGP and PTH, than the control and the sham-operated groups. These findings suggest that exercise may inhibit bone loss and prevent osteoporosis by regulating the serum levels of CT, PTH, and BGP.

Alteration of protein levels of IL-1β in the bone marrow and IL-6 and COX-2 in tibias

As shown in **Table 7 and Figure 4**, the OVX rats showed an increase in the protein levels of IL-1β, IL-6, and COX-2 compared to the control and the sham-operated groups, which were all restored to normal levels in the DES-OVX group, suggesting that estrogen deficiency is the reason behind the alteration of the expression of these proteins. Moreover, we found that the Ex-OVX group had much lower levels of IL-1β, IL-6, and COX-2 than the OVX group. These results suggest that exercise could partially inhibit the expression of IL-1β, IL-6, and COX-2, which helps to suppress bone resorption.

Alteration of mRNA levels of IL-1β in the bone marrow and IL-6 and COX-2 in tibias

To validate the above finding, we also analyzed the mRNA levels of these proteins on bone sections by in situ hybridization. As shown in **Table 8 and Figure 5**, the OVX rats showed much higher levels of IL-1β, IL-6, and COX-2 mRNA than the control and the sham-operated groups, which were restored to normal levels in the DES-OVX group. Moreover, the Ex-OVX group rats showed much lower levels of IL-1β, IL-6, and COX-2 mRNA than the OVX group. These results suggest that exercise could inhibit the expression of these cytokines at the mRNA level.

Table 7. IL-1β, IL-6, and COX-2 protein levels in the five groups.

Group	IL-1βprotein expression (%)	IL-6protein expression (%)	COX-2protein expression (%)
control group	4.84±1.17	5.32±0.92	5.04±0.94
sham-operated group	5.30±1.24	5.41±1.07	5.26±1.08
OVX group	10.76±1.80□□**	8.64±1.65□□**	11.36±2.14□□**
DES-OVX group	5.18±1.05△△	6.03±1.25△△	5.69±0.99△△
Ex-OVX group	7.48±1.37□□**△△▲▲	7.65±1.20□□**▲▲	7.99±1.50□□**△△▲▲

compared with the control group: □□$p<0.01$;
compared with the sham-operated: **$p<0.01$;
compared with the OVX group: △△$p<0.01$;
compared with the DES-OVX group: ▲▲$p<0.01$.

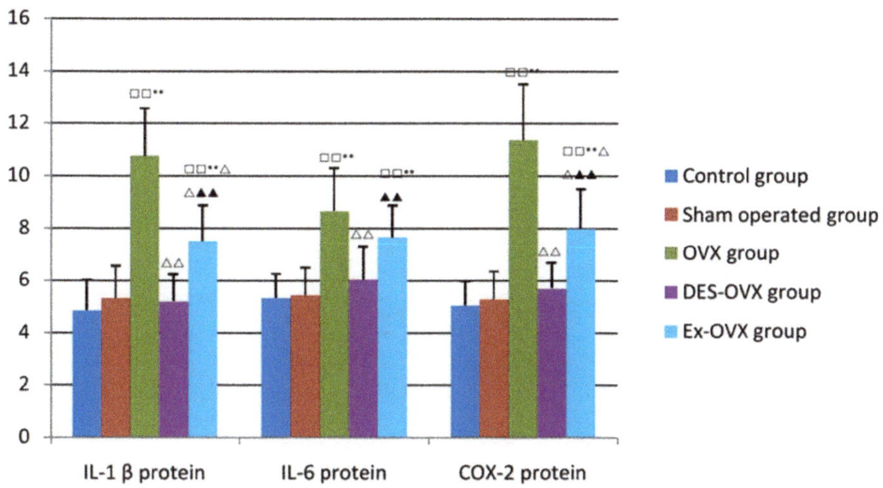

Figure 4. IL-1β, IL-6, and COX-2 protein expression in the five groups. compared with the control group: □□$p<0.01$; compared with the sham-operated: **$p<0.01$; compared with the OVX group: △△$p<0.01$; compared with the DES-OVX group: ▲▲$p<0.01$.

Discussion

Ovariectomized rats and mice are well-established models for the study of the pathogenesis of postmenopausal osteoporosis and are widely used for evaluation and development of new drugs for treatment of postmenopausal osteoporosis [23–25]. Here we used the rat model to study the possible effect of exercise on bone remodeling. Consistent with the previous results, we found that ovariectomized rats exhibited a significant decrease in bone mass, whereas bone resorption indexes TRS%, PTH, and bone formation markers TFS%, MAR, OSW, mAR, and BGP, were all significantly increased. This finding indicates that ovariectomy increases bone turnover rate, wherein bone resorption outpaces bone formation, leading to the development of osteoporosis. Moreover, DES was found to reverse all these changes in ovariectomized rats.

Previous studies have shown that osteoporosis-related bone loss in postmenopausal rat was partially prevented by moderate exercise [26–28]. Our findings support this concept and provide more histomorphometric evidence. Rats in the EX-OVX group showed higher TBV% than those in the OVX group, indicating that running wheel improves cancellous bone in ovariectomized rats. Compared to the OVX group, the EX-OVX group rats showed a modest decrease in bone resorption rate, which is correlated with an increase in serum levels of estrogen and CT. On the other hand, exercise increased bone formation, especially of trabecular bones, which is reflected by an increase in TFS%. However, bone formation rate at the endosteal surface of cortical bones in the EX-OVX group was lower than that in the OVX group, suggesting that exercise may differentially regulate bone formation in trabecular and cortical bones. It seems that exercise can partially prevent estrogen deficiency-induced bone loss by suppressing bone resorption and increasing bone formation. While it is still debated whether decreased bone resorption or increased bone formation is the main reason behind exercise-induced bone mass elevation [29,30], our results support the involvement of both events.

Estrogen exerts its anti-osteoporotic activity by directly or indirectly regulating bone resorption [31,32]. While there is convincing evidence that estrogen, acting via estrogen receptor α, stimulates osteoclast apoptosis and suppresses osteoblasts apoptosis [33], estrogen has been shown to act on MSCs and osteoblasts to regulate the expression of cytokines and growth factors that control osteoclast differentiation and activity. Since long-term HRT has adverse effects, caution is expected in choosing HRT for prevention and treatment of osteoporosis in women [34,35]. On the other hand, a number of studies have shown that appropriate intensities of exercise can increase serum levels of estradiol and testosterone, which helps to improve osteoblast proliferation and activity, leading to an increase in bone mass and density [36,37].

Table 8. IL-1β, IL-6, and COX-2 mRNA levels in the five groups.

Group	IL-1βmRNA expression (%)	IL-6mRNA expression (%)	COX-2mRNA expression (%)
control group	6.17±0.99	5.48±1.08	5.28±1.01
sham-operated group	6.14±1.10	5.68±1.13	5.14±1.13
OVX group	11.20±2.02□□**	9.07±1.33□□**	10.49±1.36□□**
DES-OVX group	6.59±1.23△△	5.53±1.10△△	5.52±1.00△△
Ex-OVX group	9.45±1.53□□**△▲▲	7.90±1.05□□**△▲▲	7.81±1.38□□**△△▲▲

compared with the control group: □□$p<0.01$;
compared with the sham-operated: **$p<0.01$;
compared with the OVX group: △$p<0.05$, △△$p<0.01$;
compared with the DES-OVX group: ▲▲$p<0.01$.

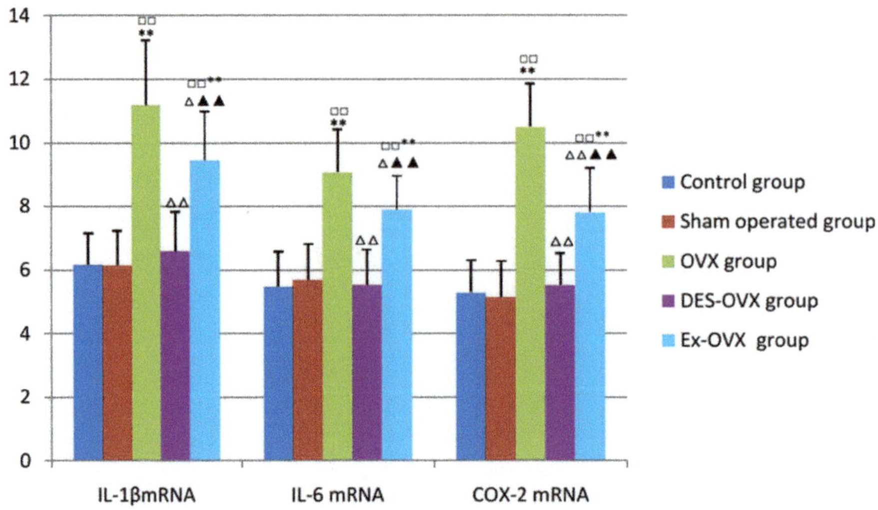

Figure 5. IL-1β, IL-6, and COX-2 mRNA expression in the five groups. compared with the control group: □□$p<0.01$; compared with the sham-operated: ** $p<0.01$; compared with the OVX group: △$p<0.05$, △△$p<0.01$; compared with the DES-OVX group: ▲▲$p<0.01$.

However, some clinical studies showed that the estrogen levels were unchanged in response to exercise [38]. This discrepancy could be caused by the difference in the intensities of exercise, the age and ethnicity of the patients, or both. Nevertheless, this study shows that wheel running increases serum E_2 in ovariectomized rats, which can slow down bone loss induced by ovariectomy. In addition, the levels of CT, an inhibitor of osteoclast differentiation and activity [5], are also decreased after ovariectomy, likely due to estrogen shortage. Indeed, previous studies have shown that estrogen stimulates the synthesis of CT [4]. We found that exercise also increases the levels of CT in ovariectomized rats, which might be a result of increased estrogen.

We found that the OVX group rats showed higher levels of BGP and PTH than the control group. BGP is a hormone-like peptide synthesized and secreted by osteoblasts and is significantly increased in the serum of postmenopausal women [9]. It has pro-minerilization function and is an indicator of in vivo bone formation rate. Thus, it is possible that estrogen regulates bone formation and bone resorption thorugh these two hormones as well. The observation that supplementation with diethylstilbestrol reversed the alteration in BGP and PTH expression in ovariectomized rats suggests that estrogen deficiency is the underlying cause for the change in BGP and PTH levels. In addition, we found that exercise decreases the levels of BGP in ovariectomized rats, which might be due to the increase in the E2 levels.

Our study further showed that the protein and mRNA levels of the bone marrow IL-1β and osteoblastic IL-6 and COX-2 were increased in ovariectomized rats. The change in the levels of these proteins was highly related to $E_{2,}$ as there is no significant difference between the DES-OVX group and the sham-operated group. Charatcharoenwitthaya et al. demonstrated that in humans, like in rodents, part of the effects of estrogen deficiency on increased bone resorption is mediated by IL-1 [39]. Moreover, IL-6 can enhance osteoclastogenesis in vivo and in vitro, which could be prevented by 17 beta-estradiol or an antibody against IL-6. Thus, IL-1 and IL-6 play critical roles in estrogen-regulated osteoclastogenesis. Moreover, IL-1 and IL-6 regulate the expression of Cox-2 and therefore the production of PGE_2, which also increases osteoclast activity and bone resorption [40]. Our study revealed that exercise could effectively decrease the mRNA and protein levels of IL-1, IL-6, and Cox-2 in ovariectomized rats. These results, taken together, suggest that exercise may regulate serum levels of the hormones and cytokines via E2, to inhibit bone resorption and to prevent further bone loss in estrogen deficiency-induced osteoporosis models.

While therapeutic HRT inhibits both osteogenesis and bone resorption, with inhibition of bone resorption being the dominant effect, we found that exercise inhibits bone resorption but increases osteogenesis. The dual beneficial effects of exercise may have positive impact on bone geometry in addition to bone mass and density. As such, an increasing number of researchers are considering using exercise or combination of exercise with drugs such as bisphosphonates to treat osteoporosis [41,42].

Conclusions

Overall, our study revealed that exercise acts on both bone formation and bone resorption to slow down bone loss in ovariectomized rat models. Exercise not only increases the serum levels of E2 but also affects the expression of hormones that play critical roles in bone remodeling, such as CT, BGP and PTH. Moreover, exercise also inhibits the expression of IL-1, IL-6, and Cox-2 to negatively regulate osteoclastogenesis and bone resorption. However, the interaction between these cytokines and hormones needs further investigation.

Author Contributions

Conceived and designed the experiments: JZ. Performed the experiments: SL MD. Analyzed the data: LZ JY. Contributed reagents/materials/analysis tools: LZ JT. Wrote the paper: LL LX YS XC. Provided suggestions and wrote most of the revised version: XC LX.

References

1. Nih Consensus Development Panel on Osteoporosis Prevention D, Therapy (2001) Osteoporosis prevention, diagnosis, and therapy. JAMA 285: 785–795.
2. Lacey JV, Jr., Mink PJ, Lubin JH, Sherman ME, Troisi R, et al. (2002) Menopausal hormone replacement therapy and risk of ovarian cancer. JAMA 288: 334–341.
3. Nelson HD, Humphrey LL, Nygren P, Teutsch SM, Allan JD (2002) Postmenopausal hormone replacement therapy: scientific review. JAMA 288: 872–881.
4. Doggrell SA (2004) Recent important clinical trials of drugs in osteoporosis. Expert Opin Pharmacother 5: 1635–1638.
5. Karsdal MA, Henriksen K, Arnold M, Christiansen C (2008) Calcitonin: a drug of the past or for the future? Physiologic inhibition of bone resorption while sustaining osteoclast numbers improves bone quality. BioDrugs 22: 137–144.
6. Gesty-Palmer D, Luttrell LM (2011) 'Biasing' the parathyroid hormone receptor: a novel anabolic approach to increasing bone mass? Br J Pharmacol 164: 59–67.
7. Carrillo-Lopez N, Roman-Garcia P, Rodriguez-Rebollar A, Fernandez-Martin JL, Naves-Diaz M, et al. (2009) Indirect regulation of PTH by estrogens may require FGF23. J Am Soc Nephrol 20: 2009–2017.
8. Nakamura M, Udagawa N, Matsuura S, Mogi M, Nakamura H, et al. (2003) Osteoprotegerin regulates bone formation through a coupling mechanism with bone resorption. Endocrinology 144: 5441–5449.
9. Price PA, Parthemore JG, Deftos LJ (1980) New biochemical marker for bone metabolism. Measurement by radioimmunoassay of bone GLA protein in the plasma of normal subjects and patients with bone disease. J Clin Invest 66: 878–883.
10. Edwards CJ, Williams E (2010) The role of interleukin-6 in rheumatoid arthritis-associated osteoporosis. Osteoporos Int 21: 1287–1293.
11. Kwan Tat S, Padrines M, Theoleyre S, Heymann D, Fortun Y (2004) IL-6, RANKL, TNF-alpha/IL-1: interrelations in bone resorption pathophysiology. Cytokine Growth Factor Rev 15: 49–60.
12. Subbaramaiah K, Marmo TP, Dixon DA, Dannenberg AJ (2003) Regulation of cyclooxgenase-2 mRNA stability by taxanes: evidence for involvement of p38, MAPKAPK-2, and HuR. J Biol Chem 278: 37637–37647.
13. Denkert C, Weichert W, Winzer KJ, Muller BM, Noske A, et al. (2004) Expression of the ELAV-like protein HuR is associated with higher tumor grade and increased cyclooxygenase-2 expression in human breast carcinoma. Clin Cancer Res 10: 5580–5586.
14. de Araujo Junior RF, Souza TO, de Medeiros CA, de Souza LB, Freitas Mde L, et al. (2013) Carvedilol decrease IL-1beta and TNF-alpha, inhibits MMP-2, MMP-9, COX-2, and RANKL expression, and up-regulates OPG in a rat model of periodontitis. PLoS One 8: e66391.
15. Going S, Lohman T, Houtkooper L, Metcalfe L, Flint-Wagner H, et al. (2003) Effects of exercise on bone mineral density in calcium-replete postmenopausal women with and without hormone replacement therapy. Osteoporos Int 14: 637–643.
16. Evans EM, Racette SB, Van Pelt RE, Peterson LR, Villareal DT (2007) Effects of soy protein isolate and moderate exercise on bone turnover and bone mineral density in postmenopausal women. Menopause 14: 481–488.
17. Kemmler W, von Stengel S, Engelke K, Haberle L, Kalender WA (2010) Exercise effects on bone mineral density, falls, coronary risk factors, and health care costs in older women: the randomized controlled senior fitness and prevention (SEFIP) study. Arch Intern Med 170: 179–185.
18. Joo YI, Sone T, Fukunaga M, Lim SG, Onodera S (2003) Effects of endurance exercise on three-dimensional trabecular bone microarchitecture in young growing rats. Bone 33: 485–493.
19. Tromp AM, Bravenboer N, Tanck E, Oostlander A, Holzmann PJ, et al. (2006) Additional weight bearing during exercise and estrogen in the rat: the effect on bone mass, turnover, and structure. Calcif Tissue Int 79: 404–415.
20. Sakakura Y, Shide N, Tsuruga E, Irie K, Yajima T (2001) Effects of running exercise on the mandible and tibia of ovariectomized rats. J Bone Miner Metab 19: 159–167.
21. Liu SQ (1996) Plastic-embedded undecalcified bone tissue glasscutter slicing technology. Chinese Journal of Pathology 25: 49.
22. Wood CE, Stavisky RC, Nowak J, Kaplan JR (2012) Stimulatory adrenocortical effects of a selective estrogen receptor modulator in ovariectomized female macaques. Toxicol Pathol 40: 55–61.
23. Saville PD (1969) Changes in skeletal mass and fragility with castration in the rat; a model of osteoporosis. J Am Geriatr Soc 17: 155–166.
24. Inada M, Matsumoto C, Miyaura C (2011) [Animal models for bone and joint disease. Ovariectomized and orchidectomized animals]. Clin Calcium 21: 164–170.
25. Chachra D, Lee JM, Kasra M, Grynpas MD (2000) Differential effects of ovariectomy on the mechanical properties of cortical and cancellous bone in rat femora and vertebrae. Biomed Sci Instrum 36: 123–128.
26. Barengolts EI, Curry DJ, Bapna MS, Kukreja SC (1993) Effects of endurance exercise on bone mass and mechanical properties in intact and ovariectomized rats. J Bone Miner Res 8: 937–942.
27. Chen Y, Wang S, Bu S, Wang Y, Duan Y, et al. (2011) Treadmill training prevents bone loss by inhibition of PPARgamma expression but not promoting of Runx2 expression in ovariectomized rats. Eur J Appl Physiol 111: 1759–1767.
28. Winters-Stone KM, Dobek J, Nail LM, Bennett JA, Leo MC, et al. (2013) Impact + resistance training improves bone health and body composition in prematurely menopausal breast cancer survivors: a randomized controlled trial. Osteoporos Int 24: 1637–1646.
29. Iwamoto J, Takeda T, Ichimura S (1998) Effects of moderate intensity exercise on tibial bone mass in mature ovariectomized rats: bone histomorphometry study. Keio J Med 47: 162–167.
30. Barengolts EI, Lathon PV, Curry DJ, Kukreja SC (1994) Effects of endurance exercise on bone histomorphometric parameters in intact and ovariectomized rats. Bone Miner 26: 133–140.
31. Gong YS, Chen J, Zhang QZ, Zhang JT (2006) Effect of 17beta-oestradiol and ginsenoside on osteoporosis in ovariectomised rats. J Asian Nat Prod Res 8: 649–656.
32. Zhao X, Wu ZX, Zhang Y, Yan YB, He Q, et al. (2011) Anti-osteoporosis activity of Cibotium barometz extract on ovariectomy-induced bone loss in rats. J Ethnopharmacol 137: 1083–1088.
33. Nakamura T, Imai Y, Matsumoto T, Sato S, Takeuchi K, et al. (2007) Estrogen prevents bone loss via estrogen receptor alpha and induction of Fas ligand in osteoclasts. Cell 130: 811–823.
34. Cummings SR, Ensrud K, Delmas PD, LaCroix AZ, Vukicevic S, et al. (2010) Lasofoxifene in postmenopausal women with osteoporosis. N Engl J Med 362: 686–696.
35. Prestwood KM, Kenny AM, Kleppinger A, Kulldorff M (2003) Ultralow-dose micronized 17beta-estradiol and bone density and bone metabolism in older women: a randomized controlled trial. JAMA 290: 1042–1048.
36. Scott JP, Sale C, Greeves JP, Casey A, Dutton J, et al. (2014) Treadmill running reduces parathyroid hormone concentrations during recovery compared with a nonexercising control group. J Clin Endocrinol Metab 99: 1774–1782.
37. Wallace BA, Cumming RG (2000) Systematic review of randomized trials of the effect of exercise on bone mass in pre- and postmenopausal women. Calcif Tissue Int 67: 10–18.
38. Campbell KL, Westerlind KC, Harber VJ, Bell GJ, Mackey JR, et al. (2007) Effects of aerobic exercise training on estrogen metabolism in premenopausal women: a randomized controlled trial. Cancer Epidemiol Biomarkers Prev 16: 731–739.
39. Charatcharoenwitthaya N, Khosla S, Atkinson EJ, McCready LK, Riggs BL (2007) Effect of blockade of TNF-alpha and interleukin-1 action on bone resorption in early postmenopausal women. J Bone Miner Res 22: 724–729.
40. Yuk TH, Kang JH, Lee SR, Yuk SW, Lee KG, et al. (2002) Inhibitory effect of Carthamus tinctorius L. seed extracts on bone resorption mediated by tyrosine kinase, COX-2 (cyclooxygenase) and PG (prostaglandin) E2. Am J Chin Med 30: 95–108.
41. Leblanc A, Matsumoto T, Jones J, Shapiro J, Lang T, et al. (2013) Bisphosphonates as a supplement to exercise to protect bone during long-duration spaceflight. Osteoporos Int 24: 2105–2114.
42. Liu M, Zhong C, He RX, Chen LF (2012) Icariin associated with exercise therapy is an effective treatment for postmenopausal osteoporosis. Chin Med J (Engl) 125: 1784–1789.

21

Spinal Loads during Post-Operative Physiotherapeutic Exercises

Antonius Rohlmann*, Verena Schwachmeyer, Friedmar Graichen, Georg Bergmann

Julius Wolff Institute, Charité – Universitätsmedizin Berlin, Berlin, Germany

Abstract

After spinal surgery, physiotherapeutic exercises are performed to achieve a rapid return to normal life. One important aim of treatment is to regain muscle strength, but it is known that muscle forces increase the spinal loads to potentially hazardous levels. It has not yet been clarified which exercises cause high spinal forces and thus endanger the surgical outcome. The loads on vertebral body replacements were measured in 5 patients during eleven physiotherapeutic exercises, performed in the supine, prone, or lateral position or on all fours (kneeling on the hands and knees). Low resultant forces on the vertebral body replacement were measured for the following exercises: lifting one straight leg in the supine position, abduction of the leg in the lateral position, outstretching one leg in the all-fours position, and hollowing the back in the all-fours position. From the biomechanical point of view, these exercises can be performed shortly after surgery. Implant forces similar or even greater than those for walking were measured during: lifting both legs, lifting the pelvis in the supine position, outstretching one arm with or without simultaneously outstretching the contralateral leg in the all-fours position, and arching the back in the all-fours position. These exercises should not be performed shortly after spine surgery.

Editor: Mohammed Shamji, Toronto Western Hospital, Canada

Funding: This study was funded by the Deutsche Forschungsgemeinschaft (project: Ro 581/18-1) and the Deutsche Arthrose-Hilfe e.V., Frankfurt. The funders had no role in the study design, data collection and analysis, decision to publish, or preparation of the manuscript.

Competing Interests: The authors have declared that no competing interests exist.

* Email: antonius.rohlmann@charite.de

Introduction

Patients with a severe compression fracture of a vertebral body are often surgically treated with an internal spinal fixation device implanted from the posterior and with a vertebral body replacement (VBR) inserted anteriorly. During the rehabilitation phase, physiotherapeutic exercises are performed to regain muscle strength and to enhance a rapid return to normal life. To improve their strength, the muscles must be activated accordingly. However, high trunk muscle forces cause high loads in the corresponding spine region, which can result in implant subsidence, pedicle screw loosening, or even implant failure. Therefore, physiotherapeutic exercises that can cause high spinal loads should be avoided, but it is unclear which exercises are most relevant.

Only a few existing musculoskeletal models [1–7] are appropriate for calculating the spinal loads during complex activities. Validation of these models for complex activities is difficult due to a lack of experimental data.

Intradiscal pressure has been measured *in vivo* for many different activities [8–11], but only a few data exist for physiotherapeutic exercises.

The loads on internal spinal fixation devices during physiotherapy were measured in 10 patients [12]. Activities while lying, sitting, standing, and kneeling on the hands and knees (all-fours position) were investigated. The highest loads were measured for walking and activities during standing. The preliminary results for the loads on a VBR, measured shortly after surgery in up to 3 patients, showed high implant forces for forward flexion of the upper body, ascension of stairs, and elevation of both arms with weights in the hands or against the resistance applied by a physiotherapist [13,14]. The implant loads during sitting, walking, whole-body vibration, and changing body position were also measured [15–18]. However, little information exists regarding the loads for exercises in lying positions or the all-fours position.

The aim of this paper is to present the loads on a VBR, measured during physiotherapeutic exercises in a lying position and while kneeling on the hands and knees. The results may help physiotherapists select the optimal exercises for patients — depending on the postoperative time point — to avoid high spinal loads, which may endanger clinical outcomes.

Materials and Methods

Ethics statement

The Ethics Committee of Charité – Universitätsmedizin Berlin approved implantation of the telemeterized VBR in patients and the subsequent measurements (registry number 213-01/225-20). Before surgery, the procedure was explained to the patients, and they provided their written informed consent for the implantation of the modified implants and the obtaining of load measurements. Measurements were permitted within a maximum period of 6 years.

Table 1. Description of the investigated exercises.

Exercise number	Body position	Exercise	Total number (range per patient) of measurements
1	Lying supine	Lifting one straight leg	94 (8 to 40)
2	Lying supine	Lifting both straight legs	41 (1 to 21)
3	Lying supine	Lifting the pelvis (Bridging)	93 (10 to 32)
4	Lying prone	Lifting one cranially stretched arm	62 (6 to 33)
5	Lying prone	Lifting one arm and the contralateral leg	44 (6 to 23
6	Lying lateral	Abduction of a straight leg	64 (2 to 33)
7	All-fours position	Outstretching one arm cranially	15 (2 to 7)
8	All-fours position	Outstretching one leg	8 (2 to 2)
9	All-fours position	Outstretching one arm and the leg on the contralateral side	23 (2 to 12)
10	All-fours position	Flexing the lumbar spine (Arching)	16 (2 to 7)
11	All-fours position	Extending the lumbar spine (Hollowing)	13 (2 to 5)

Telemeterized VBR

The clinically used VBR Synex^{TM} (Synthes Inc., Bettlach, Switzerland) was redesigned. Six load sensors (strain gauges), a telemetry unit, and a coil for the inductive power supply were inserted into a cylindrical tube, with the original implant endplate on one side. A plate was electron-beam-welded on the other side to close the tube. Screwed-on endplates of various heights allowed for intraoperative adaptation of the implant height to the defect length. Telemetry was only active within a magnetic field of 4 kHz. Before implantation in patients, the VBRs were calibrated extensively by applying 21 different load combinations [19]. The typical average measuring errors were less than 2% for forces and less than 5% for moments related to the maximum applied force (3000 N) and moment (20 Nm). The resolution was better than 1 N and 0.01 Nm. The instrumented implants are described in detail elsewhere [20].

Subjects

Telemeterized VBRs were implanted in five patients (4 male, 1 female, 62–71 years old, 60–74 kg body mass, 168–180 cm height, 19–26 kg/m^2 body mass index). Four patients (WP1–WP4) each had a compression fracture of the L1 vertebral body and one (WP5) of the L3 vertebral body. In the first step, internal spinal fixation devices, spanning 2 segments in 3 patients and 4 segments in 2 patients (WP3 and WP4), were implanted from the posterior to stabilize the spine. In a second operation, a ventrolateral

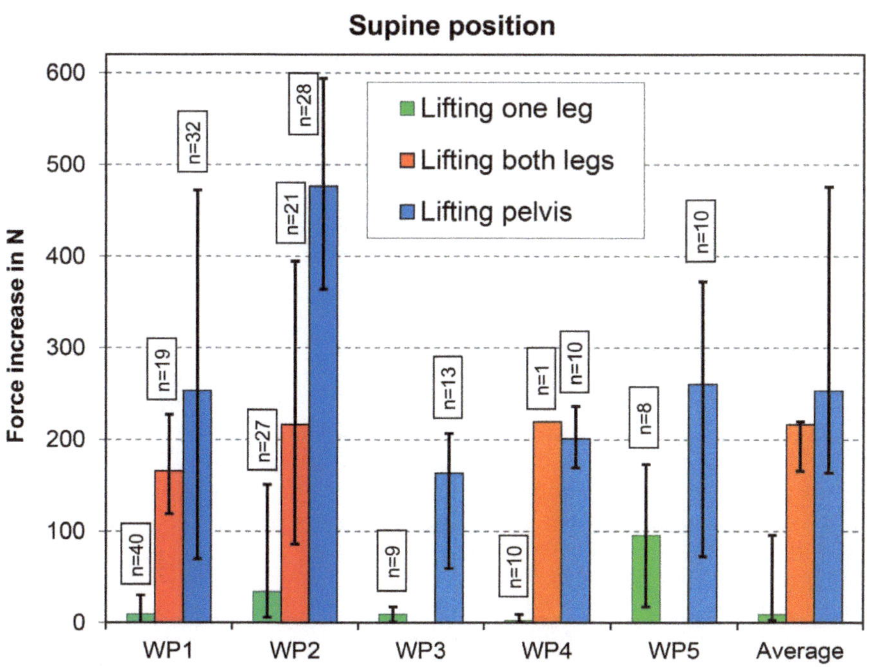

Figure 1. Supine position. Increases in peak force for three exercises. Data from 5 patients (WP1–WP5). The median values and ranges of the single patients and their averages are shown. n = number of evaluated trials. The force increase relates to the relaxed resting position.

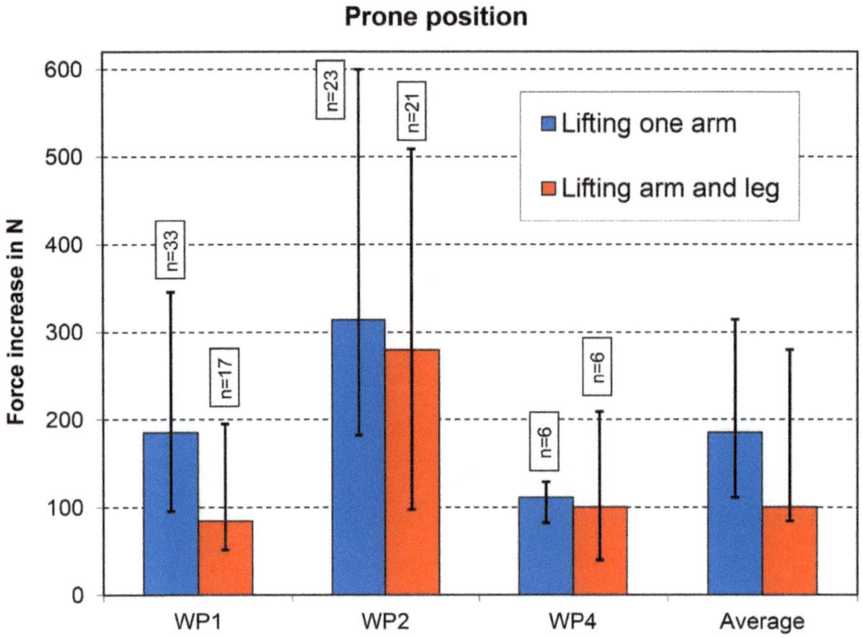

Figure 2. Prone position. Increases in peak force for two exercises. Data from 3 patients (WP1, WP2, and WP4). See also Figure 1.

approach was used to perform partial corpectomy of the fractured vertebra and to remove parts of the adjacent discs. The telemeterized VBR was inserted in the created niche. Bone material from the iliac crest and the resected rib was used to cover the implant and to enhance the interbody fusion process. The internal fixation devices remained in the patient after insertion of the VBR.

For the measurements, a power coil was placed around the patient's trunk, and a small wire antenna was placed on the patient's back; both devices were fixed with a harness [21]. The signals of telemetry were transmitted to a notebook computer, with which the loads were calculated. The patients were videotaped during the measurements, and the load-dependent signals of telemetry were stored simultaneously on the audio track of the same videotape. This process enabled a detailed analysis of implant loads later, without the patient having to be present.

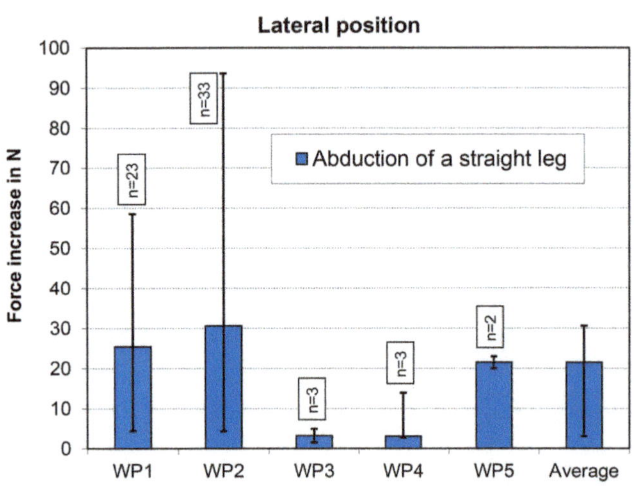

Figure 3. Lateral position. Increases in peak force for abduction of a straight leg. Data from 5 patients (WP1–WP5). See also Figure 1.

Exercises

Measurements of the VBR loads began a few days after surgery and were repeated 15–28 times at follow-up sessions over a period of up to 65 months postoperatively. Approximately 25 standard exercises, such as flexion, extension, lateral bending and axial rotation of the upper body, walking, and elevation of an arm with a weight in the hand, were performed during almost all of the 97 measuring sessions. The loads were measured during approximately 1000 different combinations of activities and parameters.

Eleven exercises performed in a lying position and the all-fours position were investigated in the present study. These exercises are described in Table 1. Only a few general instructions were given to the patients because we wanted to measure the everyday situations in which the patients would perform the exercises, without the supervision of a physiotherapist. The measurements were obtained over a time period of approximately 5 years. The number of repetitions varied greatly for the various exercises. Not all the patients agreed to perform all the exercises. In some cases, a patient was unable to perform a certain exercise due to a lack of strength.

Evaluation

The forces were measured throughout each exercise. The peak value during an exercise was compared to the mean value in the resting position. Hence, the increase in the resultant peak force on the implant due to exercise is reported here. The median values and ranges of the resultant force increases were determined. The resultant force is the geometrical sum of the three force components. For an 'average patient', the medians and the ranges of the medians for single patients are given.

Walking is the most important activity in daily life that causes higher spinal loads than lying, sitting, or standing. Loads less than those during walking are regarded as safe. Therefore, the

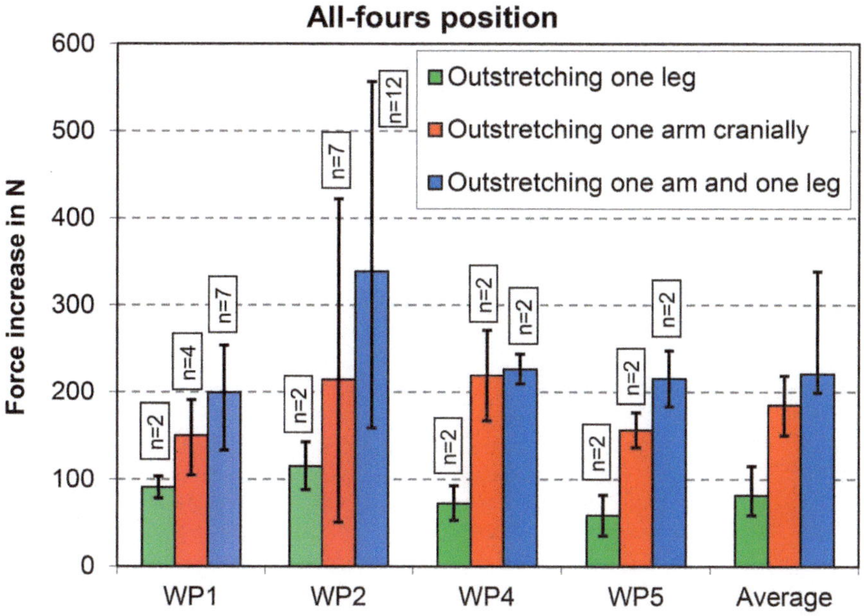

Figure 4. All-fours position. Increases in peak force for three exercises. Data from 4 patients (WP1, WP2, WP4, and WP5). See also Figure 1.

individual resultant forces for physiotherapeutic exercises are compared with those during level walking in the same patient [22].

Results

Exercises in a lying position

In the lying position, the resultant force on the VBR was usually small (less than 50 N). Due to higher muscle tension, e.g., when awaiting an arduous exercise or when lying in an uncomfortable position, the force could increase to 100 N.

Supine position. Lifting a straight leg in the supine position (exercise 1 in Table 1) led to an average force increase of only 10 N (Figure 1). However, in one patient (WP5), the increase was nearly 100 N. Lifting both straight legs (exercise 2) caused a force increase of nearly 220 N. Lifting the pelvis (exercise 3) led to an average force increase of approximately 250 N. Particularly with this exercise, there was large intra-individual variation, depending strongly on the height of the pelvis lifting.

Prone position. Lifting a cranially stretched straight arm (exercise 4) increased the force on the VBR by an average of approximately 185 N (Figure 2). Additionally, with this exercise, there were large inter- and intra-individual variations in the force increases. Surprisingly, lifting an arm and the contralateral leg (exercise 5) led mostly to a smaller force increase (100 N) than only lifting an arm.

Lateral position. Abduction of a straight leg in the lateral position (exercise 6) caused a median force increase of only 22 N (Figure 3). Additionally, with this exercise, there was large intra- and inter-individual variation.

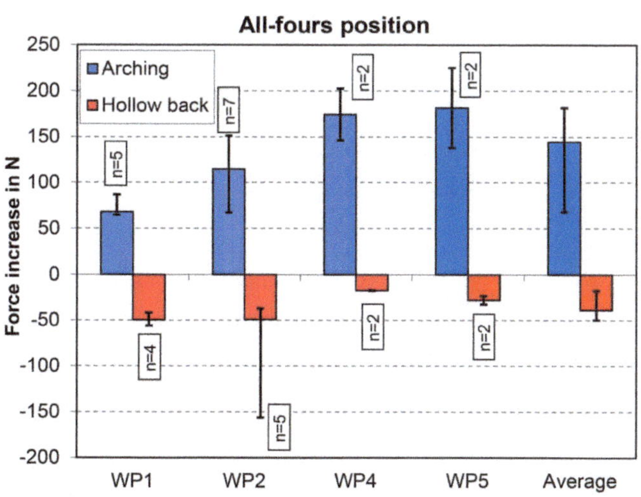

Figure 5. Changing spinal shape. Increases in peak force for arching and hollowing the back in the all-fours position. Data from 4 patients (WP1, WP2, WP4, and WP5). See also Figure 1.

Exercises in the all-fours position

In the relaxed all-fours position, the average resultant force on the VBR for patients WP1, WP2, WP4, and WP5 were 81 N, 169 N, 74 N, and 121 N, respectively.

Outstretching one arm or leg. Outstretching one leg in the all-fours position (exercise 7) usually resulted in a force increase of less than 100 N, while outstretching one arm cranially (exercise 8) increased the force on the VBR by approximately twice that value (Figure 4). Outstretching one arm and the contralateral leg (exercise 9) caused a median force increase of 220 N, but in one patient, the maximum force increase was 555 N.

Arching and hollowing the back. Arching the back in the all-fours position (exercise 10) led to a median force increase of approximately 150 N (Figure 5). In contrast, hollowing the back (exercise 11) reduced the resultant force on the VBR by approximately 40 N. Additionally, with the exercises in the all-fours position, the force increases varied greatly both intra- and inter-individually.

Discussion

The resultant forces on a VBR were measured for physiotherapeutic exercises in three different lying positions and the all-fours position. Median force increases of more than 200 N were measured for lifting both legs, lifting the pelvis in the supine position, and outstretching one arm and the contralateral leg in the all-fours position.

The average force increases for exercises in a lying position were less than 25 N for lifting one leg in the supine position and for abducting one leg in the lateral position. Therefore, from a biomechanical point of view, these exercises can be performed shortly after spine surgery. Lifting one cranially stretched arm and the contralateral leg in the prone position caused a median force increase of 100 N and is also an exercise that can be performed shortly after surgery. However, lifting both extended legs and lifting the pelvis in the supine position caused median force increases of more than 200 N. These exercises create a resultant force that might be even greater than that during walking [15,22]. Walking is considered to be the most important activity with relatively high loads that everyone should perform daily. Therefore, these physiotherapeutic exercises should not be performed shortly after spine surgery or when patients have back problems.

Outstretching one leg in the all-fours position usually increased the force on the VBR by less than 100 N. Thus, this exercise should not place the patient at risk. Outstretching an arm cranially, with or without simultaneous outstretching of the leg, led to a force increase of approximately 200 N and thus to a force on the VBR that might be greater than that during walking [15,22]. Therefore, these exercises should not be performed shortly after spine surgery. Arching the back in the all-fours position also led to resultant forces on the VBR that were similar to those during walking. In contrast, hollowing the back reduced the forces on the VBR but most likely increased the compressive forces on the facet joints. If the facet joints generate pain, then this exercise should not be performed.

For nearly all the activities studied, there were large intra- and inter-individual variations in the resultant force increases. The variations might have been due to small deviations in the surgical procedures, different performances of the exercises, different postoperative times, subsidence of the VBR, differences in body weight, and different positions of the center of mass of the upper body due to various factors, e.g., different positions of the head or of the extremities [15,16,22,23]. The manner in which the exercises were performed varied because only a few general instructions were given to the patients. Physiotherapists can influence loads by providing specific instructions. Particularly in lifting the pelvis, the lifting height had a strong influence on the force increase. Therefore, lifting the pelvis *not* up to the maximum possible level may help to avoid high spinal loads. However, the results presented here describe the spinal loads during patient training in daily life.

The following limitations should be borne in mind. The spinal load at the implant level was shared by the VBR, the internal fixation device, the remaining bone, and the added bone material. The instrumented VBR measured only the loads on the spinal implant and not the complete loads across the entire segment. Measurements could be obtained only in a small cohort of 5 patients, making it difficult to draw general conclusions from the results, particularly when they varied greatly among the subjects. The numbers of trials and the postoperative times varied among the various patients. These patients were involved in several other load-measuring studies [15,22–24]. To avoid overstressing the patients, the numbers of activities and repetitions were limited. This limitation and the large number of different exercises studied did not allow for motion analyses to be performed or for other additional parameters to be measured. Despite these limitations, this study still provided novel, unique, and helpful information regarding the loads acting on VBRs during physiotherapeutic exercises. This information may help physiotherapists to choose the most appropriate postoperative exercises for an individual patient.

In summary, the resultant forces on a VBR were measured for eleven physiotherapeutic exercises performed in lying positions or the all-fours position. Forces similar to or even greater than those for walking [15,22] were measured for lifting both legs, lifting the pelvis in the supine position, outstretching one arm with or without simultaneous outstretching of the contralateral leg in the all-fours position, and arching the back in the all-fours position. These exercises should not be performed shortly after spine surgery.

Acknowledgments

The authors greatly appreciate the cooperation of their patients. They also thank Dr. A. Bender, J. Dymke, and M. Lauks for their technical assistance.

Author Contributions

Conceived and designed the experiments: AR GB FG. Performed the experiments: AR FG VS. Analyzed the data: AR VS. Contributed reagents/materials/analysis tools: FG GB. Contributed to the writing of the manuscript: AR VS GB.

References

1. Cappozzo A (1984) Compressive loads in the lumbar vertebral column during normal level walking. J Orthop Res 1: 292–301.
2. Cholewicki J, McGill SM (1994) EMG assisted optimization: a hybrid approach for estimating muscle forces in an indeterminate biomechanical model. J Biomech 27: 1287–1289.
3. De Zee M, Hansen L, Wong C, Rasmussen J, Simonsen EB (2007) A generic detailed rigid-body lumbar spine model. J Biomech 40: 1219–1227.
4. Han KS, Rohlmann A, Zander T, Taylor WR (2013) Lumbar spinal loads vary with body height and weight. Med Eng Phys 35: 969–977.
5. Marras WS, King AI, Joynt RL (1984) Measurement of loads on the lumbar spine under isometric and isokinetic conditions. Spine 9: 176–187.
6. McGill SM, Marshall L, Andersen J (2013) Low back loads while walking and carrying: comparing the load carried in one hand or in both hands. Ergonomics 56: 293–302.
7. Shirazi-Adl A, El-Rich M, Pop DG, Parnianpour M (2005) Spinal muscle forces, internal loads and stability in standing under various postures and loads–application of kinematics-based algorithm. Eur Spine J 14: 381–392.
8. Nachemson AL (1981) Disc pressure measurements. Spine 6: 93–97.
9. Sato K, Kikuchi S, Yonezawa T (1999) In vivo intradiscal pressure measurement in healthy individuals and in patients with ongoing back problems. Spine 24: 2468–2474.
10. Wilke H-J, Neef P, Caimi M, Hoogland T, Claes LE (1999) New in vivo measurements of pressures in the intervertebral disc in daily life. Spine 24: 755–762.
11. Wilke H-J, Neef P, Hinz B, Seidel H, Claes L (2001) Intradiscal pressure together with anthropometric data - a data set for the validation of models. Clin Biomech (Bristol, Avon) 16: S111–126.
12. Rohlmann A, Graichen F, Bergmann G (2002) Loads on an internal spinal fixation device during physical therapy. Physical Therapy 82: 44–52.
13. Rohlmann A, Graichen F, Bender A, Kayser R, Bergmann G (2008) Loads on a telemeterized vertebral body replacement measured in three patients within the first postoperative month. Clin Biomech 23: 147–158.
14. Rohlmann A, Graichen F, Kayser R, Bender A, Bergmann G (2008) Loads on a telemeterized vertebral body replacement measured in two patients. Spine 33: 1170–1179.
15. Rohlmann A, Dreischarf M, Zander T, Graichen F, Bergmann G (2014) Loads on a vertebral body replacement during locomotion measured in vivo. Gait Posture 39: 750–755.
16. Rohlmann A, Petersen R, Schwachmeyer V, Graichen F, Bergmann G (2012) Spinal loads during position changes. Clin Biomech 27: 754–758.
17. Rohlmann A, Schmidt H, Gast U, Kutzner I, Damm P, et al. (2013) In vivo measurements of the effect of whole body vibration on spinal loads. Eur Spine J 23:666–672.

18. Rohlmann A, Zander T, Graichen F, Dreischarf M, Bergmann G (2011) Measured loads on a vertebral body replacement during sitting. Spine J 11: 870–875.
19. Bergmann G, Graichen F, Rohlmann A, Bender A, Ehrig R, et al. (2008) Design and calibration of load sensing orthopaedic implants. J Biomech Eng 130: 021009–021001.
20. Rohlmann A, Gabel U, Graichen F, Bender A, Bergmann G (2007) An instrumented implant for vertebral body replacement that measures loads in the anterior spinal column. Med Eng Phys 29: 580–585.
21. Graichen F, Arnold R, Rohlmann A, Bergmann G (2007) Implantable 9-channel telemetry system for in vivo load measurements with orthopedic implants. IEEE Trans Biomed Eng 54: 253–261.
22. Rohlmann A, Dreischarf M, Zander T, Graichen F, Strube P, et al. (2013) Monitoring the load on a telemeterised vertebral body replacement for a period of up to 65 months. Eur Spine J 22: 2575–2581.
23. Rohlmann A, Zander T, Graichen F, Bergmann G (2013) Lifting up and laying down a weight causes high spinal loads. J Biomech 46: 511–514.
24. Rohlmann A, Hinz B, Bluthner R, Graichen F, Bergmann G (2010) Loads on a spinal implant measured in vivo during whole-body vibration. Eur Spine J 19: 1129–1135.

PERMISSIONS

All chapters in this book were first published in PLOS ONE, by The Public Library of Science; hereby published with permission under the Creative Commons Attribution License or equivalent. Every chapter published in this book has been scrutinized by our experts. Their significance has been extensively debated. The topics covered herein carry significant findings which will fuel the growth of the discipline. They may even be implemented as practical applications or may be referred to as a beginning point for another development.

The contributors of this book come from diverse backgrounds, making this book a truly international effort. This book will bring forth new frontiers with its revolutionizing research information and detailed analysis of the nascent developments around the world.

We would like to thank all the contributing authors for lending their expertise to make the book truly unique. They have played a crucial role in the development of this book. Without their invaluable contributions this book wouldn't have been possible. They have made vital efforts to compile up to date information on the varied aspects of this subject to make this book a valuable addition to the collection of many professionals and students.

This book was conceptualized with the vision of imparting up-to-date information and advanced data in this field. To ensure the same, a matchless editorial board was set up. Every individual on the board went through rigorous rounds of assessment to prove their worth. After which they invested a large part of their time researching and compiling the most relevant data for our readers.

The editorial board has been involved in producing this book since its inception. They have spent rigorous hours researching and exploring the diverse topics which have resulted in the successful publishing of this book. They have passed on their knowledge of decades through this book. To expedite this challenging task, the publisher supported the team at every step. A small team of assistant editors was also appointed to further simplify the editing procedure and attain best results for the readers.

Apart from the editorial board, the designing team has also invested a significant amount of their time in understanding the subject and creating the most relevant covers. They scrutinized every image to scout for the most suitable representation of the subject and create an appropriate cover for the book.

The publishing team has been an ardent support to the editorial, designing and production team. Their endless efforts to recruit the best for this project, has resulted in the accomplishment of this book. They are a veteran in the field of academics and their pool of knowledge is as vast as their experience in printing. Their expertise and guidance has proved useful at every step. Their uncompromising quality standards have made this book an exceptional effort. Their encouragement from time to time has been an inspiration for everyone.

The publisher and the editorial board hope that this book will prove to be a valuable piece of knowledge for researchers, students, practitioners and scholars across the globe.

LIST OF CONTRIBUTORS

Cherie Wells
Faculty of Health, University of Canberra, Bruce, Australian Capital Territory, Australia
School of Science and Health, University of Western Sydney, Campbelltown, New South Wales, Australia

Gregory S. Kolt and Paul Marshall
School of Science and Health, University of Western Sydney, Campbelltown, New South Wales, Australia

Bridget Hill
Epworth HealthCare, Richmond, Victoria, Australia

Andrea Bialocerkowski
Griffith Health Institute, Griffith University, Gold Coast, Queensland, Australia

Plínio Santos Ramos
Exercise Medicine Clinic - CLINIMEX, Rio de Janeiro, Rio de Janeiro, Brazil
Maternity Hospital Therezinha de Jesus, Faculty of Medical and Health Sciences - SUPREMA, Juiz de Fora, Minas Gerais, Brazil

Aline Sardinha and Antonio Egidio Nardi
Panic and Respiration Laboratory, Institute of Psychiatry, Federal University of Rio de Janeiro, National Institute for Translational Medicine (INCT-TM/CNPq), Rio de Janeiro, Rio de Janeiro, Brazil

Claudio Gil Soares de Araú jo
Exercise Medicine Clinic - CLINIMEX, Rio de Janeiro, Rio de Janeiro, Brazil
Heart Institute Edson Saad, Federal University of Rio de Janeiro, Rio de Janeiro, Rio de Janeiro, Brazil

Shanhu Qiu
Division of Sports and Rehabilitation Medicine, Department of Medicine II, Ulm University, Ulm, Germany
Department of Endocrinology, Zhongda Hospital, Institute of Diabetes, Medical School, Southeast University, Nanjing, P. R. China

Xue Cai and Zilin Sun
Department of Endocrinology, Zhongda Hospital, Institute of Diabetes, Medical School, Southeast University, Nanjing, P. R. China

Uwe Schumann, Martina Velders and Jü rgen Michael Steinacker
Division of Sports and Rehabilitation Medicine, Department of Medicine II, Ulm University, Ulm, Germany

Maria Clara Noman de Alencar, Manoel Otá vio da Costa Rocha, Márcia Maria de Oliveira Lima, Henrique Silveira Costa, Giovane Rodrigo Sousa, Renata de Carvalho Bicalho Carneiro, Antonio Luiz Pinho Ribeiro and Maria Carmo Pereira Nunes
Post-Graduate Program in Infectious Diseases and Tropical Medicine, School of Medicine, Universidade Federal de Minas Gerais, Belo Horizonte, MG, Brazil

Guilherme Canabrava Rodrigues Silva and Fernando Vieira Brandáo
2 School of Medicine, Universidade Federal de Minas Gerais, Belo Horizonte, MG, Brazil

Lucas Jordan Kreuser
University of Minnesota Medical School, Minneapolis, Minnesota, United States of America

Dongshi Wang, Yanqiu Wang, Yingying Wang and Chenglin Zhou
Department of Sport Psychology, School of Kinesiology, Shanghai University of Sport, Shanghai, China

Rena Li
Department of Sport Psychology, School of Kinesiology, Shanghai University of Sport, Shanghai, China
Center for Hormone Advanced Science and Education, Roskamp Institute, Sarasota, Florida, United States of America

Ulrich S. Tran, Agnes A. Hofer and Martin Voracek
Department of Basic Psychological Research and Research Methods, School of Psychology, University of Vienna, Vienna, Austria

Ammar W. Ashor
Human Nutrition Research Centre, Institute of Cellular Medicine, Newcastle University, Campus for Ageing and Vitality, Newcastle on Tyne, United Kingdom
College of Medicine, University of Al-Mustansiriyah, Baghdad, Iraq

Jose Lara, Mario Siervo, Carlos Celis-Morales and John C. Mathers
Human Nutrition Research Centre, Institute of Cellular Medicine, Newcastle University, Campus for Ageing and Vitality, Newcastle on Tyne, United Kingdom

Richard A. Washburn, Amanda N. Szabo, Kate Lambourne, Erik A. Willis, Lauren T. Ptomey, Jeffery J. Honas and Joseph E. Donnelly
Cardiovascular Research Institute, Department of Internal Medicine, The University of Kansas Medical Center, Kansas City, Kansas, United States of America

Stephen D. Herrmann
Sanford Research, Department of Children's Health Research Center, Sioux Falls, South Dakota, United States of America

Barbara Sandor, Istvan Czuriga, Kalman Toth, Eszter Szabados, Andras Toth, Miklos Rabai and Bela Mezey
1st Department of Medicine, University of Pecs, School of Medicine, Pecs, Hungary

Alexandra Nagy and Arpad Csatho
Department of Behavioural Sciences, University of Pecs, School of Medicine, Pecs, Hungary

Eun Sung Choi, Mi Kyung Kim, Jeong Min Kim, Eun Soo Kim, Woo Jin Chung, Kyung Sik Park, Kwang Bum Cho and Jae Seok Hwang
Department of Internal Medicine, Keimyung University School of Medicine, Daegu, South Korea

Min Kyung Song
Department of Food Science and Nutrition, Graduate School,
Keimyung University, Daegu, South Korea,

Byoung Kuk Jang
Department of Internal Medicine, Keimyung University School of Medicine, Daegu, South Korea
Institute for Cancer Research, Keimyung University, Daegu, South Korea

Hai-Feng Shu, Tao Yang, Si-Xun Yu, Hai-Dong Huang, Ling-Li Jiang, Jian-Wen Gu and Yong-Qin Kuang
Department of Neurosurgery, General Hospital of the People's Liberation Army Chengdu Military Region, Chengdu, Sichuan, China

Emily A. Moker and Linda S. Pescatello
Department of Kinesiology, University of Connecticut, Storrs, CT, United States of America

Lori A. Bateman and William E. Kraus
Division of Cardiology, Department of Medicine, Duke University Medical Center, Durham, NC, United States of America

Jenna B. Gillen, Michael E. Percival, Lauren E. Skelly, Brian J. Martin, Rachel B. Tan and Martin J. Gibala
Department of Kinesiology, McMaster University, Hamilton, Ontario, Canada

Mark A. Tarnopolsky
Department of Kinesiology, McMaster University, Hamilton, Ontario, Canada,
Department of Pediatrics and Medicine, McMaster University, Hamilton, Ontario, Canada

Sandra Ortlieb
Institute of Epidemiology I, Helmholtz Zentrum Mnchen, German Research Center for Environmental Health, Neuherberg, Germany
Institute of Medical Statistics and Epidemiology, Technische Universität München, Munich, Germany

Lukas Gorzelniak and Klaus A. Kuhn
Institute of Medical Statistics and Epidemiology, Technische Universität München, Munich, Germany

Dennis Nowak
Institute and Outpatient Clinic for Occupational, Social and Environmental Medicine, Ludwig-Maximilians-Universitä t, Munich, Germany
Comprehensive Pneumology Center Munich (CPC-M), Member of the German Center for Lung Research, Munich, Germany

Ralf Strobl and Eva Grill
Institute for Medical Information Processing, Biometrics and Epidemiology, Ludwig- aximilians-Universität München, Munich, Germany,
German Center for Vertigo and Balance Disorders, Ludwig-Maximilians-Universität München, Munich, Germany

Barbara Thorand and Annette Peters
Institute of Epidemiology II, Helmholtz Zentrum München, German Research Center for Environmental Health, Neuherberg, Germany

Stefan Karrasch
Institute of Epidemiology I, Helmholtz Zentrum München, German Research Center for Environmental Health, Neuherberg, Germany
Institute and Outpatient Clinic for Occupational, Social and Environmental Medicine, Ludwig-Maximilians-Universität, Munich, Germany
Institute of General Practice, University Hospital Klinikum rechts der Isar, Technische Universität München, Munich, Germany

Alexander Horsch
Institute of Medical Statistics and Epidemiology, Technische Universität München, Munich, Germany
Department of Computer Science, University of Tromsø, Tromsø, Norway
Department of Clinical Medicine, University of Tromsø, Tromsø, Norway

Holger Schulz
Institute of Epidemiology I, Helmholtz Zentrum München, German Research Center for Environmental Health, Neuherberg, Germany

Willa D. Brenowitz
Department of Epidemiology, University of Washington School of Public Health, Seattle, Washington, United States of America

Rebecca A. Hubbard
Group Health Research Institute, Seattle, Washington, United States of America
Department of Biostatistics, University of Washington School of Public Health, Seattle, Washington, United States of America

Paul K. Crane
Department of Medicine, Division of General Internal Medicine, University of Washington, Seattle, Washington, United States of America

Shelly L. Gray
School of Pharmacy, University of Washington, Seattle, Washington, United States of America

Oleg Zaslavsky
University of Haifa, Mount Carmel, Haifa, Israel

Eric B. Larson
Group Health Research Institute, Seattle, Washington, United States of America
Department of Medicine, Division of General Internal Medicine, University of Washington, Seattle, Washington, United States of America

C. Martyn Beaven, Sarah J. Willis and Hans-Christer Holmberg
Swedish Winter Sports Research Centre, Department of Health Sciences, Mid Sweden University, Östersund, Sweden

Christian J. Cook
School of Sport, Health and Exercise Sciences, Bangor University, Bangor, United Kingdom
Holger Cramer, Romy Lauche, Gustav Dobos and Jost Langhorst
Department of Internal and Integrative Medicine, Kliniken Essen-Mitte, Faculty of Medicine, University of Duisburg-Essen, Essen, Germany

Hoda Azizi
Department of Complementary Medicine, Mashhad University of Medical Sciences, Mashhad, Iran

Vanessa Oliveira
Nephrology Division, School of Medicine, Federal University of São Paulo, São Paulo, Brazil

Eliana Hiromi Akamine, Maria Helena C. Carvalho and Zuleica Bruno Fortes
Pharmacology Department, University of São Paulo, São Paulo, Brazil

Lisete Compagno Michelini
Physiology Department, University of São Paulo, São Paulo, Brazil

Tatiana Sousa Cunha
Science and Technology Institute, Federal University of São Paulo, São Paulo, Brazil

Maria do Carmo Franco
Nephrology Division, School of Medicine, Federal University of São Paulo, São Paulo, Brazil
Physiology Department, School of Medicine, Federal University of São Paulo, São Paulo, Brazil

Mo-Yeol Kang
Occupational Safety and Health Research Institute, Korea Occupational Safety and Health Agency, Ulsan, South Korea

Department of Preventive Medicine, Seoul National University College of Medicine, Seoul, South Korea

Hyoung-Ryoul Kim
Department of Occupational and Environmental Medicine, College of Medicine, the Catholic University of Korea, Seoul, South Korea

Lihui Li, Shuang Lv, Miaomiao Dong, Li Zhang, Jiaheng Tu, Jie Yang, Lingli Zhang and Yinan Song
School of Kinesiology, Shanghai University of Sport, Shanghai, China

Xi Chen
School of Kinesiology, Shanghai University of Sport, Shanghai, China
School of Sports Science, Wenzhou Medical University, Wenzhou, China

Leiting Xu
School of Kinesiology, Shanghai University of Sport, Shanghai, China
Medical School of Ningbo University, Ningbo, China

Jun Zou
Scientific Research Department, Shanghai University of Sport, Shanghai, China

Antonius Rohlmann, Verena Schwachmeyer, Friedmar Graichen and Georg Bergmann
Julius Wolff Institute, Charite´ - Universitätsmedizin Berlin, Berlin, Germany

Index